Quality Assurance in Transfusion Medicine

Volume I
Conceptual, Serological, and Microbiological Aspects

Edited by

Gail Rock, Ph.D., M.D., FRCP
University of Ottawa
Ottawa, Canada

and

M. J. Seghatchian, B.Sc., Ph.D.
North London Blood Transfusion Centre
London, England

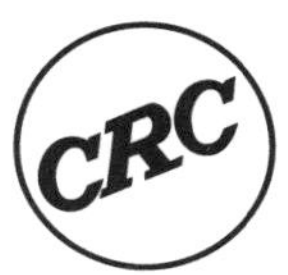

CRC Press
Boca Raton Ann Arbor London Tokyo

Library of Congress Cataloging-in-Publication Data

Quality assurance in transfusion medicine/editors, Gail A. Rock,
M. J. Seghatchian.
p. cm.
Includes bibliographical references and index.
Contents: v. 1. Conceptual, serological, and microbiological
aspects — v. 2. Methodological advances and clinical aspects.
ISBN 0-8493-4938-9 (v. 1). — ISBN 0-8493-4939-7 (v. 2)
1. Blood—Transfusion—Quality control. I. Rock, G.
II. Seghatchian, M. J.
[DNLM: 1. Blood Transfusion. 2. Quality Assurance, Health Care.
WB 356 Q12]
RM171.Q35 1992
615′.39—dc20
DNLM/DLC
for Library of Congress

92-9276
CIP

Direct all inquiries to CRC Press, Inc., 2000 Corporate Blvd., N.W., Boca Raton, Florida, 33431.

International Standard Book Number 0-8493-4938-9

Library of Congress Card Number 92-9276

Printed in the United States of America 1 2 3 4 5 6 7 8 9 0

Printed on acid-free paper

EDITORIAL

During the past few decades, major advances have been made in many areas of Transfusion Medicine. In particular, there has been a dramatic shift from the earlier preoccupation with red cell serology to the current situation in which transfusion centers operate as small pharmaceutical industries producing large numbers of blood components. Today, in modern transfusion services, more than 90% of the blood collected is made into various components and fractions. All of these fractions must be individually prepared, tested, and stored under different conditions with specified criteria for both their production and storage. Stringent quality control and assurance programs are required to assure their optimum performance and compliance with regulatory affairs. In some countries specific regulatory guidelines have been established, indicating the conceptual acceptance of quality assurance in the field of blood transfusion. The American Association of Blood Banks has had specific regulations for some time, and a European Directive is currently in preparation to develop and maintain uniformity in standards in medicinal products which may cover blood and its various components.

In respect to methodological aspects, the technologies in particular of blood and plasma collection have changed with new plastic bags permitting long-term storage and an improved storage environment, while modifying quite extensively the biochemical environment in which the cells are maintained. The introduction of automated devices for the collection of cells and plasma, and the generation of blood components by these machines, have the capability of effecting further radical changes such that the current manual methods of blood collection may well be replaced by machines within the next decade.

Apheresis is one example of a new field of medicine which originated from transfusion. This process permits collection, in very large numbers, of various blood components from a single donor during a 1- to 2-hour procedure. Alternatively, whole-body plasma exchange can be carried out with the same devices. New approaches have also been taken to freeze various cells for long-term storage and to filter blood and blood products with greater efficacy. Many new combinations of anticoagulants and preservatives are now used to prolong the storage life of the cellular components. Extended storage of both red cells and platelets has been permitted within the last decade, and this has markedly changed the logistics of blood supply, as well as making more plasma available, thus helping to achieve self-sufficiency.

With the continuous evolution of technology, considerable changes have also occurred in the methods used for testing blood and blood components. The introduction of reactive strips, microtitration procedures, automation, and the use of monoclonal antibodies in blood grouping and microbiological laboratories have all effected changes. The blood transfusion service has become a multidisciplined organization with necessary expertise in immunohematology, genetics, microbiology, and pathology.

Consequently, the principles of good laboratory practice and proficiency testing, which were well established for other disciplines, have become an essential part of quality assurance in a modern blood transfusion center. Safety being the dictating factor, the slogan of ''Quality means safety'' — safety for the donor, safety for the recipient, safety for the staff, safety for the community at large — was adopted as the policy statement at the North London Blood Transfusion Centre.

Indeed, in today's world, with the widespread threat of HIV transmission and the concern for non-A non-B hepatitis infection, patients have come to fear what was once considered only as a life-saving and relatively innocuous treatment — a blood transfusion. Now, both patients and physicians go to considerable lengths to avoid exposure to blood, and a great deal of effort and money has been committed to finding ways to avoid transfusion altogether, to use the patient's own blood, and/or to develop a substitute for blood.

Experts in Transfusion Medicine recognize a large number of other, non-infectious, complications which can derive from transfusion. These, too, have prompted widespread concern and activity in the last decade. Immune modulation by transfusion has generated great interest, and many innovative approaches have been developed to avoid or reduce such reactions. On the other hand, efforts have also been directed toward exploiting these immunological effects to benefit the patient, as in the deliberate HLA sensitization of women who repeatedly miscarry, and the collection of autologous lymphocytes and their subsequent activation by interleukin-2 to produce activated killer cells reactive against autologous tumors.

The frontiers of Transfusion Medicine have broadened greatly; where once the blood banker was mainly concerned with red cell compatibility and identification of antibodies, now the areas of component production and use, apheresis collection and therapeutics, computer science, intraoperative salvage and other autologous donations, collection and cryopreservation of stem cells, matching of unrelated bone marrow donors, and active participation in clinical therapy are among the routine activities of modern centers.

Essential to the function of a modern service also is close liaison with the public. Donor availability is essential to the entire practice. In this regard, a large number of new approaches have been taken to inform the public of the requirements for blood and to enlist their specific donation, whether it be for whole blood or for apheresis procedures. Computerization has had a marked impact in this field, facilitating transfusion practice at the donor, laboratory, and clinical levels. The use of computers has contributed to the effective implementation and monitoring of safe and efficient use of blood components, as well as the reduction of unnecessary demands on donors, and has facilitated rapid tracing between patient and donor. To optimally deliver this variety of services, each center must establish and adhere to the principles of quality assurance.

Recognizing that the code of practice varies in different countries, we felt that a detailed text describing the basics of quality assurance and transfusion methods would be of significant benefit to those concerned with Transfusion Medicine by integrating diversified activities at the international level. Quality assurance in transfusion espouses the concept of "all planned and systematic action necessary to provide adequate confidence that the product or service will satisfy specified requirements."* As such, it encompasses a number of other areas including the need for basic education, the setting of standards, and the establishment of guidelines for product and staff testing and for the use and review of product utilization. Only through a commitment to all of these activities can an optimal final product or service and compliance with regulatory affairs and specifications be guaranteed.

The primary objective of this book is to provide an up-to-date series of articles on the current state of the art of quality assurance and methods in blood transfusion. Invited experts in the field, who are familiar with both the practical aspects of transfusion and the importance of quality assurance, deal with various areas to provide a comprehensive reference text on transfusion activities describing reasons for and against certain approaches.

The first volume contains papers dealing with the concept and applications of quality assurance and methods in transfusion medicine, both in theory and in practice.

Then begins the presentation of current methodological and microbiological aspects and computerization, followed by, in Volume II, chapters dealing with instrumentation and various aspects of component therapy and the systematic presentation of different topics which reflect the spectrum of activity in this rapidly growing field, ending with a consideration of future trends in transfusion medicine.

We wish to thank the many individuals who have contributed articles to *Quality Assurance in Transfusion Medicine*. Their findings and opinions bring us state-of-the-art information combined with technical details to assure quality performance and to enhance the safety and efficacy of the products and services provided.

Gail Rock
M. J. Seghatchian

* References ISO 8402, 1986 or B5 4778 Quality Vocabulary.

THE EDITORS

Gail Rock, Ph.D., M.D., FRCP, is an Associate Professor of Medicine at the University of Ottawa and consultant to the Surgeon General's office (Canada) and the Department of Agriculture (Canada). Dr. Rock graduated in 1961 from Patrick's College at the University of Ottawa with a B.Sc., and she obtained her Ph.D. in Biochemistry in 1966 from the University of Ottawa. She then undertook 2 years of postdoctoral training at the National Research Council of Canada and 1 year at the University of Ottawa in the Department of Medicine. She subsequently entered the Faculty of Medicine and obtained her M.D. and later her specialty training in Hematopathology. Dr. Rock was the Medical Director of the Ottawa Centre of the Canadian Red Cross for 14 years and has been Chairman of the Canadian Apheresis Study Group during the 11 years of its existence. She is a member of many societies involved in the practice of Hematology and was chairman of the Scientific Program Committee of the American Association of Blood Banks for 6 years. She is a past president of both the American Society for Apheresis and the World Apheresis Association. She is currently the editor in chief of the journal *Transfusion Science*.

Dr. Rock has presented over 350 papers at various national and international meetings and has published more than 125 research papers and 50 book chapters and other articles. Her current interests involve the fields of coagulation and apheresis.

M. J. Seghatchian, B.Sc., Ph.D., is the Principal Clinical Scientist in charge of the Quality Assurance Laboratory at the North London Blood Transfusion Centre (NLBTC) and Honorary Lecturer at Guy's Hospital Medical School, London. His basic training is in Chemistry, specializing in Radiation Chemistry at the Centre National de Recherche Scientifique (CNRS, Orsay) and subsequently obtaining (in 1964) his doctorate in Physical Chemistry from the University of Paris, France. In 1972, he also obtained a Ph.D. in Medical Biochemistry from the University of London, England. Since 1973, Dr. Seghatchian's interests focused on the regulatory control of blood components, originating the integrated system of quality assurance at NLBTC, while working for several years as a visiting scientist at the National Institute for Biological Standards and Control and the MRC Epidemiology and Medical Care Unit, London, England. He has also acted as a WHO Expert Consultant on Coagulation for Mediterranean countries.

Dr. Seghatchian pioneered chromogenic and electrophoretic methods for the characterization of native and altered forms of FVIII and thrombogenic components of prothrombin complexes. He collaborated with several leading scientists and clinicians in Sweden, France, Italy, the U.S., Canada, and South America on the molecular abnormality of hemostatic components. His current research interests include characterization of the activity states of the hemostatic components implicated in hemapheresis procedures and hypercoagulability. He has recently been active in the development of simple screening tests for platelet morphological/functional integrity using automated cell counters and platelet activation/release markers by microplate techniques to facilitate standardization and harmonization in platelet function testing in the U.K. Blood Transfusion Services.

Dr. Seghatchian is an editor of the journals *Transfusion Science* and *Thrombosis Research*. He has co-edited a two-volume publication on Factor VIII/vWF (CRC Press, 1990) and also acts as referee and an editorial advisory member for CRC Press publications. He has published more than 200 scientific papers and abstracts and has delivered more than 40 guest lectures at national and international meetings. He is a founding member of both the British Blood Transfusion Society and the British Society of Haemostasis and Thrombosis and is a member of several international societies.

CONTRIBUTORS

Volume I

R. Aller
Department of Pathology
Long Beach Memorial Medical Center
Long Beach, California

J. A. J. Barbara
North London Blood Transfusion Centre
London, England

J. R. Birch
Celltech Ltd.
Slough, United Kingdom

I. M. Bromilow
Regional Transfusion Centre
Liverpool, England

R. G. Cable
ARC Blood Services
Connecticut Region
Farmington, Connecticut

P. Davies
Regional Transfusion Centre
Sheffield, England

R. Dodd
Jerome H. Holland Laboratory
American Red Cross
Rockville, Maryland

J. K. M. Duguid
Regional Transfusion Centre
Liverpool, England

C. P. Engelfriet
Department of Immunohematology
Central Lab of The Netherlands' Red Cross
Amsterdam, The Netherlands

J. Freedman
Blood Bank
St. Michael's Hospital, Toronto
Ontario, Canada

G. S. Gabra
The League of Red Cross and Red Crescent Societies
Geneva, Switzerland

D. Goldfinger
Cedars-Sinai Medical Center
Los Angeles, California

L. T. Goodnough
Washington University Medical Center
Barnes Hospital
St. Louis, Missouri

T. J. Greenwalt
Hoxworth Blood Center
University of Cinicinnati
Cincinnati, Ohio

B. Habibi
Centre National de Transfusion Sanguine
Les Ulis, France

R. J. T. Hancock
United Kingdom Transplant Service
Bristol, England

R. J. L. Klaassen
Department of Immunohematology
Central Lab of The Netherlands' Red Cross
Amsterdam, The Netherlands

W. Kline
American Red Cross
National Headquarters
Washington, DC

R. Kuijpers
Department of Immunohematology
Central Lab of The Netherlands' Red Cross
Amsterdam, The Netherlands

B. A. Lenes
ARC Blood Services
South Florida Region
Miami, Florida

J. E. Menitove
Hoxworth Blood Center
Cincinnati, Ohio

L. Messeter
University Hospital Blood Bank
Lund, Sweden

W. Ouwehand
East Anglian Blood Transfusion Service and
Division of Transfusion Medicine
University of Cambridge
Cambridge, England

S. H. Pepkowitz
Cedars-Sinai Medical Center
Los Angeles, California

P. K. Phillips
National Institute of Biological Standards and Control
Hertfordshire, England

Gail Rock, Ph.D., M.D., FRCP
University of Ottawa
Ottawa, Canada

M. L. Scott
International Blood Group Reference Laboratory
Bristol, England

M. J. Seghatchian, B.Sc., Ph.D.
North London Blood Transfusion Centre
London, England

W. E. St. Clair
Joint Commission on Accreditation of Healthcare Organizations
Oakbrook Terrace, Illinois

J. F. A. Stivala
North London Blood Transfusion Centre
London, England

D. Voak
East Anglian Blood Transfusion Service and
Division of Transfusion Medicine
University of Cambridge
Cambridge, England

A. E. G. Kr. von dem Borne
Department of Immunohematology
Central Lab of The Netherlands' Red Cross
Amsterdam, The Netherlands

W. Wagstaff
Regional Blood Transfusion Centre
Sheffield, England

D. H. Yawn
Department of Pathology
Baylor College of Medicine
Houston, Texas

T. F. Zuck
Hoxworth Blood Center
Cincinnati, Ohio

Volume II

J. Anderson
Baxter Healthcare Corporation
Fenwal Division
Round Lake, Illinois

J. P. AuBuchon
Department of Pathology
Dartmouth-Hitchcock Medical Center
Lebanon, New Hampshire

P. J. Ballem
Canadian Red Cross Society
Blood Transfusion Service
Vancouver, British Columbia, Canada

V. Blanchette
Department of Pediatrics
Division of Hematology/Oncology
The Hospital for Sick Children
Ontario, Canada

B. Brozovic
North London Blood Transfusion Centre
London, England

N. Buskard
Canadian Bone Marrow Registry
Vancouver, British Columbia, Canada

S. Chandra
Biologicals Development
Armour Pharmaceuticals
Kakakee, Illinois

H. J. Deeg
Program in Transplantation Biology
Fred Hutchinson Cancer Research Center
Seattle, Washington

J. Dutcher
Department of Oncology
Montefiore Hospital
Bronx, New York

T. N. Estep
Baxter Healthcare Corporation
Blood Substitutes
Round Lake, Illinois

F. Feldman
Biologicals Development
Armour Pharmaceuticals
Kakakee, Illinois

W. Gray
Baxter Healthcare Corporation
Fenwal Division
Round Lake, Illinois

R. J. Kaufman
HemaGen
St. Louis, Missouri

W. A. L. Heaton
Blood Services, Mid-Atlantic Region
American Red Cross
Norfolk, Virginia

M. Hrinda
Rhone-Poulenc Rorer Central Research
King of Prussia, Pennsylvania

C. Högman
Department of Clinical Immunology and Transfusion Medicine
University Hospital Blood Center
Uppsala, Sweden

S. Holme
Blood Services, Mid-Atlantic Region
American Red Cross
Norfolk, Virginia

J. Hounsell
Department of Hematology
Royal North Shore Hospital of Sydney
Sydney, Australia

J. Isbister
Department of Hematology
Royal North Shore Hospital of Sydney
Sydney, Australia

T. A. Lane
Department of Pathology
University of California
San Diego, California

V. Martlew
Regional Blood Transfusion Centre
Liverpool, England

G. Moroff
Product Development Laboratory
American Red Cross
Rockville, Maryland

W. G. Murphy
South East Scotland Regional Blood Transfusion Centre
Edinburgh, Scotland

U. Nydegger
Division of Transfusion Medicine
Hamatologische Zentrallabor Inselspital
Bern, Switzerland

E. Paietta
Department of Oncology
Montefiore Hospital
Bronx, New York

C. Politis
Hellenic Red Cross Hospital
Blood Transfusion Centre
Athens, Greece

G. Rock, Ph.D., M.D., FRCP
University of Ottawa
Ottawa, Canada

B. J. Sadoff
Product Development Laboratory
American Red Cross
Rockville, Maryland

A. Schreiber
Rhone-Poulenc Rorer Central Research
King of Prussia, Pennsylvania

M. J. Seghatchian, B.Sc., Ph.D.
North London Blood Transfusion Centre
London, England

R. G. Strauss
Department of Pathology and Pediatrics
University of Iowa Hospitals and Clinics
Iowa City, Iowa

J. Teitel
Department of Medicine
Division of Hematology
St. Michael's Hospital
Toronto, Ontario, Canada

P. Toy
Blood Bank
Moffitt-Long Hospital and San Francisco General Hospital
University of California
San Francisco, California

J. B. Welch
Center for Biologics Evaluation and Research
United States Food and Drug Administration
Rockville, Maryland

TABLE OF CONTENTS

Volume I
Conceptual, Serological, and Microbiological Aspects

Volume II
Methodological Advances and Clinical Aspects

Chapter 1

CONCEPTUAL ACCEPTANCE OF QUALITY ASSURANCE AND THE IMPLEMENTATION OF TOTAL QUALITY MANAGEMENT IN BLOOD TRANSFUSION SERVICES

M. J. Seghatchian and J. F. A. Stivala

TABLE OF CONTENTS

ISBN 0-8493-4938-9

I. INTRODUCTION

Quality in terms of transfusion practice means conformance with specified safety requirements and fitness for purpose. Attainment of quality standards has always been fundamental to the existence of blood transfusion services, from their inception. This is exemplified by the early emphasis on donor hemoglobin screening and serological testing, followed by the additional mandatory microbiological screening of the donor population. Today, transfusion microbiology deals with the provision of relevant clinical, epidemiological, laboratory, educational, and advisory services on blood transfusion microbiology, making the safety aspects the most important issue. In fact in many blood transfusion services, quality as a mission is still synonymous with safety: safety for donors, safety for recipients, safety for staff, and for the community at large.

Accordingly, blood transfusion services, apart from assessing and safeguarding the community healthcare, provide a comprehensive range of safe and efficacious blood components and products while ensuring the application of an effective program of quality assurance in all aspects of transfusion practice and science, taking an active part in appropriate research and development work, as well as maintaining relevant national and international links in support of the above.

Quality awareness in blood transfusion services is currently at an all-time high. Though some of the reasons for this observation, such as the increasingly litigious nature of patients and the spread of statutory controls, may be seen as somewhat negative influences, there is undoubtedly a positive side as well. Today, all transfusion staff are becoming fully aware of their responsibilities and commitments to both the suppliers of their staple raw material (donors) and their users and customers (clinicians and patients).

Recent statutory changes in the nature of the National Health Service in the U.K. have had a major impact on the status of the U.K. blood transfusion services. These changes have, among other things, promoted the concept of an internal market where each operational unit is considered to be either a provider or a purchaser of products or services, or both. It is in this new environment that quality in all its aspects has had a major impact.

From April 1, 1991, the U.K. blood transfusion services have for the first time been subject to licensing requirements, along similar lines to those that have existed for the pharmaceutical industry for over two decades. This is, of course, only the beginning; much remains to be done in many spheres, including standards and standardization, harmonization of planned systems of quality audit and review, staff education and training, and handling procedures and error trapping. Much of the above involves extensive improvement to documentation and record keeping, as well as reliance on computerized systems for information management.

Prioritizing the implementation of quality assurance in the blood transfusion services has been given to influencing events starting with staff education. This is not surprising as the quality of products relies heavily on the skills and commitment of staff. Training and education are constant threads that run through all aspects of quality, requiring convergence in approach.

In this chapter, it is our intention to describe the evolution of a quality philosophy and practice in blood transfusion, from its inception as a tool for analysis and testing to the present day implementation of total quality management. We shall do this by first outlining the conceptual development of quality assurance and the adoption of the tenets of good manufacturing practice and good laboratory practice in blood transfusion services generally; we also include an overview on the implications in regard to documentation. We shall then describe how we have applied these principles and practices to the implementation of a quality system at our own transfusion center. Finally, we look at quality improvements achieved and sought, including an in-depth review of standardization, and at future trends in the field of quality and transfusion practice.

No treatise such as this can ignore the established array of regulations and guidelines that relate to this field. Of particular international importance and interest are the standards originating from the International Organization for Standardization (ISO). Where there has been harmonization of standards, these ISO standards also appear as national standards, e.g., British Standards (BS), or supranational standards, e.g., European Standards (EN). A list of such documents, considered by the authors as relevant to this chapter, has been included with the References.

II. CONCEPTUAL ACCEPTANCE OF QUALITY

Quality is the totality of features and characteristics of a product or service that bear on its ability to satisfy stated or implied needs.

ISO8402: 1986

The way in which the concept of quality is adopted in an organization will undoubtedly depend considerably on the relationships established with its customers. In blood transfusion services (BTS), the safety of patients comes first and quality in this context must mean safety and efficacy. In this respect, it is the responsibility of the BTS management to take steps to ensure a proper program of quality appreciation, quality measures, and quality awareness in the whole organization — from donors to recipients. This is a tough and challenging but rewarding road as, at the end of the day, when high quality standards are achieved, clinicians develop confidence and are satisfied. The benefits of this approach are not just an increased supply, reduced waste, and improved efficiency but also the reduction of costs associated with poor quality. Such costs involve operational failure, rejects, reworks, complaints, and wasted effort, which all lead to loss of confidence both internally and externally. The underlying principles of quality assurance (QA) do not vary in substance between industries although details will vary; as such, they are equally relevant and applicable in the field of blood transfusion.

A. EVOLUTION OF THE CONCEPT OF QUALITY

Expressed simply, a quality product or service means one which is fault-free. This common-sense approach existed long before the more formalized and structured approach widely adopted in modern industry and commerce. It even existed before the onset of the Industrial Revolution and the ensuing burgeoning of the manufacturing industry. No one would dispute the fact that the artisans and craftsmen of the past had an acute sense of quality even though they would not have been aware of the current concepts of quality philosophy and awareness that have made the subject a discipline in its own right. The driving forces for quality in those days were few but powerfully persuasive. As well as the intrinsic craftsman's skill and pride in his workmanship, the effects of faulty products in a subsistence existence would have been comparatively greater and the producer would have almost certainly been known to his customers on a personal basis.

With the establishment of industries, which achieved their major impetus during the Industrial Revolution, there was a shift towards gainful employment within often hostile and somewhat dehumanizing environments. Thus a machine operator's main responsibility was to mind the machine without necessarily ever seeing the final product. In addition, customers were remote and unknown to the operators. It is into this type of environment that inspection and testing were introduced as the first formal control systems.

Early attempts at quality measures concentrated on observation and measurement, in the form of inspection and testing. In this way it was possible to measure products against a specification and allow through only those that passed these tests. This constituted a policing function to ensure that only satisfactory products reached the customer. This approach, however, offered no protection from unacceptable levels of irrecoverable rejects and would not normally result in quality improvement. More commonly, it might identify the less effective operators and result in punitive measures. Inspection and testing survive and still thrive to this day, although as more integrated functions within the area of quality control (QC).

B. QUALITY CONTROL

> *The operational techniques and activities that are used to fulfil requirements for quality.*
>
> *ISO8402: 1986*

The progression from inspection and testing to formal quality control was an evolutionary rather than a revolutionary process, where essentially the same activities were carried out in a planned and systematic way to control quality of output. The purpose of this exercise was not only to release or reject output on merit but also to monitor on-going performance and reduce waste. It is in the development of QC that one observes the growth of audit as an important tool.

In the area of the blood transfusion services, a parallel evolution may be seen with the development from the early phases, when testing was largely a matter of serology of each donation, to the subsequent extension into the various facets of quality involving, first, transfusion microbiology and then the subsequent interest in such matters as donor quality, quality of collection systems, and quality of the donation. It is symptomatic of the nature of the BTS that the growth of processing activities (''manufacturing'') was paralleled by the development of an appreciation of the need for QC rather than testing.

C. QUALITY ASSURANCE

> *All those planned and systematic actions necessary to provide adequate confidence that a product or service will satisfy given requirements for quality.*
>
> *ISO8402: 1986*

In the earlier concept of quality, effort was mainly directed towards the belief that no faulty product should leave the producer/supplier while, in the current concept of quality, effort is directed towards ensuring that no faulty products are produced in the first place. A common-sense management approach is required for both attaining and maintaining the declared levels of quality with the expected reliability and consistency.

Reliability is the time-dependent dimension of quality and consistency in a forward plan requiring regular review. The common requirements of an integrated quality system are

- Documented procedures
- Documented records of faults and errors, the records of the action "loop"
- Standardized QA based on records of training and working instructions
- Updated changes within the system
- Defined QA responsibility and managerial authority

Based on the above requirements, quality assurance is therefore neither a new discipline nor an add-on feature, but simply a predetermined, logical, procedural, and common-sense approach to work. In practice, however, QA aims to ensure that

- Policies are clearly understood
- Procedures are correctly implemented
- Instructions are clear and followed without short cuts

QA should not be misconceived as simply measurement, policing, or error trapping, although these features are part of its overall discipline.

Quality in all its totality can be assessed by observation, enquiry, inspection, measurement (analysis/testing), and comparison (evaluation/validation/auditing), all leading to improvement in performance.

D. TOTAL QUALITY MANAGEMENT

All the different strands of quality philosophy and practice reach their apotheosis in total quality management (TQM). This incorporates the various philosophies and practices of quality control and quality assurance into an all-embracing proposition that the pursuit of true quality is best achieved by attention to all the contributory aspects, whether they be clinical, practical, procedural, or managerial.

The fundamental axioms of TQM include

- Quality is not the monopoly of particular persons or units within an organization, but is the responsibility of everyone within it.
- Quality must be an intrinsic part of all processes and procedures from the start rather than inspecting/testing/controlling it out at the end.
- The quality ethos is subscribed to by everyone within an organization, including top management, who must declare its commitment in this respect and provide appropriate resources.
- Quality is about interrelationships, not only extraorganizationally, but also intraorganizationally; hence the concept of the internal customer.

Currently, the concept of the internal customer is highly relevant to many health care organizations and particularly the blood transfusion services, which rely so much on multidisciplinary workforces for the total quality of their output. The formerly monolithic state-run health services, such as the National Health Service in the U.K., have in recent years undergone reform to create a type of internal market which is highly reliant on these concepts.

III. GOOD MANUFACTURING PRACTICE IN BLOOD TRANSFUSION SERVICES

Good Manufacturing Practice is that part of Quality Assurance which ensures that products are consistently produced and controlled to the quality standards appropriate to their intended use . . .

Guide to Good Manufacturing Practice for Medicinal Products, EC 1989

It is now a matter of international recognition and agreement that any organization dealing with the production of human blood products for therapeutic purposes, such as blood transfusion services, must have in place a planned, integrated system of QA that complies with appropriate and approved good manufacturing practice (GMP). This plan forms part of licensing requirements to ensure that products are fit for their intended use and thus safe and effective. To achieve these important quality objectives there must be a comprehensively designed and correctly executed system of GMP and good laboratory practice (GLP) and quality control/quality improvement, with documented methods for monitoring their effectiveness.

Though codes of GMP emanating from different sources do vary in detail and enforcement, their basic structure and approach may be summarized as a series of questions about the product(s), as shown below:

Who makes the product?
- Organization
- Personnel

Where is the product made?
- Buildings
- Environmental control
- Cleaning and sanitation

With what is the product made?
- Equipment
- Measuring equipment
- Subcomponents

How is the product made?
- Manufacturing specifications and processes
- Reprocessing

How is the product identified?
- Labeling
- Packaging

How is the product stored?
Storage conditions
Stock rotation
How is the product supplied?
Distribution
Installation
How is the product checked?
Inspection
Control and testing
Corrective action
What records are kept?
Master documentation
History record
What is done if something goes wrong?
Failure investigation
Complaint files
Recall
How is compliance verified?
Audits

A. REGULATORY ASPECTS

As has been mentioned already, the responsibility for attaining and maintaining the quality objectives rests with required participation and commitment by all staff at all levels within an organization, as well as the company's suppliers and distributors. The definition of these quality objectives is driven by two influences, one regulatory, the other advisory. The former is GMP compliance, which is mandatory in many countries, and the latter is Quality Systems (ISO9000/BS5750), which is advisory.

Compliance with GMP principles becomes compulsory in 1992 in all countries of the European Community (EC). In line with the other package of EC principles, it is expected that GMP principles will be revised and updated, as necessary, to take into account technical and scientific progress. In order to uphold these regulatory requirements, a system of manufacturing licensing and inspection by the regulatory or other competent authorities has been introduced to enforce implementation of the basic principles.

Great efforts have been made in the U.K. by both national blood transfusion services and the national inspectors to become familiar with the current regulatory aspects and the implications for compliance in a way that is meaningful and effective in the service. The European GMP has superseded and now overrides national and other GMP requirements to facilitate standardization and harmonization. Compliance with regulatory affairs is never an easy task, but nevertheless essential.

Good Manufacturing Practice	Quality Systems
Industry-related or specific.	General and of quasi-universal applicability.
Biased towards all aspects of manufacture and control of particular types of product.	Includes all aspects of quality from design considerations to quality costings.
May have the force of law (regulations), be advisory, or voluntary guidelines.	Adherence is usually voluntary, though demand-driven either through market forces or international trade.
Produced, regulated and administered by government, professional bodies or trade associations.	Produced, regulated and administered by independent agencies responsible for setting national and international standards.
Normally country-specific although some forms of bilateral agreements may exist.	Of international standing.
Example: "Guide to Good Pharmaceutical Manufacturing Practice"	Example: "BS5750/ISO9000/EN29000 Quality Systems"

FIGURE 1. Main distinguishing features of GMP and quality systems.

B. INTERNATIONAL STANDARDIZATION OF QUALITY SYSTEMS

Quality system is the organisational structure, responsibilities, processes and resources for implementing quality management.

ISO8402: 1986

While codes of GMP were being promulgated by many national authorities for specific purposes, there was a parallel development in more general quality matters largely driven by the needs of engineering and the aerospace industries in conjunction with defence requirements. These initially led to the development of national quality standards such as the original BS5750 series published in the U.K. in 1979. Though these were essentially national, they had a degree of international compatibility necessary for the growing demands of international trade. Subsequent work on revision and harmonization in the 1980s gave rise to the internationalization of this standard into ISO9000-9004 and EN29000 to EN29004, the latter being the EC equivalents. The British equivalent, BS5750, was brought into line with ISO and republished in 1987.

There are substantial differences between GMP and Quality Systems, as may be seen in Figure 1. Essentially, however, both aim at meeting the overall objective of quality as fitness for purpose, but by different routes.

Whereas compliance with GMP is normally overseen by regulatory agencies, compliance with ISO9000-9004 is by certification through an accredited organization. In the U.K., there are several organizations that hold this accreditation, some specializing in particular market sectors. Though the standards for quality systems are more related to systems and procedures than in-depth knowledge of specialist processes, nevertheless it has been found that certification organizations with inspectors possessing specialist knowledge and expertise are used by related industries. Certification inspections are normally frequent (once or twice yearly) and of a nature to ensure that the organization being inspected is worthy to retain certification. Examples of noncompliances and their frequency are shown in Figure 2; it is interesting to note how similar these are to GMP-related noncompliance in GMP-regulated organizations. In the U.K. blood transfusion services, the impact of ISO9000-9004 has been quite considerable, as the standard provides a suitable model for a comprehensive quality management system, once it is translated and adapted to the transfusion environment. Hitherto, its main use has been as the foundation for parts of the *Guidelines for the Blood Transfusion Services in the United Kingdom.*[6] This takes, as a basis, the structure of ISO9001, Section 4, and adds specifics, such as computer systems and product recall, which are alluded to but not specified in the standard.

The structure of the International Standard itself is worthy of comment, as it is a multipart document:

- ISO9000 is the guide to the selection and use of the appropriate quality system for the purpose intended
- ISO9001-9003 are three variants of quality system, specified according to the complexity of the product/service, process, etc., it is against one of these that an organization is assessed for certification purposes
- ISO9004 provides the guidelines for the quality management and quality system elements; this part is fundamental to successful compliance with the standard and yet is often ignored in initial setting up of a compliant system
- BS5750: Part 4 does not have an ISO equivalent but is nevertheless useful in amplifying and interpreting the contents of Parts 1 to 3 in the U.K. framework.

C. DOCUMENTATION AS THE BASIS OF COMPLIANCE

No discussion on the subject of quality can afford to ignore the matter of documentation. It would be true to say that any quality system that is based on poor documentation is bankrupt and unsustainable. Therefore, it is essential that appropriate effort and resources are made available to create and control a comprehensive documentation system. In this light, it is important that all considerations of documentation systems should include specific procedures for document control. It would be inappropriate to recommend a specific system that would suit all conditions; however, in a system that complies with GMP and the quality systems standard, the following types of documentation are recommended:

1. **Quality manual**

    - Systems oriented
    - Company/organization/division based
    - Outline of compliance with a particular external standard (ISO9001-3)
    - Refers to more detailed documents
    - Not explicitly a requirement for compliance with GMP

2. **Standard operating procedures (SOPs)**

    - Detailed documents covering all GMP-compliant activities
    - Containing specifications where appropriate
    - Process/procedure based
    - Modular
    - Reflecting current practice

3. **Records**

    - Interactive documents, e.g., forms
    - Proof of compliance
    - May also act as means of interfunction communication

D. REGULATORY AUDIT AND NONCOMPLIANCE

> *A systematic and independent examination to determine whether quality activities and related results comply with planned arrangements and whether these arrangements are implemented effectively and are suitable to achieve objectives.*
>
> *ISO8402: 1986*

Within the blood transfusion services, auditing for compliance with GMP takes various forms. In the U.K., it is possible to identify at least six different types:

1. Customer audits — Customers are within their rights to ask to audit a center for compliance with agreed specifications. Though this is rare at present (albeit it is common for hospital users to visit their centers on a somewhat informal basis), relationships are changing in such a way that it may become a more common occurrence in future.
2. Internal audits — These are audits carried out by a center's own staff. They may be either a full audit or more commonly part of an audit

program covering individual functions/departments on a rolling basis. Their use is primarily to maintain a constant awareness of the need for compliance. Looked at from a somewhat negative viewpoint, it is better for deficiencies to be found by staff rather than by an inspector of the regulatory authority!

3. Peer audits — In recent years, the National Blood Transfusion Service in England and Wales has organized a program of peer audits of its constituent centers. In this program, each center is audited annually by teams drawn from other transfusion centers. This is a very effective form of GMP audit, as it is carried out by auditors who are well versed in the operations of a transfusion center but retain an element of detachment by virtue of not being members of staff.
4. Regulatory audits — These audits are mandatory in connection with statutory licensing of transfusion centers. In the U.K., these are carried out by Inspectors from the Medicines Control Agency ("Medicines Inspectors"), an executive agency of the Department of Health. Noncompliance found during the course of one of these inspections could lead to severe repercussions.
5. Certification audits — At present, transfusion centers in the U.K. are not directly affected by this type of audit which leads to certification of compliance with the quality systems standard BS5750/ISO9000/EN29000 and is carried out by accredited certification bodies. However, this situation may soon change, as it is foreseen that certification to standards ISO9001 or ISO9002 may well be sought by some regional centers.
6. Supplier audits — This may be viewed as a reverse of the above five types in that in this case, it is suppliers to a transfusion center that are inspected by staff from the transfusion center. This supplier-customer relationship is one of the fundamental tenets of the quality systems standard.

To many producers, external audit by a certification or inspection agency can be a traumatic ordeal. Receiving a noncompliance notice may mean a further visit by the certification body, which inevitably adds to the quality costs. As may be seen in Figure 2, the frequency of noncompliance varies considerably according to specific requirements. The danger of classifying a noncompliance as a low-frequency issue such as the sampling procedures, which are often not based on any sound program, is that this may result in these areas being overlooked.

E. U.K. NATIONAL GUIDELINES

In principle, it is possible to implement the industrial quality practices in blood transfusion without any major modification. The *Guidelines for the Blood Transfusion Services in the United Kingdom* are an excellent example

Frequency	High	Medium	Low
Occurrence	>50%	20 to 50%	<20%
Items	Documentation Purchased material Equipment inspection	Quality system In process inspection Inspection status Final inspection Training Corrective action Quality system review	Workmanship Purchasers supplied products Sampling procedures Organisation Alternative procedures

FIGURE 2. Noncompliance raised against BS5750 Part 2 (ISO9002) requirements grouped into three frequency ranges.

of a first attempt at taking the basis of the quality systems standard, incorporating and adapting relevant parts of the *Guide to Good Pharmaceutical Manufacturing Practice,* and finally adding specific requirements and specifications related to transfusion science and practice, to create a set of national guidelines.

It should be noted, however, that each organization nevertheless should select a set of integrated quality measures which, in combination, will satisfy the QA needs of a given situation, in line with the legal requirements of the countries and their own quality objective. The North London Blood Transfusion Center (NLBTC) quality improvements are described later in this chapter.

IV. IMPLEMENTATION OF A QUALITY SYSTEM IN A TRANSFUSION CENTER

Like other transfusion centers, the NLBTC cannot identify a particular date on which it gained quality consciousness. It is more appropriate to describe it as a quality awakening, because even in the earliest days, there was an appreciation that the product had to be fit for its intended use. This has developed and been refined over the years to today's commitment to the tenets of TQM. An expression of this is the quality mission statement. This serves as a simple expression of intent for the benefit of staff and customers alike. In slightly altered and more rigorously defined form, this statement also serves the function of a quality policy statement, as defined in the quality systems standard.

At NLBTC, we define our quality mission statement in the following terms:

> Quality has always been regarded as of paramount importance at NLBTC, from the establishment of the Quality Assurance Laboratory in the early seventies to the adoption of the concept of Total Quality Management for the nineties.
>
> The Centre aims to comply with relevant, current quality standards, in particular the Guidelines for the Blood Transfusion Services in the U.K., the Guide to Good Pharmaceutical Manufacturing Practice, and Quality Systems as represented by directives BS5750/ISO9000/EN29000, as these apply to its particular operation.

A. INITIAL STEPS TO QUALITY CONTROL

Quality consciousness at NLBTC was boosted in the early 1970s as a result of our growing awareness of "nonquality", identified by returned products from hospitals. The management of the time, appreciating the importance of design, created a small team of staff trained in quality matters to institute quality practice in the production laboratory. Initially, emphasis was placed on trials of new processes and equipment control. This team regularly got together to implement set procedures (previously tried on a small scale) for quality improvement, despite the fact that there were no proper specifications (except those based on limited in-house trials) for standards.

B. DEVELOPMENT OF QUALITY ASSURANCE

With the increasing demand for blood components, the NLBTC came to the conclusion that the only affordable way to control the quality of all the processes was to make the production groups control their own work. Production personnel have therefore been encouraged to become involved in improving the operation and communication according to a newly designed, service-oriented control program. Efforts were directed towards both in-process control (IPC) by the production team and daily inspection and final product outcome by QA assessment.

It is now clear that it is not possible to simply carry out a number of basic tests and then rely on the good intentions of the staff to provide a safe and efficacious product. Instead, everyone needs to be encouraged to become involved in the process. Accordingly, through the cooperation of both management and staff, the NLBTC has put the "quality standard" and the "performance to schedule" on its first priority list — the latter of the two had once been considered merely a secondary priority.

All problems were documented, reviewed, discussed, and diagnosed in detail by the quality team on a weekly basis. The need for follow-up action was identified and responsibility was assigned to a joint team of QC and production personnel working together as a team.

It was in this environment that the NLBTC further instituted 100% manufacturing checks at each important work station by production staff (in-process control), training them in the rudiments of auditing (what to look for, proper documentation, maintaining their tools, housekeeping, and general orderliness and cleanliness). Control teams were engaged on final control, inspections, and research/development but still remained a service group to the production of blood components.

With the introduction of the Cell Separator machine, there was a greater need for implementing the total quality system, as the cost of failure, even occasionally, was too high. In this new system, the role of QC was no longer just a service function but, in fact, an overall quality management function from the donor to final functional testing. By injecting the ''quality concept'' into the organization, in particular by educating and retraining staff in quality appreciation and quality measures, much improvement in outcome could be expected. Therefore, apart from establishing a policy of testing and inspecting the final outcome, the NLBTC injected well-thought-out and planned, practical preventative measures into the plateletpheresis system. This involved recording the blood flow rate, the volume of anticoagulant used, and the methods used to avoid clumping, activation, and fragmentation. Efforts were also directed towards on-the-job retraining of staff, workmanship standards, and GMP (especially record keeping, housekeeping, control of changes, and statistical analyses and feedback of information transfer), so that the personnel are able to react to their own performance.

Based on the above, it became apparent that ''defects'' are caused not only by faulty operation, but more seriously and frequently, by poor manufacturing design, poor specifications, poor maintenance of machines, and so on. This means that writing a formulation for quality does not necessarily become the surrogate for action; this is an absolute requirement for cooperation between apheresis machine manufacturers and the blood transfusion services when resolving nonconformance. Once again, it can be concluded that joint activity should be an essential part of QA activity and that quality should not be considered either as a monopoly of wisdom or a matter of chance, but rather as the result of daily cooperation at all levels; this includes the customer/supplier relationship.

Today at the NLBTC, the above concept of QA is still operational and all are in agreement with the progressive objectives of QA as all want to provide quality service. An important aspect of the acceptance of this concept is the belief that the quality of service is governed by the change of attitude, the quality of the staff, and the commitment of everyone involved in running the organization.

C. THE FIVE POINTERS TO TOTAL QUALITY

As already shown, the concept of total quality differs from GMP in its propounding of the philosophy of ''quality in everything''. Thus, every aspect of an organization's operations and activities is seen as an actual or potential contributor to the quality of output. Using terminology found in the British Standard on Quality Systems, it is possible to apply these specifically to the field of blood transfusion.

Quality in Procurement
- Selection of suitable donors
- Use of appropriate equipment and materials

Quality in Manufacture
- Efficient and effective separation of blood components

Quality in Testing
- Efficient and relevant testing protocols
- Use of appropriate quality indicators

Quality in Supply and Service
- Meeting the needs of the user, at the right time, and with the right product and/or service

Quality in Design and Development
- New or improved methods and processes

D. INTERNAL AUDIT

Self-inspection is the best tool to verify conformity with GMP principles and to permit corrective action. Like an external audit, self-inspection should be carried out by designated, competent staff and the results recorded. Reports should contain information on all the observations made during the inspection, as well as proposals for corrective measures and any subsequent statement on recorded actions.

It is most important in any audit, but particularly internal audits, that all noncompliances recorded are followed up and a response is elicited from the person responsible for the area/function being audited. Unless this is strictly adhered to, internal audits will go the way of other good ideas that did not quite work.

Another important aspect of internal audits is that they are required for licensing purposes. Evidence may have to be shown at a regulatory inspection that these have been carried out regularly and efficiently, even if the inspector is not empowered to demand to read the actual reports.

V. TOWARDS QUALITY IMPROVEMENT

A. JUSTIFICATION FOR CHANGE

With the introduction of new technology and the implementation of quality principles in recent years, we have seen dramatic changes in the approach of setting standards for component production and usage. The five major areas which contributed to quality improvement are listed below.

Prioritizing the parameters affecting quality — The first step for any change must be to define what we intend to regulate or monitor, i.e., the production process or the characterization of a final product. The two areas are quite different in QC terms. In either case, one must give some degree of priority to the choice of multiple parameters affecting quality. For example, in the QC of platelet concentrates, higher priorities are given to reducing the level of leukocyte content than the plasma volume in a final product, though both have a great influence on quality.

Choice of quality indicator — With advancing technology and improvement in detection limits, the methods of measuring must be continuously reassessed. For example, the demand for leukocyte-poor products has been increasing to such an extent that these products are becoming available on request. Accordingly, we need to measure or control the quality of the final product by available means reflecting state-of-the-art methodology. Again, we must select between various options:

- Prerelease testing, i.e., by measuring the leukocyte content of the finished product
- Assessing the efficiency of the available filters in terms of percentage removal of leukocytes
- Expressing leukocyte removal by quoting log removal
- Assessing filtration-induced activation or changes in the activation state of the platelet or plasma component

Each of these options will produce a different picture of the quality of the final product. For example, an efficiency of 99.9% removal of leukocytes will be a good indicator of filtration, as is a log-three removal (which is a good performance indication of a filter). Nevertheless, when the leukocyte level is initially very high, even a 99.9% or three-log removal leaves a white cell level in the product that is unacceptable. Hence, the absolute count appears to be the best option for the final criteria for fitness of the use of the leukocyte-deficient product. Filtration should be performed on the fresh preparation as the fragmentation of leukocytes during storage may lead to immunogenic substances (fragments) which pass through the filter. Fresh platelet products are more adhesive, which means that filtration may be associated with substantial removal of active and viable platelets as well. Filtration appears to induce characteristic deleterious changes in platelet morphological/functional integrity during storage.

Setting a target standard in the control parameter — Setting an "ideal standard" is not an easy task, but must be taken into consideration. The true production standard for a particular product may not be the same for other blood transfusion services. This creates two different "standards": the actual and the ideal (the latter being the target standard, requiring a transition period). As technology improves, the target standard improves.

Selecting an appropriate sensing device — Careful consideration should also be given to the choice of equipment for monitoring the control of any parameter. While the use of automated platelet counters may seem ideal as an accurate mode of analysis, with minimal human error, this equipment has not been designed for the purpose of cell counting of blood components at the upper or lower limits of linearity. In fact, we are currently using the equipment at the extreme limitations of their operational design, therefore the results are often compromised by background interference. For example, the leukocyte contamination of filtered platelet units could be more accurately monitored by flow cytometry than automated cell counting. The problem is further exasperated by lack of an appropriate reference (calibrate) for flow cytometers. Nevertheless, with the use of relevant control charts, accurate and instructive performance indicators are obtainable for detecting trends, thereby facilitating remedial action. In this respect, we need stringent QC for recommending the ''bedside filter''. This is because the nature of the platelet pool, the processing, and the nature of the filter itself all affect the efficiency of the filtration process. If accurate QC is not performed, we are failing our user (clinicians), who can be misled into believing that reactions in patients are not due to the presence of leukocytes in the product, when patients become refractory, and also we will have failed ourselves, as QA is based on the principle of a continuous assessment which provides sound data on which to base confidence in the product and its safety and efficacy. New technologies have created many advances in the production area, but their application also carries additional responsibility and changes in attitude. Changes in standards should not be made for the sake of change, but to make the system more effective with more accurate information. There is a trend towards more information exchange between producers, therefore it is essential to ensure that the exchange data is factual and not cosmetic or fictitious.

Improving transfusion practice through self-inspection — The evaluation of the appropriateness of blood transfusion and its products is a part of the requirement for discharge monitoring in some countries. For example, platelet transfusion to patients with a count of $>50 \times 10^9/l$ platelets is questionable and will be automatically flagged for review by a transfusion committee. In patients with hematological problems and a platelet count of $<20 \times 10^9/l$, transfusion is indicated but it is important that a posttransfusion count be obtained before approving a second dose of platelets. Arrangements should be made by hospital technologists or physicians for data collection and communication concerning potential refractoriness to random-donor platelets. HLA typing and antibody screening are performed to determine if HLA matched, single-donor plateletpheresis is indicated.

Apart from justification for transfusion, on the basis of the specified criteria, it is essential to create a follow-up chart to document clinical response on the basis of laboratory data. This should include a statement of any adverse reactions, complications, and final outcome, with the signature of the reviewers. In addition, a concurrent review of all blood transfusion requests, coupled with unsolicited consultation, is believed to provide the most effective method of controlling inappropriate use. The additional benefit of this system of review (audit) is the process of building trust and improving communication between blood bank personnel and clinical staff.

It is important to bear in mind that even when the transfusion occurs outside the hospital, the monitoring of all quality assurance issues remains the joint responsibility of the hospital transfusion committee and the blood transfusion services, using compatible audit criteria. Correcting the inappropriateness of transfusion practice not only serves to avoid unnecessary adverse effects in patients, but also preserves a scarce resource. Both effective audit procedures and physician education and reeducation constitute reliable means for improving the quality of service.

Traditionally, the incentives for conducting quality assurance have been negative for the most part because of the problem-focused nature (i.e., flagging the variation or deviation from the specification or criteria). However, today, effort is directed towards positive reporting of ongoing activities, which clearly reinforces good practice and openness to potential future changes.

In this respect, clinicians and managers need to develop coaching and counselling skills to improve performance when failures occur. Occasionally, a failure or problem may not be reported because of fear of losing a job; if the problem is found, the challenging approach is to make the individual involved understand that if nothing is done about the problem this will then be cause for either losing the job or closing down. The fundamental steps in attaining a desirable level of improvement in quality of service are (1) concentration on steady improvement rather than perfection and (2) concentration on modifying the system rather than attempting rapid and drastic changes in attitude or personality.

B. STANDARDS AND STANDARDIZATION

1. Commonality of Purpose with the Health Care Industries

Although there is substantial commonality of purpose (that is to attain and maintain an acceptable standard of product quality, safety, efficiency, and economy of all activities) between BTS and the pharmaceutical industry, nevertheless there are also significant procedural and technical differences. For example, while batch control and statistical sampling techniques can be applied to fractionated products as part of an overall QA strategy, these approaches are of only limited value and applicability in the blood component context. As a consequence, in the BTSs the role of procedural control and validation becomes of paramount importance, whereby the quality of individual components is inferred primarily from the ability to demonstrate compliance with clearly defined and validated procedures. This principle applies equally to the quality of all areas of service activities and includes professional integrity and competence as well as equipment, raw materials, reagents, analytical/screening procedures, and effective surveillance of staff attitude towards product safety, efficacy, and adverse reactions, where approved standards should be set.

Requirement	Reference to
Blood donor selection	Donor selection criteria
Blood/blood components	Product specification
Processing (manufacturing)	GMP
Laboratory activities and reagents for grouping and transfusion microbiology	GLP, Laboratory accreditation
Administration/management	Quality system (TQM)
Computerised release and issue	System validation and reliability

FIGURE 3. Quality requirements according to specific guidelines.

2. Minimum Quality Requirements

A good deal of work concerning quality requirements has already been achieved by international organizations and learned societies such as the Council of Europe, the World Health Organization, and the International Society for Blood Transfusion. However, it appears that there are no agreed and established systems or models for an effective quality system applicable to blood transfusion services.

It is, nevertheless, pleasing to note that many individual transfusion services now recognize the merits of an integrated quality approach and published national guidelines and standards are becoming available, though progress is still somewhat erratic.

Standardization in its strictest sense deals with the methods and systems of organization, allowing the recognition of deviations from the quality requirements. These requirements are summarized in Figure 3.

In assessing the effectiveness or standard of the above requirements, the following questions are pertinent:

- Do satisfactory quality requirements exist for every component and essential activity?
- Are the parameters used the best available indicators of quality of products and operations?
- How often is each product or operation controlled (frequency)?
- Does poor quality reflect deficient operations and what corrective action is taken?
- Is there an agreed procedure to check the adequacy of supplies, control of import/export, and even the promotion of knowledge in the entire field?

High standards are effectively achieved by first validating all existing activities/procedures, then by compliance with specification and standard operating procedures (SOPs), and finally by effective communications and exchanges.

3. Standards of Testing as Applied to Blood Components

Testing encompasses all aspects from donors and raw materials at the beginning, through involvement with in-process controls, to the QC of finished products, as well as process/system validation and evaluation of deviations and unusual events. Items which impinge on the quality of components are numerous and include donor and team care, transport, premises and facilities, equipment, documentation, validation, QC/QA, emergency supplies, long-term storage, staffing, training, excessive throughput, inadequate supervision, mishandling of samples, equipment variances and/or contamination, invalid testing, inappropriate actions or communications, and inadequate characterization of products.

In establishing standards for testing, it should be emphasized that blood components are considered biological materials that cannot be precisely characterized by physical and chemical means. Therefore, the essential requirement that must be fulfilled during collection, processing, storage, and despatch is that the chemicals used, anticoagulant and/or additives, should not be damaging, in the quantities used, to the blood collected or indeed to the donor/recipient. At the same time, any decomposition products from the components or metabolites formed during storage must not be harmful to the intended recipient.

4. Standardization Programs in Blood Transfusion Services

Unfortunately, while impressive strides have been made towards the harmonization of the procedural aspects of blood component collection, processing, and storage, there has been comparatively little progress towards standardization of the analytical aspects. This is despite the fact that there is general agreement that the quality of measurements are a potential source of disharmony between blood transfusion services, both on a national and international level.

The major objective in the standardization of blood component testing is the establishment of a group infrastructure for a core program of comparative relevant analytical measurements, along the lines of existing EQAS (External Quality Assessment Schemes). In this way, individual laboratories would be able to demonstrate the validity of their data in a comparative way and facilitate the mutual recognition of each other's analytical measurements.

The four major principles which assist in the assessment and improvement of the quality of analytical measurements are

- Use of validated methods
- Incorporation of certified reference materials in the testing system

- Participation in externally administered proficiency testing schemes
- Formal recognition that all analytical laboratories should conform to the same principles, which is the basis for accreditation or licensing

The two most significant activities in a standardization program are the collaborative strategies in the preparation and maintenance of reference materials and the validation of relevant methods which possess the desired levels of accuracy and precision.

Within blood transfusion services, the main purpose of standardization is to ensure acceptable uniformity in results while allowing for different methods in the various laboratories. Standard preparations should fulfill at least three requirements:

- They should be well defined with agreed potency
- There should be material equivalence to preclude matrix effects
- They should possess good long-term stability

Translating these requirements to blood components, it becomes immediately obvious that material equivalence is generally not possible because of the heterogeneity of the source materials which is further aggravated by the preparation procedures; decay rates differ for substantially the same products, and standardized tests are often not available. Nevertheless by conforming to GMP, it is still possible to produce components with satisfactory levels of quality, safety, efficacy, reliability, and cost effectiveness. The ensuing comments are pertinent to current testing procedures for both the cellular and the hemostatic (plasma, cryoprecipitate, and platelet concentrates) blood components.

C. NEW DEVELOPMENTS IN COMPONENT TESTING PROCEDURES

1. Standardization of Red Cell Components

Accurate assessment of red cell volume (MCV) and hematocrit is essential when attempting to ensure morphological and functional integrity of the red cell. Automated red cell counters which are increasingly being used in hematology laboratories, can provide this data rapidly and reliably. However, measurement of cellular indices in a hematology laboratory is carried out on fresh (<6 hours) samples in ethylenediaminetetra-acetic acid (EDTA) dipotassium salt, and caution is required when the same technique is indiscriminately applied for the assessment of red cells or other cellular components of blood, collected in citrate and stored for the agreed clinical shelf life. This is exemplified by the observation that the cellular indices for an EDTA sample are quite different from those for a citrated sample. Moreover, when EDTA is added to the citrated sample to simulate comparability in counting test conditions, there is a concentration-related increase in MCV. An analogous situation relates to hematocrit which is measured by automated cell counter as compared to the more traditional microcentrifugation technique where aberrant results would be generated by the absence or difference concentration of EDTA.[1]

Moreover, changes in MCV and hematocrit also occur during storage and are evident as measured by either of the above-mentioned methods. This has considerable implication when evaluating the efficacy of frozen/thawed/deglycerolized red cells on the basis of MCV where an increase of up to 18% is seen after thawing/deglycerolyzation. In both these cases, a more reliable method will be, to use in conjunction with MCV, the measurement of hemoglobin which remains reasonably constant during storage or after deglycerolyzation.[1]

2. Standardization of Hemostatic Component Testing

Apart from the problem of heterogeneity in the source preparation in respect to anticoagulant ratio, processing can introduce further heterogeneity (such as high fibrinogen, von Willebrand Factor [vWF], and fibronectin levels subsequent to cryoprecipitation) affecting the validity of certain assays and any results thus obtained. This is despite the ready availability of international standards for Factor VIII and Factor IX. In a recent collaborative study between three European centers, while good comparability was observed between one-stage clotting and two-stage chromogenic assays in all three laboratories, the values obtained by the two-stage clotting assays were more variable and differed from the chromogenic assay by up to 30%. Since coagulation assays are highly sensitive to traces of thrombin, it is suggested that an activity ratio such as one-stage clotting vs. one-stage chromogenic or vWF:Ag (FVIII carrier protein) be considered for reporting.[1,2] A standardized program which provides essential information on the activation state of the native activated or inactivated product would be a necessary requirement. This trend is already started in many transfusion services (for details, see Reference 13).

3. Standardization of Platelet Function Testing

There is an urgent need to introduce a standardized prerelease method for platelet viability indicators and storage lesion. The fundamental objective of platelet function testing in the blood transfusion services is, therefore, to ensure that platelet concentrates destined for platelet transfusion are morphologically intact and functionally viable. A comprehensive range of platelet function tests is currently available, but none appear to be particularly suitable for large-scale screening and prerelease testing, particularly in a large establishment. An innovative approach, recently introduced by one of the authors, has not only improved the reproducibility in cell counting procedure and the validity of the result, but also provided a platelet viability indicator, using an automated hematology cell counter which can be fully standardized.[3,4] This System for Enumeration, Activity, and Leukocyte content, known by its acronym "SEAL" of approval, embraces three important criteria of acceptability in one test and is based on the difference between cellular indices — in particular, mean platelet volumes (MPV) — of paired samples with and without added EDTA ($dMPV_{EDTA}$).[5] The correlation between $dMPV_{EDTA}$ and platelet age is shown in Figure 4 and is based on work carried out in the NLBTC Quality Department.

The difference in MPV using this paired sample procedure is equally applicable to various other situations associated with changes in platelet morphology, such as exposure to cold, hypotonic stress, mechanical trauma, and aging, which are associated with variable degrees of changes in platelet indices, all providing useful information on platelet functional integrity. It has been observed that $dMPV_{EDTA}$ and $dMPV_{storage}$ correlate with a host of other functions, making this family of indicators attractive for both producers and users.[6]

Evidence is accumulating that dMPV correlates with a progressive rise in glycocalicin (GC), a major segment of the glycoprotein 1b released or cleaved from platelets into the supernatant plasma during storage.[7] This is corroborated with the release of the vWF, another marker of platelet storage lesion.[5-7] With the advances in flow cytometry and microplate assays, it becomes possible to differentiate platelets in their native activated and/or secretion status, helping the assessment of quality at a cellular level.[8] Apart from the reliability of these test procedures, they readily lend themselves to large-scale prerelease testing, and by derivation could lead to the establishment of a standard procedure in the near future. These things can best be achieved by establishing a special-interest advisory group with the following tasks:

- Validation of new generation tests in order to assess their benefit as an integral part of testing program at a national/international level
- Promotion of the idea of free exchange of information and technical expertise by removing technical barriers
- Action in advisory capacity to help in troubleshooting of quality problems, providing appropriate training, workshops, and seminars in either conventional or new technology
- Provision of locally made and calibrated reference material reagents, for like-with-like assay, establishing and contributing to QA schemes on a local or national basis

VI. FUTURE TRENDS

New developments in blood transfusion science and medicine, in particular with the expected changes in European regulations in 1992, require continuous updating of blood transfusion policy and practice. In the future, it is envisaged that increasing emphasis will be placed on the areas of quality described below.

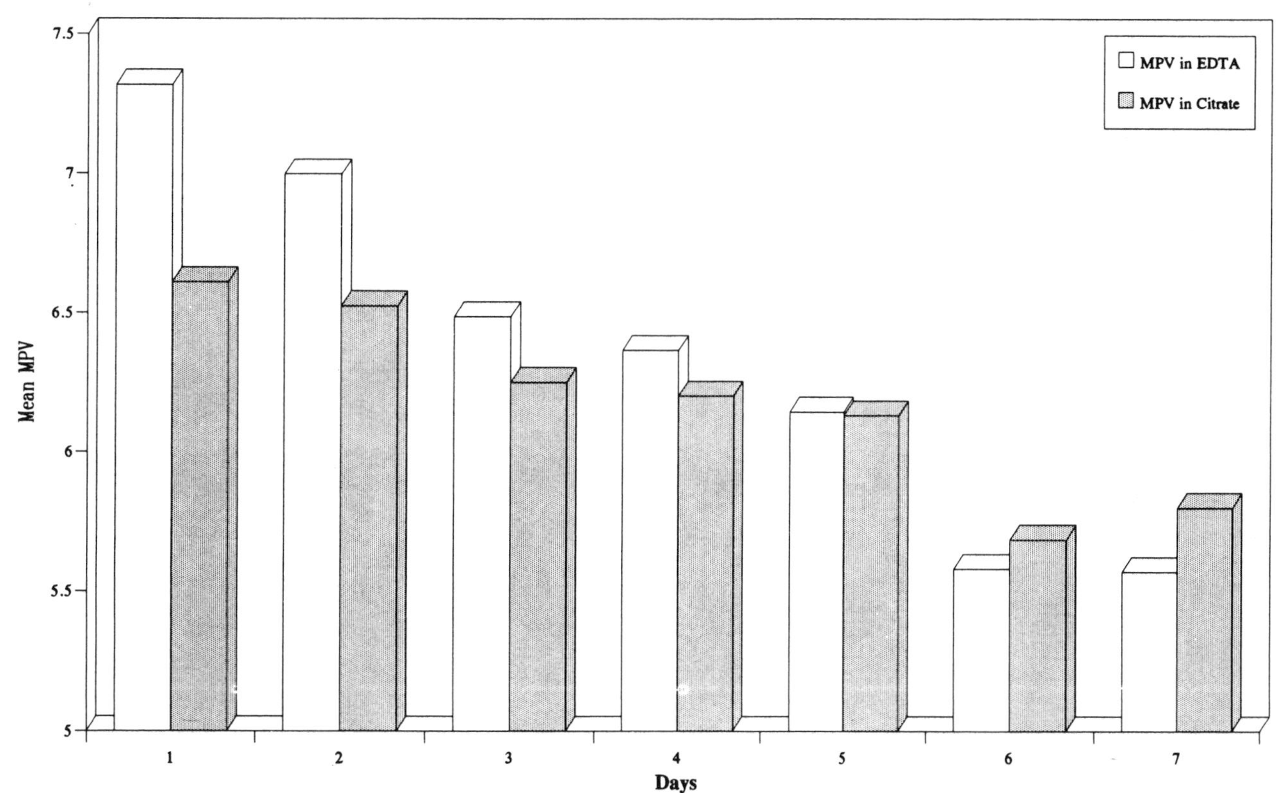

FIGURE 4. Changes in mean MPV during platelet shelf life.

Prioritizing — At the top of the priority list are professional standards, special business know how, and the technical skills required for effectively running the blood transfusion services. The need at all levels for special training in quality concept and quality awareness cannot be denied. Training must not only be documented but should lend itself to second- and third-party accreditation. Expectedly in the 1990s, laboratory managers in the blood transfusion services are required to have not only a broad spectrum of knowledge of various acts and regulations (i.e., product liability, health and safety, environmental and health care regulations, and confidentiality), but also to become effective and competent in management practice. Another top priority is to stay competitive while coming to terms with expected new laws on unification, regulations, and accreditation standards. The cost of falling behind, of not keeping up with the current momentum of innovation and initiatives wil definitely prove to be risky. This is of particular relevance as the liability risk can range from simple notice, to complete shut down of the organization, with gross penalty.

Continuous education — Blood transfusion medicine embraces a vast spectrum of public health knowledge and technology of a diversity of disciplines covering blood donor epidemiology, blood donor recruitment, motivation and selection, automated hemapheresis for collection of cells and plasma, advanced laboratory technologies essential for rapid, reliable, and accurate screening of samples and products at various stages, and critical care in formulating appropriate specifications and indications for blood product monitoring, usage, release, and recall. Each requires specialized documentation and records of competence. Equally important are the knowledge of some other special areas such as immunohematology, pharmacology, cryobiology, cellular and molecular biochemistry and biology, intensive care, and management and accountancy skills. Naturally, certain conditions should be met in integrating all diversified activities to assure safe and efficacious transfusion and to provide unequivocal support in the context of litigation and compliance. These have become mandatory in some countries.

Training — One must make sure that everyone understands that the BTS is no longer a mere institution but an enterprise which cannot escape the need to elaborate its own advanced strategic plan and to assess its own relative technological training and educational capabilities. This is best achieved by having a long-term development policy, possibly through collaborative work with other BTS and/or private sector organizations at national and/or international levels.

Cost effectiveness and competitiveness — It is important to ensure that the required levels of competitiveness, in the constraint of economic problems, are realistic. Unfortunately, medical problems are often due to economic shortcomings, and only through collaboration with other BTSs can economic gain and waste reduction be achieved. For example, the use of standardized reagents in coordination with large centers will allow lower prices, making the establishment more competitive in some other areas.

Staff enrichment and satisfaction — Staff must be encouraged in broadening and perfecting their technological capability by allowing the initiative of individuals in the team to be fully explored, instead of being stultified for the sake of uniformity. Note, however, that this must never be at the expense of full compliance.

Full regulatory compliance — This, undoubtedly, would substantially increase the cost of various products and processes. In this respect, from the regulatory standpoint, the European Directive on product licensing demands that the same level of statutory compliance for all medical products be applied (much in line with the Food and Drug Administration [FDA] regulatory practice), regardless of the status of the manufacturer (state owned or private). In fact, both the FDA and the Department of Health are seeking comments as to whether blood and blood components intended for transfusion should be exempt from the Prescription and Drug Marketing Act of 1987.

Research and development aspects — The increasing demand for plasma and its derivatives has already led to introduction of dedicated apheresis machines, which allow plasmapheresis to be performed in mobile sessions. This provides a better opportunity for donors who will have the advantage and comfort of donating near their home or work. The recent introduction of blood collection tubes with an integral sampling site is another development which helps in improving donor safety while avoiding a breach of the closed system. This also reduces accidental endangering of staff when stoppers of vacuum container systems must be pierced. Preliminary studies using this technique have revealed no significant difference in either the activation of coagulation, fibrinolysis, and complement systems, or alteration in Factor VIII or platelet yields. Such an economical sampling technique can prove useful for collection and storage of long-term samples from individual blood donations to be used either as reference or research samples. Modern automated sampling (i.e., from pilot sample tubes), in combination with computerized information transfer, offers an alternative economical solution for streamlining of collection and archiving which, inevitably, would become an adjunct to quality monitoring in support of new litigation and liability.

The extent of investment in developing new technology and the time scale for achieving the transfusion objective also depends on how soon blood and plasma derivatives will be replaced by products originating from nonhuman sources (i.e., hybridomas and recombinant processes). Both protein fractions and red blood cell substitutes are currently on the agenda, with the private sector assessing the cost of competitiveness. Product safety and efficacy will be based on clinical trials and regulations, and manufacturers' liability. With current economic constraints, and with safety being intrinsic to the process of design, it is unlikely that individual blood transfusion centers and fractionators can make great breakthroughs unless the projects are supported through joint ventures with the private sector. Similarly, extensive trials on new processes, equipment design, control and protection, and preservation of product quality during handling, storage, packaging, and delivery are essential. These require continuous updates with state-of-the-art methodology. In this respect, despite many advances in different areas of transfusion science and medicine, much remains to be resolved concerning storage stability criteria. For example, optimal storage conditions of platelets in various additive solutions or different sizes of packs and the leukocyte depletion capacity of various filters all need to be further scrutinized. The criteria of acceptability and the rate of meeting threshold limits for action-taking need to be fully established and standardized.

The feedback of QC results and failures to the manufacturers also contributes to quality maintenance and improvement. Occasionally, the high values for leukocytes in products are due to preparation and storage and may not be dependent on the efficiency of filters or the counting system used, requiring comparative analyses by the manufacturers who can reach the users, and therefore, the critical information.

Documentation archiving — New procedures to reduce workload or stress are also vital to the effectiveness of the service. In the future, it may become necessary to continuously redefine areas of affinity, based on documentation archiving. This is of particular relevance in the context of compliance with the Consumer Protection Act and product liability legislation, which would be associated with an increase in quantity and quality documentation in the use of blood and its products. This would have additional cost implications. For example, package inserts must be more comprehensive while remaining understandable to users; record keeping of product release, receipt, and maintenance must be meticulous; and labeling and accompanying forms and scrutiny of appropriate documentation must be ensured and more attention must be paid to the wording. The ultimate goal of those involved in transfusion science and medicine is, of course, to provide the patient with an effective product which must achieve maximum therapeutic effect with minimum risk. Blood, as a biological source material, would never be considered as entirely risk-free or defect-free, but maximum efforts must be directed towards reducing the risk to a minimum, through the implementation of quality systems. These must encompass not only the quality of premises, storage, equipment, reagents, staff selection, training, and continuing education, but also all of the steps involved from donor recruitment to administration of the product to the patients, including the measurement of the *in vivo* response. The buck, therefore, does not stop at the hospital door but must be shown to continue through to the bedside, involving the hospital transfusion committee and internal/external auditing for the optimal usage of this important resource.

Automation and computerization — One critical area is our increasing reliance on evolving automation. In areas of dependency on automation and computerization, a substantial investment has already been made. Computer systems help to manage the organization and ensure the integrity and safety of the blood supply, hence becoming the primary control point of the whole operation. Figure 5 shows schematically the input of computerized checking

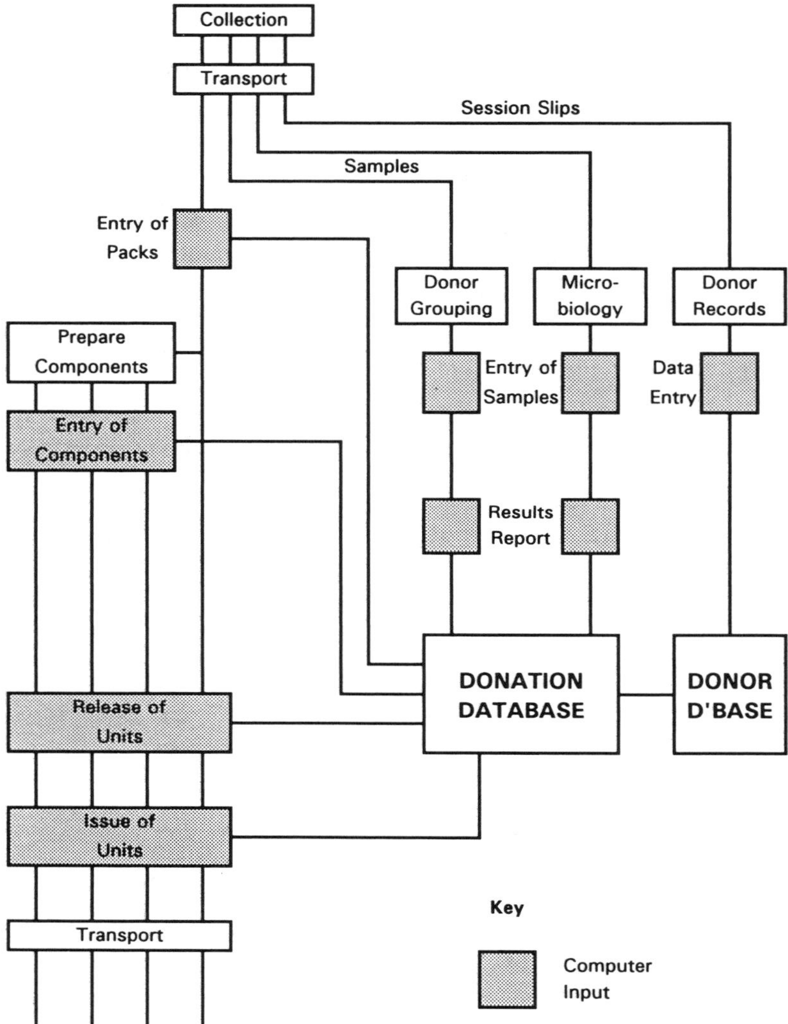

FIGURE 5. Current computerized donor/donation management system.

of suitable units (as operational at NLBTC) helping in the detection of unsuitable units from collection to issue. The shaded boxes indicate input operations which assist in the reconciliation of stock, prevent issue of a product which is subject to a hold condition, and present various action lists indicating noncompliance. This provides the quality personnel with information which must be followed up with corrective action.

Contingency planning — Disaster recovery planning is another area of critical dependence that may have evolved because of automation. Disaster recovery planning is an essential part of planning for each department and is considered essentially a business issue rather than a technical one. This should not be considered as a matter of ''just a good idea'' but as a matter of survival deserving special attention. There are many issues that managers must consider as measures of contingency planning. Undoubtedly, the ability to survive and to continue to deliver safe and effective blood products and services to the community is dependent upon the level of preparation and the level of risk determined to be acceptable.

A final thought — This chapter contains many references to licensing and certification as an integral part of the conceptual acceptance of quality assurance. It would be wise to remember that successful attainment of licensing and/or certification should not be seen as an end in itself but only the end of the beginning. Otherwise, it might just represent the beginning of the end. Perfect quality does not exist, there is always room for improvement.

This manuscript is not intended to provide the specific answers to quality needs, but rather aims at exploring some compelling areas that make quality assurance an essential approach for the blood transfusion community.

ACKNOWLEDGMENTS

The authors wish to express their gratitude to Dr. Branko Brozovic, Consultant Haematologist at the North London Blood Transfusion Center (NLBTC), for his expert advice and encouragement and to the members of the NLBTC Quality Department for their technical support and expertise. A special thanks to all the staff of NLBTC for their wholehearted support in attaining and maintaining high standards of quality.

REFERENCES

1. **Seghatchian, M. J. and Tandy, N.,** Standards and Standardisation of Blood Component Production and Testing Procedures, Newsletter No. 01, Dec. 1991, British Blood Transfusion Society, UK.
2. **Seghatchian, M. J.,** Regulatory control, standardisation and characterisation of clinical concentrates, in *Factor VIII – von Willebrand Factor,* Volume II, Seghatchian, M. J. and Savidge, G. F., Eds., CRC Press, Boca Raton, FL, 1990.
3. **Seghatchian, M. J.,** An overview of current quality control procedures in platelet storage lesion and transfusion, *Blood Coagulation and Fibrinolysis,* 2, 357, 1991.
4. **Ip, A. H. L. and Seghatchian, M. J.,** Quality monitoring of haemapheresis platelet concentrates: sampling with EDTA helps with the standardisation and improves the consistency, *Blood Coagulation and Fibrinolysis,* 2, 239, 1991.
5. **Seghatchian, M. J.,** Newer approaches to quality monitoring platelet concentrates, *Haematology Highlights,* No. 14, 1992, Speywood, UK.
6. **Vickers, M. V., Ip, A. H. L., Coutts, M., Tandy, N. P., and Seghatchian, M. J.,** Characteristics of platelet concentrates with particular reference to Autopheresis C Plateletcell™: correlation between dMPV and other tests for platelet function, *Blood Coagulation and Fibrinolysis,* 2, 361, 1991.
7. **Bessos, H., Murphy, W. G., and Seghatchian, M. J.,** Monitoring the release of glycocalicin in platelet concentrates by ELISA, *Blood Coagulation and Fibrinolysis,* 2, 373, 1991.
8. **Goodall, A. H.,** Platelet Activation during Preparation and Storage of Concentrates: Detection by Flow Cytometry, 377.

ADDITIONAL BIBLIOGRAPHY OF RELEVENT PUBLICATIONS

- BS 4778: Part 1: 1987 (ISO8402: 1986) Quality Vocabulary — International Terms, British Standards Institution, London.
- BS 5750: Part 0: Section 0.1: 1987 Quality Systems — Principal concepts and applications/ Guide to selection and use (equiv. to ISO9000: 1987, EN29000: 1987), British Standards Institution, London.
- BS 5750: Part 0: Section 0.2: 1987 Quality Systems — Principal concepts and applications/Guide to quality management and quality system elements (equiv. to ISO9004: 1987, EN29004: 1987), British Standards Institution, London.
- BS 5750: Part 1: 1987 Quality Systems — Specification for design/development, production, installation and servicing (equiv. to ISO9001: 1987, EN29001: 1987), British Standards Institution, London.
- BS 5750: Part 4: 1989 Quality Systems — Guide to the use of BS 5750: Parts 1, 2 and 3 (no ISO or EN equivalent), British Standards Institution, London.
- Guidelines for the Blood Transfusion Services in the United Kingdom, Her Majesty's Stationery Office, London, 1989.
- Guide to Good Pharmaceutical Manufacturing Practice, Her Majesty's Stationery Office, London, 1983.
- The Rules Governing Medical Products in the European Community: Volume IV — Guide to Good Manufacturing Practice for Medicinal Products, Office for Official Publications of the European Communities, Luxembourg, 1989.
- Current Good Manufacturing Practice for Blood and Blood Products (FDA Regulations in the U.S.A.), Code of Federal Regulations, 21CFR606, Office of the Federal Register, National Archives and Records Administration, Washington, DC.
- Technical Manual, 10th ed., American Association of Blood Banks, Arlington, VA, 1990.
- Requirements for the Collection, Processing, and Quality Control of Blood, Blood Components, and Plasma Derivatives (Requirements for Biological Substances No. 27, 1988), World Health Organisation, Geneva, 1988.

Chapter 2

THE ACHIEVABLE IDEAL TRANSFUSION SERVICE

Tibor J. Greenwalt

TABLE OF CONTENTS

ISBN 0-8493-4938-9

I. INTRODUCTION

I could make this the shortest chapter ever written, quoting P.J. Schmidt's prediction that " . . . by the year 2000 blood bankers will have put themselves out of business. The blood bank will be obsolete.

"We will no longer be giving blood transfusions because we will have blood substitutes that are more efficient than the real thing. We will be using hemoglobin substitutes that can carry and deliver more oxygen to the body's cells than our own red blood cells. We will have platelet substitutes that not only arrest the flow of blood in broken blood vessels, but will stabilize clotting as well.

"We will know how to transform blood from one type to another. And we'll be able to generate in tissue culture the various chemicals, enzymes, and metabolites carried in the bloodstream."[1]

Much progress has been made, but blood banks are not likely to advance into obsolescence within the foreseeable future.[2] Experimentation with hemoglobin solutions to substitute for red blood cells started in 1933.[3,4] After several hopeful innovations, promise of success still seems remote.[5] The synthesis of artificial red cells by microencapsulation has been received with some excitement and cautious optimism, but has not progressed beyond that.[6,7] Experimentation with perfluorochemical (PFC) emulsions as oxygen-carrying blood substitutes for at least three decades[8] has also eluded practical application.[5] The conclusion of Gould et al. in 1986, that the PFC emulsion Fluosol-DA, 20%, appeared to be an inadequate red cell substitute in acute anemia served to halt clinical trials at that time.[9] This product has recently been licensed only to supplement oxygen delivery to the myocardium during coronary artery balloon angioplasty.[10]

The use of hematopoietic growth factors, including erythropoietin and G-CSF, produced by recombinant DNA technology, holds immediate promise[11] to reduce requirements for red blood cells and very likely also platelet and granulocyte concentrates. A recombinant Factor VIII product is in the final phase of very successful clinical trial.[12] The generation of other coagulation factors and plasma proteins by these means will surely follow. Pharmacologic agents are also being more widely used in patients with coagulopathies.

Woodman and Harker[13] have recently reviewed the use of drugs in the management of bleeding. Included in this category are: 1-deamino-8-D-arginine vasopressin (desmopressin, DDAVP); epsilon aminocaproic acid (Amicar, EACA); prostaglandins (PGI_2, prostacyclin), and aprotinin (Trasylol). The manufacture of the formed elements in tissue culture remains a remote possibility.

The expanding and aging population and the development and expansion of the use of new therapeutic modalities (e.g., chemotherapy, transplantation of bone marrow and solid organs) promise to outstrip the sparing effects on blood resources by the application of the products mentioned above. Thus, it is timely to propose a model for the most effective delivery of transfusion services designed to be acceptable to both clinician and patient.

Discussion of donor resource development (recruitment), collection, processing, component preparation, or the details of laboratory procedures and automation will not be included.

Most appropriate appears to be discussion of a model, idealized transfusion service for the most effective utilization of what is now, or soon to be, available. Concern for the maximum safety of the patient, protection of staff, and satisfaction of the clinician are givens.

II. ORDERING

For years we have been dreaming of a way in which to influence the practices of doctors regarding the use of blood components. Education is one weapon. The Transfusion Medicine Academic Award program of the National Heart, Lung, and Blood Institute (NHLBI), which is being closed even now, was designed to support enhancements of the teaching of this discipline in medical schools, to house staff, and to clinicians. This is a worthwhile evolutionary approach. The Consensus Development Conferences of the Office of Medical Applications of Research (OMAR) focused needed attention on the use of blood components. Three such conferences dealing with Fresh Frozen Plasma,[14] Platelet Concentrates,[15] and Perioperative Red Cell Transfusions[16] have been held and the results have been widely disseminated. The importance of blood as a national resource has received further recognition by the inauguration of the National Blood Resources Education Program (NBREP) in 1986 by the Office of Prevention, Education and Control (OPEC) of the NHLBI. Briefly stated, the goals of NBREP are (1) to improve public awareness of the need and safety of blood donation and also bone marrow, and (2) to educate doctors about the utilization of these resources. It is difficult to measure the impact of these programs.[17,18] They have put useful tools into the hands of local professional staff. Local efforts must be draconian if they are to succeed. What can be done to accelerate the learning curve?

A. COMPUTERIZED ORDERING

A dedicated computer terminal on each floor for the ordering of blood components, intravenous fluids, and drugs could serve to implement transfusion triggers and also to prevent error in the use of drugs and IV fluids. The patient's diagnosis and all the updated laboratory information would have to be entered. Examples of messages that might be used are

1. This patient has a hematocrit of 24% and a hemoglobin of 8 g. Please justify your order for two units of packed red cells.
2. Caution — hemoglobin of 7.0 g after delivery may be adequate. If absolutely necessary, do not transfuse at over 1 ml/kg/hour.

3. Platelet count is ≥20,000/μl (2×10^{10}/l). Indication for platelet transfusion should be reviewed.

An important byproduct of such a system would be the capability of collecting data about the utilization of blood components by diagnosis. This would be valuable information for updating hospitals' Maximum Surgical Blood Ordering Schedules (MSBOS).[19,20] It is assumed that all sophisticated hospital transfusion services already have well established MSBOS. Pooling of such information nationally would furnish accurate data about the total use of all the major components and also much-needed information about diagnosis-related trends in utilization.

The Hospital Transfusion Committee, if properly organized and used, can serve as another effective educational tool.[21] It is important to have as members representatives of all the major blood users (including trauma surgery, cardiovascular surgery, orthopedics, obstetrics, pediatrics, anesthesiology, hematology/oncology, transplantation, and nursing). The transfusion service and laboratory medicine should be represented but the chair must be from one of the user departments or divisions. The use of blood components must be audited, as required by the Joint Committee for Accreditation of Hospitals.[22] Retrospective audits are not very effective because the auditee cannot be expected to recall details two to four months back or may have moved on, e.g., a resident.[23] The computerized ordering mechanism described above can also be adapted to serve a concurrent audit handled on a daily basis by professional transfusion medicine staff. Only flagrant violations of good transfusion medicine practice, chronic offenders, and policy matters would have to be placed on the agenda of the Hospital Transfusion Committee.

III. CLOSING THE DONOR TO PATIENT LOOP

Most serious transfusion reactions are caused by clerical errors.[24,25] Many of these errors result from the lack of understanding of the importance of identifying the patient's blood sample for the crossmatch in a foolproof manner. There is no way to know how often this happens, because, without knowing either the donor's or the recipient's ABO blood groups, approximately two thirds of the time they would be compatible by chance (A to A; O to O; O to A; O to B; O, A, AB or B to AB, etc.). Such errors may only be uncovered when it is necessary to collect another sample from the patient for additional crossmatching during the same hospital stay or on a subsequent occasion. Clearly, it is important to retain in the crossmatch laboratory computer's memory all data for screening purposes on future hospitalizations of the patient. The computer file could be purged on a prospective schedule based on the patient's age or some other acceptable plan. It is conceivably possible to close the loop between donor and patient electronically using a portable bar code reader which would match the bar code identification assigned to the patient and affixed to any laboratory blood sample and to blood components delivered for that patient's use. Prototypes of such devices have been field tested but are not considered ready for profitable marketing by the developer. A lock and key system in eight different combinations (O+, O−, A+, A−, B+, B−, AB+, AB−) is also feasible.[26] The patient would have attached to his wrist band a key which would make it possible to open the lock on the bag port only if it had the right blood group lock attached in the crossmatch laboratory. This would not be as individualized as the bar code system and would only assure that components of the right blood groups were transfused but not necessarily those which had been crossmatched with the patient.

Ideally, the intravenous service of the hospital would be staffed by and operated by the transfusion service. Thus, there can be assurance that only staff fully aware of the hazards, trained and skilled in all aspects of intravenous therapy, are involved. The responsibility for collecting all specimens, including those for the clinical pathology laboratory, would be fixed. The same trained staff would complete the loop by bearing the responsibility for all intravenous therapy. Improper handling and storage of blood components and the infusion of incompatible IV fluids would be less common. Chemotherapy for oncology patients should be left under the aegis of well-trained nurse clinicians in the division of hematology/oncology. With such a tightly controlled organization, closing the loop by bar code or lock and key is conceivable. In those places where the addressograph is used for generating labels it would be possible to generate multiple addressograph plates for each patient. One attached to the patient could be used to generate specimen labels and one could be attached to the crossmatch blood sample going to the transfusion service to be used for generating overlay identification labels for crossmatched products. The means to generate additional addressograph plates would have to be constantly available on all hospital floors with patients needing transfusions.

Another inconvenience and frequent source of trouble and annoyance is lack of control of the transporter service for blood samples and blood components. The model transfusion service should have its own transport staff for the traffic to and from the ER, OR, recovery rooms, ICU, SICU, hospital floors, and clinics.

IV. CLINICAL RESPONSIBILITIES

Transfusion medicine has become a predominantly clinically oriented discipline. The specialist in this field of medicine needs to have training in both laboratory and clinical medicine, very much like the hematologist. The director and professional staff of a model transfusion service are expected to assume the role of consultants to any physician who uses blood components, blood derivatives, or related pharmaceutical products. Only in this way can proper utilization of the available services be achieved. At one hospital, the use of fresh frozen plasma was reduced by 77% in 24 months by the intervention of one physician from the blood bank staff.[27] This cannot be achieved by sending out memos and speaking at rounds but only by aggressive consultation whenever the service is ordered. The transfusion service cannot intervene in this manner unless a formal mechanism for triggering consultation is in place and accepted by the clinical staff. Consultation on every nonemergency order for blood components, derivatives, and relevant pharmaceuticals should be automatic at the discretion of the director of the transfusion service. It would be impossible to review the chart and/or to see every patient for whom red blood cells, fresh frozen plasma, platelets, and cryoprecipitate, etc. are ordered, but selective monitoring and the transfusion medicine consultant's note in the patient's chart should be part of the system.

Clearly, it is impossible for the transfusion service staff to know when to consult unless they are notified. In my experience, one cannot rely on the hematologist, surgeon, pediatrician, or anesthesiologist to call for consultation by the transfusion specialist. In most institutions the transfusion service gets involved only when there is an alarming reaction, if there is difficulty in crossmatching or, perhaps, when a new procedure such as heart or liver transplantation or extracorporeal membrane oxygenation (ECMO) is introduced. Then usually the transfusion service is only expected to play a passive role. Ideally the transfusion experts should be involved from the start and should play an integral role in the planning.

Involvement and consultation can be enhanced if there is an early warning mechanism for alerting the transfusion service to problems of concern. I suggest, therefore, that the transfusion service take over some of the functions of the pharmacy in being responsible for inventorying and issuing plasma derivatives (albumin, plasma protein fraction, colloid plasma expanders, intravenous gamma globulin, hyperimmune anti-Rh globulin, anti-hemophilic factor concentrates); the pharmaceuticals used for the management of bleeding disorders such as DDAVP, epsilon aminocaproic acid (EACA, Amicar), and aprotinin; and the hematopoietic growth factors (erythropoietin and G-CSF etc.) which will have an impact on the future management of transfusion problems. It would be advantageous if physicians specializing in the management of patients with hemostasis and thrombosis problems would hold joint appointments in medicine and transfusion medicine. Thus, the transfusion service would be alerted to such problems by the products ordered and the clinical clotter would be part of the transfusion medicine consulting team.

A. INTERNAL AND EXTERNAL ELECTRONIC LINKS

It is not unusual for the blood bank to learn of events long after the clinicians have scheduled them. Examples are organ transplantations, especially liver, bone marrow harvesting and infusion, and ECMO. Ideally, dedicated telephone lines to be used by designated staff to give early notice would eliminate hassle and friction. Similar links to the ER and OR would be useful.

Blood bank staff spend a great deal of time telephoning around the world looking for rare donors. It would be very useful if the American Association of Blood Banks, American Red Cross, and World Health Organization lists would be placed in one electronic bank accessible to any authorized person. Only the complete blood group profiles and the blood bank locations with telephone numbers would be on line. Such a hook-up already exists for kidney donors and is being developed for bone marrow donors.

V. SPECIAL SERVICES

A. THERAPEUTIC APHERESIS

Blood banks are looked to as resources for single donor (apheresis) and random donor blood components. As a transfusion service, they should also be responsible for all therapeutic apheresis and serve as consultants to the doctors requesting these procedures.

B. TRANSPLANTATION

It is ideal to have all transplantation laboratory resources for a community centralized in one transfusion service. Paternity testing utilizes related skills and should be included. The highly skilled staff needed for these services should not be duplicated in other departments and at multiple sites.

C. SALVAGE

Intraoperative blood salvage and perioperative isovolumic hemodilution require skills possessed by transfusion service personnel. It does not appear to be logical to have independent teams trained for these services. They can best be coordinated by the transfusion service to avoid costly overlap and duplication.

VI. SUMMARY

Transfusion medicine has achieved recognition as a specialty during the past decade. Rapidly developing knowledge and technology have made it impossible for other branches of medical science to keep abreast. It is essential that this special area of medicine be recognized by our medical colleagues. I have speculated on how transfusions can be made safer for the patient and how the skills of the transfusion specialist might be better utilized. The changes suggested will not occur overnight but it is important to begin serious dialogue and planning for their implementation before we fall further behind. The responsibility has to be placed with those who are most aware of the weight of the responsibility.

ACKNOWLEDGMENT

The author is indebted to Michelle Fine for significant support in preparing the manuscript.

REFERENCES

1. **Schmidt, P. J.,** Blood banking in the year 2000: advance into obsolescence, *Med. Lab. Observer,* July, 1979, p. 2.
2. **Kahn, R. A., Allen, R. W., and Baldasarre, J.,** Alternate sources and substitutes for therapeutic blood components, *Blood,* 66, 1, 1985.
3. **Amberson, W. R., Mulder, A. G., Steggerda, F. R., Flexner, J., and Pankratz, D. S.,** Mammalian life without red blood corpuscles, *Science,* 78, 160, 1933.
4. **Cannan, R. K. and Redish, J.,** The large scale production of crystalline human hemoglobin: with preliminary observations on the effect of its injection in man, in *Blood Substitutes and Blood Transfusion,* Mudd, S. and Thalhimer, W., Eds., Charles C. Thomas, Springfield, IL, 1942, 147.
5. **Zuck, T. F.,** The quest for a blood substitute: in 1990 an unfulfilled promise, in *Transfusion Medicine in the 1990's,* Nance, S. J., Ed., American Association of Blood Banks, Arlington, VA, 1990, 181.
6. **Chang, T. M. S., Ed.,** *Microencapsulation and Artificial cells,* Humana Press, Clifton, NJ, 1984, 320.
7. **Hunt, C. A., Burnette, R. R., MacGregor, R. D., et al.,** Synthesis and evaluation of a prototypal artificial red blood cell, *Science,* 230, 1165, 1985.
8. **Clark, L. C., Jr. and Gollan, F.,** Survival of mammals breathing organic ligands equilibriated with oxygen at atmospheric pressure, *Science,* 152, 1755, 1966.
9. **Gould, S. A., Rosen, L. A., Sehgal, L. R., et al.,** Fluosol-DA as a red-cell substitute in acute anemia, *N. Engl. J. Med.,* 314, 1653, 1986.
10. Alpha Therapeutics Fluosol Oxygen Transport Fluid Approved for Use in Angioplasty, F-D-C Rep. January 8, 1990, 8.
11. **Elias, L.,** Hematopoietic growth factors, in *Transfusion Medicine,* Rossi, E. C., Simon, T. L., and Moss, G. S., Eds., Williams & Wilkins, Baltimore, 1991, 301.
12. **Kaufman, R. J., Wasley, L. C., and Dormer, A. J.,** Synthesis, processing, and secretion of recombinant human factor VIII expressed in mammalian cells, *J. Biol. Chem.,* 263, 6352, 1988.
13. **Woodman, R. C. and Harker, L. A.,** Bleeding complications associated with cardiopulmonary bypass, *Blood,* 76, 1680, 1990.
14. Consensus conference. Fresh frozen plasma: indications and risks, *JAMA,* 253, 551, 1985.
15. Consensus conference. Platelet transfusion therapy, *JAMA,* 257, 1777, 1987.
16. Consensus conference. Perioperative red blood cell transfusion, *JAMA,* 260, 2700, 1988.
17. **Lomas, J., Anderson, G., Enkin, M. et al.,** The role of evidence in the consensus process, *JAMA,* 259, 3001, 1988.
18. **Perry, S.,** The NIH consensus development program: a decade later, *N. Engl. J. Med.,* 317, 485, 1987.
19. **Friedman, B. A., Oberman, H. A., Chadwick, A. R. et al.,** The maximum surgical blood order schedule and surgical blood use in the United States, *Transfusion,* 16, 380, 1976.
20. **Henry, J. B. and Boral, L. I.,** The type and screen: a safe alternative and supplement in selected surgical procedures, *Transfusion,* 17, 163, 1977.
21. **Grindon, A. J., Tomasulo, P. S., Bergin, J. J. et al.,** The hospital transfusion committee, *JAMA,* 253, 340, 1985.
22. Accreditation Manual for Hospitals, Joint Commission on Accreditation of Hospitals, Chicago, 1984.
23. **Toy, P. T., Strauss, R. G., Stehling, L. C. et al.,** Predeposited autologous blood for elective surgery: a national multicenter study, *N. Engl. J. Med.,* 316, 517, 1987.
24. **Honig, C. L. and Bove, J. R.,** Transfusion-associated fatalities: review of Bureau of Biologics reports 1976-1978, *Transfusion,* 20, 653, 1980.

25. **Schmidt, P. J.,** Transfusion mortality with specific reference to surgical and intensive care facilities, *J. Fla. Med. Assoc.,* 67, 151, 1980.
26. **Greenwalt, T. J. and Coe, N.A.,** Device and method for preventing transfusion of incompatible blood, U.S. Patent 4,685,314, August 11, 1987.
27. **Shanberge, J. N.,** Reduction of fresh-frozen plasma use through a daily survey and education program, *Transfusion,* 27, 226, 1987.

Chapter 3

GENERAL PRINCIPLES OF QUALITY ASSURANCE IN DEVELOPING COUNTRIES

Gamal Saber Gabra

TABLE OF CONTENTS

ISBN 0-8493-4938-9

I. INTRODUCTION

Before discussing the application of quality assurance measures in developing countries, it is important to review the concepts and principles of quality assurance in general. It is only against this background of information that it will be possible to view the situation of transfusion services and their need for quality assurance.

The level at which implementation of relevant quality assurance measures are carried out depends primarily on the degree of development of the national health care delivery system. It is also affected, not only by the degree of sophistication of clinical disciplines and primary health care, but also, and specifically, by the development of transfusion medicine and technology.

Less than 40% of developing countries have national blood transfusion advisory committees and only 50% have formulated national blood policies. Countries with national or regional directors range between 33 and 62% in the different geographical regions as defined by the World Health Organization (WHO), and only about 52% of the countries have ethical codes or legislations governing blood transfusion practice. Governments in most third world countries are primarily responsible for financing the operation of blood transfusion services. This is frequently done without adequate cost recovery systems to sustain the continuity of supplies, consumables, and the quality of services in general.

Less than 20% of the countries in any region collect 30 or more blood donations annually per 1000 population. The proportion of countries that maintain systems based entirely on voluntary nonremunerated blood donations range from 0 to 23%.

There are countries that are unable to screen blood donations for HBsAg, and up to now, in 1990, blood is transfused in some places with no screening for the presence of anti-HIV because of the lack of reagents, training, or storage facilities.

The basic components of quality assurance in any blood transfusion facility should cover all activity areas, including the principal ones listed in Table 1.

All staff should be trained to consider quality assurance as a comprehensive on-going activity designed to implement the principles of good laboratory and manufacturing practice, and to ensure quality standards by quality monitoring, at the various steps of the blood transfusion service operations, from donor selection and care down the line to clinical bedside hemotherapy. Effectiveness of quality assurance programs depends on proper application of the methods and procedures that are laid down for each step in the different activities in any blood transfusion facility. Documentation of the standard operational procedures (SOP) and laboratory manuals is essential, and serves as the basis for any comprehensive quality assurance program.

TABLE 1
Activity Areas for Quality Assurance

- Blood collection
- Handling of blood donations
- Component preparation
- Laboratory procedures
- Transfusion practice
- Record keeping and inventory control

The main and basic objective of quality assurance schemes is to reduce the number of errors in the blood transfusion service. In the International Society of Blood Transfusion (ISBT) guide on quality assurance,[1] Myrhe divides errors into technical, organizational, and operational. He proposes an index of errors to be maintained by the laboratory supervisor and to be inspected frequently by the laboratory director for appropriate action to be taken. Many blood transfusion laboratories have found this system to be quite helpful.

II. QUALITY OF BLOOD COLLECTION

A. DONOR SELECTION

Procedures for donor selection and care include criteria to ensure protection of the donor and safety of the recipient of the blood. Written operative procedures for blood collection also ensure the standard quality of each blood unit collected.

B. DONOR PROTECTION AND CARE

Criteria for eligibility to give blood include the upper and lower age limits, the weight, the predonation hemoglobin level, the time period between donations, etc. These criteria are specified to ensure high quality of donor care. They are usually determined on a national level and in accordance with guidelines prepared by international organizations, such as the World Health Organization, the League of Red Cross and Red Crescent Societies, the International Society of Blood Transfusion, the American Association of Blood Banks, and the Council of Europe.

Deviation or changes in these criteria can affect the quality of donor care. They are usually introduced by government or health authority regulations and must be on a sound medical basis. The support given to blood donors who are found to be positive for markers of infectious diseases varies. Some transfusion services include donor care programs as part of the procedure of blood collection. This is becoming increasingly important in handling HIV-positive donors. The procedure of informing donors and providing them access to counselling and support reflects the quality of donor care. Written operative procedures for blood collection also specify the equipment required, the preparation of the phlebotomy site, the volume or weight of the blood collection, the handling of the blood donation during and after collection at the donor session, the initial documentation of the records of the donor and of the donation, and the care given to the donor following donation.

Collection of plasma is increasingly being used by many transfusion centers to supplement the source material used for preparation of plasma products. Although plasmapheresis is not widely practiced in developing countries, many blood transfusion services have reached the stage where they are beginning to consider modern plasma procurement techniques to acquire some degree of self-sufficiency in blood products. Collection procedures affect the safety of donors and may equally affect the safety of recipients. Detailed standard procedures of plasma collection whether manually or by machine, should be prepared in every facility where plasma is collected. The manual should outline in detail the operative procedure, starting with the donor selection criteria, the documentation, the tests required before collection, the equipment, the handling of the donor after collection, and the handling and processing of the donation. It was unfortunate that incorrect handling of plasmapheresis equipment led in 1983 to the transmission of HIV to a number of paid plasma donors.[2]

In general, all procedures for plasma, platelet, or white cell collection require the presence of a well-trained physician and it is considered imperative to provide all possible measures that would ensure the standard quality of donor care, product handling, and safety. Access to emergency medical facilities should be available, particularly when the procedure is more complicated than the one in which commonly used one-arm-procedure machines are used. Details of these measures are produced in most countries and a 1986 Council of Europe booklet was produced which provides reasonable quality assurance guidelines.[3]

C. SAFETY OF RECIPIENT

A simple questionnaire serves as a checklist to evaluate the donor's state of health, which in addition allows exclusion of donors whose blood is likely to be unsafe. Donors at risk are expected to be excluded by general education of the potential donor population. The questionnaire helps donor attendants and the donors themselves to see clearly the areas which were not sufficiently understood. The procedure of going through the questionnaire can be crucial for the elimination of dangerous donations. The effective use of these questionnaires depends on their clarity and the proper training of the donor attendant staff responsible for the predonation interview.

In developing countries, the level of literacy in the community poses the main problem. The diversity of local tribal languages complicates the approach to donor selection. Cultural beliefs and social misconceptions have to be carefully considered in the planning of any system for donor selection and for donor self-exclusion.

TABLE 2
Variables that Affect Quality of Whole Blood

- Weight of blood
- Mixing of blood
- Donor medication
- Quality of venepuncture
- Donation time

D. STANDARD QUALITY OF BLOOD UNITS

Several variables have to be monitored at this early stage to ensure standard quality of whole blood units (Table 2). The quality of blood components is determined in the first place by the degree of quality monitoring of whole blood at the early stage of collection. Regular check of the balances used in blood collection is a simple but an essential quality assurance measure.

E. HANDLING OF BLOOD DONATIONS

Clear written operative procedures in every blood collection facility will allow the staff to handle blood donations in a standard way. This includes the procedure for provision of the pilot samples, the technique for securing the sealing of the blood container, as well as the temperature and method of storage of individual blood units until they are tested, labeled, and adequately documented before issue for transfusion or for processing into components.

Manual record keeping, initiated at this stage, is being replaced increasingly by different computerized blood banking systems. The main objectives of any of these systems are to improve safety by preventing possible clerical errors and, in general, to assure the quality of stock control, donor call-up procedures, quarantine control, release of blood and its components, and follow up of previous donations involved in transfusion problems. Of course, these new systems bring with them different quality assurance requirements and problems.

Suitably constructed containers may be used for transport of units of blood collected outside a transfusion center by mobile teams in order to standardize the storage conditions during transport. The temperature of walk-in cold rooms and reach-in refrigerators is controlled by regular temperature-recording charts and battery operated or automatically chargeable audible and visual alarms to provide early warning of changes in the storage temperature. Refrigerators on vehicles have equally sensitive temperature-monitoring devices. The responsibility for supervision of storage equipment is assigned to a senior member of the technical staff who ensures that maintenance of the equipment is performed regularly following written protocols and that permanent records are kept of actual daily storage temperatures.

TABLE 3
Quality Assurance Program for Component Preparation

- Product specifications
- Design of preparation procedure
- Validation
- Revalidation under normal working conditions
- Quality monitoring and quality control
- Monitoring of therapeutic use

III. COMPONENT PREPARATION AND QUALITY OF PRODUCTS

Blood transfusion centers are increasingly processing the majority of the blood units collected to meet the demand for blood components and fractions. The quality of these products is monitored regularly to ensure that they continually meet the standards expected. Quality standards or specifications of the products are defined to meet the therapeutic effectiveness and the safety of the products. The quality standards are usually specified by the national health authorities. The quality of a product is usually defined as the degree to which it matches the specifications of a standard product whose characteristics and properties have been exhaustively studied and validated.

> "Quality assurance is the sum total of the organized arrangements made with the object of ensuring that products will be of the quality required by their intended use . . . "[4]

A quality assurance program for blood components includes written operative procedures for the processing of whole blood into the various components with special reference to all equipment used, the methods, and the special precautions required for nonsterile techniques. A comprehensive quality assurance program for component preparation can be described as consisting of several separate stages (Table 3).

Quality monitoring is effected by testing, on a regular basis, a specified sample size of the blood product during or at the end of the production procedure, to ensure that certain specific standard characteristics are achieved.

Quality control confirms that the quality of the product meets the standard specifications. This term refers to sampling and testing procedures in order to decide whether or not a certain product can be released for use.

Quality in-process monitoring tests, on the other hand, should provide day-to-day information on the quality of components to allow taking the necessary action required to correct any developing problem or undesirable trend.

In order to facilitate user feedback and to improve the quality of prescribing practices, a blood product should be properly labeled and accompanied, if possible, with a brief description of its standard features, a brief description of its method of preparation, its date of expiry, the instructions for usage, and the optimum conditions for storage and handling.

The participation of the staff in formulation of the various stages of the quality assurance program is essential for its success.

Plasma derivatives produced by fractionation are also subject to rigorous quality monitoring protocols and in-process testing. Plasma can be obtained from individual blood units (recovered plasma) or by plasmapheresis (source plasma). The quality of these two starting products varies significantly and standard specifications for the two have to be established in order to define the characteristic features of the final fractionated products prepared from them. The platelet content of plasma can, for example, affect the quality of some of the fractionated derivatives. It is therefore essential to standardize the centrifugation of whole blood and validate the performance of plasmapheresis machines to obtain source plasma with the allowable level of platelet contamination.

The availability of fractionated products in third world countries is severely restricted by the lack of resources. A very small number of countries possess fractionation facilities. It is, however, possible that with international help, plasma collection can be improved to allow, at the least, contract fractionation to develop, possibly on a regional rather than on national basis. The quality of plasma destined for fractionation would then need to meet the expected standards to yield safe and effective derivatives.

IV. LABORATORY PROCEDURES

The quality of laboratory practice in blood transfusion services and laboratories is determined by the proficiency of the staff, the quality of the reagents and equipment, and the effectiveness of internal and external quality assurance schemes. Training of the staff is one of the pillars of good laboratory practice. Continued regular training is the key to formation of proficient technical staff.

Participation of the laboratories in external quality control schemes is mandatory in developed countries and should be encouraged in less well developed services, to allow laboratory and staff self-assessment and to further introduce the necessary changes, whether in human resources, laboratory techniques and methods, equipment, or reagents. Evaluation of the performance of technical and other staff should be done regularly. This can be achieved by frequent circulation of unknown specimens, by participation in in-house proficiency exercises, and by appropriate panels of internal quality monitoring specimens inserted in the daily routine work. Poor performers may benefit from retraining and refresher courses.

Protocols for maintenance of the equipment and detailed procedures to monitor their performance should be clearly laid down and followed rigorously. Training in equipment maintenance should take priority in third world blood transfusion services. The difficulty in transport restricts access to specialized technical skills. The responsible members of staff should be identified and their tasks accurately determined. Monitoring and maintenance of equipment can be a tedious undertaking and operational errors are avoided by skillful management and supervision. These procedures become really effective when they grow to become natural laboratory discipline and not simply tasks to be performed.

Proficiency testing can be organized internally, regionally, or nationally. Each one of these systems serves specific functions and the choice of exercises should accordingly reflect the purpose of each scheme. Simple unknown sera can be used for in-house weekly or daily controls, but the choice of exercises for regional schemes is to answer specific questions about the methods or the reagents such as enzyme and enhancement additives, or antiglobulin reagents, with a view, perhaps, of harmonizing laboratory techniques. National schemes may have some of the regional functions but are basically designed to provide reassurance for some laboratories and give early warning signals for others.

All methods and techniques in use should be validated under the laboratory working conditions and documented in a laboratory manual and any changes in equipment or reagents should be evaluated and seen not to affect the performance of the laboratory tests. Quality control measures should be incorporated at every step of the procedure to ensure that the technique is performing as expected, and that the reagents are specific and sensitive and capable of providing the correct expected results from the testing procedures.

Quality control measures vary; the use of positive and negative control red cells is one example, a weak antibody can be included in antibody screening procedures to control the level of sensitivity of the method and technique used, the use of a dye in reagents provides a check to ensure that this has been added, etc. This latter measure is particularly important in automated methods.

All reagents in use should be subject to regular rigorous quality assurance checks starting from the saline and the low ionic strength solution (LISS) through the list of additives such as albumin, enzymes, polyethylene glycol (PEG), and antisera, whether plasma derived or monoclonal. The method recommended by the manufacturer should be strictly followed and any deviation thoroughly validated. Improper storage temperature and dilutions of reagents can seriously affect the standard and quality of the results; special protocols must be put in place for storage procedures, temperature, and recommended volumes for storage and the shelf life for the dilutions in use.

Documentation and accuracy of the patient and specimen records is the basis for the quality of laboratory procedures. This is particularly important in pretransfusion and compatibility testing. Checking and double-checking details on patient samples and requests must be included in the steps of the procedure and should preferably be performed by separate workers. Special procedures should be available and documented for emergency testing techniques where incubation times, centrifugation speeds, and volumes are different from ordinary routine methods.

Newer automated methods have improved and standardized the quality of laboratory practice, but at the same time have introduced new variables that require special quality assurance measures. Cell washers are complicated and automated grouping machines require special skills in monitoring the quality of their performance and in following their safety codes.

Worksheets and general organizational documentation are particularly important in the hospital blood transfusion laboratory, where a large number of investigations and compatibility testing procedures are performed at the same time by a small number of operators and where technical, organizational, and operational errors could take place. The ISBT manual on quality assurance[1] describes another cause for error resulting from deterioration in precision which takes place when a routine technique is routinely performed by a junior staff member without adequate supervision. This is quite likely to be seen in routine compatibility laboratories, where the series of negative results create a sense of an expected flow of negative readings and "deterioration of precision". Thorough training, supervision, and flexible, variable deployment of staff is often required to keep the good quality of practice in hospital blood transfusion laboratories.

V. LABORATORY SAFETY

Good laboratory practice cannot be complete without proper attention given to laboratory safety. Safety must be built into every technique and operation in any blood transfusion facility. The objective of a laboratory safety program is to improve laboratory safety performance. This is achieved in Western developed services by careful job safety analysis to identify hazards and by safety training programs designed to provide staff with new information and skills for immediate application to local situations.

The senior laboratory supervisor should be responsible for adherence to safety standards, assignment of laboratory duties, and maintenance of equipment. The designation of a special safety officer or a safety committee is an added measure to further improve the quality of laboratory safety. The principles and practices of laboratory safety have been reviewed in a comprehensive publication of the American Society for Microbiology.[5]

Precautions for preventing laboratory-acquired infections are of particular importance in the environment of resource constraints of third world countries. Specific measures have to be developed to control laboratory infections, particularly hepatitis B and HIV. Maintenance and review of accident records constitute the backbone of any safety program. Working conditions in many third world countries are difficult and technicians and laboratory aids are, as a matter of course, exposed to blood and samples from patients and donors with a high prevalence of HIV and hepatitis B. They are at increased risk of acquiring these infections through direct contact, needle stick injuries, broken glass, faulty equipment, or improper techniques such as mouth pipetting.

Employee health surveillance, including hepatitis B vaccination of laboratory staff, needs to be considered as a national priority regulation in some countries. Senior laboratory staff who are in constant contact with the employees should encourage accident reporting and supervise the implementation of infection control measures such as appropriate use of gloves and protective clothing, frequent hand washing, and effective disinfection of spilled blood.[6]

VI. HOSPITAL AND BEDSIDE TRANSFUSION PRACTICE

The concepts of quality assurance were developed in industry and used to control the quality of manufactured goods. These measures can be implemented easily in laboratory work, component preparation, and in plasma fractionation plants. Application of the principles of quality assurance and quality monitoring in hospital and clinical blood transfusion practice has not gained the required attention. Recently, the interest in quality of medical care became a focus of attention of health authorities and hospitals. Casparie describes a flow sheet for transfusion practice, starting with the physician who establishes the indication and type of blood product.[7] This request is taken by the laboratory, which supplies the correct therapeutic product. The product finally comes to the physician who treats the patient and ideally reports back to the blood transfusion laboratory on the outcome and any complications that occur. The flow sheet provides the various steps at which standard operative procedures are required. Guidelines on the choice of blood products will help improve the quality of transfusion practice. The indications for transfusion and the quality of the product must also be monitored, evaluated, and validated.

The proportion of the blood units used out of the total number matched (C/T ratio) can be calculated for each individual surgical procedure; deviations from the expected ratio require investigation and may merit introducing changes in the clinical or laboratory practices. Hospital blood transfusion committees are useful to point out the essential aspects of hospital bedside and laboratory blood transfusion practice that require monitoring, changing, or improving. Hospital transfusion committees have also been established to meet the need for physician education regarding the use of blood, blood components, and derivatives. The history, function, composition, and value of this peer review system in American hospitals was well reviewed in 1982 and presented by the American Association of Blood Banks.[8] This, however, is to be considered just as one model and a suitable version will need to be developed according to the facility and the level of health care delivery in each area.

TABLE 4
Record Keeping in Blood Transfusion Service

- Donor register and identification
- Donor profile and donation history
- Donor card system and recall
- Donation — register identification, labeling
- Donation — additional information and test results
- Blood component register — labeling
- Issues, returns, inventory control
- Patient records and compatibility forms

The hospital transfusion committee or similar audit systems should play the central role in promoting and monitoring the safe and appropriate use of blood and blood products. The objective is to ensure that the patient receives the correct blood or component as and when indicated. A successful quality assurance plan should include both collection of data on blood usage and review of records to evaluate actual practice. Comparing the data with the standard criteria supplies information on the quality of transfusion practice and highlights the need to introduce any change required to improve the standard of transfusion practice. Finally, reassessment and follow up is always necessary to ensure that the quality has indeed changed.

VII. RECORD KEEPING AND INVENTORY CONTROL

Documentation and its organization is considered of major importance in blood transfusion services. The areas of activities where good quality records are essential are summarized in Table 4.

Computer-assisted programs have replaced manual card systems in many transfusion services. This facilitates donor registry records and accumulation of personal donor files to permit access of information on donor history and for regular donor recall.

Manual donation registry systems are updated with results of laboratory procedures and accordingly units are labeled and banked for issue or discarded. Similarly, all components prepared from individual units are given the unit's unique numbered label and registries are kept of banking issues or returns.

Manual labeling systems in use in almost all developing countries have now been replaced in Western services with uniform preprinted labels for bottles, packs, and the satellite packs used for components. Some new label systems utilize machine readable bar codes and eye readable symbols. The use of unique numbering systems for these labels reduces human error. The newer labels are self-adhesive, using noninvasive materials. They are water, humidity, and smear resistant, but unaffordable in services that are hardly able to purchase plastic packs.

The procedure and control for release of blood and blood products should be clearly delineated and documented, from collection through testing, quarantine storage, and issue of red cells with or without compatibility. The flow

TABLE 5
Factors that Affect Introduction of Quality Assurance Measures

- Emergency nature of blood transfusion practice
- Absence of regular blood donor population base
- Shortage of reagents, irregularity and variability of supply
- Storage of supplies and variation in sources of energy
- Blood collection
- Absence of national reference centers and policy
- Inappropriate use of blood and limitations of hospital transfusion practice

chart (Figure 1) highlights the areas where documentation and record keeping are essential to maintain the quality and safety of transfusion practice.

Records of issues and returns along with documentation on donation and components provide the basis for inventory and stock control. Introduction of computer-assisted procedures facilitates this task and can even help to produce statistics and additional information to optimize the usage of blood and blood products and improve the safety standards of blood transfusion therapy. Simple basic personal computers are frequently used in a few developing countries with modest blood services. These steps are to be cautiously encouraged and not dismissed as an unnecessary luxury.

VIII. FACTORS THAT INTERFERE WITH EFFECTIVE QUALITY ASSURANCE MEASURES IN DEVELOPING COUNTRIES

Introduction and development of quality assurance programs are hindered in blood transfusion services of the third world countries by a variety of constraints. The list in Table 5 covers the most prominent problems but is by no means exhaustive.

A. EMERGENCY NATURE OF BLOOD TRANSFUSION PRACTICE

Blood transfusion services in many developing countries are emergency oriented. In general, blood collection results directly from immediate patient needs, with a short-term planning span. Stocks are usually nonexistent and the usage rate of blood donations, mostly earmarked for specific patients, is very high. Most blood transfusion facilities are hospital based, and developed around the clinical requirements of hospital patients. There is usually little central planning and many countries have not yet developed national policies for transfusion practice nor national standards for blood and blood products. These factors, along with severe resource limitations, force blood transfusion services to become second- or third-class clinical support services. Financial resources are further curtailed because, in many parts of the world, blood transfusion is considered as a minor part of the hospital laboratory services

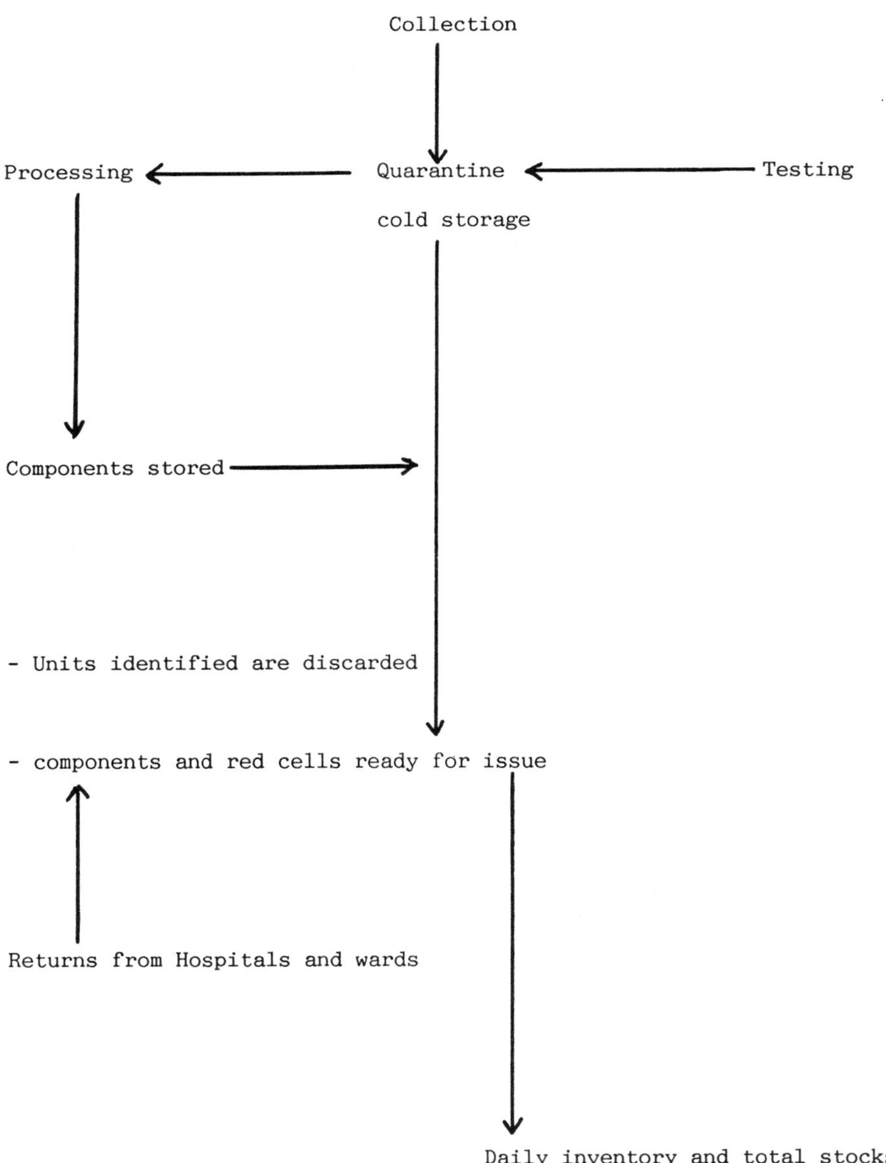
Collection
Processing
Quarantine
cold storage
Testing
Components stored
- Units identified are discarded
- components and red cells ready for issue
Returns from Hospitals and wards
Daily inventory and total stocks

FIGURE 1.

and represents an unacceptably high percentage of the total health budget. In this emergency climate, standard operating procedures are rarely followed and suboptimal quality is frequently considered as normal practice and the acceptable option.

Blood transfusion services also become preoccupied only with supply of whole blood. Because of all these constraints, whole blood is often used where only one specific component is needed. It is common practice to use fresh whole blood to supply patients requiring platelets or Factor VIII.

Regular or even occasional preparation of blood components cannot be achieved by blood transfusion services that are mostly hospital based and fragmented, with no central or national guidance or policy to ensure the quality and basic elements for blood transfusion practice.

B. ABSENCE OF REGULAR BLOOD DONOR POPULATION BASE

The vast majority of third world countries rely on family/related blood donors. In fact, the responsibility to supply blood for patients, which should be institutional — in the hands of government or hospitals — has been left to the patients and their relatives and in some places to the treating doctor. This responsibility shift results in patients relying heavily on family donors or paid donors influenced to a considerable degree by coercion or incentives that compromise the quality of the blood supply. This, in turn, leads to development of "professional" blood donor circles with the expected increased risks of transfusion-transmitted disease and unacceptable human and ethical consequences.

C. REAGENTS

Shortage of reagents and irregularity and variability of supply leads to deviation from laboratory methods and procedures. The use of control cells in grouping and compatibility testing depends on availability of hard currency or previously grouped cells, therefore checking the potency of reagents may be severely limited. The use of reagents beyond their expiry date and without control cells is often resorted to because of shortage or delay of delivery of supplies. Adverse exposure to extreme temperatures can lead to early deterioration of reagents and, consequently, the quality of laboratory practice in many services is adversely affected and compromised.

D. STORAGE OF SUPPLIES AND VARIATION OF SOURCES OF ENERGY

Temperatures can be difficult to monitor even with the use of maximum-minimum thermometers. The frequent breakdown of electricity supply and the unavailability of generators makes storage difficult. The control of temperature is also not reliable in gas- or kerosene-operated refrigerators. Reagents, and chemicals such as anticoagulants, blood, and blood products are all affected by unreliable storage conditions. The performance of sensitive equipment is also likely to be affected by temperature and environmental conditions prevailing in the working areas and laboratory premises.

Implementation of storage rules is almost impossible under these conditions and indeed it is difficult to build large stocks of fresh frozen plasma or cryoprecipitate unless the technical components of cold storage are reliably established. This may be possible in one central location where adequate, reliable freeze storage facilities can be developed using central funds.

Ideally, blood should be stored in a refrigerator having automatic-cycle dual compressors, special insulation, external temperature recording, and alarm systems. Such is unlikely to be available. If blood is collected and stored in disposable closed-system plastic bags, the risk of introducing infection is minimized. Blood may be safely stored for 21 days in a well-functioning domestic refrigerator dedicated for blood only, with a maximum-minimum thermometer. Variations from 2 to 10°C are acceptable. Visual inspection for hemolysis or discoloration is essential before issue. If blood is collected and stored in reusable glass bottles, temperature control must be strict.

E. UNAVAILABILITY OF PLASTIC PACKS

Blood collection into bottles continues in many parts of the world. This poses particular problems of quality assurance, beginning with the preparation of the collection equipment, the anticoagulant solution, and its sterile filling and sterilization. Problems may also be encountered with the quality of bottles and the unavailability of the bungs, caps, and sterile preparation of blood collection sets.

Cleaning and supply of standard quality bottles and sterile collection sets can be interrupted by a number of factors. Lack of appropriate cleaning agents can, for example, be a major problem.

The use of bottles for blood collection restricts the preparation of blood components, affects the appropriate indications for hemotherapy and lowers the standard of clinical blood transfusion practice.

F. ABSENCE OF CENTRAL OR NATIONAL POLICY

The absence of a national blood transfusion policy lowers, in general, the quality of services. Lack of resources specifically identified for blood transfusion services leads to inability to adhere to quality standards in all areas, whether in laboratory procedures, preparation and proper use of blood, or proper handling of blood donors and blood collection. The absence of a national reference center specifically leaves the fragmented services to perform without advice or reference consensus guidance and with no access to reliable external quality assurance or proficiency testing schemes.

G. QUALITY OF TRANSFUSION PRACTICE

Fragmentation in the blood transfusion services results in inappropriate use of blood and blood products, particularly since infusion fluids such as saline and synthetic colloidal plasma volume expanders are not readily available in many countries. The person responsible for the transfusion laboratory frequently has no clinical training and is unable or unwilling to give guidance to clinical colleagues on usage of blood and blood products. Training programs for blood transfusion technical and medical staff are disorganized, inadequate, or unavailable in many countries.

IX. SOLUTIONS FOR DEVELOPING COUNTRIES

What can be done to facilitate the implementation of the elements of quality assurance and improve the quality of laboratory and clinical blood transfusion practice in developing countries?

Blood transfusion needs and services vary from country to country, but the condition of some services is so poor that it is difficult to see how safety and quality standards can be improved. It is difficult to propose any measures for a transfusion service that is in a perpetual crisis situation. In many places blood transfusion services, as understood in developed countries, do not exist. The infrastructure that is necessary to permit implementation of the principles for quality assurance is lacking. Added to this is the absence of any audit of the clinical results of transfusion which becomes merely a desperate response to a desperate clinical situation. The chronic shortage aggravates the lack of quality assurance by perpetuating the emergency nature of blood transfusion services where there is no time for donor selection and care or laboratory testing and no facilities for component preparation or proper manufacturing practice.

Chronic shortage can be alleviated by the creation of panels of safe, regular donors. However, this is regularly hindered by the lack of resources. The infrastructure can be improved within the constraints of the available limited resources by creating a national blood transfusion committee that develops national policy to regulate transfusion services and practice as far as it is practically possible. Such a national body will be able to make optimum use of the available resources and explore the possibilities for regional and international cooperation. Establishment of a national blood transfusion advisory board or committee is therefore a priority for countries in which this or a similar body does not exist.[9]

The infrastructure can also be improved by proper selection of personnel and improving their skills and proficiency by relevant and regular training. The adoption of national regulations for the blood transfusion service will improve the quality of laboratory and transfusion practice. The national transfusion committee would facilitate the development of simple laboratory manuals and use of standard procedures, as well as the creation of reliable record systems for donors, patients, and blood products.

Regular review and upgrading of the manuals and standard operating procedures sustains the development of the quality of the services. Participation of the staff in the regular review of the standard procedures ensures that these remain realistic and achievable.

Using local, regional, or international resources, each country should try to develop or have access to a reference center to provide external quality assurance schemes, to provide guidance and improve the quality of laboratory practice.

The choice of appropriate equipment should take into account the local conditions and provide training of the technical staff in maintenance. This contributes to the establishment of reliable laboratory services.

The quality of clinical transfusion practice can be improved by encouraging regular monitoring of usage of blood and blood products and also by encouraging the investigation and follow up of the adverse effects of blood transfusion.

The creation of a simple audit system at the hospital level will help to monitor and analyze the pattern of usage and develop criteria for appropriate and safe use of blood and blood products.

The quality of transfusion practice will also improve if alternatives for transfusion are encouraged and facilitated, including the availability of infusion fluids and synthetic colloidal volume expanders.

Developing countries are short both in financial and human resources; most countries have no regular donor panels and, even if they had the storage facilities, the resources would not be adequate to maintain the quality of the products. It is obvious that developing countries are plagued with vicious circles, clearly reflected in several operational areas in their transfusion services. International funding of operating costs can be useful only when it is provided on a short-term basis on the understanding that systems for cost recovery are clearly planned for the predictable future. Long-term dependence is counterproductive. It leads, in most instances, to collapse of the services once external support is stopped.

A worldwide effort is required to establish integrated blood banking and transfusion systems that are capable of adopting quality assurance measures and procedures on a routine and sustained basis. The Global Blood Safety Initiative (GBSI) of the WHO was conceived in 1988 by the Global Programme on AIDS (GPA) and the unit of Laboratory Technology and Blood Safety (LBS), in association with the League of Red Cross and Red Crescent Societies (LRCS) and the International Society of Blood Transfusion (ISBT). The main objective of this international cooperative effort is to develop integrated blood transfusion services within the broad context of national health plans with special emphasis on third world countries. There are many other agencies involved in international support and development of transfusion services in developing countries. The role of these agencies and the impact of international support for blood transfusion services has been recently discussed in detail by Britten.[10]

Services in a number of countries have benefited from planned international assistance and bilateral cooperation between countries. In other areas, the regional supply of reagents and implementation of quality assurance schemes have helped maintain standard, quality services. Other avenues for international cooperation must be explored, particularly in the training of scientific and technical staff, to support the development of the infrastructure of transfusion services that can maintain good laboratory and bedside transfusion practice.

REFERENCES

1. **Myhre, B.,** *Quality Assurance in the Blood Transfusion Laboratory,* Moore, B. P. L., Friesleben, E., and Högman, C. F., Eds., International Society of Blood Transfusion, Paris, 1978.
2. **Kohloff, A. and Flessenkämper, S.,** Tenth case of HIV transmission after plasma donation, *Lancet,* ii, 965, 1988.
3. Quality Control in 'Blood Transfusion' Services, Council of Europe, Strasbourg, 1986.
4. Guide to Good Pharmaceutical Manufacturing Practice, Her Majesty's Stationery Office, London, 1983.
5. **Miller, B. M.,** *Laboratory Safety: Principles and Practices,* 1st ed., Gröshel, D. H. D., Richardson, J. H., Vesley, D., Songer, J. R., Housewright, R. D., and Emmit Barkely, W., Eds., American Society for Microbiology, Washington, D.C., 1986.
6. Guidelines on Sterilisation and Disinfection Methods Effective against Human Immunodeficiency Virus (HIV), 2nd ed., WHO AIDS Series No. 2, World Health Organization, Geneva, 1989.
7. **Casparie, A. F.,** Blood transfusion practice in hospitals: a topic for quality assurance, in *Quality Assurance in Blood Banking and its Clinical Impact,* Smit Sibinga, C. Th., Das, P. C., and Taswell, H. F., Eds., Martinius Nijhoff, Boston, 1984.
8. **Muller, V. H.,** Structure and Function of a Hospital Transfusion Committee, in *The Hospital Transfusion Committee,* 1st ed., Wallas, C. H. and Muller, V. H., Eds., American Association of Blood Banks, Arlington, VA, 1982.
9. Guidelines for the appropriate use of blood, Global Blood Safety Initiative, Geneva, WHO/GPA/INF/89.18.
10. **Britten, A. F.,** Role and Impact of International Blood Transfusion activities, Transfusion International No. 50, Geneva, 1990, 10.

Chapter 4

TRANSFUSION-ASSOCIATED HIV: MEDICAL-LEGAL ISSUES

Jay E. Menitove and Thomas F. Zuck

TABLE OF CONTENTS

ISBN 0-8493-4938-9

I. INTRODUCTION

Case reports of three hemophiliacs with the disorder now known as acquired immunodeficiency syndrome (AIDS) first appeared in the July 1982 *Morbidity and Mortality Weekly Report (MMWR)*.[1] In December, 1982, the Centers for Disease Control reported a 20-month-old infant from the San Francisco area with unexplained cellular immunodeficiency and opportunistic infections.[2] At birth, he had severe erythroblastosis fetalis and during the first month of life received blood components from 19 donors, one of whom subsequently developed AIDS.

By the fall of 1990, 3351 adults and 238 children were known to be infected with the human immunodeficiency virus (HIV), the etiologic factor for AIDS, as a result of transfusions given prior to the spring 1985 implementation of HIV antibody screening on donated blood. In addition, 1258 hemophilic patients were known to have acquired HIV infections from coagulation factor concentrates. But these cases may be only the tip of the iceberg: in 1987, it was estimated that approximately 12,000 persons then may have been infected with HIV as a result of blood transfusions received prior to the spring of 1985.[3]

AIDS is a devastating clinical illness, and, unlike other chronic or fatal conditions such as cancer, a patient cannot be provided with a reasonable prognosis; the HIV-infected patient cannot be told to a reasonable degree of medical probability what to expect and when to expect it. The illness, the uncertainty, the fear, and the social stigmatization associated with this disease, have led many HIV-infected individuals to turn to the courts for redress and compensation. Plaintiffs — those who sue blood collection agencies such as regional blood centers for transfusion-transmitted HIV (TA-HIV) infections (and there have been several hundred of plaintiffs to date) — include transfusion recipients, third parties infected with HIV as a result of contact with infected transfusion recipients, and estates of those who died from TA-HIV. Many of these cases settle for undisclosed sums. Of the dozen or so that have been fully tried before a jury, several have resulted in multimillion dollar judgments being rendered against blood centers; others have resulted in victories for blood centers.

II. CAUSES OF ACTION

Shortly after the advent of transfusion medicine during the Second World War, people with transfusion-transmitted infections (primarily hepatitis) began suing the responsible blood collection agencies. For the most part, they sought recovery based on three causes of action: breach of warranties, strict liability, and negligence.

A. BREACH OF WARRANTIES

Consumers dissatisfied with their purchases can and do sue vendors and manufacturers. If they are pursuing a contract action (and not one based on negligence), they generally argue that the defendants breached one or both of two warranties: express warranties and implied warranties.

Express warranties arise when the seller or manufacturer makes an affirmation of fact or promise (either in writing or orally) which relates to the product being sold and is part of the basis for the bargain. An express warranty will arise where, for example, the seller or manufacturer states that its spot remover removes spots and the consumer purchases the spot remover based upon this representation. (Mere opinion or advertisement puffery, however, does not count). If the spot remover does not remove spots as promised, then the consumer has a claim for breach of express warranty.

Plaintiffs with transfusion-transmitted diseases could sue for breach of express warranties if the blood collection agency told the prospective transfusion recipient that the blood was "absolutely safe" and it was not. Because it is generally known throughout the medical community that blood is an unavoidably unsafe biologic available only by the prescription of a licensed physician, express warranties regarding its safety or purity are rarely made and thus rarely breached.

So, instead of express warranties, plaintiffs more frequently pursue breach of implied warranty claims. For almost every sale, the law implies two warranties: the implied warranty of merchantability, and the implied warranty of fitness for a particular purpose. The implied warranty of merchantability means that the goods (1) pass without objection in the trade under the contract description; (2) are fit for the ordinary purposes for which such goods are used; (3) are adequately contained, packaged, and labeled; and (4) conform to the promises or affirmations of fact made on the container or label. A warranty of fitness for a particular purpose is implied if the seller or manufacturer has reason to know of any particular purpose for which the consumer goods are required and the buyer has relied on the skill and judgment of the seller to select and furnish suitable goods.

The transfusion-transmitted infection breach of implied warranty claim is best illustrated by the landmark decision of *Perlmutter v. Beth David Hospital.*[4] During the early 1950s, a patient suffering from homologous serum hepatitis sued the hospital that provided the blood. Complaining that she had purchased "bad blood", she sought recovery based upon breach of implied warranties. She alleged that the blood she received was sold to her, that the defendant hospital knew the purpose for which the blood was to be used, and that she relied upon the hospital in selecting blood that was of merchantable quality. The court rejected her claims. It stated that:

> Concepts of purchase and sale cannot separately be attached to the healing material such as medicines, drugs or, indeed, blood supplied by the hospital for a price as part of the medical services it offers. That the property or title to certain items of medical material may be transferred, so to speak, from the hospital to the patient during the course of medical treatment does not serve to make each such transaction a sale.

The court concluded that providing blood was a service and not the sale of a product. Absent a sale, there can be no implied warranties.[4]

B. STRICT LIABILITY

In 1970, an Illinois hospital was found strictly liable for a transfusion-acquired hepatitis infection.[5] Like the breach of warranty claim, the doctrine of strict liability arises from the sale of a product. But unlike a breach of warranty claim, it is not an action on a contract; rather it is the analogous tort claim. In a strict products liability case, liability may be imposed on one who sells a product in a defective condition unreasonably dangerous to the user or consumer for the harm caused to the ultimate user or consumer. The doctrine only applies if the seller is engaged in the business of selling such a product and the product is expected to and does reach the user or consumer without substantial change in the condition in which it was sold.[6] By applying the strict liability doctrine, the Illinois court accepted the notion that blood should be treated like any other commodity and that the blood collection agency can be held liable for the sale of blood in a defective condition unreasonably dangerous to the user.[5]

C. BLOOD SHIELD STATUTES

In part a result of the verdict against the Illinois hospital, significant concern was voiced that blood centers could face insolvency if strict liability or breach of implied warranty doctrines were maintained. At that time, there was no method to determine whether a unit of blood was infected with the causative agent of hepatitis.[7] Hence, blood collection agencies were continually at risk for lawsuits if blood components were treated as products. To prevent disruption and maintain an adequate blood supply, eventually 48 of 50 states passed laws known as ''blood shield statutes''. These statutes recognize that the provision of blood is a medical service rather than the sale of a product. Absent the sale of a product, there can be no strict liability and there can be no implied warranties. In 1990, Vermont became the 49th state to enact blood shield statutes, leaving New Jersey the only state that depends on case law to protect blood processors from product liability laws.

Blood shield statutes do not, however, provide an absolute shield from liability. First, some plaintiffs have attacked the statutes themselves, and second and more importantly, blood shield statutes preserve a plaintiff's right to bring a negligence action against a blood collection agency.

Plaintiffs usually attack blood shield status from one or both of two directions. Either they argue — usually unsuccessfully — that the statute is unconstitutional or that the statute is inapplicable under the circumstances. For the latter approach, plaintiffs determine whether either the statute itself (as many do), or the legislative history regarding the intent of the body enacting the statute, limits the statute's scope to cases of transfusion-transmitted hepatitis. If so, they argue that TA-HIV is outside the statute's scope and, therefore, they are not barred from maintaining strict liability or breach of warranty claims. Some states are currently resolving this issue by amending their statutes; others are relying on the courts to broadly construe the statutes.

D. NEGLIGENCE

Although blood shield statutes, in effect, eliminate strict liability and breach of implied warranties as causes of actions against blood collection agencies, they do not leave the potential plaintiff bereft of legal redress. He or she can still allege negligence, and negligence has become the predominant cause of action upon which plaintiffs rely when seeking compensatory damages from blood centers.

To establish negligence, a plaintiff must prove four elements by the preponderance of the evidence. (''Preponderance'' means that the plaintiff must show that it is more probable than not that the evidence supports the allegation.) The four requisite elements are (1) the defendant owed a duty to the plaintiff; (2) the defendant breached that duty by acts of commission or omission; (3) the plaintiff was injured; and (4) the injury was proximately caused by defendant's breach (i.e., but for the defendant's breach, the plaintiff would not be injured). Plaintiffs generally seek recovery for actual losses such as past and future earnings, medical expenses, etc. Compensation is also sought for pain and suffering, loss of society and companionship, and other noneconomic losses. If plaintiffs can prove that there was ''willful, wanton, or reckless misconduct'', the plaintiffs may be able to recover punitive damages.

III. LEGAL CLIMATE IN THE U.S.

A. LITIGATION ISSUES

Jurors, representing a cross section of society, should not have formulated opinions about the case and often are not knowledgeable about the scientific issues to be discussed.[8] Lay witnesses such as physicians and technicians affiliated with defendant blood collection agencies tell juries about the defendants' practices at the time the blood was collected and transfused. Expert witnesses, employed by both plaintiffs and defendants, tell juries about the state of medical knowledge during the relevant time period and what other blood collection agencies or allegedly comparable organizations were doing under the same or similar circumstances. In a professional negligence action, expert witnesses define the prevailing standard of care and opine whether the defendant deviated from that standard; that is, they establish the bench mark by which the defendant's actions will be judged and then state whether they, based upon their expertise, believe the defendant failed to meet that mark. Judges instruct the jurors on the law and to weigh the evidence, the opinions of the expert witnesses, and the credibility of all witnesses. They are also instructed to set aside their sympathies.

However, this is exceedingly difficult, especially in TA-HIV cases where jurors must come to grips with a devastating disease process regarded as the worst plague to afflict mankind in modern time, one that can be transmitted to innocent third parties, and one that is associated with social ostracism and rebuke. It is not surprising that juries are sympathetic to the plights of plaintiffs and award enormous sums of money. Defendants are thus faced with two options. They can pursue the legal process to trial hoping that the evidence presented on their behalf supports their position and is convincing to the judge or jury. Or, if concerned about "run-away" verdicts, they may choose to settle, since TA-HIV patients are often seen as "innocent victims".[9-13]

B. RELEASING THE IDENTITY OF HIV-INFECTED BLOOD DONORS

Plaintiffs may seek to discover the identity of volunteer blood donors. They often allege that even if the blood center's procedures met the prevailing standard of care, these procedures may have been negligently followed at the time of the implicated donation. They argue that they need to depose the donor to determine whether he was properly educated about AIDS and whether his interview was conducted according to established procedures. Blood centers argue that the donor's identity is protected by the physician-patient privilege, the donor has a constitutionally protected right to privacy and the release of donor names would have a chilling effect on the willingness of donors to voluntarily provide blood.[12,14]

Courts have been divided on this issue. Cases initially heard involved multiple donors, requiring that many donors would be asked probing questions to determine if one might have been HIV-positive.[15,16] Currently, most cases addressing the donor-identity issue involve the look-back program in which a single positive implicated donor had been identified. Hence, the issue is whether a single identified donor's privacy rights outweigh the rights of the plaintiff to discovery. In some cases the donor's identity has been protected, but he/she has been asked to answer questions.[16-18] Blood banks contend that donors may be reluctant to provide answers to sensitive questions if there is a potential that the information will not remain confidential. The countervailing argument is that fear of disclosure fosters a safer blood supply.

C. TA-HIV LITIGATION PHASES

1. 1977 through Early 1983

The initial AIDS cases occurred during this time period. The first cases of AIDS in transfusion recipients and hemophilic patients were described, the etiology of AIDS was unknown, and the initial recommendations by blood banking organizations and federal regulatory agencies about the possibility of TA-HIV were issued.[10,13,14,19]

In the cases arising during this time period, plaintiffs attempt to identify errors in donor history taking, seek to obtain the identity of donors, argue that the blood center did not educate the medical community, and argue that an unindicated transfusion is, in and of itself, sufficient to find a physician liable for all consequences resulting from that transfusion.

2. 1983 through Spring 1985

During this time, HIV-1 was identified as the etiologic agent of AIDS, antibody tests were developed, self-exclusion by high-risk donors was relied upon, directed donations were discouraged by a joint statement of the blood banking organizations, some blood centers initiated surrogate testing and confidential unit exclusion, look-back on donations by people with AIDS was stated, and patients demanded directed donations.

Plaintiffs claim that despite Joint Statements, blood banking practice is not uniform. Who knew what and when they knew it, becomes an important issue. In general, plaintiffs have been unsuccessful in claiming that surrogate testing should have been performed during this period, but the later the donation, the stronger the claim becomes that surrogate testing should have been implemented, especially in high-risk areas. Also, there is increased emphasis on strengthening donor screening procedures, including direct questions and examinations for swollen lymph glands.

3. 1985 through the Present

During this time, HIV antibody testing was implemented. Donor notification and counseling was started, look-back programs were initiated, donor exclusion criteria were defined, and confidential unit exclusion was recommended by the FDA.

Plaintiffs claim that HIV testing should have been implemented immediately and that any transfusion-transmitted AIDS subsequent to the licensure of HIV testing could have been prevented. In cases involving transmission of HIV by untested blood in inventory following HIV test implementation, plaintiffs again claim these should have been prevented. Also, plaintiffs argue that look-back should have been implemented earlier.

IV. NEGLIGENCE ISSUES

A. DONOR SCREENING

Presentations at Public Health Service (PHS) meetings in Washington, D.C. in July 1982, and at the Centers for Disease Control (CDC) in Atlanta, Georgia in January 1983, provided the background data by which the clinical syndrome known as AIDS was characterized and "risk groups" for AIDS were defined. Evidence that AIDS was transmitted by transfusion was considered "incomplete" at the time. Nevertheless, on January 13, 1983, the American Association of Blood Banks (AABB), the American National Red Cross (ARC), and the Council of Community Blood Centers (CCBC) issued the first of many "Joint Statements" about AIDS that provided information about AIDS as it related to transfusion.[20] These suggestions included donor screening questions to detect possible AIDS or exposure to patients with AIDS by donors and questions designed to elicit a history of night sweats, unexplained fevers, unexplained weight loss, lymphadenopathy, or Kaposi's sarcoma. Direct or indirect questions concerning a donor's sexual preference were considered inappropriate and were specifically not recommended.

By March, 1983, the Food and Drug Administration (FDA) issued "Recommendations to decrease the risk of transmitting acquired immune deficiency syndrome (AIDS) from blood donors.[21]" It recommended that blood centers institute "educational programs" to inform persons at increased risk of AIDS that they "should refrain from donation." Persons at increased risk of AIDS included those with "symptoms and signs suggestive of AIDS, sexually active homosexual or bisexual men with multiple partners, Haitian entrants to the United States, present or past abusers of intravenous drugs, and sexual partners of individuals at increased risk of AIDS."

Plaintiffs have criticized the Joint Statement and FDA recommendations because they did not recommend that blood donors be asked directly whether they were homosexually active. They contend that answers to such questions would have been truthful. However, leaders of gay activist organizations in late 1982 and early 1983 argued against the introduction of questions designed to disclose the sexual preference of homosexually active men. They were concerned about stigmatization and possible discrimination. Representatives from the National Gay Task Force indicated that "So called 'fast lane' gays are causing the problem, and they are just a minority of male homosexuals... [Why] stigmatize at the time of a major civil rights movement a whole group, only a tiny fraction of whom qualify as the problem we are here to address." "To identify gays as those across the board that you exclude will not eliminate AIDS from blood products." "It ignores the fact that 20%–25% of the at-risk population is not gay. Also many gays don't self-identify as such and won't respond to the questionnaire."[22]

Donor education and donor self-deferral programs were rapidly adopted throughout the U.S. and remained accepted and recognized practice until 1989. At that time, the AABB recommended that donors be questioned about activities placing them at risk for AIDS through direct questions.[23] The FDA issued similar recommendations in December, 1990.[24] A study conducted in Tampa, Florida and San Bernardino, California showed that blood donors were not offended by orally asked questions about AIDS risk activities in 1987 to 1988.[25] Evidence supporting the efficacy of the self-deferral program is derived from studies performed in New York City and San Francisco. In New York, following the institution of a self-deferral program, a statistically significant decrease in the percentage of donations from men occurred (62.6 to 61.5%). Among males 21 to 35 years of age, 12% fewer donations were made in 1983 than 1982, again a statistically significant difference.[26] In a retrospective study of blood donors in San Francisco, names of patients who had been blood donors were compared with a listing of patients with AIDS. Of 199 persons who made 634 donations, most ceased donating in 1983.[27]

B. BLOOD TESTING

At the January, 1983 CDC meeting, a variety of laboratory test results from patients with AIDS were analyzed. In the absence of an etiology for AIDS and, hence, a specific marker for infection, laboratory tests abnormal in the majority of AIDS patients were considered as surrogate or substitute tests to detect those at risk for the syndrome. Support was sought for testing blood donors with surrogate tests as a potential method for increasing the safety of the blood supply by those who believed AIDS was transmitted by transfusions. However, the Public Health Service did not recommend instituting surrogate testing. Instead, it suggested that studies be performed to determine their efficacy.[28]

The tests under consideration included T-helper/T-suppressor ratios, total lymphocyte count, antibody to hepatitis-B core antigen, circulating immune complexes, β-2-microglobulin, thymosin, and CMV testing.[22,28-33] Of these, anti-HB_c testing of T-helper/T-suppressor testing were implemented by a handful of volunteer blood collection agencies principally centered in the San Francisco Bay area.

Subsequent to introduction of HIV testing, it was found that 38% of blood donors found anti-HIV-positive in San Francisco were anti-HB_c-positive.[34] In a study performed at Stanford, California, involving 5565 consecutive blood donors, T-helper/T-suppressor ratios of 0.15 to 10.00 with a mean of 2.00 ± 0.10 (SEM) were found. Less than 2% of the donors had T-helper/T-suppressor ratios ≤0.85. They implemented T-helper/T-suppressor testing in July, 1983 and in February, 1984, considered the significance of their findings in relation to the risk of AIDS transmission as uncertain.[29] However, prior to performing anti-HIV testing, in a report submitted in November, 1984, the clinical significance of T-helper/T-suppressor ratios ≤0.85 and their relationship to AIDS risk in healthy blood donors who do not belong to AIDS high-risk groups was still considered uncertain.[30] In the U.S., T-helper/T-suppressor testing as a surrogate marker for AIDS assessment of blood donors was limited to the Stanford Hospital Blood Bank and perhaps a few others.

Anti-hepatitis B core testing was implemented by blood centers in the San Francisco Bay area in May, 1984. The Hepatitis B Core Antibody Testing Study Group, formed as a result of the FDA Blood Products Advisory Committee deliberations on surrogate testing for AIDS, met in Bethesda, Maryland on March 6, 1984.[35] The Committee, chaired by Michael Rodell, Ph.D., had a divided opinion on the appropriateness of anti-HB_c testing as a means of identifying certain population groups. A majority of the study group felt such testing was inappropriate; a minority believed otherwise. Position papers indicating the thinking of each group were developed and distributed. Those opposing the implementation of anti-core testing for source and recovered plasma did so for a variety of reasons. First, the test for anti-core was not specific for individuals at risk of AIDS. Such tests would reject blood from 3 to 10% of volunteer donors and 15 to 20% of paid plasma donors. Core antibody-positive individuals ranged from 80% of male homosexuals and bisexuals seen at venereal disease clinics in AIDS endemic areas, 38% of gay male plasma donors in the southwest, and 15% of New York Blood Center male donors who asked that their blood not be used for transfusion. Preliminary data from the CDC's investigation of possible transfusion-associated AIDS cases indicated that this marker was present in only 50% of donors suspected of transmitting HIV to recipients. Second, the loss of a significant number of otherwise healthy blood donors might adversely affect the availability of components and derivatives for patients. Third, notification and deferral of anti-core-positive donors might cause inappropriate concern and additional cost for medical evaluation. Fourth, the cost of testing was felt to be high even if done only for plasma donors, perhaps adding $140,000,000 to health care costs in the U.S. Finally, the use of anti-HB_c to screen out individuals at high risk for developing AIDS was thought to become less significant subsequently because of vaccination programs against hepatitis B; that is, male homosexuals were being urged to be vaccinated against hepatitis B and that these individuals would make anti-HB_s rather than form anti-HB_c.

Those advocating the implementation of anti-core testing believed the benefits of safer coagulation factor concentrates outweighed the disadvantages of testing for anti-HB_c. However, they thought the logistics of performing the test on whole blood donors might preclude its use on individual units of whole blood and components.

An additional argument against the use of surrogate testing is that it might have attracted persons who participated in activities placing them at risk for AIDS to donate blood to obtain a test providing them with information about their AIDS status. Since testing was not fully effective, such donors might be negative for the surrogate marker yet be capable of transmitting AIDS through transfusion.

C. INVENTORY TESTING AT THE TIME OF HIV TEST IMPLEMENTATION

HIV antibody test kits manufactured by Abbott Laboratories were licensed by the FDA on March 2, 1985. Despite guidance in memoranda issued by the PHS in January[36] and the FDA in February, 1985,[37] two issues remained inadequately addressed. The first concerned the appropriate period following test availability for training staff to become proficient in performing anti-HIV testing. The second issue involved the appropriate period to convert an inventory untested for anti-HCV to one that was fully tested.

Although the anti-HIV test format involved an enzyme immunoassay, laboratory personnel required training to assure that testing was performed accurately. In addition, test kit availability was uncertain as a result of limited supplies. The latter issue confounded the timeliness with which blood in hospital inventories could be tested.

Assuming that test kits were in short supply in early March, 1985, it would have been more effective to test newly donated blood than components in inventory. For example, testing a freshly donated unit would result in a red cell and another component that were tested, both of which would have been anti-HIV negative. Had red cells and a unit of fresh frozen plasma or a platelet concentrate been tested for anti-HIV, two tests would have been used, causing a further shortage of test kits.

Another confounding factor at the time of test kit licensure was the possibility that persons engaging in high-risk activities would donate blood to obtain an HIV test result. It should be noted that test kits were available only at blood centers. Since test kit sensitivity was less than 100%, there was concern that test implementation and the absence of alternative sites for persons to be tested might result in people who otherwise would have self deferred donating blood to obtain a test result. Since the tests may have missed some infectious donors, the net result would be a decreased safety of the blood supply.

The countervailing arguments are that following HIV test availability, a last-in, first-out policy rather than the usual first-in, first-out policy for inventory management should have been instituted. Moreover, blood should have been labeled as tested or untested. Between March and July, 1985, approximately 0.17% of blood donors tested repeatedly reactive for anti-HIV, and approximately .04% were confirmed to have antibody by Western blot analysis.[38] Hence, on a nationwide basis, approximately 4 per 10,000 donors were infected with HIV and potentially capable of transmitting it to a transfusion recipient. The risk to transfusion by untested blood in inventory or through components drawn after test kit licensure and prior to test implementation should be viewed in this context.

D. IMPLEMENTING LOOK-BACK

Subsequent to test kit introduction in the spring of 1985, some blood donors were found to be anti-HIV-positive by enzyme-linked immunosorbent assay (ELISA) and later confirmed positive by Western blot. The date when these donors became infected was unknown. Hence, persons who had donated previously may have been infected at the time of a previous donation and their blood may have transmitted HIV to previous recipients. Therefore, these recipients might be at risk for AIDS, for transmitting it to their sexual partners, or to their newborn children.

During 1985, the ELISA tests were sensitive but suffered from nonspecificity. Western blot testing was available, although interpretation was not always straightforward and wide variation was present in the ability of various laboratories to perform and interpret Western blot results. In June, 1985, the major blood banking organizations indicated that studies were needed to determine whether there was an ''adequate basis for notification of recipients of blood components from a previous donation'' by a donor subsequently found to be HIV-antibody-positive''.[39] By 1986, pilot studies demonstrated that the majority of previous recipients of blood from donors found repeatedly reactive for anti-HIV by ELISA and confirmed by Western blot had been infected, presumably as a result of the blood they received.[40]

In June, 1986, AABB, ARC, and CCBC recommended that a ''look-back'' program be established by which recipients of blood drawn prior to anti-HIV testing from a donor subsequently determined to be anti-HIV confirmed positive should be notified of the possibility they were infected with HIV. The proposed notification process had blood centers notifying transfusion services that, in turn, would contact the attending physician who ordered the transfusion.[41] It was then the attending physician's responsibility to assess the situation and determine those patients who would be notified, counseled, and tested for anti-HIV. Additional comments about look-back notification appeared in March, 1987 in a *Morbidity and Mortality Weekly Report*[42] and in recommendations stemming from the Presidential AIDS Commission in 1988.[43] However, implementation guidelines stemming from the latter report are murky.

Some plaintiffs identified through look-back programs have alleged that the blood center was negligent in failing to implement look-back programs earlier. These plaintiffs argue that more prompt notification may have prevented transmission to others, including infants conceived at a time when it was known that blood was received from a donor subsequently found to be anti-HIV-positive, or delayed their own diagnosis or treatment.

E. WARNING PATIENTS (INFORMED CONSENT)

Prior to performing operative or invasive procedures, physicians obtain consent from patients after informing them of potential benefits, risks, and alternatives. Extension of this procedure to include therapeutic agents such as blood component therapy have not been uniform. In part, this relates to the supposition that blood components are withheld unless needed, in which case, alternatives do not exist or that the risk involved with their utilization is outweighed by their benefit. The time when there was sufficient evidence to conclude that AIDS could be transmitted by transfusion and that the risk was appreciable remains controversial. It could be argued that although the hazard was significant, the remote risk was insufficient to require specific informed consent for transfusion.

In 1986, the AABB issued a statement recommending that patients who receive nonemergency transfusions be informed of the risks and benefits of blood and blood products and consent to their use.[44] The informed consent should include (1) an understanding of the recommended medical action; (2) the associated risks and benefits; (3) alternatives to the recommended therapy and their potential risks and benefits, including the risk of not receiving the recommended therapy; and (4) an opportunity to ask questions.[45] The duty to obtain informed consent rests with the physician ordering transfusion therapy. Physicians have an obligation to share their medical knowledge with the patient when the patient needs the information to make an intelligent choice regarding treatment ("Canterbury" rules).[46] Although patient contact is nonexistent or limited between blood center and patient or transfusion service and patient, respectively, medical directors of these facilities have an ill-defined role in educating those directly responsible for patient care.

F. ADVISING THE MEDICAL COMMUNITY

The Joint Statement issued in January, 1983 included a recommendation that blood centers and transfusion services provide educational materials to physicians about the risk of AIDS transmission through transfusion.[20] While specific methods were not mentioned, an expectation was created that blood centers and transfusion services had a duty to provide such information.

Quantification of risk was inaccurate in the absence of clear data enumerating TA-HIV cases and precise numbers of transfusion recipients at risk. It was not possible to determine the extent to which donors were infected with HIV prior to virus identification and donor testing. In conjunction with more precise estimates of the length of the incubation period between transfusion and illness using the Weibull model, projections about the number of patients infected with HIV as a result of transfusion increase.[47] Preliminary information in 1983 indicated the risk per recipient was less than 1 per million.

By 1986, there was an estimate that 29,000 transfusion recipients were infected between 1978 and 1984 and that 12,000 were living.[3] Interpolation to periods prior to testing should be viewed with skepticism since the scope of the epidemic expanded between 1983 and 1985, and an estimate of the number infected during this interval would be, of necessity, imprecise.

Hence, given a duty to inform the medical community about the possibility of TA-HIV, the magnitude of the risk was difficult to quantify. Confounding the issue, enormous media attention was paid to AIDS, including transfusion-associated cases, between 1983 and the present. Hence, even in the absence of specific targeted information about TA-HIV, it is inconceivable that practicing physicians were ignorant of this issue.

G. APPROPRIATE UTILIZATION OF TRANSFUSION THERAPY

Therapeutic intervention has always involved a risk/benefit analysis. When risk exceeds potential benefit, in general, the intervention is considered contraindicated. Similar admonitions apply to the utilization of blood transfusion therapy.

Precise guidelines for prescribing blood components did not become commonplace until the mid-1980s. Medical school curricula provided scant training about transfusion. House officers usually learned about transfusion through clinical experience and comments made by a more experienced house staff or attending physicians. In 1984, the first of three National Institutes of Health Consensus Conferences addressing the appropriateness of blood transfusion was conducted.[48] It considered the use of fresh frozen plasma. The second Consensus Conference was held in 1986[49] and addressed the use of platelet concentrates, and the third, held in 1988, examined the use of red cell transfusions in the perioperative period.[50] Improvement in transfusion practice as a result of these conferences has not been apparent. Concern about TA-HIV by patients and their physicians led to declines in blood usage in the mid-1980s. In addition, accrediting agencies such as the Joint Commission of Accreditation of Hospital Organizations (JCAHO) took action to foster review of transfusion practice.[51]

Since some adverse consequences of transfusion are unavoidable, it seems prudent to limit transfusions to meet established guidelines. Unfortunately, this intuitive advice defies clinical practice. Results of laboratory tests are not always available when clinical decisions about the need for transfusion are required. Also, retrospective review is insensitive to factors influencing the clinical management of a patient. Nonetheless, liability issues are raised when an adverse outcome occurs in the absence of a justified need for an implicated transfusion.

V. DEFENSE AGAINST ALLEGATIONS

A. BLOOD SHIELD STATUTES

Suits initiated against blood centers on the basis of strict liability or breach of implied warranties have generally been negated by blood shield statues that treat the provision of blood as a service rather than the sale of a product. Hence, plaintiffs generally do not pursue these causes of action to resolve disputes. Instead, they rely on negligence as a cause of action.

B. STANDARD OF CARE

Critical to the defense of negligence suits is the formulation of the prevailing standard of care. As previously mentioned, a plaintiff seeking to recover under a negligence theory must prove that the defendant owed him a duty and that the defendant breached that duty. The duty at issue is often described as the standard of care and the question is asked whether the defendant's action met that prevailing standard of care.

In a typical negligence action, such as an automobile accident, a court will apply a standard of care that is commensurate with that degree of care which a reasonably prudent person would exercise under the same or similar circumstances. If the person's conduct falls below the standard he may be liable in damages for the injuries resulting from his conduct. The court relies upon the jury — presumably composed of reasonably prudent persons — to exercise their own knowledge and set the prevailing standard of care as it relates to the subject of the law (for example, the safe operation of automobiles).

In a professional malpractice action, the standard of care measures the competence of the professional physician, attorney, accountant, etc. The prevailing professional standard of care is not what a reasonably prudent person would have done under the circumstances. Rather, the standard of care is what other members of the defendant's profession, exercising that degree of skill, care, and diligence that is generally accepted and recognized by the profession and practicing under the same or similar circumstances at the same time would have done. In other words, what the defendant was doing was accepted by his or her peers as reasonable given available knowledge. Because a jury is presumed not to know what a reasonable professional would have done under the circumstances, they are expected to rely upon experts to establish prevailing practices. Thus, a lay jury can judge a professional defendant according to the standards set by the defendant's professional peers. The jury is not expected to substitute its lay opinion for that of the experts.

There are two notable exceptions to this rule. The first is simple: if the alleged breach is obvious (e.g., a surgeon leaves a scalpel inside the patient) then expert testimony is unnecessary. The second is a bit more complex: if the defendant met the prevailing standard of care practiced by his profession, then the plaintiff may attack the entire profession. For example, the *Helling v. Carey* case (Washington State) involved an ophthalmologist who was found negligent for not performing a test for glaucoma on a patient less than 40 years of age even though it was not the standard of care to do so.[52] *Helling* is in keeping with earlier precedent allowing plaintiffs to attack an entire industry's (as opposed to a profession's) practices. During the early years of the Depression, a Federal Circuit Court of Appeals, applying a reasonably prudent person standard in an ordinary negligence case, found a tugboat company negligent for not having a radio on board even though it was not the standard in the industry for tugboats to carry radios at the time the accident occurred.[53] The court opined that "There are precautions so imperative that even their universal disregard will not excuse their omission." With *Helling*, that industry-wide attack was brought to the professional malpractice action.

In the context of TA-HIV litigation, the plaintiff would prefer that the standard of care to be applied would be that of the reasonably prudent person. Normally, it is easier to convince a jury that it can rely upon its own knowledge (and sympathy) that the defendant breached his duties. Defendants, however, prefer that the professional standard of care applied. In that instance, the jury is expected to rely upon the opinions of experts as to the existence of the prevailing standard of care and not to rely upon what a reasonably prudent person would have done. The weight of authority is that blood centers will be treated as professionals and that the professional standard of care would apply in a TA-HIV case. For example, the South Carolina Supreme Court in *Doe v. American Red Cross Blood Services*[54] held that a medical malpractice standard of care applies in a negligence action against a blood center. In *Doe* the volunteer donor had donated whole blood after AIDS screening in the form of donor education and donor self-deferral; no surrogate tests had been implemented. The *Doe* court concluded that "the standard of care that the plaintiff must prove is that the professional failed to conform to the generally recognized and accepted practices in his profession."[64] Citing a blood shield statute and "ample" other precedent, the court held, "[s]ince the transfusion of blood is characterized as a skilled medical service, then we hold that the Red Cross, as a blood collector and processor, should be treated as professional." A recent Seattle case,[55] however, was decided in favor of the plaintiff by a jury told to use the "reasonable man" test of *Helling v. Carey.*[52] In the *Quintana* case, the Colorado Supreme Court ordered a new trial to allow testimony to determine whether the practices of the national blood banking community were unreasonably deficient.[56] (See also Reference 75.)

Because of what was known at the time a policy or procedure was set in place, a chronology of significant events is helpful in assessing potential liability for TA-HIV. The standard of care at various times may be reflected in joint statements issued by the major blood banking organizations, FDA memoranda, and recommendations from the Public Health Service contained in *Morbidity and Mortality Weekly Report* articles.

For example, the Joint Statement of January 13, 1983,[20] on AIDS related to transfusion make specific suggestions about (1) extending educational campaigns to physicians to balance the decision to use each blood component against the risks of transfusion; (2) increasing the use of autologous transfusions; (3) being aware of possible increases in usage of cryoprecipitate; (4) augmenting donor history questions to detect possible AIDS or exposure to patients with AIDS; (5) not targeting donor recruitment efforts toward groups that may have a high incidence of AIDS; (6) not asking donors direct questions about their sexual preference; and (7) not advising routine implementation of surrogate tests.

The March 4, 1983 *MMWR*[28] report on interagency recommendations for prevention of AIDS indicated: (1) avoid sexual contact with persons known or suspected to have AIDS; (2) as a temporary measure, groups at increased risk for AIDS should refrain from donating plasma and/or blood; (3) conduct studies to evaluate screening procedures (including laboratory tests, history questions, or physical examinations) for effectiveness in identifying and excluding persons with a high probability of transmitting AIDS; (4) physicians should adhere strictly to medical indications for transfusion and encourage autologous transfusion; and (5) work should continue toward development of safer blood products for hemophilic patients. Also, those at increased risk of AIDS were specified.

The March 24, 1983, memorandum from the FDA[21] contained recommendations to decrease the risk of transmitting AIDS from blood donors by (1) initiating educational programs to inform persons at increased risk of AIDS to refrain from blood donation; (2) re-educating personnel responsible for donor screening about early signs and symptoms of AIDS; and (3) treating as highly infectious, quarantining and destroying blood inadvertently collected from a donor known or suspected of having AIDS.

The June, 1983 Joint Statement on Directed Donations and AIDS[57] stated that there was no evidence that directed donations were safer than those available through a community blood bank and strongly recommended against "directed donation" programs.

The January, 1984 Joint Statement reviewing AIDS and blood transfusion development[58] reaffirmed previously made recommendations and indicated that in high-incidence AIDS areas, it may be important to have confidential forms for donors to indicate whether their blood should be used for transfusion or a telephone number to call to request their blood should not be used for transfusions.

The December, 1984 Joint Statement about transfusion-associated AIDS with interim recommendations for notification of blood collecting organizations and transfusion services.[59] This statement provided guidance on what to do in the case of blood or plasma donors who develop AIDS within five years of donation, in the case of former donors who have lymphadenopathy syndrome or AIDS-related syndromes, and in the case of recipients not in high-risk groups who develop AIDS within five years of transfusion.

A December 14, 1984 FDA memo revised recommendations to decrease the risk of transmitting AIDS.[60] The signs and symptoms of AIDS were expanded to include persistent cough, shortness of breath, white spots or unusual blemishes in the mouth, and persistent diarrhea. The wording for donors asked to refrain from donation was modified to "males who have had sex with more than one male since 1979, and males whose male partner has had sex with more than one male since 1979."

The January 11, 1985 *MMWR*[36] report provided provisional Public Health Service interagency recommendations for screening donated blood and plasma for antibody to the virus causing AIDS. Included were recommendations about screening blood and plasma, notification of donors, maintaining confidentiality, medical evaluation of those with repeatedly reactive ELISA test results, and recommendations for the individuals found antibody-positive.

The February 19, 1985, memorandum from the FDA[37] about implementation of PHS provisional recommendations concerned testing blood and plasma for HIV antibodies. This lengthy memo was intended to answer questions that might arise when HIV testing was implemented. It indicated a voluntary phase-in period would exist prior to mandatory testing. It also established a working group to be contacted if additional assistance was needed.

The memo specifically addressed blood and plasma testing; medical follow-up and donor counselling; alternative mechanisms for obtaining antibody testing; informed consent, donor deferral registers, donor notifications, and confidentiality requirements; definition of reactive results; additional testing of reactive samples; standard operating procedure revision, use of outside testing laboratories, and biosafety; and blood product labeling.

The AABB sent a memo to institutional and associated institutional members on April 6, 1985 about HIV antibody testing.[61] It advised all AABB blood banks to begin HIV testing as soon as possible. It defined a positive test result and indicated donors should not be told of positive results until "the phase-in period was completed *and* community mechanisms for educating and counseling donors was identified *and* alternative test sites were available." It indicated that it was a goal to reach a position where all products in inventory were tested, that it should be reached as rapidly as possible, and that at some point, it would be appropriate to recall untested products for retrospective testing or discard. It mentioned that individual units that were tested for HIV did not have to be labeled individually. Instead, the *Circular of Information for Human Blood and Blood Products,* once amended to include HIV testing, could be used. It advised that first testing could be done with either "unlinked" samples or samples identified with a particular donor.

The American Red Cross issued a Blood Services letter on March 22, 1985.[62] It contained procedures and requirements for phase-in testing for HIV antibody. It indicated routine testing should begin within 14 days of receipt of test kits and all blood center inventory testing should be completed within 35 days of the date routine testing started. In addition, it stated that "every effort should be made to ensure that alternative facilities for obtaining HIV test results are available .... before announcing that donated blood will be tested and that donors whose blood tested positive will be notified."

The May 7, 1985, memorandum from the FDA on testing for HIV antibodies[63] clarified the terminology and current position of the PHS and FDA with respect to not making available for distribution blood products with repeatedly reactive test results for transfusion or for further manufacture into other products capable of transmitting infectious agents. It also contained updated definitions of initial tests, repeat tests, repeatedly reactive results, and retests.

The June, 1985 Joint Statement on tests for HIV antibody[64] indicated donor notification, ideally, should wait until alternative test sites were available. It noted that only donors whose tests could be verified by additional testing (e.g., Western blot) should be notified, although their blood should not be used for transfusion. It stated that notification of recipients of blood components prepared from previous donations of HIV-antibody-positive blood donors should await results of studies looking into this matter.

The September 3, 1985 memorandum from the FDA revised the definitions of high-risk groups with respect to AIDS transmission from blood and plasma donors.[65] It modified the December 14, 1984 memorandum[60] definition of at-risk donors to "any male who has had sex with another male since 1979".

The June 1986, Joint Statement about "look-back"[41] notification of previous recipients of blood and components from donors who returned to donate and had a confirmed positive test for anti-HIV was recommended.

The October 30, 1986 memorandum from the FDA[66] had additional recommendations for reducing further the number of units of blood and plasma donated for transfusion at increased risk of HIV infection. The categories for determining persons at increased risk of HIV infection were changed to include: "Men who had sex with another man one or more times since 1977," "persons emigrating since 1977 from countries where heterosexual activity is thought to play a major role in transmission" of HIV infection, and "men and women who have engaged in prostitution since 1977 and persons who have been their heterosexual partners within six months." The donor consent was expanded to include a statement that "if I consider myself to be a person at risk for spreading the virus known to cause AIDS, I agree not to donate blood or plasma for transfusion ..."

The use of a confidential unit exclusion (CUE) system was recommended. Units designated not for transfusion to others were required to be removed from inventories, strict confidentiality of the donor's decision was needed, HIV testing was to be performed on all units, donors with positive test results were to be notified, and all donors were to be assured that units confidentially excluded would be used for laboratory testing.

The March 20, 1987 *MMWR*[42] report on HIV infection in transfusion recipients and their family members estimated there were approximately 12,000 people living in the U.S. who acquired HIV infection between 1978 and 1984 as a result of transfusion. It noted "look-back" programs could not identify all infected transfusion recipients. It stated "physicians should consider offering HIV antibody testing to some patients who received transfusions between 1978 and late spring of 1985." The consideration of whom to test was relegated to those at greater risk of infection; e.g., recipients of large numbers of transfusions and if blood was collected in the years closest to screening in areas with a high incidence of AIDS.

The February 5, 1990, memorandum from the FDA[67] made recommendations for prevention of HIV transmission by blood and blood products. Modifications were made to the criteria for exclusion of unsuitable donors such that "men who have had sex with another man even one time since 1977" were asked to self-exclude. Donors were to be told that an interval during early infection was present when the HIV test was negative but transmission of the virus could occur. The names of those with positive test results would be added to donor deferral registries. Comments about use of Western blot testing and reentry of donors with "false-positive" ELISA results were included.

The December 5, 1990, memorandum from the FDA[68] revised recommendations for the prevention of HIV transmission by blood and blood products. Oral communications and direct questions about risk behavior were recommended. In addition, donors were to be deferred if they had a diagnosis of syphilis or gonorrhea in the past 12 months and the deferral for use of a prostitute was extended from 6 to 12 months.

C. NO CAUSATION

One of the four elements needed to be proven for a negligence claim is causation. If plaintiff cannot prove that a transfusion was the proximate cause (loosely meaning an event that was foreseeable) of the plaintiff acquiring HIV, the action is generally lost. For example, individuals who have participated in activities placing them at risk for AIDS that antedate the time of a putative transfusion may provide grounds for dismissal.

D. LEARNED INTERMEDIARY DOCTRINE

The duty of a regional blood center to inform patients directly about TA-HIV is probably limited to the learned intermediary doctrine. This doctrine states that because there existed a learned intermediary (usually the physician) between the center and patient, the duty to warn rests with the intermediary.

VI. CONCLUSION

The causes of action supporting lawsuits against blood centers, transfusion services, and physicians are described. The defense portions have also been presented. The Appendix contains a listing of TA-HIV lawsuits that have been pursued in litigation. The verdicts and awards and the major negligence issues are cited. TA-HIV is a tragic event: the victims gain only money if they win, and the defendants get little satisfaction if they achieve a victory over a patient they sought to help.

ACKNOWLEDGMENT

The authors thank Steven J. Labensky, Esq. for his thoughtful insights, comments, and suggestions during the preparation of this manuscript.

APPENDIX
Selected TA-HIV Cases
(presented in chronological order of initial trial)

Case	Decision	Issues	Ref.
Rasmussen v. South Florida Blood Service	State Supreme Court decision in favor of Blood Service.	Donors' rights to privacy more important than plaintiff's need for names of donors.	15
Kozup v. Red Cross & Georgetown Hospital	Appeals Court Judgment in favor of Red Cross & Georgetown. Time of blood donation deemed important. Case remanded to trial court to try for a battery claim.	Blood donated October, 1982 by male homosexual who later developed AIDS. Negligence, breach of implied warranties, strict liability, lack of informed consent against Red Cross and hospital. "Canterbury" set aside: "informed consent" different from "consent to treatment" with regard to battery.	69
Tarrant County Hospital Dist. v. Hughes	Texas Appeals Court decision to allow plaintiff access to donor identity through trial court supervision.	Donor confidentiality issue.	16
Borchett v. Irwin Blood Bank	Settled mid-trial.	72-year-old woman transfused in 1983. Administrative error by blood bank — donor history questionnaire incomplete for hepatitis.	70

APPENDIX (continued)
Selected TA-HIV Cases
(presented in chronological order of initial trial)

Case	Decision	Issues	Ref.
Quintana v. UBS	Jury decision in favor of defendant (blood bank). Physician found negligent; decision in favor of blood bank overturned by Supreme Court: trial court should have allowed testimony to determine if blood bankers, in general, were deficient.	Emergency surgery for self-inflicted gun shot wound in May 1983. Negligence claimed for failing to properly screen blood and to warn recipients of risk of AIDS transmission through transfusion.	56
Osborn v. Irwin Blood Bank	$750,000 awarded to plaintiff by jury. (Noneconomic damages later reduced to $250,000.)	Eight-week-old infant received 12 units of blood during surgery to repair congenital heart defect in February, 1983. Donor screening and surrogate test issues decided in favor of blood bank. Directed donation policy held against blood bank.	71
JAC v. Blood Center of Southeastern Wisconsin	$3.9 million awarded to plaintiff by jury. (Later out-of-court settlement reached.)	63-year-old man received a unit of cryoprecipitate during open heart surgery in April, 1985 from a donor who later tested HIV-positive. Negligence for failure to test blood donated March 6, 1985 (in inventory) claimed.	72
Shelby v. St. Luke's Episcopal Hospital	Summary judgment in favor of defendant.	July, 1984 transfusion. Strict liability, breach of expressed and implied warranties, product liability, and negligence claimed. Court stated blood center followed standard of care.	73

APPENDIX (continued)
Selected TA-HIV Cases
(presented in chronological order of initial trial)

Case	Decision	Issues	Ref.
Jane Doe v. American Red Cross, South Carolina Region	State Supreme Court decision in favor of defendant.	Jan. 1985 transfusion for gallbladder surgery, Red Cross accused of negligence for not performing surrogate tests and excluding donors at high risk of AIDS. Supreme court ruled negligence must be based on conformity with generally recognized and accepted practices; i.e., profession standard of care recognized.	54
Kirkendall v. Harbor Insurance Company	U.S. Court of Appeals decision in favor of defendant.	March 28, 1985 transfusion: HIV nontested inventory issue. Standard of care followed. Risk to disruption of blood supply felt to be greater than risk of blood contamination. Donor screening and surrogate testing issues dismissed.	74
Jane Doe v. Univ. of Cincinnati	State Court of Appeals in favor of defendant's position. (Still in litigation.)	Discovery of name of donor by plaintiff denied.	17
KW v. Bell Bonfils Memorial Blood Bank	$5.5 million awarded to plaintiff by jury (award reduced to $3.6 million post-trial).	March 22, 1985 transfusion during emergency hysterectomy for postpartum bleeding. HIV untested blood (in inventory) transfused 9 days after receipt of test kits. A general standard of care appeared to be applied.	75
Clark v. United Blood Services	$970,000 awarded to plaintiff by jury (award later reduced to $437,293).	June, 1984 transfusion following hunting accident. Donor required to answer questions in a telephone deposition — he was deferred temporarily because of history of syphilis. Plaintiff claimed negligence based on surrogate testing and donor screening issues.	18

APPENDIX (continued)
Selected TA-HIV Cases
(presented in chronological order of initial trial)

Case	Decision	Issues	Ref.
Edwards v. Samaritan Health Service	$28.7 million awarded to plaintiff by jury from physician (later settled for $6 million plus medical expenses).	March, 1985 transfusion to neonate with respiratory distress. Transfusion given "routinely". Informed consent not obtained.	76
O'Rourke v. Irwin Memorial Blood Bank	Jury decision in favor of defendant.	Premature infant transfused in October, 1982. Plaintiff claimed donor screening efforts inadequate, surrogate testing should have been performed, and directed donation policy not administered uniformly.	77
Hoemke v. New York Blood Center	Federal Court of Appeals decision in favor of defendants.	Nov. 1981 transfusion. Court held that doctors not required to contact and inform past patients of possible harms they did not know. Date of transfusion was considered an important factor in reaching this decision.	78
Eik v. Irwin Memorial Blood Bank	Jury decision in favor of blood bank; $180,000 awarded from hospital.	Nov. 1983 transfusion. Jury found in favor of blood bank on plaintiff's claims of failure to use surrogate tests, warn about transfusion-AIDS risk, and properly screen donors. Monetary award based on informed consent issues.	79
Judy Jeanne v. Hawkes Hospital of Mt. Carmel	$15 million awarded to plaintiff by jury. Blood bank settled out of court.	25-year-old woman infected during cosmetic surgery by unit of blood donated the day HIV antibody test kits were received. Plaintiff claimed transfusion was unnecessary and given without attending physician's permission.	80

REFERENCES

1. **Centers for Disease Control,** *Pneumocystis carinii* pneumonia among persons with hemophilia A, *MMWR,* 31, 365, 1982.
2. **Centers for Disease Control,** Possible transfusion-associated acquired immunodeficiency syndrome (AIDS) — California, *MMWR,* 31, 602, 1982.
3. **Peterman, T. A., Lui, K.-J., Lawrence, D. N., and Allen, J. R.,** Estimating the risk of transfusion-associated acquired immune deficiency syndrome and human immunodeficiency virus infection, *Transfusion,* 27, 371, 1987.
4. **Perlmutter v. Beth David Hospital,** 308, N.Y. 100, 123 N.E. 2d 792 (App. 1954).
5. **Cunningham v. MacNeal Memorial Hospital,** 226 N.E. 2d 897 (Ill. 1970).
6. Restatement (Second) of *Torts,* Section 402A (1965).
7. **Hutchins v. Blood Services of Montana,** 161 Mont. 359, 506 p. 2d 449 (1973).
8. **Sugarman, S. D.,** The need to reform personal injury law leaving scientific disputes to scientists, *Science,* 248, 823, 1990.
9. **Lipton, K. S.,** Blood donor services and liability issue relating to acquired immune deficiency syndrome, *J. Legal Med.,* 7, 131, 1986.
10. **Zuck, T. F.,** Legal liability for transfusion injury in the acquired immunodeficiency syndrome era, *Arch,. Pathol. Lab. Med.,* 114, 309, 1990.
11. **Gostin, L. O.,** The AIDS litigation project. A national review of court and Human Rights Commission decisions. I. The social impact of AIDS, *JAMA,* 263, 1961, 1990.
12. **Gostin, L. O.,** The AIDS litigation project. A national review of court and Human Rights Commission decisions. II. Discrimination, *JAMA,* 263, 2086, 1990.
13. **Jenner, R. K.,** Professional Negligence. Transfusion-associated AIDS cases, *TRIAL,* May, 1990, p. 30.
14. **Jenner, R. K.,** Identifying HIV-infected blood donors. Who is 'John donor'?, *TRIAL,* June, 1989, p. 47.
15. **Rasmussen v. South Florida Blood Service Inc.,** 500 So.2d 533 (Fla. 1987).
16. **Tarant County Hospital District v Hughes,** 734 S.W.2d 675 (Tex. Civ. Appl. 1987), *cert denied,* 108 S.Ct. 1027 (1988).
17. **Doe v. University of Cincinnati,** 42 Ohio App. 3d 227, 530 N.E.2d 419 (1988).
18. **Clark v. United Blood Services,** Cause No. CV 88–6981 (Nev. 2d Jud. Dist. Ct. April 27, 1990).
19. **McKay, J. E.,** AIDS and blood transfusions, *Verdicts, Settlements & Tactics,* March, 1990, p. 74.
20. **Joint Statement of the American Association of Blood Banks, American Red Cross, Council of Community Blood Centers,** On acquired immune deficiency syndrome related to transfusion, 1983.
21. Recommendations to decrease the risk of transmitting acquired immune deficiency syndrome (AIDS) from blood donors, in Memorandum to All Establishments Collecting Human Blood for Transfusion, Office of Biologics, National Center for Drugs and Biologics, Food and Drug Administration, Washington, D.C., 1983.
22. **Check, W. A.,** Preventing AIDS transmission: should blood donors be screened?, *JAMA,* 249, 567, 1983.
23. Statement and Recommendations of the American Association of Blood Banks Regarding Donor History Questions Approved by the Board of Directors, AABB, August 9, 1989.
24. Memorandum, Revised Recommendations for the Prevention of Human Immunodeficiency Virus (HIV) Transmission by Blood and Blood Products—Section I, Parts A & B only, Center for Biologics Evaluation & Research, Department of Health & Human Services, Public Health Service, Washington, D.C., December 5, 1990.
25. **Silvergleid, A. J., Leparc, G. F., and Schmidt, P. J.,** Impact of explicit questions about high-risk activities on donor attitudes and donor deferral patterns. Results in two community blood centers, *Transfusion,* 29, 362, 1989.

26. **Pindyck, J., Waldman, A., Zang, E., Oleszko, W., Lowy, M., and Bianco, C.,** Measures to decrease the risk of acquired immunodeficiency syndrome transmission by blood transfusion, *Transfusion,* 25, 3, 1985.
27. **Perkins, H. A., Samson, S., and Busch, M.,** How well has self-exclusion worked?, *Transfusion,* 28, 601, 1988.
28. **Centers for Disease Control,** Report of interagency recommendations. Prevention of acquired immune deficiency syndrome (AIDS), *MMWR,* 32, 101, 1983.
29. **Fishwild, D. M., Lifson, J. D., and Engleman, E. G.,** Human T-lymphocyte subsets defined by monoclonal antibodies: functional analysis and application to a blood donor screening program for the AIDS carrier state, in *Acquired Immune Deficiency Syndrome,* Gottlieb, M. C. and Groopman, J. E., Eds., Alan R. Liss, New York, 1984, 247.
30. **Lifson, J. D., Finch, S. L., Sasaki, D. T., and Engleman, E. G.,** Variables affecting T-lymphocyte subsets in a volunteer blood donor population, *Clin. Immunol. Immunopathol.,* 36, 151, 1985.
31. **Simon, T. L. and Bankhurst, A. D.,** A pilot study of surrogate tests to prevent transmission of acquired immune deficiency syndrome by transfusion, *Transfusion,* 24, 373, 1984.
32. **Hersh, E. M., Reuben, J. M., Rios, A., Mansell, P. W. A., Newell, G. R., McLure, J. E., and Goldstein, A. L.,** Elevated serum thymosin α, levels associated with evidence of immune dysregulation in male homosexuals with a history of infectious diseases or Kaposi's sarcoma, (letter), *N. Engl. J. Med.,* 308, 45, 1983.
33. **Zolla-Pazner, S., William, D., El-Sadr, W., Marmor, M., and Stahl, R.,** Quantitation of β_2-microglobulin and other immune characteristics in a prospective study of men at risk for acquired immune deficiency syndrome, *JAMA,* 251, 2951, 1984.
34. **Zuck, T. F.,** Silent sequences and the safety of blood transfusions, *Ann. Intern. Med.,* 108, 895, 1988.
35. **Rodell, M.,** Interim summary statement of hepatitis B core antibody testing study group. Final report: hepatitis B core antibody testing study group, Food and Drug Administration, Bethesda, MD, 1984.
36. **Centers for Disease Control,** Provisional Public Health Service inter-agency recommendations for screening donated blood and plasma for antibody to the virus causing acquired immunodeficiency syndrome, *MMWR,* 34, 1, 1985.
37. Implementation of Public Health Service provisional recommendations concerning testing blood and plasma for antibodies to HTLV–III, in Memorandum to All Registered Blood Establishments, Office of Biologics Research and Review, Department of Health and Human Services, February 19, 1985.
38. **Schorr, J. B., Berkowitz, A., Cumming, P. D., Katz, A. J., and Sandler, S. G.,** Prevalence of HTLV–III antibody in American blood donors (letter), *N. Engl. J. Med.,* 313, 384, 1985.
39. **Joint Statement of the American Association of Blood Banks, American Red Cross, Council of Community Blood Centers,** Tests for HTLV–III antibodies, 1985.
40. **Menitove, J. E.,** Status of recipients of blood from donors subsequently found to have antibody to HIV (letter), *N. Engl. J. Med.,* 315, 1095, 1986.
41. **Joint Statement of the American Association of Blood Banks, American Red Cross, Council of Community Blood Centers,** Look-back: Notification of previous recipients of blood and components from donors who now have a confirmed positive test for anti-HTLV–III, June 16, 1986.
42. **Centers for Disease Control,** Human immunodeficiency virus infection in transfusion recipients and their family members, *MMWR,* 36, 137, 1987.
43. Report of the President's Commission on the human immunodeficiency virus epidemic, U.S. Government Printing Office, Washington, D.C., 0–214–7–1:QL3, 1988.
44. **Berkman, E. M.,** Informed consent for blood transfusion, American Association of Blood Banks Memorandum, July 10, 1986.

45. **Willett, D. E.,** The duty to warn about transfusion risks, *Arch. Pathol. Lab. Med.,* 113, 307, 1989.
46. **Canterbury v. Spence,** 464 F.2d 772 (D.C. Cir.), *cert denied,* 409 U.S. 1064 (1972).
47. **Lui, K.-J., Lawrence, D. N., Morgan, W. M., Peterman, T. A., Haverkos, H. W., and Bregman, D. J.,** A model-based approach for estimating the mean incubation period of transfusion-associated acquired immunodeficiency syndrome, *Proc. Natl. Acad. Sci. U.S.A.,* 83, 3051, 1986.
48. **Office of Medical Applications of Research, National Institutes of Health,** Fresh frozen plasma: indications and risks, *JAMA,* 253, 551, 1985.
49. **Office of Medical Applications of Research, National Institutes of Health,** Platelet transfusion therapy, *JAMA,* 257, 1777, 1987.
50. **Office of Medical Applications of Research, National Institutes of Health,** Perioperative red cell transfusion, *JAMA,* 260, 1700, 1988.
51. **Van Schoonhoven, P., Berkman, E. M., and Lehman, R.,** Medical staff monitoring functions blood usage review. Fromberg, Ed., Chicago, JCAH, 1987, pp. 1–35.
52. **Helling v. Carey,** 519 P.2d 981 (Wash. 1974).
53. **The T. J. Hooper,** 60 F.2d 737 (2d Cir. 1932).
54. **Doe v. American Red Cross Blood Services,** 297 S.C. 430, 377 S.E.2d 323 (1989).
55. **Doe v. Puget Sound Blood Center.**
56. **Quintana v. United Blood Services, et al.,** Cause No. 86–CV–11750, (Colo. Dist. Ct. 1988). SS–CA–1057 (1990).
57. **Joint Statement of the American Association of Blood Banks, American Red Cross, Council of Community Blood Centers,** Directed donations and AIDS, June 22, 1983.
58. **Joint Statement of the American Association of Blood Banks, American Red Cross, Council of Community Blood Centers,** Acquired immune deficiency syndrome (AIDS) and blood transfusion, January 3, 1984.
59. **Joint Statement of the American Association of Blood Banks, American Red Cross, Council of Community Blood Centers,** Transfusion associated AIDS: Interim recommendations for notification of blood collecting organizations and transfusion services, December 10, 1984.
60. Revised recommendations to decrease the risk of transmitting acquired immunodeficiency syndrome (AIDS) and other procedures related to blood product preparation, Memorandum to All Registered Blood Establishments, Office of Biologics Research and Review, Department of Health and Human Services, December 14, 1984.
61. **American Association of Blood Banks,** Member communication on HTLV-III antibody testing, in Memorandum to AABB Institutional and Associate Institutional Members, April 6, 1985.
62. **American Red Cross National Headquarters,** Phase-in of HTLV III antibody testing, in Memorandum, March 22, 1985.
63. Testing for antibodies to HTLV-III, in Memorandum to All Registered Blood Establishments, Office of Biologics Research and Review, Department of Health and Human Services, May 7, 1985.
64. **Joint Statement of the American Association of Blood Banks, American Red Cross, Council of Community Blood Centers,** Tests for HTLV III antibodies. Recommendations for notification of HTLV III antibody positive donors and for recipients of products form previous donations, June 7, 1985.
65. Revised definition of high-risk groups with respect to acquired immunodeficiency syndrome (AIDS) transmission from blood and plasma donors, in Memorandum to All Registered Blood Establishments, Office of Biologics Research and Review, Department of Health and Human Services, September 3, 1985.

66. Additional recommendations for reducing further the number of units of blood and plasma donated for transfusion or for further manufacture by persons at increased risk of HTLV-III/LAV infection, in Memorandum to All Registered Blood Establishments, Office of Biologics Research and Review (OBRR), Center for Drugs and Biologics, Food and Drug Administration, Department of Health and Human Services, October 30, 1986.
67. Recommendations for the prevention of human immunodeficiency virus (HIV) transmission by blood and blood products, in Memorandum to All REgistered Blood Establishments, Center for Biologics Evaluation and Research, Department of Health and Human Services, February 5, 1990.
68. Revised recommendations for the prevention of human immunodeficiency virus (HIV) transmission by blood and blood products-Section I, Parts A & B only, in Memorandum to All Registered Blood Establishments, Center for Biologics Evaluation and Research, Department of Health and Human Services, December 5, 1990.
69. **Kozup v. Georgetown University,** 663 F. Suppl. 1048 (D.C.D.C. 1987), *aff'd in rel. part,* 851 F. 2d 437 (D.C.Cir. 1988).
70. Borchett v. Irwin Blood Bank.
71. **Osborn v. Irwin Memorial Blood Bank,** Cause No. 89–1–642 Cal. Superior Ct. (City and County of San Francisco 1988).
72. **Carroll V. Blood Center of Southeastern Wisconsin,** Cause No. 753–411 (Wis. Cir. Ct. Milwaukee County Branch 18, 1988).
73. **Shelby, V. St. Luke's Episcopal Hospital,** Civil Action No. AH–86–3780, 1988 WL 288996, 56 U.S.L.W. 2680 (S.D. Tex. 1988).
74. **Kirkendall v. Harbor Insurance Co.,** 698 F.Suppl. 768 (W.D. Ark. 1988).
75. **KW, RW v. Belle Bonfils Memorial Blood Center,** Cause No. 87–CV–4127 (Colo. D.Ct. Denver County 1989).
76. **Edwards V. Samaritan Health Service, et al.,** Cause No. CV–87–35695 (Ariz. Super. Ct. June 12, 1990).
77. **O'Rourke v. Irwin Memorial Blood Bank,** Cause No. 887431 (Cal. Super. Ct. July 24, 1989).
78. **Hoemke v. New York Blood Center,** 912 F.2d 550 (2d Cir. 1990); 720 F.Suppl. 45 (S.D.N.Y. 1098).
79. **Eik v. Irwin Memorial Blood Bank, et al.,** Cause No. 898251 (Cal. Super. Ct July 24, 1989).
80. **Jeanne v. Hawkes Memorial Hospital of Mount Carmel,** Cause No. 87–CV–1669 (Ohio County Ct. March 8, 1990).

Chapter 5

EDUCATIONAL ASPECTS OF TRANSFUSION MEDICINE

Bruce A. Lenes and Lawrence Tim Goodnough

TABLE OF CONTENTS

ISBN 0-8493-4938-9

I. INTRODUCTION

The rapid expansion and increased complexity of transfusion medicine demands continuous dissemination of accurate and up-to-date information in order to provide excellent transfusion support to patients. In recent years, blood banking, now called transfusion medicine, has undergone significant changes due to (1) advancements and improvements in pretransfusion testing which have made the provision of compatible blood for transfusion routine; (2) technical advances, such as the development of plastic blood bags and of apheresis instruments; and (3) the availability of blood component therapy, in which transfusion of packed red blood cells, plasma, platelets, and/or cryoprecipitate has replaced transfusion of whole blood units. At the same time, however, increasing concern about the risks of transfusion requires more frequent and more intense interactions between transfusion specialists and the transfusing physician. It has become increasingly evident that the education of transfusing physicians has not kept pace with these technologic advances. For example, the use of fresh frozen plasma has increased tenfold nationally over the 10 years from 1970 to 1980, a period of time in which no new indications for plasma transfusion emerged.[1,2] Similarly, transfusion of platelet concentrates has increased markedly so that unit requirements of this product now exceed that of red blood cells;[2] the source of platelets is no longer just a byproduct of blood donation but often requires plateletpheresis to meet demand.[3] Although some of the increased blood component use can be attributed to the transfusion support of increasingly complex patients in therapy of cancer, trauma, transplantation, and the intensive care setting, one inescapable conclusion is that many patients are receiving combinations of red blood cells, plasma, platelets, and/or cryoprecipitate at the cost of exposure to the blood of many donors.

The recognition of these changes has led to a national effort to educate physicians and to effect changes in transfusion practice. In 1983, the National Heart, Lung, and Blood Institute established a Transfusion Medicine Academic Award Program.[4] To date, 35 schools of medicine and 5 schools of veterinary medicine have been funded to establish multidisciplinary undergraduate transfusion medicine curricula and educational programs. The National Institutes of Health (NIH) has sponsored consensus conferences on the use of fresh frozen plasma,[5] platelet transfusion therapy,[6] and perioperative red blood cell transfusions.[7] The Joint Commission on Accreditation of Health Care Organizations (JCAHO) has mandated the audit of every transfused patient against established transfusion guidelines, and requires education of physicians who transfuse outside those guidelines, with a re-audit to show improved transfusion practice.[8]

This chapter will discuss transfusion medicine education by looking at the impact of these efforts, by designating who is responsible for the quality of transfusion practice, by evaluating what guidelines are available to monitor practice, and by discussing what educational interventions can be instituted to improve transfusion support.

II. SETTING STANDARDS OF CARE

Who is responsible for the quality of the transfusion practice at your facility? The answer to this question is more complex than it appears at first glance. Arguments could be made that the primary attending physician, consulting physician, the hospital blood bank medical director, the medical director of the regional blood center, the Medical Advisory Committee, the Transfusion Audit Committee, the Quality Assurance Committee, the hospital administration, the blood bank technologist, the phlebotomist, the transfusing nurse, the risk manager, and others may all have a role. In order to achieve excellent transfusion practice, each of these people must work together as a team to ensure that patients receive the highest quality transfusion support. Each person on this team must do their part for the whole system to work correctly.

Legally, the standard of care is defined differently for medical malpractice cases than for other negligence claims. For medical malpractice, the standard of care is defined as what like physicians would do in like circumstances. For other cases it is defined as what a reasonable man would have done in like circumstances. The difference in this legal standard is extremely important in litigation but is not relevant to the concepts presented in this chapter. Regardless of the legal issues, there are transfusion practices which are clearly appropriate and those which are clearly not. However, most transfusion decisions are not black and white, and therefore the decision to transfuse, or not to transfuse, requires analysis and judgment. Even though many people have attempted to define rules of transfusion,[5–7,9–13] for practical purposes no rules exist. Each patient and each circumstance is unique and requires analysis and thought to decide what is the optimum transfusion support.

Given this background, who is responsible for transfusion support of patients, and what role does each person play? The ultimate responsibility for the patient's therapy (transfusion support and other) lies with the primary attending physician. Like an orchestra's conductor he should direct and oversee all the players to produce the best performance. He/she must synthesize all the information from all sources and make the final decision about what is best for a particular patient at a particular time in a particular situation. He/she must consider the underlying diagnosis, the prognosis, the projected course of the patient, the signs and symptoms which may or may not be related to the proposed indication for transfusion, the coexistence of diseases which may exacerbate or ameliorate the ability of the patient to tolerate, or not tolerate, transfusion, the severity and frequency of consequences of not transfusing, the availability of evaluation and support if transfusion is withheld, the standard of care in the community, etc. It becomes clear that rules

rules cannot be generated to cover each situation which may require transfusion. Furthermore, it is clear that the attending physician must make a clinical decision about whether the benefits outweigh the risks of transfusion in each case. All other individuals involved in transfusion support of patients act as consultants to the ordering physician.

The blood bank medical director, like the attending physician, must know the principles of transfusion practice and how to apply them to particular patients. In addition, he/she should (1) provide the medical community with the most up-to-date information available about transfusion medicine; (2) monitor the literature and ongoing research in transfusion medicine and be responsible for the timely dissemination of this information to transfusing physicians; (3) assist the hospital in setting standards in transfusion practice and also in monitoring whether those standard are being met.

The medical director of the regional blood center has a similar role to that of the hospital blood bank medical director, except his/her relationship is to the hospital blood bank medical director and not to the transfusing physician. He/she (1) provides consultations on complex cases and in cases where the availability of blood components may play a role; (2) develops a consensus on transfusion-related issues and policies which form the basis for the standard of care for a community; (3) monitors transfusion-transmitted disease and adverse consequences of transfusion in the community; and (4) monitors related literature and ongoing research in the field and ensures that appropriate information is provided to the hospital blood bank community in a timely fashion.

The blood bank technologist assists the blood bank medical director in providing compatible and appropriate transfusion components. He/she (1) is accountable for performing appropriate tests to ensure safe transfusion of components; (2) plays a major role in monitoring transfusion practice and identifying potentially inappropriate practices which require evaluation and physician peer review; and (3) provides technical advise on transfusion questions to transfusing nurses and other paramedical personnel.

The hospital administration and medical staff committees are critical in monitoring transfusion practice and ensuring that policies and procedures are appropriate and are followed by transfusing physicians. These committees are charged with monitoring policies, procedures, and practices which relate to the quality of transfusion practice in the hospital. They should identify problems, assess the scope of the problem, make recommendations for corrective actions, measure the results of the corrective actions, and document the effect of the actions on patient care.[9] Table 1 is a list of appropriate activities for these committees.

In summary, there are many professionals involved with the decision to transfuse. Each one has a role to play in making sure that the patient receives the highest quality transfusion support. Each individual has to do their part in order for the system to work correctly.

TABLE 1
List of Appropriate Activities for Transfusion Audit Committee

1. Establishment of audit criteria for blood component therapy.
2. Alteration of poor transfusion practices identified by audit through personal and peer consultation and review.
3. Investigation of all transfusion reactions, including post-transfusion hepatitis, and possible review of massive transfusion and single-unit transfusions.
4. Review and analysis of the statistical reports of the blood bank.
5. Reaudit of previously identified problem areas.
6. Promotion of the development and maintenance of continuing education in transfusion practice.
7. Promotion of blood procurement efforts.
8. Assurance of compliance of written hospital policies with JCAHO and FDA standards.[a]
9. Reporting to the hospital committee charged with overall responsibility for quality assurance and recommendation of corrective action when indicated. Reports to the Medical staff and executive committee of the medical staff are also recommended.

[a] JCAHO, Joint Commission on Accreditation of Health Care Organizations; FDA, Food and Drug Administration.

III. GUIDELINES FOR MONITORING TRANSFUSION PRACTICE

In order to effect change in transfusion practice, the transfusion specialist must monitor and audit transfusion practice and identify situations which have a high probability of representing less than optimum transfusion support. He/she must then construct an appropriate intervention to correct identified deficiencies. It is important to understand that criteria for the audit of transfusion practice do not themselves provide or establish standards of care. They are designed only to select charts which require further peer review. The criteria selected are designed to define a level of performance which is clearly acceptable to the audit committee and local medical community, so that charts meeting these criteria are not further reviewed. The selection of a chart for review does not necessarily mean that the transfusion practice provided to the patient was deficient, it means only that further peer review must occur.

The process in which the criteria are developed offers an opportunity to initiate good communications and a sound relationship between the transfusion specialist and the transfusing physician. The criteria should not be imposed, but all involved should have ample opportunity to review, criticize, and offer suggestions on alterations in the audit criteria. Such a process will not only influence the acceptance of the system by those being monitored but should afford feedback about current transfusion practice and attitudes, and begin the educational process concerning advances and changes in transfusion practice. By emphasizing the educational aspects of audits, and by including the transfusing physician in the process, the chances that transfusion behavior can be modified without confrontation and without stimulating a reactive attitude in monitored physicians will be increased.

The oversight function of monitoring transfusion practice can be accomplished through retrospective, and/or concurrent (prospective) audits.

IV. RETROSPECTIVE AUDITS

Retrospective chart review is the classical format for audit of transfusion practice. Both ''systems'' audit and ''medical practice'' audits have traditionally been performed to identify problems which require further peer review. Systems audits deal with the operational effectiveness of the clinical and laboratory staff. They monitor trends in any of the following areas: the number of units transfused, the number of patients receiving each component, units transfused per patient transfused, relative percent of whole blood vs. red cells used, the crossmatch-to-transfusion ratio, the outdate rate, the transfusion reaction rate, measures of workload and productivity, hours worked per unit transfused or patient transfused, number of uncrossmatched units issued, number of fresh unit requests, the turnaround time between receipt of a transfusion request and the availability of the unit for transfusion, the number of urgent requests, the number of units returned unused, the age distribution of units used, the number of late requests for preoperative crossmatches, etc. With this type of audit, corrective actions not only include education of the transfusing physician but also changes in administrative policy and procedures.

The second type of retrospective audit (medical practice audit) deals with evaluation of the therapeutic appropriateness of specific transfusion events. These audits monitor such things as indications for transfusion, chart documentation, and transfusion outcome. Corrective action usually involves changes in physician transfusion practice through physician education and consultation.

Scientific evidence that retrospective audits are effective in altering transfusion practice is sparse and inconclusive. One study using audit with feedback failed to produce a significant change in total hospital charges.[14] The authors speculated that failure to reduce costs could have been because the education was not directed at those who set standards of care. Other reasoning may be that the transfusion decision-maker cannot always be identified or because the ''long-after-the-fact'' education effort may not be very effective in altering behavior.[13]

V. CONCURRENT (PROSPECTIVE) AUDITS

Retrospective audits monitor trends and patterns of transfusion practice after they have occurred. They are designed to identify problems that can be corrected to improve subsequent transfusion therapy. Concurrent or prospective audits, on the other hand, are designed to evaluate the appropriateness of transfusion practice in a time frame which allows intervention before poor practice actually occurs. This method may be more effective than retrospective audits in altering physician behavior.

The first method to accomplish concurrent auditing would be to have a transfusion medicine physician prescreen all orders for blood components. One institution reported that less than 5% of all plasma and platelet transfusion were identified as inappropriate (during audit 1 to 3 days post-transfusion) using this method.[15] The contrast with retrospective audit (unaccompanied by education) results, in which 84 and 43% of plasma and platelet transfusion, respectively, were identified as inappropriate[16] is instructive; if prospective audits are accompanied by an educational intervention, inappropriate blood use can be reduced. Preliminary results using a prospective audit mechanism for ordering blood and blood components without educational intervention, suggests that blood utilization is not reduced in this setting.[17] The major drawback of this method is that it is physician intensive, and may be impractical given current resources in medicine today.

A second method would be to create a system of special case consultations to identify orders from transfusing physicians that have a high likelihood of leading to inappropriate transfusion therapy.[18–22] The systems can monitor orders both in the hospital and in the regional blood center. One study was effective in reducing fresh frozen plasma use by 77% over a 2-year period.[22] Inappropriate red cell transfusion practice[23] and platelet transfusion practice[15,24] have also been reduced using such an approach. In another article[19] a system is described where the transfusing physician who has placed an order outside the routine, receives an unsolicited consultation from a transfusion medicine specialist to clarify the intent of the order and help construct optimum transfusion support. These consultations must be handled in a positive, constructive, and nonjudgmental fashion so as to be effective and accepted by the ordering physician. A list of circumstances which might provoke a special case consultation is reproduced as Table 2.

A final approach to concurrent auditing is the use of written justification of blood orders on the physician's ordering sheet.[13,17] This method encourages the physician to analyze the rationale and justification for transfusion at the time of the order, and ensures documentation of indications in the chart. The system can be simplified so that frequent indications can be listed in a check-off format, making it convenient for physicians to use the system. Whenever an appropriate indication is not documented on the ordering sheet, a transfusion medicine physician can initiate a consultation.

TABLE 2
Situations which may Require Automatic Consultation

A. Inventory Management
1. There is a request for the emergency release of uncrossmatched blood.
2. Inventory dictates that Rh-negative patients receive Rh-positive blood or platelets.
3. Blood less than 7 days old is requested for an adult patient.
4. Washed red cell preparations are requested.
5. Blood products screened for antibodies to the cytomegalic inclusion virus are requested.
6. Irradiated blood products are requested.
7. A patient receives platelet transfusions on 3 consecutive days.
8. HLA matched platelets are requested.
9. Fresh platelet concentrates are requested.
10. Granulocyte concentrates are requested.
11. Varicella-zoster immune globulin is requested.
12. There is an unusual or extraordinary request for blood.

B. Transfusion Practice
1. A patient suffers a transfusion reaction.
2. An adult patient's red cell transfusions exceed 8 units in 8 hours.
3. A patient receives more than 6 units of fresh-frozen plasma in 24 hours.
4. A patient has severe reactions to platelet concentrates.
5. A request is made for cryoprecipitate in a patient with a diagnosis other than hemophilia A or von Willebrand's disease.

C. Dosage Consideration
1. Fewer than 3 or more than 12 units of platelets are requested for an adult patient.
2. Two or fewer plasma units are requested for an adult patient.

VI. EDUCATIONAL INTERVENTIONS TO IMPROVE BLOOD TRANSFUSION PRACTICE

A. UNDERGRADUATE

The Transfusion Medicine Academic Award (TMAA) program provides grants from the National Heart, Lung, and Blood Institute of the NIH for the purpose of creating and strengthening educational activities related to transfusion medicine. Principal investigators representing 40 medical and veterinary schools have developed and organized a comprehensive transfusion medicine curriculum.[25] The curriculum is organized into three sections: overall curriculum goals, specific educational goals, and specific educational objectives. The curriculum goals describe, in general terms, the desired impact of curriculum use. The overall goals include "to help students to develop an understanding of the basic science that underlies transfusion medicine, and to develop the basic clinical skills related to transfusion medicine that are needed for medical practice." The specific educational goals represent a general statement of what students should understand about the discipline of transfusion medicine. Primary goals are "to understand the basic principles and concepts of transfusion medicine and to be able to use a fund of basic knowledge in the field." Specific educational objectives are presented under 12 topic headings written as performance-based statements of postinstructional

TABLE 3
Student Objectives of the Transfusion Medicine Academic Award Curriculum

Topic	Curriculum time (%)
History of transfusion medicine	0.5
Scientific basis of transfusion	14.0
Management of blood donation and preparation of blood components	6.0
Pretransfusion testing	4.0
Transfusion of blood components	47.0
Adverse effects of blood transfusion	14.0
Autoimmunity	4.0
Transplantation	6.0
Therapeutic apheresis and phlebotomy	2.5
Blood substitutes	1.0
Organization and function of regional blood services and hospital transfusion services	0.5

competency. These major topic areas and the estimated percentage of the total transfusion medicine undergraduate curriculum time that should be directed to each topic, are shown in Table 3. In addition the curriculum, the awardees developed an instrument for cognitive evaluation of student knowledge. The instrument is a multiple choice test that has been validated, computerized, and administered to selected student groups at awardee institutions.[26] Using this and other evaluation instruments, evaluation of the impact of the TMAA programs on transfusion practice is on-going.

Another transfusion medicine educational program has been demonstrated to be effective in influencing transfusion practice in undergraduate core clinical clerkship rotations. An educational intervention at Case Western Reserve University was instituted which taught concepts of informed consent within a framework of transfusion medicine.[27] The American Association of Blood Banks Transfusion Practice Committee[28] has recommended documentation of informed consent prior to elective blood transfusion. However, physicians have been unable to deliver effectively the medical-legal elements (risks, benefits, alternatives, opportunity to ask questions, and consent) of informed consent to patients who are scheduled for elective blood transfusion.[29] The intervention at Case Western Reserve University[27] was designed to teach physicians how to communicate effectively these elements of informed consent for blood transfusion. The project consisted of two parts. The first part consisted of a one-hour didactic session in which blood transfusion risks and benefits were reviewed, along with alternative options that were available: i.e., autologous (patient's own) blood, designated (from a blood donor known to the recipient) blood, and no transfusion. The material used as a syllabus for this presentation has been previously published.[30] The second part was a 90-minute small-group session in which the ethical, legal, medical, and patient educational issues were reviewed by faculty members, along with student role playing (in which students practiced obtaining informed consent for elective blood transfusion from each other). The intervention was given to students at one hospital only; students at other hospitals served as nonintervention controls. The evaluation instrument for the intervention was an objective standardized clinical evaluation (OSCE), consisting of a format in which the student was asked to obtain informed consent for blood transfusion from a patient who was scheduled for elective orthopedic surgery. The transfusion medicine OSCE results were significantly different for the intervention group compared to the nonintervention group (65.8 ± 2.2 vs. 54.1 ± 1.8, m $\pm$ sem, $p < 0.001$, respectively). This informed consent intervention model demonstrated that students exposed to a transfusion medicine curriculum within a medical core clerkship had an increased knowledge base and clinical skills for discussing blood transfusion risks and options with patients when compared to students with serendipitous experiences related to blood transfusion over a 12-week medical core clerkship.

Another article[31] discusses educational techniques to teach transfusion medicine. A "progressive problem analysis" technique was shown to be effective in raising student awareness of the elements involved in the decision to transfuse. Case studies were presented as a teaching aid.

B. RESIDENT EDUCATION

Residents in training are important potential recipients of transfusion medicine education programs, since the nature of their service responsibilities insures that they have a primary role in the ordering of blood products. One of the unique educational problems of academic institutions is to identify the transfusion decision-maker; this may be the resident, the attending physician, or both. The attending physician, as an educator role-model, may be poorly qualified to deliver transfusion medicine education and in fact is himself/herself an important potential recipient of education. For example, one study of intraoperative communication during open heart surgery identified the surgical team as the transfusion decision-maker.[32] Since the senior surgeon participated most often in transfusion-related communications, educational programs designed to affect transfusion during open heart surgery may be most effective if directed at these senior surgical staff members (see below).

A multi-institutional survey of resident's perceived needs, resources, and opportunities to learn about transfusion medicine revealed that residents recognized the relevance of transfusion medicine to patient care but felt that their knowledge and educational opportunities could be improved.[33] Residents with more training self-rated their knowledge higher than did the first- and second-year residents, although they did not view their learning opportunities as greater. Surgery and anesthesiology residents expressed more knowledge than did internal medicine residents. One must be especially cautious in distinguishing between residents' opinions of their competence and an actual evaluation of competency and knowledge. For example, one survey indicated that 88% of anesthesiologists in 1249 institutions required a preoperative hemoglobin level of greater than 9 g/dl and 44% stipulated that it be above 10 g/dl,despite evidence that this practice may be unwarranted.[34]

C. POST-GRADUATE

Post-graduate educational activities traditionally encompass disparate activities such as regularly scheduled grand rounds, targeted continuing medical education programs, and published literature as a means of influencing physician knowledge and/or practice. The problem of the effectiveness of these approaches in issues related to blood transfusion is best illustrated by a recently published survey of surgeons and anesthesiologists in which only 31% of physicians interviewed could correctly answer four basic questions about when a transfusion is required.[35] This lack of knowledge was demonstrated despite publication of the results of consensus development conferences on the use of red cells,[7] plasma,[5] and platelets,[6] as well as distribution of a transfusion alert by the National Blood Resource Education Program.[36] These findings confirm that these methods fail to stimulate changes in physician knowledge, attitude, or practice.[37] One limitation of this approach may be due to a lack of consensus.[38] Previous studies of variation in utilization of medical and surgical services have suggested that the degree of variation is related to the degree of medical consensus concerning the indications for its use[39,40] rather than inappropriate use.[41] Another limitation may be that the educational information does not reach the targeted audience. To address these potential problems, transfusion practice guidelines developed by the Transfusion Practices Committee of the American Association of Blood Banks have been published in the subspecialty journals pertinent to the targeted audiences.[11,12]

Another example of the limitations of published literature as an educational intervention is the use of preoperative autologous blood donation. This practice has been demonstrated to be underutilized,[42] despite its widespread endorsement as a good transfusion practice.[43,44] Despite estimates that potentially 10 to 14% of blood transfused could be autologous,[42,45] a national survey indicated that while autologous blood transfusion increased from 1982 to 1987, only 3% of blood transfused in 1987 was autologous.[3] One study indicated that while knowledge about autologous blood donation varied among 118 surgeons from three different areas of the country,[46] the use by 44 surgeons who managed the largest number of patients correlated well with their knowledge and attitude. Single institutions have been able to show that physician transfusion practice and utilization of autologous blood donation can be altered by local education programs targeted for orthopedic[47] and open heart surgeons.[48]

The effectiveness of continuing medical education (CME) programs in changing physician practice has been controversial. Despite negative conclusions on CME effectiveness,[49] controlled studies provide strong evidence that properly planned CME programs can modify physician behavior.[50,51] CME has been shown to affect positively the transfusion practice of physician via both regional blood service[52] and hospital-based transfusion service[53] educational programs. One study showed that a CME intervention using a grand rounds format was effective in altering physicians' utilization of a hospital-based autologous blood procurement program.[53] To be effective, CME programs must first identify transfusion decision makers.[54] Another study used a CME workshop format to survey transfusion service directors' attitudes towards hospital-based autologous blood procurement programs and to develop an analytical model of the economic viability of such programs.[55] This model can then be used by transfusion service directors to help hospital administrators to resolve budget issues related to autologous blood donor programs. This one example serves to illustrate the increasing dependence of transfusion practice decisions on economic and budgetary factors, and how CME educational programs must take these factors into account.

D. PATIENT EDUCATION

The recognition and identification of the acquired immunodeficiency syndrome (AIDS) as a disease transmissible by several routes, including the transfusion of blood and blood products, has resulted in a need for transfusion medicine specialists to increasingly interact with patients.[56] More than 3000 cases of AIDS attributable to blood transfusion were reported through 1989.[30] Although AIDS has brought blood safety into focus for the public, the medical community has long been aware that while the blood supply is as safe as know-how can make it, blood transfusion has always carried a risk. The need for dialogue between the transfusing physician and the potential transfusion recipient concerning these risks has led to a recommendation by the American Association of Blood Banks (AABB) that informed consent be obtained and documented before an elective or anticipated blood transfusion.[28] If this process is to be effective, then early involvement of the patient in a dialogue concerning informed consent is necessary. An example of this, again, is autologous blood procurement. The rapidly increased utilization of autologous options over a 3-year period can be ascribed, in part, to patient demand for this service.[47,55] Another example, though controversial, is designated blood donation. This patient-driven transfusion practice must be addressed by patient-education programs designed to make this alternative complementary, rather than competitive with autologous blood donation[57,58] and with the concept of a national blood program.

VII. CONCLUSION

Blood Banking has evolved from a laboratory-based specialty into the multidisciplinary field better described as transfusion medicine. This change has been accompanied by an increased awareness that education must play a key role in preparing medical personnel to cope with this rapidly burgeoning field. New expectations have arisen from accreditation, regulatory, and funding agencies as well as transfusing physicians, their patients, and the blood donors who generate the blood inventory. Regional blood centers and transfusion services that effectively incorporate educational programs into their mission will be most successful in meeting these expectations and helping transfusion medicine continue its evolution.

REFERENCES

1. **Silbert, J. A., Bove, J. R., Dubin, S., and Bush, W. S.,** Patterns of frozen plasma use, *Conn. Med.*, 45, 507, 1981.
2. **Blumberg, N., Laczin, J., McMican, A., Heal, J., and Arvan, D.,** A critical use of fresh-frozen plasma use, *Transfusion,* 26, 511, 1986.
3. **Surgenor, D. M. N., Wallace, E. L., Hao, S. H. J., and Chapman, R. H.,** Collection and transfusion of blood in the United States, 1982–1988, *N. Engl. J. Med.*, 322, 1646, 1990.
4. Program guidelines, Transfusion Medicine Academic Award (first competition), National Heart, Lung, and Blood Institute, Bethesda, MD, March 30, 1982.
5. National Institutes of Health Consensus Conference. Fresh frozen plasma: indications and risks, *JAMA,* 253, 551, 1985.
6. National Institutes of Health Consensus Conference. Platelet transfusion therapy, *JAMA,* 257, 1777, 1987.
7. National Institutes of Health Consensus Conference. Perioperative red cell transfusion, *JAMA,* 260, 2700, 1988.
8. Joint Commission on Accreditation of Health Care Organizations. Accreditation manual for hospitals (AMH). Blood Usage Review 120, Chicago, IL, 1988.
9. **Grindon, A., Tomasulo, P. A., Bergin, J. J., Klein, H. G. et al.,** The Hospital Transfusion Committee, Guideline for Improving Practice, *JAMA,* 253 (4), 540, 1985.
10. **Simpson, M. B.,** Audit criteria for transfusion practices, in *The Hospital Transfusion Committee,* American Association of Blood Banks, Arlington, VA, 1982, 21.
11. **Goodnough, L. T., Johnston, M. F. M., Ramsey, K. C. et al.,** Guidelines for transfusion support in patients undergoing coronary artery bypass grafting, *Ann. Thor. Surg.*, 50, 675, 1990.
12. **Kruskall, M. S., Mintz, P. D., Bergin, J. J. et al.,** Transfusion therapy in emergency medicine, *Ann. Emerg. Med.*, 17, 327, 1988.
13. **Toy, P. T. C. Y.,** Use of medical audits for educational purposes, in *Education Programs in Transfusion Medicine,* Wallas, C. H. and Simon, T., Eds., American Association of Blood Banks, Arlington, VA, 1985, 47.
14. **Gullion, D. S., Adamson, T. E., and Watts, M. S.,** The effect of an individualized practice-based CME program on physician performance and patient outcome, *West J. Med.*, 138, 582, 1983.
15. **Simpson, M. B.,** Prospective-concurrent audits and medical consultation for platelet transfusions, *Transfusion,* 27, 192, 1987.
16. **Mozes, B., Edstein, M., Ben-Bassat, I., Modan, B., and Halkin, H.,** Evaluation of the appropriateness of blood and blood product transfusion using present criteria, *Transfusion,* 29, 473, 1989.

17. **Hopkins, E., Yomtovian, R., Shurin, S., and Goodnough, L. T.,** The prospective "transfusion appropriateness" order form as a method to reduce utilization, *Proc. of the 1990 Joint Congress,* ISBT/AABB, 1990, 219.
18. **Silverstein, L. E., Kruskall, M. S., Stehling, L. C. et al.,** Strategies for the review of transfusion practices, *JAMA,* 262, 1993 1989.
19. **Tomasulo, P. T., Lenes, B. A., Noto, T. A., Klein, H. G., and Menitove, J. E.,** Automatic special case consultations in transfusion medicine, *Transfusion,* 26, 183, 1986.
20. **Popovsky, M. A., Moore, S. B., Wick; M. R., Devine, P., Pineda, A. A., and Taswell, H. F.,** A blood bank consultation service: principles and practice, *Mayo Clin. Proc.,* 60, 312, 1985.
21. **Lichtiger, B., Fischer, H. E., and Huh, Y. O.,** Screening of transfusion service requests by the blood bank pathologist: impact of cost containment, *Lab. Med.,* 19, 228, 1988.
22. **Shanberge, J. N.,** Reduction of fresh-frozen plasma use through a daily survey and education program, *Transfusion,* 27, 226, 1987.
23. **Giovanetti, A. M., Parravicini, L., Baroni, D. et al.,** Quality assessment of transfusion practice in elective surgery, *Transfusion,* 28, 166, 1988.
24. **McCullough, J., Steeper, T. A., and Connelly, D. P.,** Platelet utilization in a university hospital, *JAMA,* 259, 2414, 1988.
25. **Simon, T. L. et al.,** Comprehensive curricular goals for teaching transfusion medicine, *Transfusion,* 29, 438, 1989.
26. **Price, T. H. and Strand, D. A.,** Cognitive evaluation, in *Educational Programs in Transfusion Medicine,* American Association of Blood Banks, Wallas, C. H. and Simon, T., Eds., Arlington, VA, 1985, 199.
27. **Goodnough, L. T., Hull, A., and Kleinhenz, M. E.,** Informed consent for blood transfusion as an education intervention in medical clinical clerkships, *Accad. Med.,* 67, 348, 1992.
28. **Campbell, S., Ed.,** AABB issues recommendations on informed consent for transfusion, *AABB Newsbriefs,* July, 1986, p. 1
29. **Meisel, B., Roth, L. H., and Lioz, C. W.,** Toward a model of the legal doctrine of informed consent, *Am. J. Psychiatry,* 134, 285, 1977.
30. **Goodnough, L. T. and Shuck, J.,** Blood transfusion in elective surgery: review of risks, options, and informed consent, *Am. J. Surg.,* 159, 602, 1990.
31. **Lenes, B. A.,** Teaching transfusion medicine by progressive problem analysis, in *Alternative Educational Methods for Continuing Education,* Summers, S., Macpherson, C., and Kennedy, M., Eds., American Association of Blood Banks, Arlington, VA, 1987, 83.
32. **Goodnough, L. T., Brennan, P. F., Shah, T., Hull, A., and Martin, B.,** Intraoperative communication in open heart surgery: implications in the decision to hang blood, *Academic Med.,* 65, 681, 1990.
33. **Eisenstaedt, R. S., Glanz, K., and Polansky, M.,** Resident education in transfusion medicine: a multi-institutional needs assessment, *Transfusion,* 28, 536, 1988.
34. **Kowalyshyn, T. J., Prager, D., and Young, J.,** A review of the present status of preoperative hemoglobin requirements, *Anesth. Analg. (Cleveland),* 51, 75, 1972.
35. **Salem, S. R., Avorn, J., and Soumerai, J. B.,** Influence of clinical knowledge, organizational context, and practice style on transfusion decision making, *JAMA,* 264, 476, 1990.
36. Transfusion Alert: Implications for the Use of Red Blood Cells, Platelets, and Fresh Frozen Plasma, NIH Publication No. 89–29749, National Blood Resource Education Program, U.S. Department of Health and Human Services, Bethesda, MD, May, 1989.
37. **Kosecoff, J., Kanouse, D. E., Rogers, W. H., McCloskey, L., Winslow, C. M., and Brook, R. H.,** Effects of the National Institutes of Health Consensus Conference development program on physician practice,
38. **Welch, H. G., Meehan, K. R., and Goodnough, L. T.,** Prudent strategies for red blood cell transfusion, *Ann. Int. Med.,* 116, 393, 1992.

39. **Chassin, M. R., Brook, R. H., Park, R. E. et al.,** Variations in the use of medical and surgical services by the medicare population, *N. Engl. J. Med.,* 290, 285, 1989.
40. **Vayda, E.,** A comparison of surgical rates in Canada and in England and in Wales, *N. Engl. J. Med.,* 289, 1224, 1973.
41. **Chassin, M. R., Kosecoff, J., Winslow, C. M. et al.,** Does inappropriate use explain geographic variations in the use of health care services?, *JAMA,* 258, 2533, 1987.
42. **Toy, P. T. Y. C., Strauss, R. G., Stehling, L. C. et al.,** Predeposit autologous blood for elective surgery: a multicenter study, *N. Engl. J. Med.,* 316, 517, 1987.
43. Council on Scientific Affairs: Autologous blood transfusions, *JAMA,* 256, 2378, 1986.
44. **Campbell, S., Ed.,** AABB established national autologous resource center, *AABB Newsbriefs,* May, 1987, p 1.
45. **Kruskall, M. S., Glazer, E. E., Leonard, S. S. et al.,** Utilization and effectiveness of a hospital autologous preoperative blood donor program, *Transfusion,* 26, 335, 1986.
46. **Strauss, R. G., Ferguson, K. J., Stone, G. G. et al.,** Surgeon's knowledge, attitude, and use of preoperative autologous blood donation, *Transfusion,* 30, 418, 1990.
47. **Goodnough, L. T., Shaffron, D., and Marcus, R. E.,** The impact of preoperative autologous blood donation on orthopedic surgical practice, *Vox Sang.,* 59, 65, 1990.
48. **Owings, D. V., Kruskall, M. S., Thurer, R. L., and Donovan, C. M.,** Autologous blood donations prior to elective cardiac surgery. Safety and effect on subsequent blood use, *JAMA,* 262, 1963, 1989.
49. **Bertram, D. A. and Brooks-Bertram, P. A.,** The evaluation of continuing medical education: a literature review, *Health Educ. Manage.,* 5, 330, 1977.
50. **Sibley, J. C., Sackett, D. L., Neufeld, V. et al.,** A randomized trial of continuing medical education, *N. Engl. J. Med.,* 306, 511, 1982.
51. **Avorn, J. and Soumerai, S. B.,** Improving drug-therapy decisions through educational outreach, *N. Engl. J. Med.,* 308, 1457, 1983.
52. **Hillman, R. S., Helbig, S., Howes, S. et al.,** The effect of an educational program on transfusion practices in a regional blood program, *Transfusion,* 19, 153, 1979.
53. **Hull, A. L., Wasman, J., and Goodnough, L. T.,** Effect of a CME program on physicians' transfusion practices, *Academic Med.,* 65, 681, 1990.
54. **Goodnough, L. T., Hull, A. L., Brennan, P. F., and Martin, B.,** Targeting continuing medical education on decision makers: Who decides to transfuse blood? *J. Cont. Ed. Health Professions,* in press.
55. **Hull, A. L., Neuhauser, D., and Goodnough, L. T.,** Prevalence and correlates of hospital-based autologous blood procurement programs, *Am. J. Med. Sci.,* 303, 285, 1992.
56. **Bryant, L. R.,** Transfusion medicine: the pathologist's ''brave new world'', *Am. J. Clin. Pathol.,* 91, 744, 1989.
57. **Chambers, L. A., Kruskall, M. S., Leonard, S. S., and Ellis, A. M.,** Directed donor programs may adversely affect autologous donor participation, *Transfusion,* 28, 645, 1988.
58. **Goodnough, L. T.,** Predeposit of designated blood does not protect against homologous blood exposure in patients who predeposit autologous blood for elective surgery, *Am. J. Clin. Pathol.,* 92, 484, 1989.

Chapter 6

CONDUCTING THE BLOOD DONOR MEDICAL INTERVIEW

Ritchard G. Cable

TABLE OF CONTENTS

ISBN 0-8493-4938-9

I. INTRODUCTION

A. GENERAL APPROACH TO BLOOD DONOR SCREENING

Blood collection requires the determination of donor suitability by a medical interview prior to the initiation of phlebotomy. The purposes of blood donor screening are threefold: first, the interviewer must ascertain that the donor is able to give an accurate medical history and that the donor understands and consents to the blood donation process. Second, the interviewer must ascertain that the donor is safely able to donate 450 cc of whole blood, a "unit" of blood in the U.S. Finally, the interviewer must exclude a history of infectious disease or a relevant history of exposure to infectious diseases which may be transmissible by transfusion.

To accomplish the first goal, it is necessary that the medical interviewer have a good understanding of the medical factors which determine donor eligibility, that he or she is trained in effective communicating and interviewing techniques, and that he or she is able to communicate well with a variety of educational levels. As appropriate to the population screened, the interviewer may also need to be fluent in appropriate alternative languages or sensitive to cultural and dialect nuances in the communication of sensitive personal information by donors from a variety of backgrounds.

The second objective of the donor medical interview is to ensure that blood donation will not harm the donor. In the U.S., collection of a full 450 cc of blood is limited to donors who weigh 110 lbs (50 kg) or more.[1] Lesser amounts of blood can be collected from donors who weigh less than 110 lbs, although this requires adjustment of the amount of anticoagulant in standard blood collection containers.[2] Collection containers designed for collection of one half a standard unit are also available.

The age of the donor is important only to the extent it requires special care in obtaining legal consent or requires additional medical evaluation. Although blood can be collected safely from larger adolescents, their inability to legally consent to donate and their relative immaturity at conveying medical information has led many blood centers to require that donors must be 18 years old. Some jurisdictions allow 17-year-old donors to consent to donate and some blood centers collect blood from 17-year-old donors with written parental permission.

At the other end of the spectrum, older age, per se, is not a valid donor criterion. Many blood collection agencies impose more rigorous screening on older donors. Some also preclude older first-time donors but allow regular donors to continue as long as their health is maintained. Certainly, the recent increase in autologous donation has demonstrated that people can safely donate blood well into their 80s.

The collection of 450 cc of blood represents a loss of up to 13% of the donor's blood volume. It also has a risk of initiating a vaso-vagal reaction in approximately 3.5% of donors.[3] Serious reactions are rare, but can include seizures.[4] In order to safely donate, therefore, the donor must be free of serious cardiovascular disease, have no history of seizure disorders or have seizures under good medical control, and have no acute illnesses at the time of donation.

The most common complication of blood donation is iron depletion. The assessment of hemoglobin prior to blood donation serves to ensure sufficient red cell mass for the recipient, but also serves as an indirect measure of iron status as well as of the possibility of hematologic disease. Thus, the measurement of hemoglobin serves both to protect the donor as well as the recipient. In the U.S., an 8-week interval between whole blood donations is required, which is primarily designed to limit the rate of iron loss of the donor.[5] Other countries have adopted even more stringent requirements for the frequency of whole blood donation. Pregnancy is also a contraindication to homologous donation, primarily because of the borderline iron status of the pregnant woman. A more extensive discussion of donation frequency, donor hemoglobin screening, and donor iron depletion is beyond the scope of this chapter.

The final purpose of blood donor screening is the identification of diseases that may be transmissible through transfusion. Although the sequelae of certain transmissible diseases may be obvious in the blood donor, more frequently donor screening focuses on risk factors which may lead to an asymptomatic carrier state for infectious agents. Specific donor screening criteria for commonly transmissible diseases will be discussed later in this chapter. Since virtually any agent which can appear in the blood is theoretically transmissible by blood transfusion, it is important that the prospective blood donor be free of symptoms of acute disease, afebrile, and not on therapeutic antibiotics which may suppress infectious symptoms. Donors should answer "yes" to a general question such as: ''Are you feeling well today?'' and should have no general constitutional symptoms or acute upper respiratory infection which may be the prodrome of a more serious illness. Finally, the donor's temperature should not exceed 37.5°C or 99.5°F.

B. TESTING VS. MEDICAL HISTORY SCREENING

The provision of a safe blood supply requires the initial selection of a safe population of blood donors. Although extensive testing of donated blood is carried out, the impossibility of achieving 100% sensitivity in testing for transmissible agents requires the blood collection agency to make every effort to preclude blood donations by donors who have a higher than acceptable risk of disease transmission.

The risk of transfusion is calculated by the prevalence of a given transmissible disease agent multiplied by one minus the sensitivity of the test being used to detect that agent. Therefore, for example, an intervention which decreases the registration of donors who are at high risk for the human immunodeficiency virus (HIV) may be more effective in preventing transfusion-transmitted HIV than an improvement in test methodology for the virus. Interventions which prevent the collection of high-risk donor blood will also preclude the adverse impact of clerical, computer, or testing errors in the blood center which might lead to release of a contaminated, high-risk unit.

C. SELECTION OF A SAFE DONOR POPULATION

Effective methods must be designed to increase the safety of the donor population. These methods can range from demographic approaches, to donor motivational research and design of confidential approaches to convey sensitive personal information at blood drives, and finally to methods identifying dangerous donors after the blood donation, such as donor deferral registries.

Although not a fool-proof method, the use of disease marker frequencies to characterize the safety of any donor population has been generally accepted. Most useful are specific disease markers such as HIV antibody or hepatitis B surface antigen. Because of their low frequency, however, they are of limited value since the size of the populations studied needs to be large to show statistically significant differences. Anti-HBc (''anti-hepatitis B core'') antibody frequency has the advantage of being a more frequent marker in donor populations. Thus, it is easier with reasonable study sizes to demonstrate statistical differences between donor populations using this marker.

Demographic approaches are currently in place in the U.S. For example, emigrants from malarial endemic areas are precluded from blood donation for 3 years after leaving the endemic area, because of the risk of malaria transmission.[6] Collection of blood from prisoners is not allowed by the American Red Cross[7] because the rate of transmissible diseases such as HIV is many times higher in such populations (and, of course, the voluntary nature of the donation may be difficult to ascertain).

It has been demonstrated in several studies in the U.S. that volunteer blood donors cause a lower incidence of post-transfusion hepatitis[8] in blood recipients. Infectious disease marker frequencies are higher in paid blood donors as well.[9] The explanation of this finding may be both demographic (paid donors are more likely to be from lower socioeconomic circumstances), and motivational (paid donors are less likely to give accurate health histories).

While some have argued that safe populations of paid donors can be identified, paid blood donors are not allowed in Canada and most European countries. In the US., blood obtained from a paid donor must be so labeled.[10] Such blood should only be used when voluntarily donated blood is unavailable.

Educating the donor population regarding blood donor requirements is another approach to improving the safety of the blood supply. If high-risk activity for disease transmission can be identified and effectively described to prospective donors with the right donor motivation, such donors will avoid blood donation. Since the voluntary blood donors in the U.S. who test positive for HIV usually give a history of high-risk activity similar to those presenting at HIV testing sites,[11] better communication with the donor before donation should eliminate these donors, thus enhancing the safety of the blood supply.

Education and motivation of donors regarding high-risk activity can take the form of publicity, brochures, predonation consent forms, direct questioning at blood drives regarding high-risk practices,[12] and confidential exclusion forms.[13]

The American Red Cross has combined the two forms into a single multipart document, which is part of its medical history form. ''What You Should Know Before Giving Blood'' (Figure 1) explains high-risk behavior to donors and asks such donors to self-defer.[7] The Confidential Unit Exclusion (CUE) form (Figure 2) allows the donor who cannot or will not self-defer, and who is unwilling or unable to give an accurate donor history, the opportunity to donate, but to designate his or her blood not for transfusion. A bar code ''ballot'' which is part of the CUE form accommodates those donors who, for example, feel obligated to be seen donating at a company blood drive or who feel unable to give an accurate history regarding their personal behavior.

Direct questioning of donors regarding sexual practices has recently been implemented in the U.S.[14] and is the most direct way to eliminate donors who are at high risk for HIV from blood donation. Direct questioning regarding intravenous drug use, country of origin, exposure to other parenterally transmitted viruses, and recent transfusions has been in place for many years in the U.S.

II. STANDARD SETTING — ORGANIZATION OF DONOR SERVICES

Blood donor standards result initially from professional standards of practice. That is, a standard is derived from the prevailing practice of blood banks

American Red Cross

WHAT YOU MUST KNOW BEFORE GIVING BLOOD

THANK YOU FOR COMING IN TODAY

It is important that you read this information before you decide whether you should give blood. If you have any questions, please ask Red Cross staff. You will be asked later to sign a statement saying that you have read and understood this information today.

■ YOUR SAFETY

To make sure that you are healthy enough to give blood we will:

- check your temperature, pulse and blood pressure.
- test a drop of your blood to be sure you have enough red blood cells to give safely today.
- ask you questions about your health.

What you tell us about your health will be kept confidential.
It is important that you provide truthful information. If you are able to give, we will take about a pint of blood from your arm. We always use a new, sterile needle for each donor.

You cannot get AIDS or any other disease by giving blood.

■ PATIENT SAFETY

Some people must not give because their blood might spread an infection to the people who receive it.

Do not give blood if you - -

- have ever had hepatitis (liver disease caused by a virus).
- have had malaria or have taken drugs to prevent malaria in the past three years. (Plasma donations may be acceptable.)
- have had or been treated for syphilis or gonorrhea in the last twelve months.

Do not give blood if you are at risk for getting and spreading any AIDS virus. You are at risk if:

- you are a man who has had sex with another man since 1977, even one time.
- you have taken ("shot up") illegal drugs by needle, even one time.
- you have taken clotting factor concentrates for a bleeding disorder such as hemophilia.
- you have ever had a positive test for any AIDS virus or any AIDS antibody.
- you have AIDS or one of its symptoms, which include:
  - weight loss (10 pounds or more in less than 2 months) that you can't explain.
  - night sweats.
  - blue or purple spots on or under the skin.
  - white spots or unusual sores in your mouth that last a long time.
  - lumps in your neck, armpits, or groin that last more than a month.
  - fever higher than 99 degrees that lasts more than 10 days.
  - diarrhea that lasts more than one month.
  - persistent cough and shortness of breath.
- you have had sex with any person described above.
- you have been given money or drugs for sex since 1977.
- you are a man who has had sex with a female prostitute or a woman who has had sex with a male prostitute in the last twelve months.

Do not give blood to find out whether you have a positive AIDS test. The tests we use are very good, but they are not perfect. A person may be infected and have a negative test result. That's why you must not give blood if you are at risk for getting AIDS or other diseases. We maintain a confidential list of individuals who may be at risk for spreading infectious diseases. Red Cross staff can tell you where you can get an AIDS test without giving blood and without giving your name.

If you decide that you should not give blood, you may leave now. If you're not sure, ask to talk privately to Red Cross staff. If you decide to give blood today, you will be given a form to let us know whether your blood is safe to be given to another person. You will be told how to use the form so that no one at the blood drive will know what you have said. If your blood should not be given to another person, you must let us know with this form.

If you give blood today, but decide later that your blood may not be safe for another person, call the telephone number on the card we will give you as soon as possible and state that your blood should not be given to another person.

■ YOUR BLOOD WILL BE TESTED

We will test your blood for hepatitis viruses, syphilis, AIDS antibodies, and certain other viruses. If tests show that any part of your blood might make someone sick, that part will not be used. In some cases, a sample of your blood may also be used now and in the future to evaluate new and experimental blood screening tests. If you would prefer not to have your blood used for experimental testing or you have any questions about the specific tests we perform, please speak with Red Cross staff.

If our tests show that you may be unhealthy, we will let you know now or in the future as new tests become available. When required, we report test results to health departments and military medical commands. We keep a confidential list of people we find who should not give blood.

■ WHILE YOU GIVE BLOOD

Most people feel fine while they give blood and afterward. A small number of people may have -

- an upset stomach.
- a faint or dizzy feeling.
- a "black and blue" mark, redness, and pain where the needle was.

Very rarely, a person may faint, have muscle spasms, and/or suffer nerve damage.

FIGURE 1. ''What You Must Know Before Giving Blood''. This form was in use at the time this chapter of the text was written, and it is subject to significant modification as circumstances require. (Reproduced with permission, American National Red Cross.[7])

and their medical directors. For the more medically important issues and to assist individuals blood banks, standard-setting bodies have also been established in the developed countries.

In the U.S., the major blood collecting organizations are the American Red Cross, the American Association of Blood Banks (AABB), and the

Choose a sticker to let us know if we should use your blood

Step 1: Please read

Even though we test all blood for AIDS and the tests we use are very good, they are not perfect. You can help us by confidentially telling us to use or not to use your blood. No one at this donation site can read the sticker you choose.

Step 2: Please review

Please review one more time the reasons we cannot use your blood because of possible exposure to an AIDS virus. If you can answer "yes" to any one of the items listed below, you are considered to be at risk for having an AIDS virus in your blood.

MALE DONORS:
- had sex, even once, with another male since 1977.
- had sex with a female prostitute in the last twelve months.

FEMALE DONORS:
- had sex, even once, with a male who has had sex with another male since 1977.
- had sex with a male prostitute in the last twelve months.

ALL DONORS:
- ever tested positive for or been diagnosed with AIDS.
- taken street drugs by needle, even once.
- been treated with a clotting factor concentrate for a bleeding disorder such as hemophilia.
- have had sex with any person described above.
- had or been treated for syphilis or gonorrhea in the last twelve months.
- been raped in the last twelve months.
- have been given money or drugs for sex since 1977.

Step 3: Peel off one of the stickers and put it on your blood donation record in the Donor Bar Code sticker box

If you answered **"no"** to all of the items listed in Step 2, place the **"USE my Blood"** bar code sticker on your blood donation record. This means you consider your blood safe to use. If you answered **"yes"** to any one of the items listed in Step 2, place the **"Do NOT use my blood"** bar code sticker on your blood donation record. Your name will NOT be placed on a list of donors who should not give blood in the future simply because you have chosen this sticker. You should consider whether to avoid donating blood in the future.

REMOVE BLACK BAR CODE STICKER ONLY
USE my blood.
I have not done anything that means I might have an AIDS virus in my blood
Do NOT use my blood.
I have done something that means I might have an AIDS virus in my blood
F6628-9
F6628-9
Bend paper & lift bar code sticker
Bend paper & lift bar code sticker

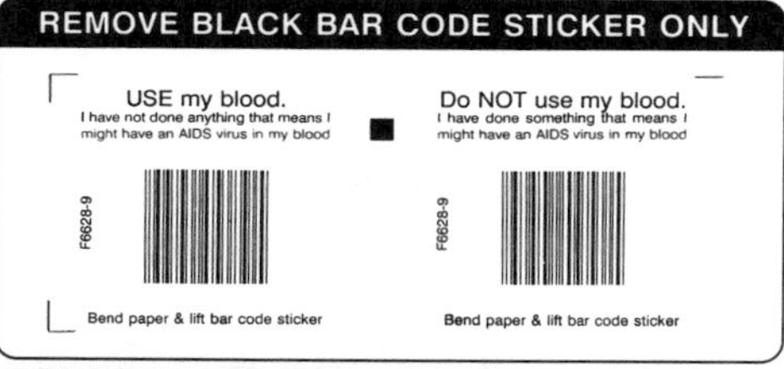

Step 4: Fold this paper and throw it away

Regardless of how you respond, your blood will be tested for exposure to AIDS viruses and you will be notified if our tests indicate you may have a health problem. If required by law, positive test results will be reported to state/federal agencies.

FIGURE 2. American Red Cross Confidential Unit Exclusion (CUE) form. This form was in use at the time this chapter of the text was written, and it is subject to significant modification as circumstances require. (Reproduced with permission, American National Red Cross.[7])

Council of Community Blood Centers. The American Red Cross is a single organization comprised of 50 blood service regions operating under centrally developed procedures called Blood Services Directives or BSDs.[15] The American Association of Blood Banks is both an organization of independent blood centers and hospital transfusion services. It is also the major professional organization of blood bankers. For its member organizations it publishes *Standards* to which member institutions must adhere. The Council of Community Blood Centers (CCBC) is a trade association of blood centers in the U.S. which, although it does not regularly set standards, has made recommendations on controversial blood bank issues to its membership.

Other countries have similar private organizations involved in standard setting. In addition, governmental regulations in each country have a significant influence on standards of professional practice. In the U.S., the Food and Drug Administration (FDA) establishes regulations that represent a minimum standard of practice. Individuals states also have blood bank regulations, often as part of their clinical laboratory regulations.

Since this is a confusing and rapidly evolving system, readers are cautioned to consult the relevant and current government regulations and blood bank standards before making decisions. This chapter will focus on current U.S. FDA regulations and American Red Cross BSDs, cross referencing them to AABB standards when the latter differ from the former.

III. RESOURCES AND FACILITIES REQUIRED

A. STAFF

An adequate and trained staff is very important to ensure accurate donor health assessment. None of the standard-setting bodies has established credentials for blood bank staff who perform medical interviews, although some states have regulations regarding who can perform phlebotomy. The FDA regulations require the suitability of donors be determined by a physician "or by persons under his supervision and trained in determining suitability."[16] In practice, however, this requires that standard operating procedures (SOPs) (under which the medical history is conducted) be approved by the medical director and be acceptable to the FDA.

Most blood collection agencies in the U.S. use a combination of trained technicians and licensed nurses at blood drives, both for medical history as well as blood collection. The American Red Cross requires a Head Nurse, who is a licensed R.N., to supervise the other staff involved in medical history and phlebotomy and to be responsible for caring for donor complications.[17] Arrangements must also be made for comprehensive medical care in the event of a serious donor reaction.[18] For whole blood donation from healthy donors outside of a health care institution, it is sufficient to have staff trained in first aid and cardiopulmonary resuscitation and to prearrange for emergency transportation to a hospital emergency room.

Facilities for a donor room should be designed to ensure adequate privacy, smooth donor flow, adequate toilet facilities, and convenient employee hand washing facilities. Adequate donor canteen facilities are needed to allow refreshments and supervised recovery for approximately 15 minutes after phlebotomy. In addition, proper storage facilities for collected blood need to be available until the blood can be transported to the processing location. The donor facility also should have adequate parking, proper visibility and signs, and be pleasant and attractive to the lay person.

In the U.S., fixed collection facilities must be approved by the FDA and, for licensed facilities, must be registered in advance with the FDA.[19]

Mobile collection sites must have the same basic elements as fixed sites. In practice, this means adequate space, temperature control, an insect-free environment, and reasonably convenient access for loading and unloading equipment. Emergency communication to call an ambulance must be available, which can be accomplished via a sponsor's phone, cellular telephone, or two-way radio. This also allows consultation with the medical director on donor eligibility questions that the Head Nurse cannot answer.

In practice, it is best to review the site plan and the proposed mobile furniture set-up before the day of the drive. This will clarify the blood center's needs for the space and ensure it will be accessible for set-up and breakdown before and after the drive and will be properly heated and lighted during the drive. It is most important to ensure that there will be adequate space for donor flow, a recovery area for donor reactions, and adequate privacy at the medical history and confidential unit exclusion station area. The impression of privacy is at least as important as the fact of privacy, in obtaining an accurate medical history.[20]

B. SOPs AND GUIDELINES

All activities conducted to establish donor suitability must be covered by detailed SOPs.[21] In addition, it is helpful to have ancillary materials available to staff conducting the donor interview such as suitable drug references,[22,23] a map of geographical exclusions (for malaria), a medical dictionary, and a brief reference on common medical conditions and treatments.[24] These will allow the staff to reference the nature of the donor's history, and to efficiently characterize its relevance to blood donation eligibility. Various algorithms have proven useful for commonly encountered histories such as those of cardiopulmonary disease, cancer, degree of exposure to infectious diseases, etc. Such algorithms, although not all part of established standards, can serve as the medical director's detailed instructions to the staff. They should be reviewed regularly to ensure they stay in compliance with evolving regulation and medical practice and new information on epidemiology.

C. EDUCATIONAL MATERIALS AND PUBLICITY

Given the importance of an informed donor population for the safety of the blood supply, blood collection agencies have a responsibility to ensure that all their efforts (from publicity on blood drives, to promotional material, to training of volunteer donor recruiters within donor groups) be consistent with discouraging donation by persons with high-risk behavior. In addition to providing recruiters with the list of risk behaviors, recruiters should also be trained to deemphasize the "mini-physical" aspect of donating blood. Blood donor medical screening and testing is of limited health maintenance value. It is important to discourage those prospective donors whose motivation to give blood is to reassure them regarding a health concern. The need for this precaution became extremely clear after the testing for HIV was implemented in the U.S., because some persons with a history of risk behavior were found to be using blood donation as a means of obtaining HIV testing.

Publicity and donor brochures can also screen out clearly ineligible donors (such as those of inadequate age or weight). The availability of trained health history personnel to support donor recruitment by answering questions before the blood drive is very helpful to a smooth-running blood drive. It does not seem helpful to provide detailed medical criteria to lay recruiters or donors, since this can lead to over-deferral with eligible donors being permanently, but inappropriately, deferred as blood donors.

D. LANGUAGE DIFFERENCES, HEARING AND VISUALLY IMPAIRED, AND OTHER HANDICAPPED DONORS

In order to obtain an adequate health history, it is necessary to adequately communicate with donors. Donors who are hearing or visually handicapped and donors who speak different languages represent a special challenge to the blood bank staff. In general, staff may rely on translators (and sign language interpreters) to conduct a verbal interview. It is the medical director's responsibility to assure that the translators are competent and able to communicate medical and sensitive personal information during the interview. The translator should not be known to the donor, so as to ensure confidentiality and accurate history giving. Thus, prearrangement for the donation is necessary, since friends, relatives, or co-workers of the donor should not be recruited to translate. The availability of written material for the donor is desirable, but the translation must be validated as accurate. In practice, bilingual staff are necessary in areas where there is a high frequency of dual language donors. The Confidential Unit Exclusion procedure needs to be explained by the translator. The donor is then left to make his or her election privately. Blind donors require the availability of braille Confidential Unit Exclusion forms or alternative procedures so that the choice can be made confidentially.

Special arrangements are necessary for donors who are mildly mentally impaired. The medical interviewer needs to determine the ability of the donor to give an accurate history and ensure that the donor understands the high-risk activities that would preclude their being an eligible donor. There is no firm guidance available on this difficult topic.

E. PREDONATION LABORATORY TESTING AND PHYSICAL EXAM

The logistical impossibility of performing a comprehensive assessment of each blood donor prevents conducting an extensive physical or laboratory assessment of donors prior to donation. The standard blood donor physical exam consists only of the general appearance, temperature, self-reported weight, pulse, and blood pressure. Only a sphygmomanometer and thermometer (usually electronic) are necessary. A scale is a useful adjunct for donors of borderline weight.

A hemoglobin determination is required prior to blood donation. This is usually performed by the van Slyke[25] method, using whole blood density determination. This method requires only alcohol wipes, lancets, capillary tubes, and copper sulfate solutions of the appropriate density (e.g., a specific gravity of 1.053 corresponds to a hemoglobin of 12.5 gm/dl). Blood banks have also found it useful to use more quantitative measures of hemoglobin, usually for donors who fail the copper sulfate screening test. A variety of portable devices exist which provide accurate results. These include a portable microhematocrit device, a portable hemoglobinometer,[26,27] and a portable whole blood conductivity device.[28]

Although theoretically desirable, in practice the concept of performing other laboratory tests prior to donation (for the more prevalent disease markers such as ALT and anti-HBc) has been difficult to achieve. Studies have demonstrated the feasibility of predonation ALT screening at blood drives,[29] but predonation anti-HBc is not available. To date, this approach has been used (with standard lab testing methods) on a limited basis for pheresis and other special donations but has not been implemented in routine blood collection.

F. DONOR RECORDS AND DONOR DEFERRAL REGISTRIES

The donor history interview and physical assessment are usually recorded, along with information regarding the phlebotomy, on a single form, called the blood donation record, which is cross-referenced to a unique whole blood identification number. (For an example of a blood donation record, see Figure 3.) The whole blood identification number will be used to track subsequent blood components prepared from that donation. This form (or a microfilm or electronic media copy of it), should be retained at least 5 years after expiration of the longest dated component[30] or longer, as dictated by the record retention policy and requirements of the blood collection agency.

In the U.S., the FDA requires maintenance of a donor deferral registry,[31] which is a list of all donors ineligible to donate blood because of recipient safety. The maintenance of this list requires development of an accurate method of donor identification on subsequent donations. This registry can be maintained by paper records, microfiche, or electronic media and can be used at the blood drive prior to donation to identify previously deferred donors, or can be checked after the blood donation for donations by persons who should be deferred.

Quality control of donor deferral registries has been a difficult problem, particularly for larger blood collection agencies. Elements of quality control include adequate donor identification methods, notification of deferred donors not to donate again, confidentiality of data, validation of computer programs, and computer security issues.

G. STAFF TRAINING

All staff conducting donor medical histories require a structured and documented training program. Blood banks need to train the staff in interviewing techniques, a conceptual understanding of the important disease processes, and a detailed knowledge of the specific SOPs. The author's blood

American Red Cross Blood Donation Record CD

Last Name | First | Middle Initial | Social Security No. | 9.1 Birth Date

Mailing Address | Apt. No. | Employer | Business Phone ( ) | Ext.

City | State | Zip Code | Home Phone ( ) | Sex M F | 9.2 Last Donation | New Card Y N

Miscellaneous Use/Change | Collection Site | Donor Group/Chapter | First Time Donor Y N

Blood Type

Donor: H A D T | Procedure: W B P P L P P L S/O

WHOLE BLOOD NUMBER

DONOR BAR CODE STICKER

Today's Date

A DONOR IF INSTRUCTED PLEASE ANSWER ONLY SHADED QUESTIONS BELOW

	In the past three years have you:		
2.2	been outside the U.S. (except for Canada)?	Y	N
2.1	had malaria or taken antimalarial drugs?	Y	N
3.1	Have you ever had a serious illness such as: cancer, heart or lung disease, convulsions, chest pain etc?	Y	N
3.2	In the past six months have you had surgery, been treated by a health professional, or been pregnant?	Y	N
3.3	Are you feeling well today?	Y	N
3.4	Have you:		
a.	had any dental work in the last three days?	Y	N
b.	taken any medications in the last month?	Y	N
3.5	Have you ever been deferred as a donor or had problems donating?	Y	N
4.1	Have you had any vaccinations (shots) or immunizations in the last year?	Y	N
5.1	Do you have a cold, flu, sore throat or trouble breathing?	Y	N
5.2	Have you ever donated under another name?	Y	N

B RED CROSS USE ONLY

1.1	Have you ever had yellow jaundice (except as a newborn), liver disease, hepatitis, or a positive test for hepatitis?	Y	N
1.2	Have you:		
a.	ever taken street drugs by needle, even once?	Y	N
b.	been a sex partner of anyone who has taken street drugs by needle?	Y	N
	In the past year have you:		
1.3	received blood transfusions, blood injections, tattoos, organ or tissue transplants?	Y	N
1.4	been exposed to anyone with yellow jaundice or hepatitis?	Y	N
3.9	Have you ever taken human growth hormone or Tegison?	Y	N
5.4	Have you:		
a.	to your knowledge, had a positive test for HIV (any AIDS test)?	Y	N
b.	been exposed to or had sex with anyone with AIDS or with a positive test for HIV (the AIDS antibody)?	Y	N
c.	been given money or drugs for sex since 1977?	Y	N
d.	taken clotting factor concentrates for a bleeding disorder such as hemophilia or had sex with someone who has?	Y	N
5.6	For men, have you:		
a.	had sex, even once, with another man since 1977?	Y	N
b.	had sex with a female prostitute in the last twelve months?	Y	N
5.7	For women, have you:		
a.	had sex, even once, with a man who has had sex with another man since 1977?	Y	N
b.	had sex with a male prostitute in the last twelve months?	Y	N
5.8	In the last year have you had or been treated for syphilis or gonorrhea?	Y	N

PHYSICAL FINDINGS

8.1 Weight | 8.2 Temp. | 8.3 Pulse | 8.4 B / P | 8.5 Hb/Hct S U g %

8.7 Arms S U | 8.8 Skin Disease Y N | Deferral Code | Date Elig. Next Donation | 8.9 AI C A B H O

PHLEBOTOMY

Lot # | Pack: D Q S T Quint | Arm L R

Time Started | Time Completed | Phleb S U | V / DVP | 9.3 Reaction SL M SEV

1. VP Signature / ID | 2. VP Signature / ID

Lab Use

REMARKS

C DONOR CONSENT I have read What You Must Know Before Giving Blood today and have had a chance to ask any questions about the information it contains. I understand that information fully and have answered all the questions on this form truthfully. In particular, I understand if I am at risk for spreading the AIDS virus or other diseases, my blood or plasma must not be given to another person. I also understand that my blood will be tested for AIDS and for other diseases. If these tests or the information recorded on this form indicate that I should no longer donate blood my blood will not be used and my name will be entered on a list of deferred donors. All the information I have given for this donation and recorded on this form is true to the best of my knowledge and I donate my blood and blood products for use as needed.

Signature HH/ID | Donor Signature X | Reviewer Initials/ID

F6628 2/92 COMBO

FIGURE 3. American Red Cross: Blood Donation Record. This form was in use at the time this chapter of the text was written, and it is subject to significant modification as circumstances require. (Reproduced with permission, American National Red Cross.[7])

center has found it helpful to train technicians first in phlebotomy and then, as a promotional opportunity, successful staff are eligible to be trained in medical interviewing.

Use of licensed nurses (RN or LPN) does not lessen the importance of training. Although licensed nurses are usually trained in interviewing techniques and are more sophisticated medically, they often have little under-

TABLE 1
Sample Medical Interviewer Training Checklist: Documentation Skills

- Requests and verifies accuracy and legibility of approved donor identification information if available.
- If the donor does not have approved identification, verifies donor's name, date of birth, and social security number as recorded on the Blood Donation Record.
- Verifies accuracy and legibility of information documented at the Temperature Station.
- Reviews all donor responses to questions and accurately documents this information in appropriate section of Blood Donation Record.
- Accurately documents each parameter required during physical assessment.
- Ensures donor has read and understands informed consent and signs his/her name.
- Checks donor signature for legibility and completeness and verifies it with registered name.
- Signs name and status once health history interview is completed.
- Enters correct date for next eligible donation.
- All documentation is concise, legible, and accurate.
- Inserts Call Back Card in appropriate space.
- Explains Confidential Unit Exclusion (CUE) procedure, gives donor the CUE information and directs donor to CUE station.
- Conducts final review of donors name, social security number, and date of birth for accuracy.

standing of transmissible diseases. Further, they need to be trained to follow SOPs strictly. Finally, phlebotomy technique, particularly for whole blood collection, is usually not part of their past experience.

The author has found it helpful to develop and use a competency-based training program. In this program, staff are evaluated for their specific competency on elements of the SOPs, utilizing a checklist approach. (For an example, see Table 1.) This insures adequate training and has been invaluable in today's highly regulated blood bank environment.

IV. PUBLIC HEALTH CONSIDERATIONS

Since blood drives operate in the general community, blood collection agencies have a responsibility to respond to the public health implications of their blood collection activities. These include referral to physicians or clinics when abnormalities are detected on physical exam (especially blood pressure) or medical history. Health educational opportunities present themselves at several points in the health interview and include nutritional counselling (for donors who fail the hemoglobin screen); AIDS, sex, and drug education (for questions which arise during the health history interview); and alerting donors to other potentially serious problems revealed by the interview. Hemoglobin screening by copper sulfate is rather nonspecific, but follow-up quantitative testing can reveal pathological hemoglobin levels that require physician referral.

The extensive infectious disease screening performed on donated blood results in detection of a significant number of abnormal test results. Each of these requires a responsible policy of donor notification, counseling, and medical care referral. The obligation to inform the donor of important test results arises not only from the possible importance for the donor's health care, but also from the risk that certain diseases detected may be transmissible to other family members and social contacts. Some test results must also be reported to governmental agencies. Finally, the entry of donors into a donor deferral registry requires donor notification for ethical and legal reasons, as well as to preclude repeat donations from the same donor. All blood collection agencies need carefully developed policies to carry out their obligations to report significant health findings to their donors, as well as to meet their public health responsibilities.

V. DONOR SCREENING STANDARDS

A. DONOR SELF-SCREENING

Donors should be encouraged to self-defer for two reasons. First, when the deferral is obvious to a lay person, self-deferral avoids needless time and effort on the part of the donor and blood bank alike. Second, when the donor is concerned about an aspect of his history that he is reluctant to share with the blood collection agency, he should self-defer. Examples of histories that donors may not wish to reveal that are important to their status as blood donors are a history of high-risk sexual activity or a history of illicit intravenous drug use.

However, for most health questions, blood banks should encourage donors to undergo a medical history interview with a trained interviewer. In this way, misconceptions of the donor will not result in inappropriate failure to present for blood donation. This is especially true for donors who have been deferred some time in the past, since older blood bank standards were often needlessly conservative, particularly regarding donor safety issues.

The author has found age, weight, and donation interval to be the only donor criteria easily used for prescreening by lay recruiters. This also has the advantage of simplicity and uniformity over time.

Publicity by the blood collection agency, as well as promotional brochures should emphasize high-risk activities for disease transmission. This assists the high-risk donor in self-deferring at a time when peer pressure is manageable and allows an opportunity for public education. The high-risk activities for disease transmission are summarized in Table 2.

Unfortunately, the effectiveness of this measure can only be generally estimated, since such donors are unlikely to reveal their motivation to a study protocol. The best indicator that self-deferral is working is the reduction of the HIV seroprevalence rate in blood donors[32] and the striking difference in HIV seroprevalence between U.S. blood donors and estimates of HIV seroprevalence in the adult population.[33]

B. CONFIDENTIAL UNIT EXCLUSION

Early in the HIV epidemic, it became clear to blood banks in the areas of highest prevalence for HIV that seropositive donors were donating who

TABLE 2
Patient Safety

Some people must not give because their blood might spread an infection to the people who receive it.

Do not give blood if you:

- Have ever had hepatitis (liver disease caused by a virus)
- Have had malaria or have taken drugs to prevent malaria in the past three years (plasma donations may be acceptable)
- Have had or been treated for syphilis or gonorrhea in the last 12 months

Do not give blood if you are at risk for getting and spreading any AIDS virus. You are at risk if:

- You are a man who has had sex with another man since 1977, even one time
- You have taken (''shot up'') illegal drugs by needle, even one time
- You have taken clotting factor concentrates for a bleeding disorder such as hemophilia
- You have ever had a positive test for any AIDS virus or any AIDS antibody
- You have AIDS or one of its symptoms, which include:
  - Weight loss (10 pounds or more in less than 2 months) that you can't explain
  - Night sweats
  - Blue or purple spots on or under the skin
  - White spots or unusual sores in your mouth that last a long time
  - Lumps in your neck, armpits, or groin that last more than a month
  - Fever higher than 99 degrees that lasts more than 10 days
  - Diarrhea that lasts more than 1 month
  - Persistent cough and shortness of breath
- You have had sex with any person described above
- You have been given money or drugs for sex since 1977
- You are a man who has had sex with a female prostitute or a woman who has had sex with a male prostitute in the last 12 months

were aware of their risk behavior. Their failure to defer was sometimes caused by a desire to obtain a free HIV test, sometimes by reluctance to risk stigmatization by not participating in their employer's blood drive, and sometimes by reluctance to have their risk activity in the records of the blood collection agency.

Early studies demonstrated that allowing a donor to indicate confidentially by secret ballot that their blood should not be used for transfusion resulted in a significant number of confidential deferrals by donors who had higher infectious disease marker rates than the general donor population.[13] Keys to a successful program included consideration of privacy in the balloting, successful education about the risk behaviors involved, giving the donors a choice to use the donated blood ''for studies'' or ''for research'', a commitment to maintain the donor's deferral confidential and without explanation, and a commitment to complete full testing on the donated unit and to inform the donor of the results.

The U.S. FDA[34] now recommends that donors be given the opportunity to confidentially exclude donated units at the blood donation site. There have also been proposals to use pictorial descriptions of risk behavior to better communicate with donors around cultural and language barriers.

Over time, the method of the Confidential Unit Exclusion (CUE) process has been refined and many blood centers now use a bar code sticker which can be used to mark the blood donation record with the donor's ballot (See Figure 2). The bar code ensures confidentiality (a number of bar codes are used for each choice); the donor can be verified to have made a choice; and the recording of the donor's choice can be automated, efficient, and accurate.

Data from the Connecticut Red Cross Blood Center continues to reaffirm that donors choosing the CUE option "Do NOT use my blood" are more likely to be male, young, and have higher anti-HBc marker rates, than are donors who choose the option "USE my blood".

As a final measure to allow self-deferral, donors should be informed that they should call the blood center if they have second thoughts about the safety of their blood donation. Such call-back numbers can also be used to report donor complications from phlebotomy, and to report illnesses emerging shortly after the blood donation. Care needs to be taken in setting up SOPs for the phone lines which must be covered 24 hours a day by knowledgeable staff. Documentation of such call-backs should be maintained, and a rapid response to retrieve components from the donation is necessary to prevent their inadvertent transfusion.

C. PHYSICAL ASSESSMENT OF BLOOD DONORS

The donor's pulse and blood pressure must be determined prior to blood donation. In the U.S., a blood pressure over 180 systolic or 100 diastolic requires physician assessment prior to donation.[35] Although concern may exist regarding hypertension in blood donors, there has not been an increase in donor reactions in donors with hypertension.

Brady- or tachycardia, as well as an irregular pulse, are quite common in healthy blood donors. Unfortunately, it is usually difficult to exclude pathology at a blood drive, where an EKG is unavailable. Tachycardia (above 100 beats per minute) often responds to rest. Bradycardia in young athletes is common. Standards in the U.S. require additional assessment if the pulse is under 50 or over 100 beats per minute.[36] Blood collection staff should have clear local guidelines for assessment of donors for pulse rate and irregularities. These guidelines need to take into account the availability of medical facilities, the age and health history of the blood donor, and the sophistication of the blood collection staff.

The temperature of the donor should be determined and should be 99.5°F or 37.5°C or less. Higher temperatures may indicate a subclinical infectious disease process.

The general appearance of the donor should be noted and should be compatible with good health. Obvious sequelae of alcoholism or illicit drug use should preclude blood donation. The donor's arms and skin should be inspected for puncture marks or scars which may be evidence of intravenous drug use. Any unexplained finding requires the deferral of the donor.

The mental status of the donor as well as his or her fluency in the interviewer's language(s) should be assessed. If the donor appears emotionally disturbed, intoxicated, or mentally retarded the donor should be deferred from blood donation, since the safety of the donation is dependent on obtaining an adequate health history and on the donor's ability to understand and act on donor self-deferral instructions. The special problems of donors who are blind or deaf, or have language difficulties have been previously addressed.

D. AUTOLOGOUS AND DIRECTED BLOOD DONATIONS

The remainder of this chapter will discuss specific homologous donor standards. Autologous blood donation, including the medical history, is beyond the scope of this chapter. It should be noted, however, that if an autologous blood donor is to be considered for homologous donation of an unused autologous unit (''cross-over''), the donor must meet all donor standards for homologous donation. It is important for the donor to recognize that they must answer all questions fully and truthfully. It has been argued that autologous donors are so focused on their own donation that they may not be able to give an accurate history. Blood banks who wish to cross-over autologous blood donations should be able to present data to refute this allegation.

Donations from friends and relatives (directed donations) present similar problems. Since the deferral of the donor will probably be known to the recipient, the same degree of confidentiality attending homologous blood donation does not exist. It is a matter of considerable debate if, under these circumstances, the donor is safer, less safe, or the same as a routine homologous blood donor. Obviously, in an individual situation it depends on the individual donor. Programmatically, however, it has not been possible to answer this question definitively.

This chapter will consider directed donor standards to be the same as routine homologous donor standards, although the AABB Standards[37] allow certain directed donors (who are part of a program to limit the recipient's donor exposure) to donate blood up to every three days if they meet all other homologous standards. The author recommends that homologous donor standards not be altered for routine directed donors, even those standards for donor protection, unless the donation has some unique medical value (e.g., a rare red cell donor). In the latter case, individualized decisions should be made by the medical director. In addition, the risk of graft-versus-host disease from related donors may be greater than from unrelated homologous donors, unless such products are irradiated. This transfusion complication is discussed later in this chapter.

E. DONOR MEDICAL HISTORY: MEASURES FOR DONOR PROTECTION

The medical history must be performed on the day of donation and the donor accepted or deferred that day on the basis of the information then available. In cases where a complete medical history cannot be obtained, the donor should be deferred. In these cases, the author has found it useful to establish a mechanism to ask donors to have their physicians send additional information to the blood bank medical director, who can then establish the donor's eligibility to donate in the future. Providing the donor with some documentation of this determination allows the donor to establish his or her eligibility at future donations and insures consistent determination of eligibility by blood drive staff.

1. Cardiovascular and Respiratory Status

Donors should be asked if they have had previous cardiac or unexplained chest pain or respiratory disease. The significance of a questionable history can often be elicited by questioning the donor regarding significant restrictions on his or her physical activity. Donors should not be accepted if they have had a recent history of a myocardial infarction or angina or symptoms suggestive of angina. Exceptions can be made for donors who are uniquely valuable to the recipient (such as a rare phenotype donor) but the donation should occur under direct medical supervision and the need for the donation should be documented in advance of the donation.

Donors who have had successful repair of congenital heart disease, rheumatic valvular disease, or who have other cardiac conditions need to be evaluated as to their ability to safely donate a unit of blood. A history of acute cardiac disease such as pericarditis should not cause deferral after the donor is completely recovered.

Donors who have had acute respiratory disease, including asthma, are acceptable if they are not currently symptomatic or on antibiotic therapy. Donors with chronic pulmonary diseases which cause restriction of physical activity should be deferred. Some state regulations in the U.S. specifically exclude donors with a history of tuberculosis, although this author sees no rationale for excluding donors who have been successfully treated.

Donors currently suffering from an acute upper respiratory infection should be deferred until recovered, primarily because the nonspecific symptoms may represent the prodrome of a more important transmissible disease.

2. Seizure Disorders

The underlying etiology of the seizures should be ascertained. Significant neurologic disease should cause the donor to be deferred. Donors with idiopathic seizure disorders may donate blood unless their seizures are not well controlled by medication. The seizures which sometimes occur with vasovagal reactions do not appear to be closely correlated with a history of seizures.

3. Pregnancy

Pregnant women should not donate blood, primarily because of their marginal iron status. (There also is little evidence on the safety of blood donation for the fetus.) Following normal delivery, a woman can donate as soon as 6 weeks, although many blood banks impose a longer waiting period. Complicated deliveries and Caesarean sections should be evaluated according to local guidelines for surgical procedures, with particular attention to the possibility of receipt of blood transfusions.

4. Other Medical Conditions

Other medical conditions exist which may cause concern for the donor's safety. These may include other chronic diseases, recent medical care, etc. In general, local guidelines need to be developed that take into account the sophistication of the health history interviewer and their access to medical supervision and advice. Some donors' medical conditions may also present a component of concern regarding recipient safety.

The author has found it best to allow the blood collection staff broad latitude on decisions on donor safety, while carefully defining SOPs for donor histories related to recipient safety. It also has proven useful to have two sets of guidelines, one set for the health history interviewer and a more detailed set of guidelines for the Head Nurse on the blood drive. The latter instructions can be very detailed and altered as necessary without the need to retrain the entire blood collection staff. Finally, providing access by phone to a physician greatly enhances the staff's willingness to accept donors with more complex medical histories.

It should be emphasized that any guidelines must be constantly reviewed and updated to accommodate the rapid changes in medical diagnoses, treatment, and terminology. Yesterday's medical guidelines are quickly obsolete.

F. DONOR MEDICAL HISTORY: MEASURES FOR RECIPIENT PROTECTION

Much of the medical history examination of the donor is designed to elicit information regarding transmissible diseases. Since this subject is covered extensively elsewhere, the following presentation is organized to give an overview of the process. For additional information see Chapter 5. The questions asked in the text are those of the American Red Cross[7] (see Figure 3). These are compatible with the AABB Standards.[1]

1. General Questioning

General questioning is designed to elicit serious medical problems and serve both to protect donor and recipient. In some cases, diseases and/or therapy such as blood transfusion may be identified that would not be elicited elsewhere in the interview. The open ended questions also invite the donor to think of his or her entire health history as they answer more specific questions. Positive answers must be investigated. The Red Cross asks the following general questions that may elicit information important to recipient safety:

- Have you ever had a serious illness such as cancer, heart or lung disease, convulsions, chest pain, etc.?
- In the past six months have you had surgery, been treated by a health professional, or been pregnant?
- Are you feeling well today?
- Have you ever been deferred as a donor or had problems donating?
- Have you taken any medications in the last month?
- Have you had any vaccinations (shots) or immunizations in the last year?
- Do you have a cold, flu, sore throat, or trouble breathing?

2. Viral Diseases

Blood donor medical interviewers should ask specific questions regarding high-risk behavior. These questions should repeat the self-deferral information the donor has been given (Table 2). Questions also should be asked regarding symptoms of HIV, previous tests for HIV, and specific sexual and parenteral exposure. The latter questions serve as precautions against HIV as well as other blood-borne diseases.

The following *questions* are included in the Red Cross questionnaire. They are used here to organize the following discussion of specific donor standards. The discussion following each question is the author's own rationale for the question and is not meant to represent Red Cross policy.

HIV-1 and HIV-2 — *Have you ever taken street drugs by needle, even once? Have you been a sex partner of anyone who has taken street drugs by needle?* Positive responses should cause permanent deferral of the donor because of the very high incidence of HIV and hepatitis B and C in the IV drug user, the known recidivism of IV drug users (so that the exposure may be ongoing despite the history), and the known efficiency of HIV transmission by sexual contact.

In the past year have you received blood transfusions, blood injections, tattoos, organ or tissue transplants? This deferral is 12 months based primarily on the apparently longer period for seroconversion to hepatitis C[38] than for hepatitis B and HIV, which previously had dictated a 6-month deferral period for this exposure. The deferral is not permanent because the dates of exposure and the veracity of the history are much clearer than for sexual exposure or IV drug use.

Have you, to your knowledge, had a positive test for HIV (any AIDS test)? A confirmed positive test requires permanent deferral. An apparently false positive test must be investigated. In the U.S. the FDA requires a formal "re-entry" test algorithm[34] be satisfied before such a donor is acceptable.

Have you been exposed to, or had sex with anyone with AIDS or with a positive test for HIV (the AIDS antibody)? Here the exposure must be evaluated against the known epidemiology of HIV. Deferral is indefinite if the exposure was sexual. Lesser degrees of exposure, such as sharing toothbrushes, or razors, require a 12-month deferral. Since this is a frequently changing area of regulation, readers should consult current FDA regulations and AABB or ARC Standards for details.

Health care workers warrant special consideration. Current Red Cross BSDs[7] require a deferral of 12 months for health care workers who have had a documented exposure to blood by needle stick or by blood contamination of mucous membranes or nonintact skin. This deferral applies despite the HIV serological status of the patient whose blood caused the exposure. This is primarily because of the usual lack of reliable information on the patient's HIV serological status and because of the high prevalence of hepatitis B and C in patients.

Since 1977 have you exchanged sex for drugs or money? This permanent deferral is based on the high HIV seroprevalence in prostitutes.

Have you taken clotting factor concentrates for a bleeding disorder such as hemophilia or had sex with someone who has? This deferral is based on the high seroprevalence of hepatitis and HIV in patients with hemophilia and their sexual partners.

For men, have you had sex, even once, with another man since 1977? For women, have you had sex, even once with a man who has had sex with another man since 1977? These donors are permanently deferred based on the known epidemiology of HIV in the U.S. The wording of this question avoids the term homosexual, which is widely misunderstood. It emphasizes by "even once" the high HIV seroprevalence in male homosexuals and that sexual activity with someone with HIV is high risk.

Have you had sex with a prostitute in the last 12 months? These donors are temporarily deferred. This deferral is based on the relatively high seroprevalence in prostitutes balanced against the unacceptable impact on the blood supply of permanent donor deferral for sexual contact with a prostitute. The 12-month interval allows for seroconversion in the overwhelming majority of exposed individuals. Such donors can then be screened out by the HIV test.

In the last year have you had or been treated for syphilis or gonorrhea? The rationale for this temporary deferral is the known association of these venereal diseases with HIV infection. The rationale for temporary rather than permanent deferral is similar to that for sex with prostitutes.

Hepatitis A, B, C, and others — Many of the HIV questions also serve to defer donors at high risk of transmitting hepatitis. Additional questions are specifically designed to detect hepatitis exposure. Hepatitis B and C appear to be much more easily spread by nonsexual and non-parenteral routes than HIV, although the epidemiology of hepatitis C is poorly understood.

The following questions are asked by the American Red Cross. Again, the rationale for the standards is the author's and is not meant to represent Red Cross policy.

Have you ever had yellow jaundice (except as a newborn), liver disease, or a positive test for hepatitis? Positive responses need thorough investigation. Any history of hepatitis or unexplained jaundice or liver disease requires permanent deferral. Recent proposals[39] to allow donation by those whose hepatitis history was before 10 years of age have been made. The rationale for deferring donors with a history of hepatitis is not entirely clear, but this donor standard is time-honored. Scientific proof of the safety of accepting such donors will not be available until we have a much better understanding of the epidemiology of hepatitis C and of post-transfusion non-A, non-B hepatitis.

A history of a positive test for hepatitis needs to be investigated. A documented history of a positive HBsAg or an anti-HCV test is cause for indefinite deferral, as are two positive tests for anti-HBc. Standards for deferral for ALT elevation are somewhat less standardized in the U.S.

In the past year have you been exposed to anyone with yellow jaundice or hepatitis? Exposure is generally regarded as routinely sharing common kitchen and toilet facilities, as well as sexual or parenteral exposure. Thus, persons residing in the same household or in group residency situations, such as dormitories or military barracks, are deferred for 12 months following the diagnosis of hepatitis in the household or living facility. Prisons or custodial facilities, such as institutions for the mentally handicapped, have such high prevalence rates of hepatitis that all persons residing in such institutions should be deferred as blood donors until 12 months after leaving the institution. Group homes require individual decisions based on the apparent epidemiologic conditions in each setting. The special problems of the homeless (who also present themselves to donate blood) require attention to local epidemiologic data.

In the past, it was standard practice to defer certain high-risk health care workers, such as dialysis workers, from donating blood because of the risk of hepatitis B. The availability of hepatitis B vaccine and the imposition of better nursing practice over the past decade has drastically altered this risk and it now seems safe to evaluate health care institutions, such as dialysis centers, on a case-by-case basis[40] when deciding on the donor eligibility of their employees.

HTLV-I/II — The epidemiology of HTLV-I/II in this country is not confined to immigrants from endemic areas. Intravenous drug use or sexual contact with IV drug users is more important.[41] As such, no other specific questions regarding HTLV I/II are asked on the health interview. Deferral of immigrants from endemic areas does not appear necessary based on the sensitivity of the ELISA screening test.

Cytomegalovirus — Cytomegalovirus (CMV) is endemic in the U.S. Screening for CMV is not routinely performed except for blood transfused to certain neonates and immunosuppressed patients. No specific donor screening questions have been proposed, although since the seroprevalence of CMV is higher in HIV risk groups, it is likely that the emphasis placed on HIV screening has, in fact, reduced the number of CMV-positive donors. When screening for CMV sero-negative donors, it is helpful to screen younger and female donors since they have a lower seroprevalence.

Slow viruses — Creutzfeld-Jakob disease has been transmitted by dura transplantation. Slow viruses have not been shown to be transmissible by blood transfusion. However, since human pituitary extracts have been used as a source of therapeutic growth hormone, donors who have taken human pituitary-derived growth hormone should be deferred as a precaution against the possibility of slow virus transmission.[42] Donors who have taken recombinant growth hormone are eligible donors.

3. Bacterial Diseases

Asymptomatic donor bacteremia — Asymptomatic donors have donated blood contaminated with a variety of bacteria. Investigation has sometimes revealed the donor to have been bacteremic. A fairly broad spectrum of organisms, including *Salmonella choleraesuis, Yersinia enterocolitica,* and *Staphylococcus aureus*, have been implicated.[43] Bacteria can, of course, also contaminate the blood unit at collection, and the epidemiology in reported cases has not always been clear. In general, although some donors have been shown, in retrospect, to have some subtle history or physical finding, it is not possible to devise donor-screening policies for detecting bacteremia that are more sensitive and specific than the donor's temperature and asking the question: *Are you feeling well today?* Encouraging donor "call back" (originally devised for HIV) may be shown to be another useful strategy since, in retrospect, some donors who have been bacteremic have become ill immediately after the implicated donation.

A variety of dental maneuvers, such as tooth brushing, have been shown to induce donor bacteremia. For this reason, a time-honored donor screening question has been: *Have you had any dental work in the last 3 days?* This question is no longer required by the AABB. In addition, specific deferral policies based on the type of dental work are, because of the limited data available, somewhat arbitrary. At present, the Red Cross practice is to accept donors with recent routine dental work, but defer donors with dental abscesses or oral surgery for 72 hours. Oral surgery should be evaluated as for any minor surgery and such donors accepted only after the surgery site is completely healed.

Syphilis — It has been known for years that syphilis is transmissible by blood transfusion. Because the syphilis spirochete does not survive in cold storage, recent cases have been reported only with platelet transfusion or transfusion of fresh blood.[44] Recently, blood banks in the U.S. have asked donors: *In the last year have you had or been treated for syphilis or gonorrhea?* This question is primarily designed as a screen for sexual activity as a surrogate marker for HIV.[14] A more remote history of syphilis does not require deferral as long as the donor has been adequately treated.

Blood is routinely screened for syphilis, primarily by cardiolipin-based screening tests. More recently, some blood banks have implemented a specific treponemal screening test.[45]

Lyme disease — Lyme disease, although caused by a spirochete, *Borrelia burgdorferi*, may not be transmissible by blood transfusion because its spirochetemic phase is quite short. Unlike syphilis, however, *Borrelia burgdorferi* survives well under blood bank storage conditions.[46] Given its long incubation time and vague symptoms, a case of post-transfusion Lyme disease would not be easy to detect. Current efforts should be on surveillance, however, rather than on efforts at donor screening. As for babesiosis, a history of tick bite does not seem a useful donor-screening device. When a history of Lyme disease is obtained in the health interview, the donor should be deferred until considered adequately treated by their physician, and on no medication for Lyme disease for a year.

4. Parasitic Diseases

Malaria — Malaria transmission by blood transfusion is well described. Since there is no laboratory screening test for malarial parasites suitable for routine blood bank use, donor history is the primary screening tool. *In the past three years have you been outside the United States (except for Canada), had malaria or taken anti-malarial pills?* Travel to or emigration from an area of the world considered endemic for malaria is a cause for temporary deferral. The accepted source for endemic areas comes from the Centers for Disease Control.[47] Current regulations require temporary deferral for 6 months for travel to a malaria area, unless malaria prophylaxis (which can suppress clinical malaria) was taken, in which case the deferral is for 3 years. Brief stops during daylight hours such as cruise ship ports or changing planes can be excepted from this requirement.

Immigrants from endemic areas and persons who have had malaria are deferred for 3 years after entering the U.S. or completing malaria treatment, respectively. The latter deferral reflects the tendency for recurrence of malaria after treatment. In all cases the donor can be accepted only if they have had no unexplained febrile illness in the 6 months or 3 years of the deferral period.

Donors who are deferred for malaria can donate plasma, since only the red cells can transmit malaria. Plasma prepared from such donors must be scrupulously free of red cells.

Babesiosis — *Babesia microti* is a tick-borne parasite endemic in many areas of the world. In the U.S. it is transmitted by the same vectors (deer ticks) and has the same reservoirs (deer and white-footed mice) as does Lyme disease. Although seven cases of transfusion-transmitted babesiosis have been reported in the U.S.,[48] the disease seems to occur only in splenectomized or immunosuppressed transfusion recipients. Long periods of asymptomatic parasitemia have been documented among the seven implicated blood donors. Consequently, a history of a tick bite would be a very broad deferral criteria and does not seem practical. The current babesia antibody tests do not appear to be useful for blood donor screening.[49] The Red Cross[7] and AABB Standards[1,50] do not require deferral for a tick bite but do require indefinite deferral of donors with a history of babesiosis.

Chagas' disease — Chagas' disease has been transmitted by transfusion in South and Central America for years. Several recent cases have been documented in North America from blood donors immigrating from endemic areas.[51] Current discussion focuses on the potential use of geographical exclusion (selected immigrants from Central and South America). A screening test is not currently available. Donors with a history of Chagas' Disease are indefinitely deferred.[7]

5. Other Infectious Diseases

A variety of other infectious agents have been transmitted by blood transfusion. In general, these have been isolated occurrences and do not require donor screening.

6. Other Measures to be Considered in Preventing Recipient Complications

Donor allergy — Although a historically important donor standard, there is little evidence that donors who have allergies can transmit them to the blood recipient. Theoretical considerations would argue that one unit of plasma is not likely to cause serious recipient complications. However, some urticaria following transfusion could conceivably be caused by the donor's IgE antibodies interacting with a recipient allergen (such as a drug). Anaphylactic reactions to transfusion have usually been attributed to IgA deficiency with anit-IgA antibody in the recipient.

In special circumstances, such as the repetitive infusion of plasma from a single donor into a recipient, it may be wise to consider the donor's allergies and the recipient's drug exposure. For routine blood bank practice, however, there is no reason to obtain or act on an allergy history in the donor.

Donors who have allergic rhinitis need to be distinguished from donors who have an upper respiratory infection. The latter may not donate.

Donor medication — Drugs have, in the past, been a source of concern in that donor drug levels have been thought to be hazardous to the recipient. Current thinking is that, with specific exceptions, drug history should be used to ascertain an underlying medical condition and that deferral or acceptance should be based on that underlying condition. In the U.S., the only drugs which currently require donor deferral because of drug levels in the donated blood are retinoid derivatives such as isotretinoin (Accutane®, a 4-week deferral is required) and etretinate (Tegison®, a 4-year deferral is required).[7] These retinoids belong to a class of drugs which, because of their potent teratogenicity and their use in treating healthy donors with skin disease, are the subject of a specific Food and Drug Administration recommendation.[52]

Of course, treatment with potent cardiac drugs; antimetabolites, alkylating and immunosuppressive agents; insulin; etc. would often lead to deferral of the donors for their underlying diseases.

Antibiotic therapy requires temporary deferral if it has been prescribed to treat an acute infectious disease. This ensures full recovery from the infectious process following discontinuation of the drug before the donor is again eligible. Chronic use of antibiotics for acne is compatible with blood donation. Other uses of prophylactic antibiotics, such as chronic urinary tract infections, need to be evaluated by the medical director of the blood collection agency.

Aspirin and other anti-platelet drugs should not be used by plateletpheresis donors within three days of donation.[53] The same precaution should apply to donors giving whole blood for production of a platelet concentrate which is the sole source of platelets for a patient (i.e., a neonate).

Donor vaccinations — Immunizations and vaccinations need to be evaluated to ascertain if live viruses have been used. Since viremia is common from live vaccines, a donor deferral of 2 weeks is required for most live virus vaccines (e.g., oral polio, measles, mumps, and yellow fever). A deferral for 4 weeks is required for donors who have received rubella vaccine and for 1 year for donors who have received rabies vaccine following the bite of a suspected rabid animal.[54] Vaccination or immunization with toxoid or killed virus is not a cause for deferral unless there has been a reaction to the inoculation.

The reason for vaccination for hepatitis B needs to be investigated. Hepatitis B vaccine is not a live vaccine and does not need to cause deferral, unless it is given in conjunction with a recent hepatitis exposure, in which case a 12-month deferral is required. Passive inoculation with hepatitis B Immune Globulin (for exposure to hepatitis B) or with Immune Serum Globulin (for exposure to hepatitis B) or with Immune Serum Globulin (for hepatitis exposure other than hepatitis B) requires a 12-month deferral because of the presumed significant exposure to hepatitis.

Cancer and other serious illnesses — Cancer is still a disease of unknown etiology. At least some human cancers are caused by viruses. Many blood banks defer donors who have a history of cancer, even if cured. Exceptions can be made at the discretion of the blood bank medical director for such borderline conditions as skin cancers, premalignant conditions such as intestinal polyps, and carcinoma-*in-situ*. In the absence of any data, any practices are necessarily arbitrary. There are no prevailing blood bank standards.

Many other illnesses are of unknown etiology, particularly the rheumatologic and neurologic diseases and other diseases such as sarcoidosis. Unfortunately, there is no consensus on donor standards and little or no science to guide the medical director in making these practical decisions.

Graft-versus-host disease and related donors — Recently, graft-versus-host disease has been reported to have been caused by related blood donors in recipients who are not immunosupressed.[55,56] The presumed etiology is that the related donor was HLA homozygous and the recipient shared the same HLA haplotype. Consequently, the recipient did not recognize the donor lymphocytes as foreign. Although nonrelated donors can also be HLA homozygous, it is less likely they will be transfused to a recipient who has the same HLA haplotype.

For this reason the AABB has recommended that blood donations from first-degree relatives be irradiated before they are transfused to the related recipient.[57] It thus becomes necessary to ascertain the relationship between the donor and recipient when collecting directed donations and to so label the blood components from such donations.

VI. CONCLUSION

Blood transfusion safety requires that donors are informed and motivated to give an honest and accurate health history. As such, well-educated volunteer blood donors represent the ideal population for recruitment.

Conducting the blood donor medical interview requires knowledge of donor and recipient safety issues. It requires sensitivity to issues of communication and requires a structured set of SOPs and guidelines developed for the staff by the medical director of the blood collection agency. Safety of collected blood is enhanced also by educational material allowing appropriate donors to self-defer, to confidentially exclude their blood for transfusion, or call back after donating blood if they have second thoughts regarding their eligibility.

Careful recruitment, donor interview, and deferral of ineligible donors identifies a population of safe blood donors. Only then can laboratory testing be optimally effective, serving as a double check of the safety of blood components destined for transfusion.

REFERENCES

1. Standards for Blood Banks and Transfusion Services, 14th ed., American Association of Blood Banks, Arlington, VA, 1991.
2. **Walker, R., Ed.,** Technical Manual, 10th ed. American Association of Blood Banks, Arlington, VA, 1990.
3. Donor Reaction Statistics, American Red Cross Blood Services, Connecticut Region, unpublished data, 1990.
4. **Brugger, J., Andrews, A., Rutman, R. et al.,** Quality assurance in the collection of blood and the care of the donor, in *Transfusion Therapy, Principles and Procedures,* 2nd ed., Rutman, R. C. and Miller, W. V., Eds., Aspen Publications, Rockville, MD, 1985.
5. United States Code of Federal Regulations, Title 21, Part 640.3 (b) 1990.
6. Standards for Blood Banks and Transfusion Services, Part B1.262, 14th ed., American Association of Blood Banks, Arlington, VA, 1991.
7. Blood Services Directive 51.110: Blood Donor Interview, Processing, and Management, American Red Cross, Washington, D.C., March 1992.
8. **Walsh, J. H., Purcell, R. H., Morrow, A. G. et al.,** Posttransfusion hepatitis after open-heart operation: incidence after administration of blood from commercial and volunteer donor populations, *JAMA,* 211, 261, 1970.
9. **Cherubin, C. E., Prince, A. M., and Brotman, B.,** Serum Hepatitis specific antigen (SH) in commercial and volunteer sources of blood, *Transfusion,* 11, 25, 1971.
10. United States Code of Federal Regulations, Title 21, Part 606.121 (c) (5), 1990.
11. Publicly funded HIV counseling and testing - United States, 1985–1989, *MMWR,* 39, 137, 1990.
12. **Silvergleid, A. J., Leparc, G. F., and Schmidt, P. J.,** Impact of explicit questions about high-risk activities on donor attitudes and donor deferral patterns, *Transfusion,* 29, 362, 1989.
13. **Pindyck, J., Waldman, A., Zang, E. et al.,** Measures to decrease the risk of acquired immunodeficiency syndrome transmission by blood transfusion. Evidence of volunteer blood donor cooperation, *Transfusion,* 25, 3, 1985.
14. Revised Recommendations for the Prevention of Human Immunodeficiency Virus (HIV) Transmission by Blood and Blood Products, Section I, Parts A & B Only, United States Public Health Service, Center for Biologics Evaluation and Research. December, 1990.
15. Blood Services Directives, American Red Cross, Washington, D.C., 1992.
16. United States Code of Federal Regulations, Title 21, Part 640.3 (a), 1990.
17. Blood Services Directive 19.104: Assignment of Personnel in Blood Donor Management, American Red Cross, Washington, D.C., February, 1981.
18. Blood Services Directive 51.123: Medical Coverage of ARC Blood Collection Operations, American Red Cross, Washington, D.C., June, 1990.
19. Blood Services Directive 12.202: Acquisition, Construction, or Alteration of Licensed Blood Services Facilities, American Red Cross, Washington, D.C., April, 1980.
20. Blood Services Directive 32.001: Current Good Manufacturing Practices Related to Blood Collection, American Red Cross, Washington, D.C., September, 1977.
21. Standards for Blood Banks and Transfusion Services, Part A6.000, 14th ed., American Association of Blood Banks, Arlington, VA, 1991.
22. *Physicians' Desk Reference,* 46th ed., Medical Economics Data, Oradell, NJ, 1992.
23. *Drug Handbook,* Springhouse Corp., Springhouse, PA, 1990.
24. *Merck Manual,* 15th ed., Merck, Sharp, and Dohme, Rahway, NJ, 1987.
25. **Van Slyke, D. D. et al.,** Calculation of hemoglobin from blood specific gravities, *J. Biol. Chem.,* 183, 349, 1950.
26. **Carlson, D. A., Daigneault, R. W., and Statland, B. E.,** Evaluation of the Hemocue photometer for measurement of blood donor hemoglobin, American Association of Blood Banks (Abstract), *Transfusion,* 27, 553, 1987.

27. **Mills, A. F. and Meadows, N.,** Screening for anemia: evaluation of a haemoglobinometer, *Arch. Dis. Child.,* 64, 1468, 1989.
28. **Kalish, R., Sataro, P., and Kiraly, T.,** Donor hemoglobin testing and evaluation of $CuSO_4$ and Stat-Crit methodology, *Transfusion,* 24, 443, 1984.
29. **Gimble, J., Kline, L., and Friedman, L.,** Evaluation of technical and behavioral issues in predonation alanine aminotransferase testing, *Transfusion,* 29, 584, 1989.
30. United States Code of Federal Regulations. Title 21, Part 606.160. 1990.
31. United States Code of Federal Regulations. Title 21, Part 160.160 (e). 1990.
32. **Ness, P. M., Douglas, D., Koziol, D. et al.,** Decreasing seroprevalence of human immunodeficiency virus type 1 in a regional donor center population, *Transfusion,* 30, 201, 1990.
33. **Kuritsky, J. N., Rastogi, S. C., Faich, G. A. et al.,** Results of nationwide screening of blood and plasma for antibodies to human T-cell lymphotropic III virus, *Transfusion,* 26, 205, 1986.
34. Recommendations for the Prevention of Human Immunodeficiency Virus (HIV) Transmission by Blood and Blood Products, United States Public Health Service, Center for Biologics Evaluation and Research. February, 1990.
35. Standards for Blood Banks and Transfusion Services, Part B1.170, 14th ed., American Association of Blood Banks, Arlington, VA, 1991.
36. Standards for Blood Banks and Transfusion Services, Part B1.160, 14th ed., American Association of Blood Banks, Arlington, VA, 1991.
37. Standards for Blood Banks and Transfusion Services, Part B1.131, 14th ed., American Association of Blood Banks, Arlington, VA., 1991.
38. **Alter, H. J., Purcell, R. H., Shih, J. W. et al.,** Detection of antibody to hepatitis C virus in prospectively followed transfusion recipients with acute and chronic non-A, non-B hepatitis, *N. Engl. J. Med.,* 321, 1494, 1989.
39. FDA Blood and Blood Products Advisory Committee, Meeting Minutes. September, 1991.
40. **Badon, S. J., Sataro, P. A., and Cable, R. G.,** Acceptance of hemodialysis employees as blood donors (Abstr.), American Association of Blood Banks, Annual Meeting, 1990.
41. **Williams, A. E., Fang, C. T., Slamon, D. J. et al.,** Seroprevalence and epidemiological correlates of HTLV-1 infection in U.S. blood donors, *Science,* 244 (4906), 757, 1989.
42. Standards for Blood Banks and Transfusion Services, Part B1.264, 14th ed., American Association of Blood Banks, Arlington, VA, 1991.
43. **Goldman, M. G. and Blajchman, M. A.,** Blood product-associated bacterial sepsis, *Transfusion Med. Rev.,* 5, 73, 1991.
44. **Risseeuw-Appel, I. M. and Kothe, F. C.,** Transfusion syphilis: a case report, *Sex. Transmitted Dis.,* 10, 200, 1983.
45. **Roberts, S. C., Dowd, J. C., and Savalonis, J. M.,** An automated test for detection of *Treponema pallidum* antibodies using the Olympus PK7000 Analyzer, Association of Clinical scientists, Ninety-second Meeting (Abstract), 1990.
46. **Badon, S. J., Fister, R. D., and Cable, R. G.,** Survival of *Borrelia burgdorferi* in blood products, *Transfusion,* 29, 581, 1989.
47. Health Information for International Travelers, Centers for Disease Control, 1991.
48. **Mintz, E. D., Anderson, J. F., Cable, R. G. et al.,** Transfusion-acquired babesiosis: a case report from a new endemic area, *Transfusion,* 31, 365, 1991.
49. **Popovsky, M. A., Lindberg, L. E., Syrek, A. L. et al.,** Prevalence of babesia antibody in a selected blood donor population, *Transfusion,* 28, 59, 1988.
50. Changes in the Standards, *AABB News Briefs,* November/December, 1990, American Association of Blood Banks, Arlington, VA, 1990.
51. **Skolnick, A.,** Does influx from endemic areas mean more transfusion-associated Chagas' disease?, *JAMA,* 262, 1433, 1989.

52. Deferral of Blood Donors who have received the drug Accutane, United States Public Health Service, Center for Biologics Evaluation and Research. February, 1984.
53. Standards for Blood Banks and Transfusion Services, Part B1.280, 14th ed., American Association of Blood Banks, Arlington, VA, 1991.
54. Standards for Blood Banks and Transfusion Services, Part B1.230, 14th ed., American Association of Blood Banks, Arlington, VA, 1991.
55. **Thaler, M., Shamiss, A., Orgad, S. et al.,** The role of blood from HLA-homozygous donors in fatal transfusion-associated graft-versus-host disease after open-heart surgery, *N. Engl. J. Med.*, 321, 25, 1989.
56. **Juji, T., Shibata, Y., Ide, H. et al.,** Post-transfusion graft-versus-host disease in immunocompetent patients after cardiac surgery in Japan, *N. Engl. J. Med.*, 321, 56, 1989.
57. Standards for Blood Banks and Transfusion Services, Part J3.413, 14th ed., American Association of Blood Banks, Arlington, VA, 1991.

Chapter 7

AUTOLOGOUS BLOOD TRANSFUSION PROGRAMS

David H. Yawn

TABLE OF CONTENTS

ISBN 0-8493-4938-9

I. INTRODUCTION

The fear of lethal viruses, especially the human immunodeficiency virus (HIV), caused revolutionary changes in transfusion medicine practices during the last decade. The rapid expansion of autologous blood donation programs has had obvious beneficial effects on reducing homologous blood exposure but has also introduced a variety of problems and controversies regarding autologous blood donation and transfusion. Section II will review current concepts related to indications for autologous blood donation, donor suitability, and standards. The use of autologous blood donations for patients with cardiovascular disease and pregnancy deserves special consideration. The lack of utilization of all autologous blood donated preoperatively has raised the controversial issues of crossover and infectious disease marker testing. What is the correct procedure for labeling autologous blood? When is liquid storage vs. cryopreservation of autologous blood components appropriate? Quality assurance is a vital part of any autologous blood transfusion program.

Section III of this chapter will deal with perioperative autologous blood salvage. A review of the indications for perioperative blood salvage, current instrumentation and technology, and quality of salvaged blood will be contrasted with hazards and complications of intraoperative blood salvage.

II. PREOPERATIVE AUTOLOGOUS DONATIONS AND TRANSFUSIONS

A. INDICATIONS FOR PREOPERATIVE AUTOLOGOUS BLOOD DONATION

Yomtovian and Yawn[1] have reviewed the 1991 College of American Pathologists Comprehensive Blood Bank Survey. This survey included 2915 institutions and focused on the percent of autologous blood components which were wasted.[1] Almost 25% of these institutions reported that >90% of autologous blood donated preoperatively was wasted! Approximately 40% of the institutions wasted or discarded less than 50% of the autologous blood. This data indicates that a major problem related to autologous blood donation is appropriate patient selection. It is important to analyze blood usage for a given surgical procedure and patient population. The following guidelines may be helpful in determining who should actually be a candidate for preoperative blood donation:

1. The surgical procedure involved should be expected to have a blood loss in excess of 500 to 1000 ml of blood.
2. Homologous blood usage for that particular surgical procedure should typically be an excess of 2 units of blood (if autologous blood is not available).
3. The surgical procedure should be elective, so that adequate planning and time can be provided for adequate preoperative blood donation.

4. There should be a documented review of the need for the preoperatively donated autologous blood for that particular surgical procedure.

Most institutions have shown that preoperative autologous blood donation is effective for the following surgical procedures:

1. Elective cardiovascular procedures, including coronary artery revascularization, cardiac valve replacement, peripheral vascular procedures, and aortic aneurysm repair
2. Major orthopedic procedures, including scoliosis correction, total knee and total hip replacements
3. Major urologic procedures, including radical resection of the prostate
4. Major plastic surgical procedures, especially reconstructive procedures
5. Major neurosurgical procedures, including treatment of intracranial aneurysms, arteriovenous malformation, and resection of intracranial neoplasms
6. Donation of bone marrow for autologous or homologous transplantation
7. Other surgical procedures in which there is an expected blood loss of 1000 cc of blood or more

Collection of autologous blood is labor intensive and expensive. In the U.S., there are serious problems for reimbursement with this activity. The procedure should not be undertaken unless it can be shown to reduce homologous blood exposure and that there is a frequent need for the donated autologous blood component.

B. DONOR SUITABILITY AND STANDARDS

Both the American Association of Blood Banks (AABB) and the United States Food and Drug Administration (FDA) have allowed the standards for homologous blood donation to be considerably relaxed and altered for the autologous blood donor. The 14th Edition of the *Standards for Blood Banks and Transfusion Services,* published by the AABB, clearly states "rigid criteria for donor selection are not applicable."[2] These standards include a requirement that preoperative autologous blood donation be with the consent of the donor/patient physician and the Blood Bank physician. The Blood Bank physician and the patient's physician together may establish a consensus regarding the volume of blood collected and the frequency of phlebotomy.In general, these patients should have a pre-phlebotomy hemoglobin of 11 g/dl (hematocrit of 33%). Phlebotomy ideally should be within 72 hours of the anticipated surgery. There are no age limits set for autologous donation procedures by the AABB. We have successfully collected autologous blood components from children as young as 8 years of age and from elderly patients in their 9th decade. The volume of blood collected can be adjusted with proportionate removal of anticoagulant from the donor bag. The two greatest risks of autologous blood transfusion therapy are clerical errors (the wrong component being transfused into a patient due to misidentification of patient or blood component) and the risk of bacterial contamination. Patients who have bacteremia or who are currently being treated for systemic bacterial infections should not be autologous blood donors.

C. SPECIAL CLINICAL CONSIDERATIONS

1. Pregnancy

We and others have found that autologous blood donation during pregnancy is a safe procedure for the patient.[3] We collect autologous blood from pregnant patients with isovolemic replacement of normal saline. An intravenous line is started in one arm while the phlebotomy is performed on the opposite arm. At the conclusion of the phlebotomy we complete the infusion of a volume of normal saline equal to the amount of blood removed. After several years of this practice we have not seen any significant donor reactions or fetal morbidity. In spite of the apparent safety of autologous blood donations during pregnancy, there is rarely a need for this blood. Therefore, we discourage this practice, except in pregnancies known to have high risk for bleeding. These conditions include: placenta previa, history of placental abruption, and women having elective caesarean sections. It should be noted that even in these cases, these patients require transfusions in less than 10% of the cases.

There is one group with a logical need for maternal blood collection: those women whose fetus may require intrauterine transfusions. The most common indication for this is isoimmune hemolytic disease of the newborn. Maternal blood is collected for possible intrauterine transfusions to the fetus. Some of this blood can also be cryopreserved (see below) for possible future need by the fetus or mother. A careful working relationship and communication with the obstetrician is important. Complete infectious disease marker (including for cytomegalovirus antibodies) testing is done, of course, prior to the utilization of maternal blood for the fetus. This blood is also irradiated with 3000 rads prior to transfusion into the fetus.

2. Cardiovascular Surgery Patients

Autologous blood collection in the patient with cardiovascular disease is a safe procedure provided (1) there is no cardiovascular instability, which we consider a contraindication for collection of autologous blood, and (2) there is no main left coronary artery disease, unstable angina, or critical aortic valve stenosis. We do not consider collection of autologous blood components from patients with main left coronary artery disease or patients with severe aortic stenosis to be safe or appropriate.

A history of angina is not an absolute contraindication for autologous blood collection. This procedure can be done safely after the appropriate consultation between the blood bank physician and the patient's cardiologist. As with the pregnant patient, it is our practice to use isovolemic saline replacement at the time of phlebotomy for our cardiovascular surgery patients. Owings and associates[4] have done an excellent analysis of the safety and indications for collection of preoperative autologous blood components in patients undergoing first-time coronary artery revascularization. Their study indicated that the collection of 3 units of autologous blood prior to coronary artery revascularization was extremely effective in reducing homologous blood usage. This is the very type of analysis that should be undertaken with all patient populations to determine: (1) Should autologous blood be collected? (2) What is the optimal amount of autologous blood to be collected?

Just as autologous blood donation can be inappropriately utilized, there can also be underutilization of this procedure. In our institution, emergency or semiurgent cardiovascular surgery most often is the reason that preoperative autologous blood donations are underutilized for this patient population. Many of our patients live far away from our medical center. Autologous blood donations can be accomplished efficiently by donation at remote Donor Centers with intrastate (or international) transportation of the autologous blood components, but this obviously requires significant planning and communication. The goals of preoperative autologous blood donations should be (1) to reduce homologous blood exposure, and (2) to provide blood components that are actually needed for the surgical procedure involved.

3. Non-Red Cell Autologous Components

After implementation of an efficient intraoperative autologous blood salvage program at our hospital, we noted that we had successfully reduced the use of homologous red cells more than 50% for the repair of complex aortic aneurysms. However, these patients still required substantial homologous blood exposure due to the transfusion of platelets and plasma. We and others have analyzed the possible benefit of other autologous blood components, especially autologous platelet-rich plasma for patients undergoing major cardiovascular procedures.[5,6] We believe that this technique, if applied with careful patient selection, can be efficient and cost effective in reducing homologous blood exposure. In our institution, suitable patients are those who are undergoing redo coronary artery revascularization, redo cardiac valve replacement, ascending aortic aneurysm repair, and descending thoracic aortic aneurysm repair. Procedures which seldom need platelet or plasma replacement, such as first-time coronary artery revascularization, first-time cardiac valve replacement, and uncomplicated abdominal aortic aneurysm repair are not logical candidates, since less than 10% of these patients require platelets of plasma to achieve hemostasis. On the other hand, patients who typically receive 20 or more units of homologous platelets, such as our thoracoabdominal aneurysm surgery patients or aortic arch repair patients, are not logical candidates. Autologous platelet-rich plasma cannot be expected to have a significant impact on total reduction of homologous exposure in these massively transfused patients. Selection of autologous platelet-rich plasma by apheresis preoperatively or perioperatively in the operating room deserves continued attention and investigation.

Fibrin surgical glue, or so-called fibrin surgical adhesive, has a variety of clinical applications.[7,8] These include use as a topical hemostatic agent at suture lines, as a sealant for cerebrospinal fluid leaks, and as an adhesive in reconstructive otologic and plastic surgical reconstructive procedures. We have used fibrin glue successfully as a mortar for hydroxylapatite.[9] Hydroxylapatite is a granular synthetic bone mineral (calcium salt) substitute which is used mainly in mandibular and maxillary surgical procedures. The fibrin glue is easily obtained by freezing freshly collected plasma at −40°C or colder. The frozen plasma is thawed at 4°C the following day. After concentration by centrifugation, the cryoprecipitate is transferred into a sterile syringe and refrozen until needed. The glue is applied simultaneously with a thrombin solution (usually 50 to 100 units per milliliter) at the surgical site needed. The fibrin glue is nothing more than concentrated cryoprecipitate. It contains fibrinogen, fibronectin, factor VIII, Von Willebrand's factor, and factor XIII. Since most of the clinical applications of fibrin glue adhesive involve elective procedures, this blood derivative should be made from an autologous source whenever possible.

D. UTILIZATION OF AUTOLOGOUS BLOOD

1. Controversy of Crossover

Should autologous blood be converted to homologous use if the patient/donor does not need it? A recent College of American Pathologists survey indicated that less than 15% of reporting institutions would convert autologous units into homologous use.[10] This issue of crossover of autologous blood components into routine homologous use has been extremely controversial. The trend in the U.S. is toward not crossing over these components. Is an autologous blood component collected from a patient/donor who meets all homologous blood donor standard, statistically less safe than that collected from a routine volunteer homologous blood donor? Kruskall emphasizes several problems related to autologous blood donors:[11]

1. Many are patients who have been previously transfused with homologous blood.
2. They have had more hospitalizations than homologous volunteer donors.
3. Like the designated blood donor, they are not true "volunteers".
4. The standards for homologous blood donors are relaxed; the quality of the component, especially red cell mass, may be inferior.

In spite of these concerns, Kruskall and associates have not shown an increase incidence in infectious disease markers in autologous donors compared to routine volunteer homologous blood donors.[12] We have seen a slight increase in the rate of seropositivity for antibodies to hepatitis C (anti-HCV) in autologous donors, but this has not reached statistical significance (unpublished data). A recent report by Connover and associates, however, has failed to show an increase incidence of antibodies to hepatitis C in autologous vs. first-time homologous blood donors.[13] Even though previously transfused autologous blood donors had a higher incidence of anti-HCV reactivity than nontransfused autologous donors, the difference was not statistically significant. Both the FDA and the AABB require that blood collected from autologous donors be specifically labeled for "autologous use only", segregated and stored initially solely for the purpose of the donor/patient. If the blood component is to be made available later for homologous transfusion, the autologous donor label cannot be removed or be obliterated (although the labeling information that indicates the patient's name and identity must of course be removed for the sake of confidentiality). The issue of having a separate label on autologous blood converted into homologous use implies this is a different class of donor from "a true volunteer donor" and therefore, there could be increased legal liability for crossing over autologous blood components. Regardless of the objective data regarding infectious disease marker testing on autologous blood components, the consensus is that autologous blood components should not be crossed over. If we achieve our goals of correct patient selection for autologous blood donation and correct number and type of autologous blood components to be collected for the given surgical indication, the issue of crossover will cease to exit because of a high utilization rate of the blood by the patient who donated it.

2. Infectious Disease Marker Testing

Standards published by the AABB requires that ABO and Rh types must be determined by the facility collecting autologous blood components. If the component will be transfused outside the collecting facility, the first unit collected from a given patient during a one-month period must also be tested for Hepatitis B Surface Antigen, anti-HIV-1, anti-HCV, and any other test recommended and required by the FDA. Infectious disease marker testing, however, is not required if the autologous blood component will be used within the institution where it was collected.

Should all autologous blood components be tested routinely for infectious disease markers? Yomtovian et al.[14] have done an excellent analysis of the expense related to autologous blood collection. A study by Forbes and associates showed that autologous and directed blood components cost approximately 50% more than routine volunteer donor blood.[15] This increased cost of autologous blood collection primarily reflects the increased work of correct labeling, tracking, segregation, and transfusion of specific blood components to specific patient/donors. In addition, the autologous donor often requires much more attention during the phlebotomy phase and the direct attention of the physician responsible at the blood donation facility. Some of the increased costs of autologous blood components could certainly be reduced by eliminating infectious disease marker testing. Current infectious disease marker testing for blood components in the U.S. include Hepatitis B Surface Antigen, anti-HIV 1 and 2, alanine-amino transferase, antibodies to hepatitis B core, anti-HTLV-I (human T-cell lymphotropic virus), anti-HCV (since May or June, 1990), and a serologic test for syphilis. From an economic standpoint, it would seem reasonable to omit infectious disease marker testing for autologous blood components (provided they are not to be shipped outside the collecting facility). Holland gave several arguments against testing autologous blood components in a national conference related to autologous blood transfusion. These arguments included the following:[16]

1. If testing of an autologous blood component leads to a discovery of an infectious disease marker such as hepatitis B Surface Antigen or anti-HIV, the blood components may not be retained for the patient who donated it. Autologous blood components with confirmed Hepatitis B Surface Antigen positivity or Western Blot-confirmed anti-HIV and anti-HTLV-I will be discarded and the donor will not be allowed to give additional blood components. Recently, the FDA has clarified the recommendations related to autologous components that test positive for anti-HCV. Blood components testing positive for anti-HCV may be retained for autologous use only (labeled "biohazard" and properly segregated). The attending physician should be notified of the anti-HCV positivity but does not have to respond with written permission for the unit to be retained for the autologous donor.
2. If autologous blood components are not going to be crossed over into homologous use, testing adds unnecessary expense to the processing of autologous blood.
3. Discovery of significant infectious disease markers in the autologous blood component should create no more hazard for those handling the blood component than other blood components in the blood bank inventory (all of which should be considered a potential biohazard, regardless of testing result).

Dr. Silvergleid and others have emphasized that complete testing of autologous blood components enables the blood center to dispose of dangerous blood components, especially those that might be infectious for hepatitis or retroviruses.[17] Will testing autologous blood help protect patients and health care workers handling the blood component?

We believe that routine processing of autologous units (in the same manner as other blood components) avoids a break in standard operating procedure. Although minimum processing of autologous blood components may reduce cost, may simplify record keeping, and avoid the complications from abnormal laboratory results to the patient/donor, the national trend is toward testing of autologous blood. The FDA has recommended that autologous blood with confirmed positive markers for Hepatitis B Surface Antigen, anti-HIV, and anti-HTLV-1 be discarded. These donors should not give additional autologous components. The discovery of a significant infectious disease marker in an autologous donor may improve that patient's future care. In our region all autologous blood components are now fully tested. Autologous blood components that are reactive for Hepatitis B Surface Antigen, anti-HIV, and anti-HTLV-1 (the latter two confirmed by Western Blot) are discarded. These individuals are not allowed to make additional blood donations. Unfortunately, there is still no national standardized procedure for handling and processing of autologous blood components. This lack of standardization is especially a problem when patients attempt to donate autologous blood components outside of the region in which their surgery will be done. Units with positive infectious disease markers may be difficult for outside centers to ship across state boundaries. Components with infectious disease markers such as anti-hepatitis B core, elevated alanine-amino transferase, reactive serologic test for syphilis, and/or anti-HCV seropositivity can be retained and/or shipped with the appropriate packaging and biohazard labels applied to the blood components. Correct and precise labeling of autologous blood components is an important quality assurance and legal issue. As noted above, any autologous unit crossed over to homologous units must still be clearly labeled that it was derived from an autologous source.

More important, it is necessary to have a labeling system that helps to assure that this blood component will be retained and transfused to the correct patient/donor. Our procedure is to have a label that indicates the blood component is for autologous use only. The patient's name, hospital number and/or social security number, the patient's physician, date of surgery, and patient's signature are affixed to this label. A sample of our label as well the labels and tags from our Regional Blood Center are included as Figures 1 and 2. Since we do not cross over autologous blood components, great care is taken to have these components labeled distinctly from routine homologous blood components. After completion of all testing, including those for infectious disease markers, the autologous blood components are brought to the Transfusion Service where they are retained in alphabetic order in a special refrigerator reserved only for autologous blood components. Segregation of autologous blood components from routine homologous blood components is extremely important.

E. STORAGE OF AUTOLOGOUS RED CELLS

1. Liquid Storage

Current red cell preservative solutions typically allow 35- or 42-day storage. The blood preservative solution systems containing additional adenine and glucose allow the packed autologous cells to be stored for a period of 42

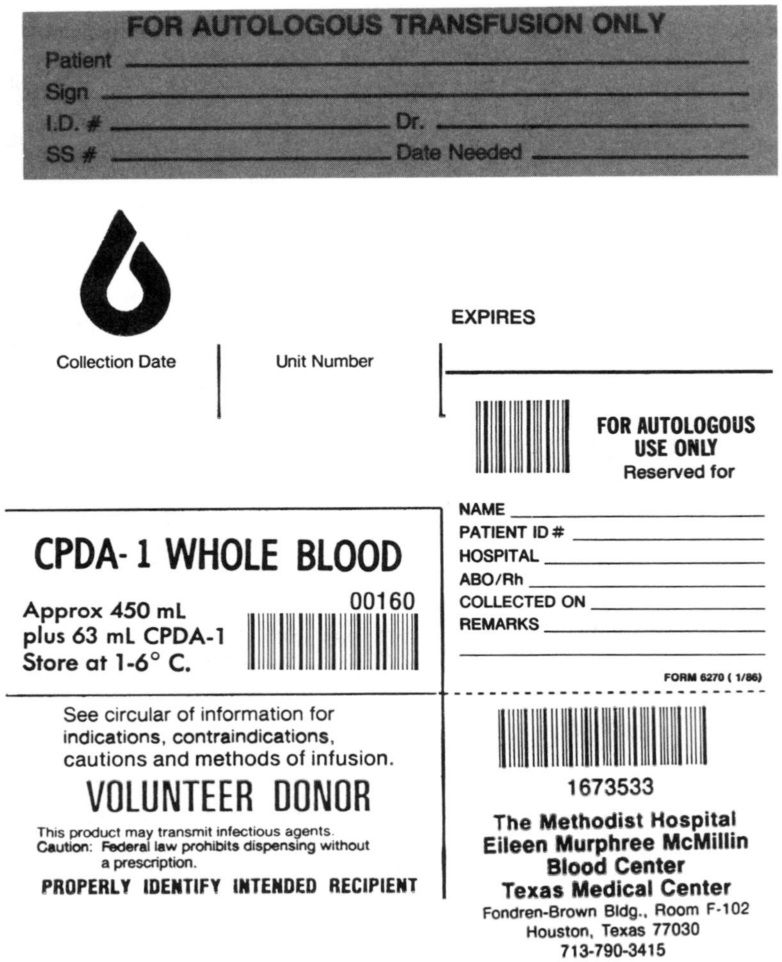

FOR AUTOLOGOUS TRANSFUSION ONLY

Patient ____________________
Sign ____________________
I.D. # ____________ Dr. ____________
SS # ____________ Date Needed ____________

Collection Date | Unit Number | EXPIRES

FOR AUTOLOGOUS USE ONLY
Reserved for

NAME ____________
PATIENT ID # ____________
HOSPITAL ____________
ABO/Rh ____________
COLLECTED ON ____________
REMARKS ____________

FORM 6270 (1/86)

CPDA-1 WHOLE BLOOD

Approx 450 mL
plus 63 mL CPDA-1
Store at 1-6° C.

00160

See circular of information for indications, contraindications, cautions and methods of infusion.

VOLUNTEER DONOR

This product may transmit infectious agents.
Caution: Federal law prohibits dispensing without a prescription.

PROPERLY IDENTIFY INTENDED RECIPIENT

1673533

The Methodist Hospital
Eileen Murphree McMillin
Blood Center
Texas Medical Center
Fondren-Brown Bldg., Room F-102
Houston, Texas 77030
713-790-3415

FIGURE 1. Labels for autologous blood collected in our donor center. All labels are applied to the collection bag.

days. The disadvantage of the latter preservative system is that the plasma removed from the autologous blood component must either be discarded, frozen, or retained in some manner to assure that it is available for the autologous patient/donor if needed. Because of the problems of tracking the autologous plasma and because of the rare breakage of an autologous blood component in the centrifuge during component separation, the majority of our autologous blood components are collected as whole blood in citrate phosphate dextrose adenine 1 (CPDA-1) preservative. This preservative solution is approved for 35 days storage. Most patients for major surgical

AUTOLOGOUS DONATION

Patient Name:__________

Hospital:__________

SSN #:__________

Component needed: ☐ Whole blood

☐ Other__________

Blood Unit I.D.:__________

Date of donation:_____ Exp. Date:_____

Date of Surgery:__________

X__________
PATIENT SIGNATURE

Present This Card to Hospital Blood Bank on Admission.
A Unit of Blood was Collected From

____

For Autologous Transfusion.

Blood Unit I.D.:__________

SSN #:__________

Date of donation:_____ Exp. Date:_____

Date of surgery__________

X__________
Patient Signature

Gulf Coast Regional Blood Center GC307

AUTOLOGOUS DONOR

FOR AUTOLOGOUS TRANSFUSION USE ONLY

Gulf Coast Regional Blood Center
Houston, Texas

PATIENT NAME:__________

HOSPITAL:__________

SOCIAL SECURITY NO.:__________

DATE OF USAGE:__________

PHYSICIAN'S NAME:__________

GC 240-306 Rev 3/91

ABO GROUP
LABEL

FIGURE 2. Labels for autologous blood collected at our regional blood center. The left label is used as a tag with a detachable card given to the patient/donor. The right label is applied to the collection bag.

procedure can donate the required number of blood components within this 35-day interval. If the plasma is not desired at the time of transfusion, it is removed before issue of the blood component by the simple plasma separation bag compression device available in the Transfusion Service. (The satellite bags are maintained with the whole blood in case it is necessary to remove the plasma from the closed multibag system.)

Most surgeons and anesthesiologists appreciate whole blood for major cardiovascular procedures and other major procedures where there is substantial blood loss. There is growing concern about cryophilic bacterial overgrowth (especially *Yersinia enterocolitica*) in units of blood older than 25 days.[18] Autologous donors with unexplained diarrheal illness should be carefully evaluated before being allowed to donate.

2. Cryopreservation

Glycerol is an excellent red cell cryoprotective agent. Most transfusion services and regional blood centers have the capability of glycerolization and cryopreservation of autologous red cells. Cryopreservation of autologous red cells adds considerable expense (in our institution, approximately $100.00 of additional expense). Furthermore, there is increased risk of breakage of the component at many stages during the preparation for cryopreservation, thawing, and deglycerolization. Many logistical problems complicate thawing the cryopreserved red cells. If all the units are thawed at the time of surgery and not needed, then these components should be outdated or discarded 24 hours after deglycerolization. Because of the limited shelf life of deglycerolized red cells and added expense related to cryopreservation of autologous red cells we have discouraged this practice, except in cases where large numbers of blood components are needed for elective surgery. These procedures include major plastic surgical reconstructive procedures, some neurosurgical procedures, and maternal blood that is collected for possible use both by the mother or her fetus or neonate.

Patients who have produced multiple allo-antibodies or who are immunized to high-frequency antigens are logical candidates for autologous red cell cryopreservation. Frequently these individuals have had previous surgery and may need repeat procedures in the future. They are encouraged to donate cryopreserved autologous red cells, even though there is no certain or known anticipated surgical need. Only a small percentage of our total autologous blood red cell transfusions are derived from cryopreserved red cells.

F. SPECIFIC QUALITY ASSURANCE ISSUES AND PREOPERATIVE AUTOLOGOUS DONATION

Yomtovian has emphasized some of the common and very important quality assurance issues related to autologous blood components.[1] The blood component may be outdated because surgery is postponed. Instead of the autologous blood component, directed or other homologous blood components may be given prior to utilization of all autologous blood components available.

The autologous blood component may be left in a remote operating room refrigerator and become lost or outdated. The glycerolized frozen autologous blood component can be prematurely thawed and outdated. The blood bank may mistakenly release homologous blood when autologous blood is available or the blood bank may release the autologous blood component to the wrong recipient. This most often occurs when two patients with the same last name have given autologous blood components. Autologous blood components collected outside the region arrive after the surgery has been completed. Autologous blood components are damaged or broken during processing or transportation, or at the time of the attempted transfusion. Autologous blood components may be collected by a facility that does not perform infectious

AVAILABLE AUTOLOGOUS AND DESIGNATED UNITS

October 7, 1991 Page 1

PATIENT NAME	PT.ID#	PT	TY	UNIT#	COMPO	UN	TY	SUR DA	S
Allen, Mary Jo	32485985	B	POS	M1284	AUWB1	B	POS	911007	Y
Bodie, Annie	14532671	AB	POS	M4032	AUWB1	AB	POS	911007	Y
Braun, Christy	48596689	B	POS	M3568	DDRBC	B	POS	911001	Y
Cole, David	52879863	0	POS	M4583	DDRBC	0	POS	911019	Y
Dole, Pine	35276918	A	POS	M5698	AUWB1	A	POS	911010	Y
Green, Eva	98346712	0	NEG	M8900	AUWB1	0	NEG	911029	Y

FIGURE 3. Sample of a portion of our database tracking system for autologous and directed donors. The list is generated daily from an IBM-compatible personal computer. Patient name is followed by hospital number **(PT. ID#)**, patient's blood type **(PT TY)**, blood component, e.g., designated donor red blood cells etc., autologous whole blood CPDA-1 etc. **(DDRBC, AUWB1)**, blood type of unit **(UN TY)**, date of surgery (**Year/month/day — SUR DA**). **S** stands for storage fee being applied. The names and hospital numbers are fictitious in this exhibit.

disease markers. The patient may change physician or hospital. The blood is sent to the new facility, it is tested and found to have a positive marker and then is discarded. In institutions which allow crossover autologous blood component, it may be used as homologous blood, but the patient may return later and expect the component to be available. All of these problems require notification of the patient and attending physician.

A careful tracking system is necessary to avoid the above errors and problems related to autologous blood components. Our technologists developed a personal computer program which tracks the availability and disposition of autologous blood components[19] (Figure 3: fictitious names and hospital numbers). The medical technologist processing blood components each day updates the computerized list of autologous and directed donors. Some institutions use special stickers or alerts to both the attending physician and the nursing staff that a particular patient has autologous components of blood available.

Inappropriate collection and utilization of autologous blood is a major quality assurance issue. Should we have the same audit and review criteria for the use of autologous red cells as for homologous red cells? Should an elderly, weakened lady with a hemoglobin of 8.5 g/dl after major cardiovascular surgery be denied transfusion with 2 units of autologous blood because of the small risk of clerical error, bacterial contamination, or volume overload? Should the same standards be applied for the use of autologous blood components in this patient as the use of homologous blood component? There is no clear-cut answer to this question. In our institution, we review all homologous red cell transfusions given when the patient's hemoglobin is 8.5 g/dl or greater.

We do not review autologous blood transfusions unless they are given at a hemoglobin of 10 g/dl or greater. Therefore we do have different criteria for monitoring the use of autologous vs. homologous red cells. We believe this is justified because of the increased safety of autologous blood components. On the other hand, many experts believe that the use of autologous blood should be reviewed with the same set of criteria as the use of homologous blood. Some institutions have attempted to help physicians develop guidelines for the collection and transfusion of autologous blood. Goldfinger at Cedars Sinai Hospital in Los Angeles has produced what he terms a ''schedule of optimal preoperative collection of autologous blood (SOPCAB).''[19a] This set of guidelines is designed to reduce under- and overcollection of blood components for specific surgical procedures. For example, this SOPCAB recommends 5 units of autologous blood be collected for coronary artery bypass surgery and cardiac valve replacement, 3 units for total hip replacement and prostatectomy, 2 units for laminectomy and hysterectomy, and 1 unit for transurethral resection of prostate. The schedule recommends no units be collected for procedures such as knee arthroscopy, Burch repair, dilatation and curettage of the uterus, nasal sinus repair, etc. Even though the schedule may not precisely predict the actual need for blood usage for these particular surgical procedures, it at least shows that this institution is facing the important questions of who should donate autologous blood and how much. The schedule can be modified easily after data is accumulated to validate or invalidate the recommendations for each surgical procedure. A similar set of guidelines can be developed for the use of perioperative autologous transfusion and the collection of specialized autologous components, such as platelet-rich plasma, plasma, and autologous fibrin glue. As with all blood components, the transfusion service dealing with autologous blood should have a clear record of the final disposition of the units. In response to a large number of inquiries about FDA guidelines and recommendations for handling of autologous blood components, a memorandum from the FDA was issued in February of 1990. This memorandum, entitled ''Autologous Blood Collection and Processing Procedures: January 1990'', is an additional important current reference for those facilities handling autologous blood components. Many of the controversies and questions related to the development of this FDA memorandum can be avoided by fully testing all autologous blood components, avoiding crossover of autologous blood components, and discarding autologous blood components with confirmed infectious disease markers for Hepatitis B Surface Antigen, anti-HIV, and anti-HLTV-1.

G. FUTURE TRENDS

Preoperative autologous blood donation is only worthwhile if it reduces or totally eliminates the need for homologous transfusion therapy. An important development in transfusion medicine is the concept of minimal donor exposure. The Mayo Clinic group has been a leader in promoting this concept. Patients who are candidates for certain surgical procedures can meet with a transfusion medicine representative for counseling to map out a strategy which will best reduce the need for homologous blood transfusion.[20] Several centers, including ours, have realized that sometimes it is impossible for the patient to give adequate amounts of autologous blood for the intended surgical procedure. A directed blood donor can give multiple components to supplement autologous blood donors. We call these individuals "surrogate autologous donors". These donors not only provide serial donations of whole blood but also can be called upon to provide platelet-rich plasma and other blood components. Using this strategy, many of our young patients undergoing orthopedic surgery (especially young girls having scoliosis correction) can avoid homologous exposure except for one parent. A designated donor giving whole blood and apheresis platelet concentrates can greatly reduce homologous blood exposure for cardiovascular surgery patients. As long as the directed donor meets complete homologous blood standards, including all infectious disease marker testing, we believe that this donor is as safe as any routine volunteer donor and that multiple donations from this individual increase the safety of transfusion therapy by limiting donor exposure. Within the past few years, one documented threat of directed blood donations has been clearly defined.[21] There is a small risk of graft-vs.-host disease when closely related directed blood donors (first-degree relatives such as siblings, parents, and their children) are used as directed blood donors. Irradiation with 1500 to 5000 rad will almost eliminate this risk of this rare complication. Therefore it is now standard practice in most centers to irradiate directed blood donations from all first-degree relatives. Another recent and controversial practice related to autologous blood donation is whether or not pharmacologic doses of recombinant human erythropoietin (rHEPO) can improve our success with autologous transfusion practice.

Goodnough and Brittenham[22] found that 30 out of 175 patients attempting to donate blood for elective orthopedic surgery were deferred for anemia with hematocrits below 34% when they attempted to donate the required amount of blood preoperatively. Anemia is a relatively common reason for elderly patients requiring major orthopedic surgical procedures not to be able to donate the full amount of autologous blood requested for the intended procedure. Endogenous release of erythropoietin apparently does not occur until the hematocrit is well below the minimum standard (33%) established for autologous blood donation. Would supplemental erythropoietin be useful for this population of patients? Some groups suggest that erythropoietin may improve the ability for some patients to donate the required amount of blood.[23] Furthermore, the red cell mass found in the number of units donated tends to be higher in those patients receiving erythropoietin. This, of course, is because many of the erythropoietin-treated patients had a higher hematocrit and red cell mass at the time of donation of teach autologous unit of blood. A report published in 1991 in the *New England Journal of Medicine* failed to show a statistical reduction in homologous blood exposure in patients receiving erythropoietin compared to a placebo group of autologous donors who did not receive this agent.[24] In addition to possible lack of efficacy in some patients, erythropoietin will add a marked increase in the cost of obtaining autologous blood.

New technologic developments benefit autologous blood transfusion programs. One such development in the last decade is the availability of the so-called "sterile docking device". This instrument (manufactured by Dupont and marketed by Haemonetics) is able to make sterile welds or splices in plastic tubing. This allows customized alteration of closed multiple blood collection bag systems. For example, for many of our patients receiving isovolemic saline replacement, we weld in a side port into the multibag blood collection system. After the phlebotomy is completed, intravenous saline can be administered through this side port. This avoids a second venepuncture. Many of the pregnant patients from whom we collect autologous blood are alloimmunized and their fetuses are at risk for hemolytic disease of the newborn. We have used the sterile docking device to make aliquots of the maternal blood for cryopreservation into a quadruple bag system (50 cc per bag). These aliquots can be deglycerolyzed individually for multiple intrauterine fetal transfusions.

III. PERIOPERATIVE AUTOLOGOUS BLOOD SALVAGE AND TRANSFUSION

A. INDICATIONS

Preoperative donation of autologous blood and blood components is only one part of a comprehensive program of blood conservation. Many patients requiring major cardiovascular surgery are unable to donate adequate blood components preoperatively. They may require surgery on an emergency basis or their clinical condition may not allow adequate preoperative blood component donation. Cardiovascular surgery patients are a complex group. Patients undergoing first-time coronary artery revascularization or first-time cardiac valve surgery usually require much fewer blood components than patients undergoing repeat operations. Long periods of cardiopulmonary bypass, excess hemodilution, profound hypothermia and circulatory arrest (utilized for aortic arch repair), antiplatelet and anticoagulant therapy can all dramatically increase perioperative blood loss and the need for blood component replacement.

We have had extensive experience with blood salvage for complex aortic aneurysms. Intraoperative blood salvage in this patient population greatly reduces homologous red cell exposure. However, many other major cardiovascular procedures and orthopedic procedures benefit much less from intraoperative blood salvage. In general, unless the surgical blood loss is expected to exceed 1000 cc, intraoperative blood salvage may add little to reduction of homologous blood use and may in fact increase the cost of blood replacement.[25] As in preoperative autologous blood donation, intraoperative blood salvage should be used selectively for those patients in whom a definite benefit (significant reduction of homologous blood transfusion) can be documented. In our institution, intraoperative blood salvage is most effective for repeat cardiovascular procedures, major orthopedic procedures (total hip and total knee replacements), and occasional neurosurgical procedures, such as repair of intracranial arteriovenous malformations.

Immediate preoperative or perioperative collection of autologous platelet-rich plasma may also be of benefit to some patients undergoing cardiopulmonary bypass procedures. Customizing a comprehensive autologous transfusion program requires focused interaction between the transfusion medicine specialist, the patient, the attending surgeon, and the anesthesiology team.

B. CURRENT INSTRUMENTATION AND TECHNOLOGY

There are numerous manufacturers of intraoperative and postoperative blood salvage systems. These devices fall into two main categories: canister-type collection containers which allow harvest of shed blood and transfusion with or without processing, and semiautomated blood salvage systems. The prototype of the canister-type system is the Sorenson device developed by Noon and associates in the 1970s.[26] This device uses a rigid, nondisposable plastic outer canister to which a vacuum is applied. Blood is collected into a disposable plastic inner liner. Blood is aspirated from the surgical field through double lumen tubing. Anticoagulant is added through the smaller lumen to anticoagulate the harvested blood. The anticoagulant used in these systems is most often citrate solution, but heparin can also be used. When sufficient blood has been harvested, it can be transfused to the patient directly by removing the inner liner and connecting it to a filter and blood administration set. Alternatively, the inner liner can be labeled and sent to a remote processing site (usually the transfusion service) where the salvaged blood can be concentrated and washed with a cell-washing system. Most institutions use the COBE 2991 for this purpose. Direct infusion of salvaged blood from these canister systems has the obvious advantage of increased simplicity and decreased cost, but with some of the disadvantages of infusing nonprocessed salvaged blood (see below). Since the development of the Sorenson system, many other manufacturers have developed disposable canister-type devices from which shed blood can be harvested both during surgery and in the postoperative period. These devices can be connected directly to a surgical wound (for example: to drain the site of a major orthopedic procedure) or can be placed in series with chest tube systems for patients having intrathoracic cardiovascular and pulmonary procedures. From an economic standpoint, these canister devices appear best suited to procedures from which the equivalent of one to three units of red blood cells are harvested.[25]

A number of manufacturers market semiautomated blood salvage systems. Many features are common to all of these systems. The blood shed during surgery is aspirated through a double lumen tubing similar to that used for the canister-type systems. A solution of heparin, citrate, or combination of heparin and citrate is added through a small tube into the larger-diameter tube into which the shed blood is aspirated. Aspiration of the shed blood is accomplished by a cardiotomy-type reservoir, to which a vacuum is applied.

Most of these reservoirs have either a macro- or microaggregate filter to remove gross particulate material from the salvaged blood. Blood harvested into the cardiotomy reservoir is then transferred using a roller pump into a disposable centrifuge bowl. The centrifuge bowl permits for concentration and then washing of the salvaged blood. Supernatant plasma and excess saline used in washing is diverted into a waste bag. After concentration and washing, the salvaged red cells are pumped into a sterile bag for infusion to the patient. Some particulate material is always present in this salvaged blood and most centers recommend transfusion through a microaggregate filter. These blood salvage systems have been well described in a recent review.[27]

The semiautomated systems are capable of producing salvaged red cells of good quality. However, they are somewhat complex to operate. There are a number of potential hazards both to the users of the devices and to the patient. Furthermore, the capital cost of acquiring this technology is expensive (currently typically in excess of $25,000). The disposables required for each patient can cost more than $150.00. We believe that a trained dedicated operator should be available to operate the system. The operation of this system should not be delegated to individuals with other duties during the surgical procedure. The operator should understand the technical aspects of the device and understand the potential risks and hazards. Because of the economic considerations, we believe these devices are best suited for surgical procedures such as cardiovascular cases and major orthopedic surgery where blood loss is expected to exceed 1000 cc during the perioperative period.

C. QUALITY OF SALVAGED BLOOD

We and others have noted that aspiration of salvaged blood from tissue surfaces causes increased hemolysis and trauma to red cells.[28] Aspiration of shed blood from pools of blood with elimination of an air-blood interface reduces trauma and injury to red cells. Furthermore, excessive vacuum used during aspiration will hemolyze red cells. We recommend −100 mmHg vacuum. We have examined the characteristics of blood salvaged from complex aortic aneurysms. We believe the best possible quality of salvage blood is available from this type of procedure. Large amounts of blood are shed rapidly; the surgeon can aspirate blood from pools. The blood is quickly accumulated into the reservoir and is immediately processed and returned to the patient.

In these cases most of the blood is shed during the early part of aneurysm repair procedure (in other words, after aortic clamping and opening of the aneurysm). Once mechanical hemostasis is achieved, blood loss in these cases declines. Even so, blood harvested from these cases typically has a lower than normal hemoglobin, usually in the rang eof 7 to 8 g/dl. It has a considerably elevated free hemoglobin. Potassium content is usually within normal limits or only slightly elevated. The blood is somewhat alkaline. Anticoagulant (either heparin or citrate, or combination thereof) is always present in the unprocessed blood. This blood typically is low in total protein, including coagulation proteins. Concentration and washing in the semiautomated devices has the beneficial effect of removing most of the anticoagulant, most of the free hemoglobin, and achieving a uniform or standardized hematocrit, usually well above 50%. Concentration and washing will not remove particulate debris with specific gravity equal to or greater than erythrocytes. As noted above, we recommend transfusion of this blood through a microaggregate filter. Blood salvaged from orthopedic cases always has a higher fat content, lower initial hemoglobin, higher free hemoglobin, and more tissue debris. Blood from these cases is usually collected much more slowly and by skimming of tissue surfaces. Washing of salvaged blood greatly reduces procoagulant protein levels and functional platelets. Therefore, patients receiving massive amounts of salvaged blood may develop a severe dilutional coagulopathy if supplemental platelet-rich plasma is not given. Patients undergoing massive transfusion of salvaged blood should be monitored with routine coagulation tests and platelet counts.

D. HAZARDS AND COMPLICATIONS ASSOCIATED WITH SALVAGED BLOOD

There are risks both to the operator, surgical team, and patient when intraoperative blood salvage is employed. Hazards to the operator and surgical team include: implosion of the cardiotomy reservoir due to the application of excess negative pressure, breakage and rupture of the disposable centrifuge bowl, and accidental needle sticks due to careless or improper handling of the salvaged blood as it is transferred or transfused. Hazards to the patient are potentially fatal. A poor-quality component can result due to lack of understanding of the function of the centrifuge bowl. If insufficient red cells are added to the bowl, the salvaged blood component will have a reduced hematocrit. Furthermore, since the red cells contribute to the efficiency of washing by volume displacement, inadequate red cells in the bowl will mean a poorer washout of anticoagulant and other undesirable materials in the salvaged blood. Improper use of the devices can also lead to inadequate washout of anticoagulant. A dreaded and disastrous complication with any semiautomated blood salvage device is air embolism due to careless transfer of air into the infusion bag.[29] Because of this, many centers ask that the technician operating the device transfer the salvaged blood into a sterile bag which can be handed to the anesthesia team for infusion. Additives to the surgical field such as microfibrillar collagen, toxic antibiotics, amniotic fluid, and methylmethracrylate pose additional hazards, since these materials are not completely washed out. The presence of neoplastic cells and bacterial contamination are also contraindications for the use of intraoperative blood salvage. We are concerned about *ex vivo* sickling of red cells, so patients with sickling hemoglobinopathies are not allowed to have intraoperative red cell salvage (or to donate blood preoperatively).

Recently Brian Bull and associates at Loma Linda have investigated the existence of "salvaged blood syndrome".[30] This syndrome is attributed to trapping of leukocytes and platelets on the inner surface of the disposable plastic centrifuge bowl. Leukocytes and platelets caught beneath the layer of packed erythrocytes undergo activation with release of leukoattractants and vasoactive materials. The syndrome has features of disseminated intravascular coagulation. Noncardiogenic pulmonary and generalized edema result from endothelial cell injury. Excessive dilution of the salvaged blood and the presence of calcium ions appear to aggravate the tendency for this syndrome to develop in an experimental model studied by Bull and his associates. We have performed thousands of cases of intraoperative blood salvage and have not recognized this syndrome in our institution. Nevertheless, we have recommended avoiding excess dilution of the salvaged blood (for example, excessive use of irrigation into the operative field during blood salvage) and we have recently added citrate to our heparin anticoagulant solution.

E. QUALITY ASSURANCE ISSUES OF INTRAOPERATIVE BLOOD SALVAGE

We believe that the first step in quality assurance and quality improvement of intraoperative blood salvage is to form a team of carefully trained and dedicated individuals who can operate the device. This team can be supervised by the transfusion service, the perfusion service, anesthesiology, surgery, the nursing service, or even an outside agency, such as a regional blood center. This activity should be coordinated with the transfusion service and have input with the supervisory staff and medical directors of the hospital's blood bank. Monitoring of the following parameters by the hospital transfusion committee or quality assurance committee can greatly improve and maintain the quality of this service:

1. Is intraoperative blood salvage being used for the appropriate case? Do the procedures usually yield more than one bowl of salvaged blood?
2. Periodic checking of the hematocrit and free hemoglobin of salvaged blood will help assure proper processing of the salvaged blood. We also periodically monitor residual free heparin level.
3. Monitoring of total transfusion requirements of patients undergoing intraoperative blood salvage. This indicates whether or not intraoperative blood salvage has made a significant impact on reducing homologous red cell exposure.

4. Did the patient have any pulmonary, renal infectious disease, or hemostasis problems which could be linked to the intraoperative blood salvage procedure?

IV. CONCLUSIONS

Autologous blood transfusion is most effective when a specific program is tailored for the patient's particular needs. For example, patients undergoing major orthopedic surgery (total knee or total hip replacement) may best benefit by an effective program of preoperative autologous blood donation. Patients requiring repair of thoracoabdominal aneurysms will benefit most by intraoperative blood salvage. Perioperative autologous platelet-rich plasma collected by apheresis may be indicated in carefully selected patients. Some patients will require supplementation of preoperative donations with perioperative blood salvage. The role of recombinant erythropoietin for selected autologous blood transfusion programs is still not clear. Cost containment with monitoring of under- and overutilization of autologous transfusion modalities should be critically analyzed in every institution offering autologous blood programs. Careful labeling and tracking of autologous blood components should be a major quality assurance focus.

REFERENCES

1. **Yomtovian, R. and Yawn, D. H.,** Autologous and Directed Blood Transfusion Therapy: Developing a Strategy for the 1990's, presented at the American Society of Clinical Pathologists Meeting, New Orleans, September 29, 1991.
2. **Widman, F. K., Ed.,** Standards for Blood Banks and Transfusion Services, 14th ed., American Association of Blood Banks, Arlington, VA, 1991.
3. **Kruskall, M. S., Leonard, S., and Klapholz, H.,** Autologous blood donation during pregnancy: analysis of safety and blood use, *Obstet. Gynecol.*, 70, 938, 1987.
4. **Owings, D. V., Kruskall, M. S., Thurer, R. L. et al.,** Autologous donations prior to elective cardiac surgery: safety and effect on subsequent use, *JAMA*, 262, 1963, 1989.
5. **Noon, G. P., Jones, J., Fehir, K. et al.,** Use of preoperatively obtained platelets and plasma in patients undergoing cardiopulmonary bypass, *J. Clin. Apher.*, 5, 91, 1990.
6. **Giordano, F. G., Rivers, S. L., Chung, G. K. T. et al.,** Autologous platelet rich plasma in cardiac surgery: effect on intraoperative and postoperative transfusion requirements, *Ann. Thorac. Surg.*, 46, 416, 1988.
7. **Rosou, J. A., Engelman, R. M., and Breyer, R. H.,** Fibrin glue: an effective hemostatic agent for nonsutarable intraoperative bleeding, *Ann. Thorac. Surg.*, 90, 766, 1986.
8. **Stark, J. and DeLeval, M.,** Experience with fibrin seal (Tisseel) in operations for congenital heart disease, *Ann. Thorac. Surg.*, 38, 411, 1984.
9. **Maldonado, O. and Yawn, D. H.,** An Alveolar Ridge Implant Composed of Hydroxylapatite, Autologous Fibrin Glue and Collagen, presented at Second International Congress on Preposthetic Surgery, Palm Springs, May, 1987.

10. College of American Pathologists AABB/CAP Donor Module of Survey, College of American Pathologists, Northfield, IL, 1991.
11. **Kruskall, M. S.,** Autologous blood collection and transfusion in a tertiary care center, in *Autologous Transfusion and Hemotherapy,* Taswell, H. F. and Pineda, A. A., Eds., Blackwell Scientific, Boston, 1991, chap. 3.
12. **Kruskall, M. S., Popvsky, M. A., Pacini, D. G. et al.,** Autologous vs. homologous donors: evaluation of markers for infectious disease, *Transfusion,* 28, 286, 1988.
13. **Connover, P. T., Fang, E., Lam, N. V. et al.,** Antibodies to hepatitis C in autologous blood donors, *Transfusion,* 31, 616, 1991.
14. **Yomtovian, R. A., Shrank, J. Y., Betts, J. M. et al.,** Transfusion of previously donated blood in a community hospital, in *Autologous Transfusion and Hemotherapy,* Taswell, H. F., and Pineda, A. A., Eds., Blackwell Scientific, Boston, 1991, chap. 4.
15. **Forbes, J., Anderson, M., Anderson, G. et al.,** Blood transfusion costs: a multicenter Study, *Transfusion,* 31, 318, 1991.
16. **Holland, P. V.,** Why test autologous units?, in *Autologous Blood Transfusions: Current Issues,* Maffei, L. M. and Thurer, R. L., Eds., American Association of Blood Banks, Arlington, VA, 1988, 167.
17. **Silvergleid, A. J.,** All blood collected should be tested for infectious disease markers, in *Autologous Blood Transfusions: Current Issues,* Maffei, L. M. and Thurer, R. L., Eds., American Association of Blood Banks, Arlington, VA, 1988, 177.
18. **Wright, D. C., Selss, I. F., Vintonk, J. et al.,** Fatal Yersinia enterocolitica sepsis after blood transfusion, *Arch. Pathol. Lab. Med.,* 109, 982, 1985.
19. **Burrough, J. and Riggan, L.,** A Computer Database Method for Tracking Autologous and Designated Blood Units, presented at the American Association of Blood Banks Annual Meeting, Kansas City, Oct., 1988.
19a. **Axelrod, F. B., Pepkowitz, S. H., and Goldfinger, D.,** Establishment of a schedule of optimum preoperative collection of autologous blood, *Transfusion,* 29, 677, 1989.
20. **Brecher, M. E., Moore, S. B., and Taswell, H. F.,** Minimal exposure transfusion: a new approach to homologous blood transfusion, *Mayo Clin. Proc.,* 63, 903, 1988.
21. **Anderson, K. C. and Weinstein, H. J.,** Transfusion associated graft versus host disease, *N. Engl. J. Med.,* 323, 315, 1990.
22. **Goodnough, L. T. and Brittenham, G. M.,** Limitations of the erythropoietic response to serial phlebotomy, *J. Lab. Clin. Med.,* 115, 28, 1990.
23. **Kruskall, M. S., Chambers, L. A., Goldberg, M. A. et al.,** Daily Subcutaneous Recombinant Erythropoietin (rHEPO) Facilitates Blood Donation, Presented at International Society of Blood Transfusion/American Association of Blood Banks, Los Angeles, Abstracts, 1990, 188.
24. **Erslev, A. H.,** Drug therapy: erythropoietin, *N. Engl. J. Med.,* 324, 1339, 1991.
25. **Solomon, M. D., Rutledge, M. L., Kane, L. E. et al.,** Cost comparison intraoperative autologous versus homologous transfusion, *Transfusion,* 28, 379, 1988.
26. **Noon, G. P., Solis, R. T., and Natelson, E. A.,** A simple method of intraoperative autotransfusion, *Surg. Gynecol. Obstet.,* 143, 65, 1976.
27. **Williamson, K. R. and Taswell, H. F.,** Intraoperative blood salvage: a review, *Transfusion,* 31, 662, 1991.
28. **Yawn, D. H.,** Properties of salvaged blood, in *Autologous Transfusion and Hemotherapy,* Taswell, H. F. and Pineda, A. A., Eds., Blackwell Scientific, Boston, 1991, chap. 10.
29. Air embolism from autotransfusion units, *ECRI Rep.,* 10, 239, 1986.
30. **Bull, B. S. and Bull, M. H.,** Enhancing the safety of intraoperative RBC salvage, *Br. J. Trauma,* 29, 320, 1989.

Chapter 8

QUALITY ASSURANCE FOR DIRECTED DONATIONS

Samuel H. Pepkowitz and Dennis Goldfinger

TABLE OF CONTENTS

ISBN 0-8493-4938-9

I. INTRODUCTION

Directed blood donation programs allow blood and blood components to be donated by the friends and family of patients and to be reserved for use, at least for a period of time, by only the specified patient. The fear of contracting AIDS through transfusion of components from random community blood donors was no doubt the moving force behind the initiation and growth of these programs in the 1980s: our program opened in February, 1983 and averaged 86 donations per month for the first half year; for the same 6 months in 1990, we averaged 358 collections per month. Proponents of directed donor programs held that patients could select specific donors whose blood would be safer for them to receive than would be the "anonymous" donations in the community supply. Prior to explicit self-exclusion of donors whose environmental-social histories placed them into groups known to be at high risk for carrying the human immunodeficiency virus (HIV), and prior to the introduction of tests for exposure to HIV, it was logical to many health care workers and patients living in AIDS-endemic areas that patients might indeed be able to choose such suitable donors. The desired donor characteristics thought to make directed donor blood safer than a random collection included a spousal or nuclear family relationship with the intended recipient, female gender, being a sexual partner of the intended recipient, or being beyond middle age. In areas with low levels of HIV infection, physicians often held an opposite opinion, namely that directed donation was not only unnecessary, but a waste of limited donor room and transfusion service personnel and time. Furthermore, it was postulated by some that directed donations would actually provide transfusion components having a greater probability of disease transmission than did the community supply, because donor coercion and peer pressure would not allow high-risk individuals to decline gracefully. Also, the likelihood of there being an increased number of first-time donors might result in an increased percentage of deferrals and false-negative tests.

This dichotomy of approaches to directed donation has continued, and somewhat by geographic areas, has solidified to become fixed policy. For example, in California there is now a law stipulating that directed donations must be allowed at donor centers,[1] and the units so obtained must be accepted by transfusion services. Meanwhile, in other locales, for example, Chapel Hill, North Carolina, there may be no provision for drawing, storing, or transfusing directed donations.

The purpose of this chapter is not to rehash the rationale for and against directed donor programs[2-9] or attempt to render a definitive judgment on the validity of the concept. Instead, we will explore aspects of the day-to-day functioning of a directed donor program and elaborate on operational problems we have encountered and approaches we have employed in our own hospital-based program.[10] The quality assurance so addressed will, therefore, focus on developing an effective program, but not whether such a program is

TABLE 1
High-Risk Donor Exclusions By History

1. Present or past gay (homosexual and bisexual) males
2. Any man who has had sex with another man even one time since 1977 — this includes even those individuals who have had only a single homosexual experience and may not regard themselves as homosexual or bisexual
3. Individuals with signs and symptoms of AIDS or laboratory evidence of HIV infection (anyone with a positive "AIDS test")
4. Past or present intravenous drug users
5. Persons born in, or emigrating to the U.S. from, Sub-Saharan African countries and islands located near these areas of Africa where heterosexual activities are thought to play a major role in the transmission of HIV-1 and HIV-2 infection
6. Persons living six (6) months or more in Sub-Saharan Africa since 1977
7. Hemophiliacs or others with blood clotting disorders
8. Sexual partners of any of the individuals at increased risk of AIDS as listed above
9. Sexual partners of individuals with AIDS or with symptoms of AIDS
10. Men and women who have engaged in sex for money or drugs since 1977 (i.e., any form of prostitution)
11. Persons who have had any sexual relations with *men* or *women* who have engaged in sex for money or drugs during the preceding twelve months (i.e., sex with prostitutes)

essential in all communities. Of course, we do consider these programs to be beneficial, especially when they are used to limit the number of donors to which a patient is exposed: a patient receiving three units of red cells and a platelet apheresis product, each originating from a different donor, has a fourfold increased probability of acquiring transfusion-transmitted disease than the patient who receives all four components from a single dedicated donor. The benefits of such a program are patently evident.

An appendix to this chapter contains our current procedures for administering this program. The pertinent sections will be referenced in the test to facilitate an understanding of our procedures in the context of the problems they are designed to alleviate.

II. PROGRAM GOALS

The basic premise of a directed donor program must be that the transfusion-transmitted infectious disease rate can be reduced by a patient's participation in donor selection. The blood supply has certainly become safer now that criteria defining high-risk donors have been expanded (Table 1), and since testing for not only HIV exposure, but also for hepatitis C virus and human T-cell lymphotropic virus (HTLV)-1 has become routine. Indeed, except for directed donors who are sexual partners, spouses, children, parents or close family members, we generally counsel prospective recipients that other less well known or intimate individuals (e.g., a second cousin or neighbor) are not necessarily better donors than are the donors who provide our community supply. However, the modification of directed donor programs to become limited-exposure donor programs by obtaining multiple products from one or several donors provides a much increased level of safety, especially if committed donors with a personal interest in the recipient are utilized. Furthermore, if at all possible, autologous donation should be utilized to provide the safest blood components. These tenets of transfusion medicine are not obvious to patients or medical personnel with unrelated specialties.[11,12] The consultative role of blood bank specialists is an essential part of an optimally run directed donor program and should integrate multiple aspects of transfusion medicine for that patient's well being.

III. COLLECTING AND ALLOCATING PRODUCTS

A. LOCATION OF DONATION

Usually, the site of anticipated transfusion is obvious since most donations are for use in a specific predesignated surgical setting, for example "for radical prostatectomy on February 6, 1991 at Pitt County Memorial Hospital". If the site of intended usage has its own donor facility, it is preferable that the donations take place there. This avoids added problems of shipping, identification, double inventory entry, timeliness of deliver, ascertaining appropriateness of blood types, and double billing for services. Patient identification for both directed and autologous donations assignment can be difficult with units transported from outside facilities because a unique identifier, the hospital identification number of that patient used to issue blood, was not an intrinsic part of the donation. The patient's name and birthday are not sufficient and the social security number is not always included in patient demographic data (see Appendix, Sections I and II).

However, for a variety of circumstance directed donation may have to be at a location different from that of the expected transfusion. This would of course be unavoidable if the hospital had no donor facility. Additionally, the most appropriate donor may reside at a distant location but be close to a donor center capable of providing suitable packaging and shipping. Such drawing sites must be appropriately licensed to ship blood. For interstate transport the shipping facility must be licensed by the Food and Drug Administration. Even if the hospital has a donor facility, it may be closed on weekends or evenings when a patient's changing medical status precipitates a search for donors. If shipping is necessary, detailed communication between the donor center and transfusion service is essential. Deliveries should not arrive unexpectedly. Knowledge of the intended recipient and appropriately drawn blood samples for pretransfusion testing should reach the transfusion service before donated units arrive so that allocation of units is not postponed after their arrival. Once put aside, their presence may be forgotten.

As mentioned, to transport blood or blood products across state lines a Federal license is required. However, private individuals can carry units as personal property without official interference. It is then up to the transfusion service whether or not the units should be transfused. We have had overseas patients arrive at our hospital carrying eight units of blood, some of autologous and some of directed donor origin. At times, the units are unfit for transfusion because of inappropriate packaging, lack of needed testing, or because they were drawn in an unlicensed facility.

B. APPROPRIATENESS OF BLOOD TYPE

When allocating units for red cell transfusion, we require that the donor's blood type be compatible, by major crossmatch, with that of the recipient. A recipient blood type must have been performed in our blood bank before units are assigned for his or her potential use (Appendix, Section I). Before units are issued, a current patient sample must have a type and screen performed to determine if any unexpected antibodies are present and to serve as a final clerical check of the historical data.

For the first three years of our directed donor program, only type-specific red cells were allocated. The decision to allow type-compatible rather than type-specific directed donor transfusions was based on three considerations: (1) the directed donations have extended shelf life additives added to achieve a 42-day shelf life and in processing have had much of the plasma removed; (2) a review of the medical literature revealed that transfusion of even significant volumes of O plasma to A, B, or AB recipients infrequently results in clinical sequelae or shortened red cell survival;[13–17] and (3) all other institutions we polled in our geographic area were already allowing the use of compatible red cells without recognized difficulty. Nevertheless, it should be remembered that a unit with an extremely high titer of anti-A or anti-B can occasionally be expected to cause hemolysis.[18]

C. ARRANGING FOR DONATION

A medical decision to obtain directed donor units must be made by the physician or surgeon who will later be responsible for ordering that transfusions be given. Knowledge of available levels of autologous and directed donor products should be routine preinterventional preparation at the time of surgery. The need for directed donation and the number of units to be assigned should be documented in the form of an order or written instruction (Appendix, Section II). This is an essential procedure for the collecting facilities' records, but may not be so obvious to many prospective donors, patients, or patients' families. We require a telephone or written order stipulating date of surgery, the patient's identifying demographics (name, hospital number, social security number, telephone number, address) and the number of units desired to be made available for the patient. Without such medical authorization an unnecessary number of units could be drawn, or even the wrong products obtained. Donors have come of their own volition to give whole blood when in fact platelets were the required product.

A second logistical part of arranging for donations should be the intended recipient's acknowledgment that a specific potential donor is indeed deemed acceptable. We require that the recipient, or an appointed family member or friend, contact our donor center with a list of names of prospective donors that have been recruited. This attempts to avoid the situation in which 15 people from a patient's workplace or church arrive at the donor facility wanting to donate. The patient in question may find some of these well-intentioned people acceptable, some not. Moreover, it is impractical and unnecessary to allocate an excessive number of units to one patient, especially if there is a directed donor charge levied for each assigned unit. Unless stipulated as an acceptable recruit, a friend or even a family member is not used by us as a directed donor. Most unsolicited donors are happy enough, once they arrive in the facility, to serve as random community donors.

D. TIMING OF DONATION

As mentioned above, directed donor red cells are processed in our facility to have a 42-day shelf life. Once a specified surgical date exists, we allow donation to occur within the preceding three weeks. Our directed and autologous donor coordinator monitors the operating schedule to be certain the surgery actually occurs when expected. If the surgery is delayed the units are released for general use, or if requested by the patient, they can be frozen for long-term storage. If not used in the week following surgery, or by hospital discharge, the directed donor units are transferred into our general pool. This policy enables us to have very few units expire unused.

E. ALLOCATION OF UNITS

At the time of surgery, requested units are delivered to the operating room blood refrigerator. If four units are requested to be crossmatched, and that patient has one autologous donation and two directed donor units, we deliver only the autologous unit to the operating room refrigerator. If this unit is transfused, then we deliver the two directed donor units. If these are transfused, only then do we deliver additional random units as needed. In this way, the blood bank assumes responsibility to assure that the units of blood are transfused in the proper order. The alternative of delivering a mixture of autologous, directed donor, and random allogeneic units places the responsibility of determining the order of transfusion on operating room personnel.

Unused directed donor and autologous components remaining in the operating suite following surgery must be returned to the blood bank without delay when the patient is transferred to the floor. Otherwise, inappropriate units (directed or allogeneic) may be issued from the blood bank to the floor should transfusions subsequently be ordered from that location.

A not uncommon request is for the transfer of units assigned to one intended recipient to a different recipient. The clinical scenario is usually that families of two patients have become friendly. After, or sometimes even before surgery is completed on the patient who has directed units in storage, his family altruistically offers to share this blood with the other patient. We do not permit this sort of transfer. Often the first patient's perioperative period of potential transfusion has not elapsed, the blood in question may be compatible but not identical in type, logistically it is difficult to accomplish, and as mentioned in the introduction, a safer directed donor for one person (e.g., a spouse) may not be a safer donor for others.

An additional issue regarding allocation is a patient's desire to stipulate the exact order in which units of directed donor blood are transfused. This is difficult to allow while maintaining donor anonymity and confidentiality. After testing is completed and units are labeled they are allocated, if appropriate, to the intended recipient by unit number. As is true for all allogeneic products, the donor's name is not on the label, and is not part of the transfusion service data. Only by connecting source data (donor service data) with blood bank inventory data can this identification be achieved. We only perform this function and prioritize the order of transfusion when multiple donations are available from a limited-exposure donor. Otherwise, units are issued in order of expiration.

IV. DONOR CONFIDENTIALITY

A. MAINTAINING CONFIDENTIALITY

Our program does not pretype prospective donors for ABO and Rh status. Donors schedule an appointment for donation and either arrive with the requisite authorization slip from the intended recipient or have had their name already listed by the intended recipient in his or her donation folder. The predonation donor interview and blood processing are identical to that for any community donor. Appropriate predonation information is read, a donor card is filled out and signed, the nurse's history and physical performed, a confidential unit exclusion card filled out, and the unit is then drawn and subsequently tested (Appendix, Section V). In the donor facility the unit is tagged with a blue directed donor age and after component processing entered into the quarantine inventory. Only after all tests are negative and the unit is found to be compatible with the recipient is the unit assigned to the designated recipient and removed from quarantine. At this juncture, a notation is made in the donor-room's "intended recipient file" that a directed donor unit (or 2nd or 3rd, etc.) is available (Appendix, Section VI). The cumulative number of suitable units in stock is made available to the recipient or ordering physician, but the identities of the acceptable and unacceptable donors is not, nor is the reason for which a unit was deemed unacceptable. This confidential exclusionary information is released only to the actual donor, often by telephone after positive identification. Nonallocation because of incompatible blood type is information that can be related by our donor facility staff, but medical testing results must be given only by a transfusion medicine physician.

Notification may be delayed pending confirmatory tests. Notification of HIV exposure is done discretely by telephone with a follow-up letter.

Providing notification for the patient and ordering surgeon as to the number of acceptable units available is difficult for us to accomplish. Should it be done two days before surgery, or a week ahead? We do not know if more donors have already been recruited or not. We try to shift this responsibility to the patient. Our written instructions stipulate that the patient or family should call to check on the number allocated, but often they do not do so, or wait until just prior to surgery when it might be found out that although five individuals donated, only one unit is acceptable for an Rh negative patient. Optimally, the blood bank would have sufficient personnel to initiate twice-a-week notification of patients and surgeons. We do not have sufficient people to do so. Perhaps the patient's physician should be responsible. Recent legislation in California requires that when circumstances permit, a physician or surgeon must inform patients of their transfusion options and allow adequate time for predonation to occur.[19] Such legislation implies that knowledge of the number of available directed donor blood components suitable for the patient should also be an adjunctive responsibility of the attending physician.

If the donor center is not directly affiliated with the transfusion service, the usual practice is to deliver all directed donor units found to be acceptable for allogeneic use to the hospital. The transfusion service, knowing the patient's blood type and screen results, must decide which units can be directed and which will be placed into random stock. The donor center would bill the hospital for all the units delivered.

B. DISCLOSING THE IDENTITIES OF ACCEPTABLE DONORS

The desire to limit donor exposures by accomplishing repeat transfusion from one donor does occasionally prompt us to release donor identities. If three relatives donated for a patient six months ago and only one unit was transfused, and now further surgery is planned and directed donor blood is again requested, we will release the name of the donor of the initially transfused unit.

V. ADVERSE EFFECTS OF DIRECTED DONATION

From an immunohematologic standpoint, there are several potential untoward effects of directed donor transfusion. Theoretically, if only random community components are transfused it is unlikely there will be a subsequent exposure to a very infrequent antigen (a "private antigen") to which an alloantibody has been induced by a prior blood exposure. Such an antibody may not be detected on a routine blood bank antibody screen. If directed donors repetitively donate for one patient, reexposure to low-frequency antigens may occur. Because of this possibility, our group has raised the possibility of requiring a complete antiglobulin crossmatch for repeat direct donor transfusions.[20] The occurrence of febrile nonhemolytic transfusion reactions or urticarial reactions from antibodies directed against soluble protein constituents or white cells would be a parallel phenomenon. Other similar outcomes would be hemolytic disease of the newborn or neonatal isoimmune thrombocytopenia due to prior maternal transfusion with paternal blood products or blood products from paternal relatives. For this reason, we discourage the use of husbands' blood for women in the childbearing age group, although we do not prohibit this practice when proper informed consent is obtained.

The possibility of producing anti-HLA antibodies that would complicate subsequent organ or bone marrow transplantation from a family member donor has been raised.[6] We do not consider this to be a problem of sufficient magnitude to warrant discussion with prospective patients who request directed donations.

The potential for developing transfusion-associated graft-vs.-host disease (TA-GVHD) after exposure to directed donor blood from genetically related donors is much higher than would be the case when genetically unrelated donors are used.[21] This nearly uniformly fatal condition can arise even in nonimmunocompromised patient recipients when HLA homozygous lymphocytes are transfused to an HLA heterozygous recipient whose HLA phenotype includes the HLA haplotype of the transfused blood: the host (recipient) immune system will not recognize the transfused cells as foreign, but the transfused cells will perceive at least half of the host's HLA antigens as foreign and mount an immune response. This complication can be avoided by the pretransfusion irradiation of cellular blood components.

Many patients believe that directed donor blood is a safe substitute for autologous blood and may choose to provide directed donors instead of donating their own blood prior to elective procedures. This is a mistaken assumption and the process must be discouraged.[12]

VI. SALUTARY EFFECTS OF DIRECTED DONATION

Discounting the obviously hoped-for reduction in transfusion-transmitted disease, there are several additional beneficial aspects of directed donation.

1. Unrelated donors of the same racial or ethnic background, or family members, may be able to supply blood that is less likely to produce alloimmunization to red cell antigens.[22] This has recently been addressed for patients with sickle cell disease.[23]
2. The use of repeat directed donors for a specific patient lessens the number of overall allogeneic exposures and may thereby decrease possible immune modulation accompanying transfusion.[24] This benefit will occur whether the blood is transfused years apart, or as part of a limited donor-exposure program involving repeated directed donation over a short period of time.

3. The "peace of mind" issue should not be ignored. Patients feel much better knowing they have either autologous or directed donor units available. Conversely, the thought of receiving random blood will be strongly resisted by some patients. We recently encountered a lady who, from postpartum hemorrhage, bled to a hematocrit of 13%, was highly symptomatic, and yet refused transfusion for two days until directed donor blood became available.

VII. DIRECTED DONOR IN A LIMITED DONOR EXPOSURE PROGRAM

Certainly the greatest medical benefit of directed donation is achieved when a committed donor agrees to donate repetitively for one patient, thereby supplying all or a significant amount of a patient's transfusion requirements. Where long-term storage is possible (i.e., for frozen red cells, cryoprecipitate, and frozen plasma) and sufficient advance notice is available, the pattern of donation can adhere to older American Association of Blood Banks (AABB) standards that required 56 days between red cell donations, and stipulated that apheresis should not follow whole blood donation for 56 days. However, in most cases for which repeated directed donation is desired, there is not the luxury of such infrequent donations. Recent modifications of donor requirements have resulted in published changes in AABB standards so that now in "Directed Donor programs, at the request of the recipient's physician, with the approval of the blood bank physician and informed consent of the donor... (the) frequency of donation should not be (less) than every three days and the (hematocrit) shall be no less than 36% for women and 38% for men."[25] Federal requirements still mandate 38% hematocrit for both men and women. In our program, while we follow the Federal restrictions, we make medical exceptions regularly when it is in the best interest of the patient and is not dangerous to the donor's health.

Our program and other similar programs have of necessity had to focus the resources available for limiting donor exposure on groups most likely to benefit from this practice (e.g., patients with limited requirements for allogeneic blood) or to situations where donor commitment, availability, and flexibility are especially strong (e.g., parents or other relatives donating for infants and children undergoing cardiac surgery). A recent evaluation of our limited exposure direct donor program's impact on 41 pediatric heart surgery patients demonstrated that 21 children (51% of those participating) received only dedicated donor products and averaged 2.8 products transfused per case. No transfusions were used by 14 children (34%). Only six children (15%), who averaged 9.4 products transfused, utilized both dedicated and random donor products.

Neonatal directed donor programs can be arranged in which donations of half units (250 cc) at frequent intervals provide a constant source of fresh red cells (Appendix, Section VII.1). A theoretical concern that maternal high-titer anti-HLA or anti-granulocyte specific antibodies may result in infant granulocytopenia has caused us to evaluate the transfusion of maternal plasma to neonates (Appendix, Section I.9).

Liver transplant candidates often spend months on a waiting list after acceptance into a transplant program. During this waiting period, most candidates are unsuitable to participate in autologous donation programs because of anemia and inadequate production of coagulation factors. Our dedicated donor program has been used in these instances to harvest single donor plasma by apheresis from one or two donors. Several patients have had up to 14 units of fresh-frozen plasma (FFP) of single donor origin available for their use at the time of surgery. We have not stored frozen red cells for these donors because of the time required to deglycerolize frozen red cells when surgery is imminent. Thus far, nine patients transplanted and surviving to discharge have participated in this dedicated donor frozen plasma storage program. Dedicated products have accounted for a mean of 20% (range 9 to 50%) of total products transfused to these nine patients in the perioperative period.

Patients benefiting most from dedicated repeat donors are those with low-level transfusion requirements. Often these individuals are undergoing treatment for malignancy, have primary hypoproductive hematologic disorders, or have received autologous or allogeneic bone marrow transplantation. We have found that one or several dedicated donors can support these patients over extended time periods, except in times of increased transfusion frequency. A similar strategy for intrauterine transfusion uses maternal donation to provide the safest treatment for the unborn infant with hemolytic disease.[26]

The routine provision of this service for all patients for whom autologous participation is impossible would be the next logical extension of this program were adequate human resources available. If patients scheduled for orthopedic, urologic gynecologic, and cardiac surgery are referred to the transfusion medicine department well in advance of the surgical date, their ability to autologously donate the requested products can be assessed in time to arrange for repeat dedicated donations if necessary.

The benefit of such a program is readily apparent if we consider a specific case: a 70-year-old gentleman is found to have prostatic cancer and is scheduled for retropubic prostatectomy in four weeks. His urologist wishes for the patient to donate four autologous units prior to surgery. At his first visit to the autologous donor center he is found not only to have a hematocrit of 32% but also, over the weekend, to have been placed by his internist on an oral broad-spectrum antibiotic for urinary tract infection.

Instead of donating himself, it is arranged that his son will donate for him, and by the time of surgery he was able to donate four times. During the hospitalization, the patient received the four transfusions. If we estimate the risk of transfusion-transmitted infectious disease to be about 1 in 500 per donor exposure, his chance of *not* receiving an infection from his son's units is 499/500 or 99.8%. Were he to have received four transfusions from four different donors, his chances of not receiving an infection is $(499/500)^4$, or 99.2%. The chance of his acquiring an infection from his son's donations (assuming his son's chance of carrying a transmissible disease is the same as that of a random donor) is 0.2%; from the four random units it is 0.8%. His risk of acquiring a transfusion-transmitted disease is four times as great when four donors are involved as when one donor is involved.

VIII. DIRECT DONATION OF NON-RED CELL PRODUCTS

Directed donations need not be limited to whole blood or packed red cells. Fresh frozen plasma or cryoprecipitate can be prepared from the plasma removed from a whole blood donation or can be obtained by plasmapheresis. We have recently begun providing both autologous and directed donor cryoprecipitate for use as "fibrin glue".[27] This is an expedient way to limit the number of donor exposures, and has been especially effective in orthopedic and neurosurgical procedures.

Single donor platelet concentrates obtained by apheresis have long been used for the support of patients with malignancies. The expanded use of this harvesting technique is appropriate to provide directed donor platelets for single-occurrence use in cardiac surgery, splenectomy, and perhaps for any surgery in which the patient has transiently or permanently dysfunctional platelets. For platelet donors we require acceptable laboratory screening tests prior to harvest. This testing can be accomplished through a minimal phlebotomy for "pre-pheresis screening" or derive from a recent whole blood or plasma donation.

IX. DIRECTED DONOR LOGISTICAL CONSIDERATIONS

Directed donor programs may have helped maintain hospital inventories as the donor base has been subjected to erosion during current societal concerns about AIDS. Yet in some fundamental aspects the donor base has not changed as the shift occurred. Our hospital transfuses approximately 1600 units of whole blood and packed red cells per month to nonpediatric patients. Autologous donations account for 9% of this total, and essentially all of the whole blood transfused. Directed donations, actually used by the original intended recipient, account for approximately 8% of the 1600 units. To support this practice our donor facility draws approximately 360 units/month of directed donor blood, and 40% of these units are indeed transfused to the initially intended recipient. The remainder are either discarded because of positive test results (only 7%), or are eventually entered into our random stock for community use. It is interesting to realize that when one examines our donor base it is probable that the units transferred to community use are not dissimilar in "quality" to the community units transfused prior to our directed donor program. This is because we previously had an active "replacement program" soliciting family members and friends to replace blood used by a patient during hospitalization. From 1979 through 1983 we averaged 3447 replacement donations per year in this replacement program. Our directed donor program began in 1983, and from 1987 through early 1991 we have averaged 4031 directed whole blood donations per year. (Replacement donations have dropped to 441 per year.) These two volumes are very comparable and suggest that these donor pools, replacement and directed, include individuals with very similar donor characteristics.

X. SUMMARY

Our involvement in directed donor programs and commitment to their evolution and growth is based really on one premise: unit for unit, a directed donor is very comparable to a random donor regarding the chance of disease transmission, but well-informed donors and intended recipients can often provide donors who may be slightly better on an individualized patient basis; all other factors being equal my wife is a better donor for me than is a randomly selected individual of similar blood type. The direct corollary of this is that limited donor exposure programs can significantly reduce the risk of transmissible disease spread through transfusion therapy.

Directed donor programs require an exceptionally high level of communication among all those involved. Quality assurance is possible when a sufficient number of dedicated, knowledgeable, and competent program personnel are integrated into the process and adhere to formal policies.

APPENDIX
POLICIES, DIRECTED DONOR PROGRAM, CEDARS-SINAI MEDICAL CENTER

I. DIRECTED DONATION PROGRAM REQUIREMENTS

1. All directed donations are to be collected in the Cedars-Sinai Medical Center (CSMC) Taft B. Schreiber Blood Donor Facility (BDF) per physician order.
2. Directed donations are to be collected no more than 21 days prior to surgery or intended use (10 to 14 days and no less than 48 hours is recommended for adequate collection time and testing). Exceptions to this policy will be confirmed with the Blood Bank physician.
3. Each directed donor (DD) is to donate one (1) unit of whole blood, at a maximum frequency of every eight (8) weeks. Exceptions to this are to be made with authorization of the Blood Bank physician and so documented on the Blood Donor Card. Suitability of the directed donor unit will be determined by the Blood Bank following collection.
4. The directed donor recipient is to have his/her blood type determined at Cedars-Sinai Medical center (CSMC) Taft B. Schreiber Blood Donor Facility, if possible. There is no pre-typing of directed donors by the Blood Donor Facility personnel.
5. Criteria for directed donor selection is that required by the Blood Donor Facility Policy and Procedure, ''Blood Donation, Whole Blood, Donor Registration, History and Physical'', Volume I, Policy and Procedure Manual.
6. Directed donors who are married to child bearing age female recipients (up to 45 years of age) are not acceptable as directed donors for their wives. Exceptions to this are at the discretion of the Blood Bank physician.
7. It is the responsibility of the recipient or his/her designate to do an acceptability check for his/her directed donor units with the Blood Donor Facility personnel.
8. Blood Donor Facility personnel reporting acceptability of directed donor units to the recipient or his/her designate are to report the number of acceptable units only. Questions concerning acceptability are to be referred to the Special Programs Coordinator, ext. 5417.
9. Mothers of Neonatal Intensive Care Unit (NICU) patients are not to donate for their infants for three (3) months following delivery. Exceptions to this are to be made with authorization of the Blood Bank physician.
10. All directed donors for NICU patients are to be negative for cytomegalovirus. The Blood Bank Liaison is to contact NICU directed donors as to acceptability.

11. Directed donor units are not to be collected for a specific recipient if the recipient's hospital identification number is not available in the Blood Donor Facility.

II. DIRECTED DONATION COLLECTION ORDERS

1. Directed donations require either a written or telephone order which specifies (1) the number of unit(s) of whole blood to be withdrawn for a specific patient (recipient), (2) if a type and screen specimen is to be drawn, and (3) the date of surgery or if it is for nonsurgical transfusion needs.
2. The attending physician is to complete the "Request for Directed Donation Collection" which is obtained from the Blood Donor Facility. This is forwarded to the Blood Donor Facility, and is to become a permanent part of the directed donation recipient's file in the Blood Donor Facility.
3. Telephone orders for directed donor collection are to be called to the Blood Donor Facility personnel by the physician or his designate.
4. Inpatient orders for directed donor collection written in the patient's hospital chart are to be telephoned to the Blood Donor Facility personnel by the Patient Care Clerk or Registered Nurse caring for the patient. The recipient's hospital identification number and date of birth are to be obtained form the clinical personnel. Family members or friends may bring an actual copy of the order to the Blood Donor Facility reception area.
5. Written documentation is to be attached to the DD donor card documenting the intended recipient's (or next of kin/legal guardian) request for the donor (by name) to donate blood for their use. The request may be made by telephone by the recipient or next of kin/legal guardian to Blood Donor Facility personnel. Personnel taking verbal requests are to sign their initials and date, after placing a "V.O" followed by the recipient's or next of kin/legal guardian's name. Only first time directed donors for a specific recipient require a consent form.

PROCEDURE

III. DIRECTED DONOR RECIPIENT REGISTRATION

1. The intended directed donor recipient is to call the Blood Donor Facility for pre-registration and recipient specimen collection for blood typing information.
2. Registration and specimen collection are to be done prior to DD blood collection.

IV. DIRECTED DONOR REGISTRATION

1. The Staff Assistant is to welcome and identify directed donors and ask the name of the recipient. The Staff Assistant is to verify the DD

order and that the date of donation is within at least 21 days of surgery. The donor is to be rescheduled if donation is too soon.

2. The directed donor is to read the "Information Sheet for Recipients and Donors of the Directed Donor Program" after reading the "Information for Individuals About Routine Donor Tests".
3. The directed donor is to complete the Blood Donor Card and sign the "Directed Donor's Consent Regarding Utilization of Their Donated Unit". The directed donor also completes the Directed Donor Recognition Card.
4. The Staff Assistant is to write "DD" and recipient's name in the "REPL/DR. NAME" section of the Donor Record Card. Repeat directed donors, donating in less than eight (8) weeks, are to have "Repeat Donation" written in the "Remarks" section.
5. The Staff Assistant is to initiate the Directed Donor Record Card (Attachment VI) and Directed Donor Recipient Envelope and complete, at least, the sections for recipient's name, I.D. number and date of birth, if available, and date of surgery, if appropriate on the Directed Donor Record Card and front of envelope.
6. The Staff Assistant is to complete one (1) Directed Donation Blood Bank Recipient I.D. tag with the following:

   Recipient's name
   Medical record number
   Date of birth (if available)
   Donor unit number
   Date of surgery or write "transfusion only", as appropriate
   Recipient's physician's name

   The tag will be attached to the Blood Donor Card prior to the screening process.
7. The Staff Assistant is to give the Directed Donation Recognition Card to the Replacement Office volunteers after the whole blood unit has been collected.

V. DIRECTED DONATION COLLECTION

1. See "Blood Donation — Whole Blood, Donor Registration, History and Physical", *Blood Donor Facility, Vol. Policy Procedure Manual.* The Registered Nurse/Medical Technologist (RN/MT) screening the directed donor is to ask the directed donor whom they are donating for and the relationship of the donor to the prospective recipient. (See Directed Donation Program Requirements 6., above.) The hematocrit is to be spun on repeat directed donors attempting to donate in less than eight (8) weeks. A hematocrit of 38% or greater is acceptable for repeat donation following notification and approval of a Blood

Bank physician; Blood Donor Card authorization by the Blood Bank physician may follow actual collection. Exceptions to this are at the discretion of the Blood Bank physician.

2. The Blood Donor Facility RN/MT collecting the directed donation is to check the spelling of the recipient's name on the Directed Donation Blood Bank Recipient ID tag with the directed donor and compare the unit number on the Blood Donor Card with the unit number on the I.D. tag for correctness.
3. The RN/MT is to witness the ''Directed Donor's Consent Regarding Utilization of Their Donated Unit''. If the directed donor refuses to sign the consent, the RN/MT is to write the reason for refusal on the consent and inform the donor that the recipient will be charged the processing fee plus the directed donor fee.
4. The primary bag is to be labeled with the Directed Donation Blood Bank Recipient I.D. Tag prior to collection.

VI. DIRECTED DONATION ACCEPTABILITY RECORD

1. The Blood Bank Supervisor or designate will send the Blood Donor Facility a copy of the ''Directed Donor Sheet'' with the directed donor recipient's names, medical record numbers, and the number of acceptable units for each recipient.
2. The Staff Assistant in the Blood Donor Facility is to transcribe the number of suitable units and date drawn to the recipient's Directed Donor Record.

VII. SPECIAL SITUATIONS

1. Neonatal Intensive Care Unit (NICU) Directed Donors
   - 1.1. First time directed donor units for the NICU patient are to be collected in 500 cc triple CP2D blood packs with one blue Directed Donor (DD) I.D. tag. The Staff Assistant will print ''NICU'' in the ''Remark Section'' of the Blood Donor Card and on each DD tag. (This is to be done for all NICU DD units.)
   - 1.2 Repeat directed donations are to be collected in 250-cc quadruple CPDA-1 blood packs with one DD I.D. tag.
   - 1.3 NICU patients going to surgery are to have Directed Donor Units collected in 500-cc triple CP2D blood packs with a single DD tag.
2. Pediatric Cardio-Thoracic Surgical Directed Donors
   - 2.1. Directed donor units for the Pediatric Cardio-Thoracic Surgical Program are to have a single DD ID tag plus a ''Spec. Product Prep Tag'' with unit number written in the designated line and ''DD/Auto FFP'' section checked.
   - 2.2. Directed donor units for the Pediatric Cardio-Thoracic Surgical Program are to be drawn in 500-cc triple CP2D blood packs.

VIII. DIRECTED DONATION UNIT STORAGE TIME

1. Directed Donor units collected for surgical procedures will be retained in the Blood Bank for 21 days following the date of surgery.
2. Directed donor units utilized for transfusion only, will be stored for 21 days following the date of collection.
3. Directed Donor Units collected for NICU patients will be retained for 21 days.

IX. DIRECTED DONATION CHARGE

1. A charge will be added to the intended recipient's account for each directed donor unit found to be suitable for the recipient's use, whether or not the blood is used.
2. No charge is to be generated for unsuitable units.

REFERENCES

1. State of California, Senate Bill 2673 Amending Section 1628 of the Health and Safety Code.
2. **Goldfinger, D.,** Directed blood donations: pro, *Transfusion,* 29, 70, 1989.
3. **Page, P. L.,** Directed blood donations: con, *Transfusion,* 29, 65, 1989.
4. **Cordell, R. R., Yalon, V. A., Cigahn-Haskell, C., McDonough, B. P., and Perkins, H. A.,** Experience with 11916 designated donors, *Transfusion,* 26, 484, 1986.
5. **Yalon, V. and Perkins, H. A.,** The arguments for directed donations, *Transfus. Sci.,* 10, 139, 1989.
6. **Collins, M. L. and Churchill, L. R.,** The case against directed donations, *Transfus. Sci.,* 10, 139, 1989.
7. **Goldfinger, D. and Pepkowitz, S. H.,** Directed blood donations and the concept of individualized case in transfusion medicine, *Am. J. Clin. Pathol.,* 92, 516, 1989.
8. **Sandler, S. G., Naiman, J. L., and Fletcher, J. L.,** Alternative approaches to transfusion: autologous blood and directed blood donations, *Prog. Hematol.,* 15, 183, 1987.
9. **Goldfinger, D.,** The community blood supply and patients' choice: the case for directed blood donations, *Hastings Center Rep.,* 17, 7, 1987.
10. **Pura, L. S., Smith, L. E., and Goldfinger, D.,** Establishment of a directed donor blood program in a hospital based blood bank, in *Autologous and Directed Blood Programs,* Garner, R. J. and Silvergleid, A. J., Eds., American Association of Blood Banks, Arlington, VA, 1987, chap. 3.
11. **Goodnough, L. T. and Shuck, J.,** Risks, options and informed consent for blood transfusion in elective surgery, *Am. J. Surg.,* 159, 602, 1990.
12. **Chambers, L. A., Kruskall, M. S., Drago, S. S., and Ellis, A. M.,** Directed-donor programs may adversely affect autologous donor participation, *Transfusion,* 30, 246, 1990.
13. **Aubert, E. F., Boorman, K. E., Dodd, B. E., and Loutit, J. F.,** The universal donor with high titre iso-agglutinins, *Br. Med. J.,* 659, 1942.
14. **Ervin, D. M. and Young, L. E.,** Dangerous universal donors. I, *Blood,* 5, 61, 1950.
15. **Ervin, D. M. and Young, L. E.,** Dangerous universal donors. II, *Blood,* 5, 553, 1950.
16. **Crosby, W. H. and Akeroyd, J. H.,** Some immunohematologic results of large transfusions of group O blood in recipients of other blood groups, *Blood,* 9, 103, 1954.
17. **Ebert, R. V. and Emerson, C. P.,** A clinical study of transfusion reactions: the hemolytic effect of group-O blood and pooled plasma containing incompatible isoagglutinins, *J. Clin. Invest.,* 25, 627, 1946.
18. **Pierce, R. N., Reich, L. M., and Mayer, K.,** Hemolysis following platelet transfusions from ABO-incompatible donors, *Transfusion,* 25, 60, 1985.
19. State of California Health and Safety Code, Section 1645 as amended by Senate Bill 2239.
20. **Smith, L., McQuiston, D., Nagin, S., Ehrlich, H., and Goldfinger, D.,** Increased risk of missed incompatibility with repeat directed donor transfusion (Abstract), *Transfusion,* 29 (Suppl.) 475, 1989.
21. **Kruskall, M. S., Alper, C. A., Awdeh, Z., and Yunis, E. J.,** HLA-Homozygous donors and transfusion-associated graft-versus-host disease (letter), *N. Engl. J. Med.,* 322, 1005, 1990.
22. **Kanter, M. H. and Hodge, S. E.,** The probability of obtaining compatible blood from related directed donors, *Arch. Pathol. Lab. Med.,* 144, 1013, 1990.
23. **Vichinsky, E. P., Earles, A., Johnson, R. A., Hoag, M. S., Williams, A., and Lubin, B.,** Alloimmunization in sickle cell anemia and transfusion of racially unmatched blood, *N. Engl. J. Med.,* 322, 1617, 1990.

24. **Triulzi, D. J., Heal, J. M., and Blumberg, N.,** Transfusion-induced immunomodulation and its clinical consequences, in *Transfusion Medicine in the 1990's,* Nance, S. T., Ed., American Association of Blood Banks, Arlington, VA, 1990, chap. 1.
25. Holland, P. V., Ed., Standards for Blood Banks and Transfusion Services, American Association of Blood Banks, Arlington, VA, 1989, Section B.1.
26. **Gonsoulin, W. J., Moise, K. J., Milam, J. D., Sala, J. D., Weber, V. W., and Carpenter, R. J.,** Serial maternal blood donations for intrauterine transfusion, *Obstet. Gynecol.,* 75, 158, 1990.
27. **Spotnitz, W. D., Mintz, P. D., Avery, N., Bithell, T. C., Kaul, S., and Nolan, S. P.,** Fibrin glue from stored human plasma, *Am. Surgeon,* 53, 460, 1987.

Chapter 9

SEROLOGICAL THEORY AND PRACTICE

Imelda M. Bromilow and Jennifer K. M. Duguid

TABLE OF CONTENTS

ISBN 0-8493-4938-9

I. INTRODUCTION

Modern serology was founded in 1901 with Landsteiner's[1] original description of the ABO blood group system. Agglutination of red blood cells had been described previously by Creite[2] and Landois,[3] but it was Landsteiner who not only observed but also interpreted the reactions occurring between red cell antigens and antibodies present in serum.

The development of the direct antiglobulin test[4] introduced the refinement of being able to detect antibodies capable of binding to red cell antigenic determinants but incapable of producing cell lysis or agglutination. The discovery of further blood group systems and the continuing occurrence of transfusion reactions led to the realization that more refined techniques were required to detect all blood group antigen-antibody interactions. This led to the development of a multiplicity of ''enhancing'' techniques to improve antibody detection. However, it has become increasingly realized that the ability to detect and identify all antibodies using all available techniques with the attendant increased time and costs incurred is not necessarily associated with improved patient care and well-being. It is now obvious that many antibodies are of no, or limited, clinical significance, and techniques are now increasingly aimed at detecting only relevant antibodies. Other methodologies may then be used to determine their likely clinical significance. A knowledge and understanding of red cell antigen/antibody systems and their relevance to clinical practice is therefore essential for the interpretation of test results.

II. RED CELL ANTIGENS AND ANTIBODIES

Human red cells exhibit extensive antigenic polymorphism. There are more than 640 characterized antigens within the various blood group systems.[5] A blood group system is comprised of immunochemically distinct antigens produced by alleles at a single genetic locus or at loci closely linked so that crossover does not occur.[6] Blood group antigens are composed of glycoproteins secreted in biological fluids and adsorbed onto cells, or glycoproteins

TABLE 1
ABO Blood Group System in Caucasians

Red cell phenotype	Antibodies in serum	Incidence %
O	Anti-A,B	44
A	Anti-B	42
B	Anti-A	10
AB	None	4

and glycolipids synthesized by the red cell. Clinically, the ABO blood group system is the most important, and ABO compatible (although not necessarily ABO identical) blood must be selected for all recipients.

A. THE ABO BLOOD GROUP SYSTEM

There are four common phenotypes within the ABO system: A, B, O, and AB, the frequencies of which, for a population of Caucasian origin, are shown in Table 1. Interracial variations are notable; for example, the group B phenotype is more common among the Chinese (up to 26%) with a corresponding decline in the frequency of group A individuals.

Genetically, an individual may be AA, AO, BB, BO, AB, or OO. The alleles determining blood groups A and B are said to be codominant, with a "silent" allele coding for phenotype O.

A functional H gene is a prerequisite for the formation of ABO blood groups. The H gene codes for the transferase enzyme responsible for adding L-fucose to the terminal of the precursor chain, as shown in Table 2.

The ABO alleles code for the production of transferase enzymes which determine the addition of the immunodominant sugar for each blood group to the L-fucose. The immunodominant sugar defining blood group A antigen is *N*-acetyl-galactosamine, and for blood group B antigen definition, the sugar is D-galactose, with both being present to define blood group AB. The O gene is a nonfunctional allele which fails to encode a protein similar to the A and B transferases and therefore does not add another sugar to the L-fucose product of the H gene-specified transferase. Group O individuals therefore have H antigen only.

B. ABO SUBGROUPS

The majority of A and AB phenotypes belong to the subgroup A_1, with about 20% of group A and AB individuals expressing the A_2 subgroup phenotype. The immunodominant sugar (*N*-acetyl-galactosamine) is identical for both A_1 and A_2 subgroups, so that the distinction between the two antigens is largely quantitative, with A_2 having fewer antigen sites per red cell than

TABLE 2
Structure of Precursor Substance and ABH Antigens

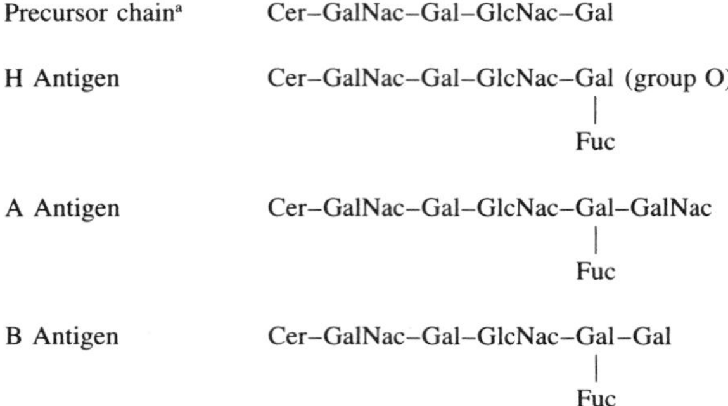

Precursor chain[a]	Cer–GalNac–Gal–GlcNac–Gal
H Antigen	Cer–GalNac–Gal–GlcNac–Gal (group O) | Fuc
A Antigen	Cer–GalNac–Gal–GlcNac–Gal–GalNac | Fuc
B Antigen	Cer–GalNac–Gal–GlcNac–Gal–Gal | Fuc

Note: Cer, ceramide; GalNac, *N*-acetyl-galactosamine: Gal, galactose; GlcNac, *N*-acetyl-glucosamine; Fuc, fucose.

[a] Precursor chains may be type 1 or type 2, differing in the linkage of the terminal galactose to *N*-acetyl-glucosamine. Type 1 chains possess a beta 1–3 linkage, and type 2, beta 1–4. Both types are found in secretions, body fluids, and various tissues, type 1 chains can be adsorbed onto red cells from the plasma, but only type 2 is actually synthesized by the red cells.

A_1. However, there are qualitative differences as defined by several serological or biochemical characteristics. The A_1 red cells react specifically with the lectin from *Dolichos biflorus*,[7] when properly diluted, and individuals of A_1 subtype do not produce anti-A_1, whereas about 2% of A_2 and up to 25% of A_2B individuals do. There are also differences in antigenic structure and antigenic determinants associated with the two subgroups. Transferase studies have also shown qualitative distinctions, the A_1 transferase being optimal at pH 6 and more active than the A_2 transferase which is optimal at pH 8.[8]

Many other, rare, subgroups of A that carry even weaker expression of the A antigen than the A_2 subtype have been characterized. These are classified by virtue of their serological activity with anti-A, anti-A_1, anti-A, B, and anti-H, as summarized in Table 3. Saliva inhibition studies, serum transferase investigations, and family studies are often necessary to elucidate a subgroup as well as the mode of its inheritance.

The characteristic mixed-field agglutination of an A_3 subgroup must be distinguished from other causes of a mixed-field hemagglutination pattern. Other serological causes include blood group chimeras and A_{mos} subgroups. Clinical causes of mixed-field agglutination in ABO blood grouping tests can be due to detection of red cells from an antigen-different blood transfusion,

TABLE 3
The Most Commonly Encountered Subgroups of A

	Grades of reactions with red cells				
Subgroup	**Anti-A**	**Anti-A_1**	**Anti-A,B**	**Anti-H**	**Remarks**
A_1	4+	4+	4+	–	
A_2	4+	0	4+	2+	May contain α_1 in serum
A_{int}	4+	2+	4+	3+	
A_3	$2+^{mf}$	0	$2+^{mf}$	3+	May contain α_1 in serum
A_x	$+^{w}$	0	2+	4+	Usually contains α_1 in serum
A_m	–/w	0	–/w	4+	

Note: 0, Negative reaction; mf, mixed-field agglutination; subgroups of A are also associated with group AB individuals.

bone marrow transplantation, feto-maternal hemorrhage or Tn polyagglutination.

Subgroups of B are not as commonly encountered as those of group A, though B_3, B_x, and B_m have been described. The percentage agglutination with anti-B has been used to classify such subgroups when they are termed B_{60}, B_{20}, and B_0.[5]

A rare genetic abnormality in the biosynthetic pathway for ABO antigen formation can produce a ''Bombay'' phenotype. Absence of a functional H gene (Table 2) prevents the products of normal A and/or B genes from effecting the addition of further terminal sugars, resulting in the absence of A, B, and H antigenic determinants. The A and B genes are inherited and expressed normally in the next generation if one H gene is present. The red cells of a ''Bombay'' phenotype react serologically as group O, but the serum contains anti-H as well as anti-A and anti-B. This phenotype is found in India at a frequency of about 1 in 13,000, but it only rarely presents in other populations.

C. ANTIBODIES OF THE ABO SYSTEM

Anti-A and anti-B are predominantly immunoglobulin M (IgM) antibodies, reacting optimally at low temperatures. They are potent antibodies that fix complement, so that transfusions must be ABO compatible to avoid intravascular red cell destruction of the transfused cells.

Anti-H formed by the ''Bombay'' phenotype is a potent hemolysin reactive at 37°C. As all other blood groups carry at least some H antigen, finding blood compatible for transfusion to these patients can be problematic.

Anti-A and anti-B are not readily demonstrable in newborns. They can be detected by about 3 to 6 months and reach their maximum level between 5 and 10 years.

TABLE 4
Investigation of Polyagglutinable Red Cells

	Polyagglutinable Red Cells			
	T	Tk	Tn[a]	Cad[b]
Normal serum (human)	+	+	+	+
Anti-T (peanut lectin)	+	+	−	−
Dolichos biflorus lectin[c]	+	+	−	+
Vicia cretica lectin	+	−	−	−
Salvia sclarea lectin	−	−	+	−

[a] Nonmicrobial polyagglutination possibly due to somatic stem cell mutation.
[b] Inherited antigen.
[c] Only if cells are group O or B.

D. PROBLEMS AND SOURCES OF ERROR IN ABO GROUPING

1. Antigenic Anomalies

In the majority of cases, ABO typing gives clear and unequivocal results. However, grouping anomalies can occur, and when a discrepancy is found, several causative factors must be considered. Subgroups of A or B, inherited mosaic groups, chimeras, or genetic anomalies can produce ambiguous results.

Weakened expression of A or B antigens can occur in the elderly, and in neonates. Alteration of ABO antigens can be acquired in disease states; for example, it has been found that partial or complete loss of A or B antigen occurs in patients with hypoplastic or sideroblastic anemia. This is of significance because there is an increased incidence of progression to acute leukemia in this group of patients.[9] Mixed-field agglutination has been reported in acute leukemia and preleukemia and specific ABH anomalies have also been found in these conditions. ABH antigenic alteration in hemopoietic disorders has been found to correlate with the activity of the gene-specified H enzyme, which decreases with disease progression, but rises again during clinical remission.

The acquired B phenotype is sometimes found in association with leukemia, and is also associated with gastrointestinal malignancies and alimentary infections. In the latter, bacterial enzymes appear to produce B substance from ABH precursor chains in a similar manner to normal B antigen production.

Bacterial infections can also cause red cells to become polyagglutinable, for example by the action of the bacterial enzymes exposing the crypt-antigens T or Tk. The red cells then react with anti-T or Tk present in most human sera used as grouping reagents. Polyagglutinable cells may be investigated and identified by the use of various lectins (Table 4).

Because monoclonal antibodies are specific for antigenic epitopes, their use overcomes the problem of grouping polyagglutinable red cells due to T or Tk antigen exposure.

2. ABO Antibody Anomalies

The normally expected alloantibodies are lacking in neonates and are often reduced in the elderly as well as in many acquired immunodeficiency states.

Problems can occur when a serum containing irregular antibodies produces false-positive serum grouping tests, which may be misinterpreted as part of the ABO typing reactions. Certain clinical conditions, notably myeloma, cause the sera being tested to promote rouleaux formation of red cells which can also subsequently cause misinterpretation of results.

Other causes of possible error result from technical or clerical mistakes, the latter being the most common.

E. THE RH BLOOD GROUP SYSTEM

The Rh system is possibly the most complex of all blood group systems, containing over 46 characterized antigens. The Rh D antigen is the most immunogenic of all non-ABO blood groups and is thought to be the product of one of a series of three closely linked alleles. The antithetical antigens C and c, and E and e are the products of the other two alleles. No antithetical partner to D has been found to date, so that it is accepted that ''d'' indicates the absence of D. The D, c, and E antigens have been shown to be proteins with a molecular weight of 32 kDa, and the Rh antigens Cc, D, and Ee are carried on three different but closely related molecules.[10] The principal Rh molecules are roughly globular in shape and deeply embedded in the lipid membrane of the red cell with only one surface of the antigen exposed for antibody attachment.[11]

Another recent speculative genetic concept for the Rh blood group system proposed by Tippett,[12] is based on two closely linked structural Rh loci, D and CcEe.[10] Biochemical data suggesting that the Rh antigens are associated with two groups of related polypeptides[13,14] complement and possibly confirm Tippett's model. D and ''non-D'' are found at the first locus, and four alleles (ce, Ce, cE, CE) are found at the second. Rare or unusual Rh gene complexes are accounted for by mutations or unequal crossing over.

An individual inherits one Rh gene complex or haplotype from each parent. The Rh genes are codominant, and therefore, the products of both inherited gene complexes will be expressed on the red cells. The most commonly encountered genotypes in the Caucasian population are shown in Table 5. Probable genotypes are obtained by testing red cells with five Rh antisera to detect the D, C, c, E, and e antigens which determine the Rh phenotype. The probable genotype is ascertained from the known frequencies of genes and their products. Determination of probable Rh genotypes can be useful in

TABLE 5
Rh System — Commonly Encountered Genotypes

Probable genotype (1 × haplotype from each parent)	Rh (D) Type	Fisher-Race notation	Frequency %
CDe/cde	Positive	R_1r	32
CDe/CDe	Positive	R_1R_1	18
CDe/cDE	Positive	R_1R_2	12
cDE/cde	Positive	R_2r	11
cDE/CDE	Positive	R_2R_2	2
cDe/cde	Positive	R_0r	2[a]
cde/cde	Negative	rr	15
Cde/cde	Negative	r′r	1
cdE/cde	Negative	r″r	1

[a] 42% in U.S. black population.

predicting the risk of hemolytic disease of the newborn (HDN), providing typed red cells for transfusion to alloimmunized recipients, paternity or forensic testing, and population studies.

1. G Antigen

The G antigen was first described in 1958,[15] and is present on almost all red cells that possess either a D or C antigen. When anti-D or anti-C are made apparently without exposure to the D or C antigen, then anti-G should be considered as the specificity. The rare r^G cells are phenotypically D- and C-negative but G-positive.

2. The Rh-Positive D^u Phenotype

The D^u phenotype denotes a weakened expression of the D antigen, and in serological tests a D^u phenotype can exhibit extensive variable reactivity with anti-D sera. This phenotype can result from a gene coding for weakened quantitative expression of D (for example, there can be as few as 600 D antigen sites per cell; a "normal" D expression possesses 1 to 3 × 10^5 sites per rbc) or resulting from gene interaction whereby the D carried on one haplotype is depressed by the C antigen of the Cde haplotype in the *trans* position. In the latter case, the D^u phenotype is not passed on to the next generation, but is expressed as a normal D antigen.

The frequency of the D^u antigen is relatively low (less than 1%), and is more common in black populations. D^u is a poor immunogen, however, Rh immunoglobulin is generally given to Rh-negative mothers who deliver an infant found to carry the D^u phenotype. Prophylactic administration of Rh immunoglobulin to D^u antigen-positive mothers is not required.

3. Partial D Phenotypes

The D antigen is comprised of genetically separate subdivisions or epitopes; to date, eight epitopes have been identified. Rarely, individuals may lack one or more of these components and can produce an alloanti-D to the missing component. Tippet and Sanger[16,17] classified these into categorized I to VI on the basis of the reactions obtained when tested with anti-Ds from other partial D individuals. A further category (VII) has been proposed and category I is now considered obsolete. Each of the categories has been demonstrated using monoclonal anti-D antibodies, and results indicate that other epitopes must also exist.[18] Each category lacks one or more epitopes, and this absence could be explained on the basis of a single amino acid alteration, occurring at a site which is common to several D epitopes.

Antenatal patients exhibiting partial D phenotypes are generally treated as Rh (D)-negatives and given anti-D prophylaxis after miscarriage, amniocentesis, or delivery of an Rh (D)-positive infant.

4. Variant Antigens of the Rh System

C^w antigen appears to be a low-incidence marker antigen rather than an allele of C/c. It is fairly rare, occurring in less than 2% of whites and even less in blacks. Antibodies to C^w are usually naturally occurring; however, they have been implicated in both hemolytic transfusion reactions and HDN. Other variants include C^u, C^v, and c-like (Deal). There are also some E/e variants such as E^t, E^w, E^u, hr^s, and hr^B.[15]

5. Deletion Phenotypes

Alleles at the CDE locus can code for absence of the normal gene product. The missing Rh antigens are denoted using a dash or dot. –D– red cells show enhanced reactions with anti-D sera and have the largest number of D antigen sites of all D-positive haplotypes. Individuals displaying the –D– phenotype are easily immunized and so can present transfusion and antenatal problems. ·D· is similar to –D– but the D activity is not as enhanced, there being fewer D antigen sites per cell.

6. Rh_{null} Phenotypes

An individual displaying an Rh_{null} phenotype lacks expression of all Rh antigens, due to one of two genetic mechanisms. The regulator type of Rh_{null} results from homozygous inheritance of X^0r suppressor genes instead of the normal X_1r genes. The normal Rh genes are present but are unable to be expressed. Offspring who are heterozygous for X^0r exhibit partial expression of Rh antigens.

The second, even rarer type of Rh_{null} results from homozygosity for a silent or amorphic allele at the Rh locus denoted by the symbol $\overline{\overline{r}}$. Offspring heterozygous for $\overline{\overline{r}}$ will exhibit only antigens inherited from the parent with normal Rh genes. Rh_{null} cells also exhibit suppressed S, s, and U antigens, possibly due to the structural membrane abnormality associated with the Rh_{null} phenotype. Decreased red cell survival is common in Rh_{null} individuals and the phenotype is associated with a hemolytic anemia of varying severity, with the presence of stomatocytes and spherocytes in the peripheral blood.

F. ANTIBODIES OF THE RH SYSTEM

Rh antibodies are mainly produced due to immunization through transfusion or pregnancy, and are generally IgG, requiring laboratory test systems that potentiate agglutination. Most of these antibodies have been implicated in hemolytic transfusion reactions and HDN. However, because Rh(D)-negative individuals are invariably transfused with Rh(D)-negative blood, transfusion reactions are rarely due to anti-D.

Anti-D is still the most common single cause of severe HDN, despite Rh immunoglobulin (RhIG) being administered routinely to Rh(D)-negative mothers after delivery of Rh(D)-positive infants.[19] Concurrent developments in obstetric and neonatal care and improvements in laboratory techniques have, however, reduced mortality due to HDN by about 90%.

Anti-E is by far the most common Rh antibody and can often be found as a naturally occurring IgM antibody. Anti-c is usually IgG and is the second most common cause of HDN. Ic is also implicated in transfusion reactions. Anti-e is fairly rare, as only 2% of the population are e antigen-negative and therefore able to form the antibody. Anti-C does not usually occur on its own in serum, and is most often found with anti-D. Most ''anti-C'' antibodies are mixtures of anti-C and anti-Ce.

G. PROBLEMS AND SOURCES OF ERROR IN RH TYPING

Errors involving mistyping Rh(D)-negative patients as Rh(D)-positive are potentially serious. A potential transfusion recipient mistyped as Rh(D)-positive may be given Rh(D)-positive cells, and this will result in anti-D production in the majority of cases. There can be serious consequences of such an action, particularly if the recipient is a woman of child-bearing age. Antenatal patients wrongly typed as Rh(D)-positive would not be given RhIG and may become sensitized by fetal Rh(D)-positive cells.

Such errors may result because of the use of anti-G-contaminated human anti-D typing sera. Red cells that are C+, D−, and G+, therefore, could be mistyped as Rh(D)-positive. Errors also occur because anti-D antisera can be contaminated with other antibodies, particularly anti-C. Polyagglutinable red cells are a further potential cause of Rh mistyping, as are direct antiglobulin test (DAT)-positive cells. Problems may be avoided by the use of monoclonal antibodies in conjunction with appropriate controls.

H. OTHER BLOOD GROUP SYSTEMS

Kell blood groups — The Kell system has 24 characterized antigens. Kell (K) and Cellano (k) antigens are the product of two alleles at one locus and are the most important antigens in this system. K is a potent immunogen, and transfusion of K-positive blood has around a 5% chance of inducing the formation of anti-K in Kell-negative recipients. As only about 10% of the population are K-positive, finding compatible blood does not present much difficulty. Conversely, anti-k produced by rare homozygous Kell individuals who represent less than 1 in 500 (0.2%) of the population, when present, does cause problems in finding compatible blood. Kell antibodies are usually non-complement-fixing IgG antibodies, detected most effectively by the antiglobulin test. The Kell antigens are well developed at birth, so that antibody production in antenatal patients can cause HDN. Anti-K is thought to cause HDN by suppression of erythropoiesis as well as by red cell destruction. This can present problems in assessing severity of HDN using spectrophotometric analysis of amniotic fluid and direct fetal blood sampling is preferable in these cases.

Duffy blood groups — The Duffy system is composed of five red cell antigens. The two most significant alleles code for the antigens Fy^a and Fy^b. The Fy(a+b−) phenotype occurs with a frequency of about 17% in the European population and individuals homozygous for Fy^a can form anti-Fy^b. Anti-Fy^b does not appear to be a potent antibody in terms of eliciting hemolytic transfusion reactions or HDN. Individuals expressing the Fy(a−b+) genotype can be stimulated by transfusion or pregnancy to produce anti-Fy^a, which can subsequently cause serious hemolytic transfusion reactions and which has been implicated in cases of HDN. About 49% of Europeans are phenotypically Fy(a+b+), but Fy(a−b−) is extremely rare in this population. Conversely, the Fy(a−b−) type is common in blacks (69% of American blacks and almost 100% of the West African population), and anti-Fy3 may be produced by these individuals, which reacts with red cells possessing either Fy^a or Fy^b antigens, causing compatibility problems. The high frequency of Fy(a−b−) blacks is now known to be related to resistance to malarial infection, the Duffy antigen site being necessary for malarial parasites, particularly *Plasmodium vivax*, to enter and parasitize the red cells.[20,21]

Kidd blood groups — The Kidd system is composed of the antigens Jk^a, Jk^b, and Jk3. The most important alleles of the Kidd system are Jk^a and Jk^b. The possible phenotypes are Jk(a+b−), present in 27% of the population; Jk(a+b+), present in 50%; and Jk(a−b+), present in 23%. The rare Jk(a−b−) phenotype is found mainly in Chinese and Polynesian populations (about 1%). Phenotyping for Kidd antigens utilizes rare, and often unsatisfactory antibodies; however, recently IgM human monoclonal antibodies to Jk^a and Jk^b have been produced.[22] The Kidd system is important in transfusion because antibodies, particularly anti-Jk^a, are often implicated in cases of delayed, but serious, hemolytic transfusion reactions. Kidd antibodies are usually IgG and fix complement, but can be difficult to detect. They are often identified in antiglobulin tests by virtue of their complement-fixing characteristics but may remain undetected if antiglobulin reagents lacking anti-complement activity are used. Fresh samples are required when testing for

Kidd antibodies before the complement level present in the sample falls and because the antibody itself deteriorates on storage. Kidd antibodies, mainly anti-Jk^a, have also been implicated in HDN.

Other blood group systems such as MN, Lewis, P, Ii, and Lutheran systems are less critical from the point of view of patient care in transfusion or antenatal serology. Antibodies of these systems are rarely significant but can interfere with the efficient supply of compatible blood as they are frequently detected during antibody screening procedures.

III. ANTIBODY SCREENING AND IDENTIFICATION

Antibody screening procedures are designed to detect the presence of antibodies in a patient's serum which could cause either a hemolytic transfusion reaction if blood were transfused or hemolytic disease of the newborn (HDN) in an antigen-positive foetus. Unfortunately, there is no single serological technique which can selectively detect antibodies of such significance. Identification of irregular (non-ABO) antibodies is performed after their detection in an antibody screening system.

In an effort to be more clinically relevant and cost effective, most laboratories select methods which will predominantly detect antibodies of pathological significance, using reagent cells expressing the clinically most significant antigen systems, preferably in the homozygous state.[23]

Of all the techniques available, the indirect antiglobulin test (IAT), enhanced by the use of low ionic strength saline (LISS), is the most important procedure for recognition of clinically significant antibodies. Good laboratory practice should encourage the use of a sensitive two-stage enzyme technique as an adjunct to the antiglobulin test, particularly as it can detected some Rh antibodies more readily than the LISS IAT.[24]

There is little evidence to support the necessity of using an albumin-enhanced screening procedure, and it is now widely recognized that antibodies reacting at room temperature alone are unimportant.

A. THE INDIRECT ANTIGLOBULIN TEST (IAT)

IgG antibodies sensitize red cells of the appropriate antigenicity, but are unable to promote agglutination. The addition of anti-human globulin (AHG) directed against the antibody coating the red cells is required to visually demonstrate the presence of such an antibody.

The subsequent introduction of LISS as an incubation medium improved both the speed and sensitivity of the IAT technique for most antibodies.[25] The low ionic concentrations of LISS solutions reduces interference by charged ions and vastly speeds up antibody uptake. Disadvantages of LISS include enhancement of some nonsignificant antibodies, such as anti-I and anti-P_1, and not all clinically important antibody reactions are enhanced, notably some examples of anti-E and anti-K. Polyspecific antiglobulin reagents should contain anti-C3c and anti-C3d in addition to anti-IgG, in order to assure that antibodies best detected by virtue of complement coating of red cells are not missed in the screening procedure — of particular importance in this respect are anti-Jk^a, anti-Fy^a, and some examples of anti-K. Quality assurance of IAT results depends on eliminating the potential for errors. Inadequate washing of the test prior to AHG addition may cause a false-negative result due to neutralization of the AHG by unbound immunoglobulin. Control cells weakly sensitized with antibody added to all apparently negative tests will ensure that adequate washing has taken place by promoting agglutination of the control cells by the free AHG. Neutralized AHG will fail to promote agglutination and the test should be repeated after assessing and correcting the wash procedure. False-negative results may also be due to elution of weak antibodies during the wash phase, or from inappropriate agitation of the completed test. IAT are most sensitive when performed as a spin-tube method, with careful microscopic reading of results. Red cell suspensions should not exceed 3%, and for LISS techniques a 2:2 serum to cell ratio is recommended. The IAT method for antibody screening and identification may also be performed in microplates; however, these techniques require considerable expertise.[26,27]

B. ENZYME METHODS

Red cells may be treated with proteolytic enzymes which effect removal of some negatively charged surface glycoproteins, and thus allow antibody molecules easier access to antigen sites which may otherwise be inaccessible due to steric hindrance. Enzyme treatment also produces "clustering" of certain antigen sites, which further facilitates antibody binding. Commonly, the enzyme used for manual serological techniques is papain, while automated procedures generally employ the enzyme bromelin, as this does not require the presence of an activator, which is necessary when papain is used. Although pretreatment of cells using such enzymes enhances antibody detection rates, not all antibodies detected and identified by this method are clinically important, and false-positive rates can be high. Nevertheless, early detection of some specific weak antibodies by enzyme-treated cells can be important in antenatal serology, enabling regular monitoring of the antibody throughout pregnancy. Some red cell antigens are destroyed or weakened by treatment with proteolytic enzymes, notably the Duffy, MN, and S antigens, and so may remain undetected by a two-stage enzyme method.

C. THE CLINICAL SIGNIFICANCE OF RED CELL ANTIBODIES

An antibody is considered to be clinically significant if it causes hemolysis *in vivo*, either destroying transfused red cells or fetal red cells after transplacental passage. The two most important serologic characteristics for predicting *in vivo* significance are the antibody specificity and its ability to react at 37°C. *In vitro* functional bioassays may be more accurate than serological characteristics alone in determining the amount and rate of *in vivo* red cell destruction likely to be caused by a particular antibody.

Intravascular hemolysis — Intravascular antibody-mediated red cell destruction is complement dependent, and occurs by way of the classical pathway of complement activation, from Cl uptake through to the C789 complex which damages the red cell membrane. Not many alloantibodies are able to destroy red cells intravascularly, anti-A and anti-B being the best examples; anti-Kidd, anti-Vel, anti-Tj^a, and some examples of anti-Fy^a and anti-Le^a can sometimes also activate the complement cascade with subsequent intravascular hemolysis.

Extravascular hemolysis — Red cell destruction can also be mediated by a mechanism of sequestration of erythrocytes by macrophages of the reticuloendothelial system (RES), particularly in the liver and spleen. The IgG Rh, Kell, and Duffy antibodies are the best examples of antibodies which cause hemolysis by this mechanism. The functional activity of these IgG antibodies depends on the Fc part of the molecule, which binds to mononuclear phagocytes and placental membrane. The red cells, sensitized with IgG antibody, are destroyed by phagocytosis within the RES. In some instances, red cells may be only partly engulfed by the phagocytic cell, and damaged red cells return to the circulation, as poikilocytes and spherocytes.

Macrophages and possibly lymphocytes may also destroy sensitized red cells by extracellular cytotoxicity, brought about by lysosomal enzymes released from macrophages in addition to phagocytosis. Thus cells may be destroyed either outside the macrophage, or within the cytoplasm. These two mechanisms of extravascular red cell destruction are used as the basis for *in vitro* assays to determine the clinical significance of antibodies.

Antibody-dependent cell-mediated cytotoxicity (ADCC) — The principle of this assay is the measurement of lysis of ^{51}Cr-labeled red cells sensitized with the IgG antibody under test, with monocytes acting as effector cells. The radioactivity released by lysed cells is recorded and the percentage lysis indicates the ability of the antibody to promote red cell destruction. It has been shown that the degree of red cell lysis using ADCC correlated better with clinically significant hemolysis in infants with Rh(D) HDN than other methods of antibody quantitation.[28,29]

Phagocytosis assays — The basic phagocytosis assay consists of a monolayer of peripheral blood monocytes adhered to a plastic or glass surface. Red cells sensitized with the antibody under test are added to the monolayer, and the number of red cells adhering to and/or phagocytosed by the monocytes are counted. The number of red cells phagocytosed by 100 monocytes is known as the phagocytic index of the antibody and interpretation of a phagocytosis assay is optimized by using this as the measure of antibody activity. A phagocytic index of greater than 2 is said to be a significantly elevated value for an antibody and would indicate decreased survival of incompatible red cells if transfused.[30] When the assay is used to predict severity of HDN, there has been good correlation between pregnancy outcome and positive assay results.[31,32] The assay is also a good predictor of a benign clinical course.

Chemiluminescence assays — The chemiluminescence test (CLT) is based on a reaction mixture of monocytes, luminol, and red cells sensitized with the antibody under test. Occupation of cellular Fc receptors effects the release of large amounts of reactive oxygen intermediates, which, in the presence of luminol, can be converted to light and measured in a luminometer. The amount of light is therefore a measure of the phagocytic/adherence activity taking place. Results using IgG anti-D-sensitized red cells have shown good correlation with clinical outcome of alloimmunized pregnancies[33,34] and CLT assays are easier to perform, slightly more sensitive, less labor-intensive, less subjective, and more easily standardized than manually interpreted phagocytosis assays.

Quantitation of antibodies — This technique is routinely used in the U.K. to measure the level of anti-D antibody in maternal sera. Quantitation is undertaken against a National Standard preparation of anti-D, using an autoanalyzer, continuous flow technique according to the recommended method as defined by the *British Pharmacopeia*. Quantitated levels of anti-D greater than 4 IU/cm^3 are generally accepted as the level at which amniocentesis or cordocentesis is indicated. Anti-c antibodies may also be quantitated in the same way. Levels of less than 10 IU/cm^3 are usually considered to indicate little risk to the fetus of HDN.[35]

Antibody titers — Clinically significant antibodies other than anti-D (and anti-c if quantitated) that are demonstrable by indirect antiglobulin testing are assessed for activity/strength by titering against antigenically heterozygous cells. Results are expressed either as a reciprocal of the final dilution at which a positive reaction was obtained or as a titer score where graded reactions are numerically valued.[23] Unfortunately, although the prognostic value of antibody titers is not very good, there being little correlation with pregnancy outcome, this method is still the best routinely undertaken technique for antenatal antibody assessment. The main problems associated with antibody titers are the subjective nature of the reading and interpretation of the hemagglutination reactions, and the fact that an antibody titer may increase due to an anamnestic response rather than secondary immunization by fetal red cells. Paternal phenotyping for the appropriate antigen can be helpful in some cases.

D. AUTOANTIBODIES

The majority of blood group antibodies are alloantibodies. Sometimes, however, autoantibodies are produced. Different mechanism are known to be responsible for production of these autoantibodies, resulting in a variety of clinical pictures, but all cause problems in routine serological testing and difficulty in providing compatible blood if transfusion is required. Difficulties arise because of red cell-bound antibody and free antibody in the patient's serum.

Red cell-bound immunoglobulin is demonstrated by the finding of a positive direct antiglobulin test (DAT). The specific component bound to the red cell can be determined by using monospecific antiglobulin reagents and most commonly is IgG but may be IgM, IgA, or may consist of complement components only. The type of cell-bound immunoglobulin may help in elucidating the cause of the immune process but quantitation of bound immunoglobulin does not appear to be related to the extent of the hemolytic process.[36] A negative DAT in AIHA may be due to low-affinity autoantibodies or cell-bound IgG being below the threshold of the sensitivity of the test system.

The amount and specificity of free antibody in serum shows wide variation. High-affinity, warm-reacting antibodies are often largely cell bound, whereas cold-reacting antibodies are often present in serum at a high titer. The specificity of autoantibodies is often difficult to elucidate. Cold antibodies may show specificity such as anti-H, anti-I, or anti-i; warm antibodies often show broad patterns of reactivity, reacting with all test cells although sometimes specificity within the Rh system occurs, particularly auto-anti-e. Drugs can cause immune hemolysis by a variety of mechanisms. This may be also associated with the production of red cell autoantibodies, as seen classically with the antihypertensive drug α-methyl dopa.[37]

E. SEROLOGICAL PROBLEMS ASSOCIATED WITH AUTOANTIBODIES

In the presence of cold autoantibodies which cause direct agglutination of all cell suspensions, it is often difficult to determine ABO grouping. To overcome this problem, blood and all reagents used should be kept warm during testing. Treatment of red cells with 0.01 *M* dithiothreitol (DTT) prior to ABO typing may occasionally be necessary. Rh typing can pose a problem when warm autoantibodies are present, particularly if albumin, enzyme, or antiglobulin methods are used, when saline reacting typing sera may be required. Sometimes modifications of the red cells by heating or chemical treatment with ZZAP (0.1 *M* DTT plus 0.1% cysteine-activated papain)[38] or an acid solution of chloroquinine diphosphate[39] is needed, particularly if full Rh genotyping or typing for other red cell antigen systems is required. Occasionally, differential absorption techniques using cells heterozygous, homozygous, and negative for a particular antigen need to be performed in order to type a patient's red cells.[9]

IV. ROUTINE COMPATIBILITY TESTING

The main aim of red cell compatibility testing is to prevent hemolytic transfusion reactions. It is essential, therefore, that consideration is given to a variety of factors as part of pretransfusion testing. The patient's previous serological history — transfusions, pregnancies, drugs — is important. It is also essential that prior to transfusion a final check on ABO compatibility is made, though whether this should be a paper (or computer) check of previously recorded findings, a rapid compatibility check such as an immediate spin technique, or a formal crossmatch, is debated.[24,40,41]

A. MAXIMUM BLOOD ORDER SCHEDULE

Increasingly maximum blood order schedules incorporating a group and antibody screen procedure and an immediate spin cross-match are being used. Advantages of a pretransfusion antibody screen are that it can (and should) be carried out well in advance of transfusion, allowing sufficient time to detect and identify alloantibodies and to select compatible donors. Data suggest that 99.6% of irregular antibodies can be detected by antibody screen alone[42] when appropriate screening cells are selected. By combining this with an immediate spin technique prior to transfusion to ensure ABO compatibility, it is possible to omit a major cross-match from the majority of compatibility testing procedures. Confidence in this approach depends on a high standard of proficiency in antibody detection techniques.

If a major crossmatch is to be undertaken it should always include an antiglobulin test. This may be undertaken in normal or low ionic strength media. The use of other enhancing techniques such as albumin or enzyme techniques is not warranted.[43,44]

B. COMPATIBILITY TESTING IN THE PRESENCE OF AUTOANTIBODIES

Compatibility testing in the presence of autoantibodies can be problematic. Fortunately, the majority of patients with immune hemolysis do not require transfusion as they adapt to the chronic anemia or respond to specific therapy. Compatibility problems may arise, however, during both antibody screening and cross-matching. Antibody screening should be performed using both serum and an eluate. Absorption techniques ought to routinely be used when investigating patients width autoantibodies in order to be confident that alloantibodies do not coexist, as up to 40% of patients with autoantibodies also possess alloantibodies.[45] Warm autoabsorption using enzyme-treated cells or differential absorption may be performed using an enzyme-treated cell negative for non-Rhesus antigens commonly associated with hemolytic transfusion reactions, i.e., Kell-negative, Jk^a-negative, Jk^b-negative, or Fy^a-negative.[9] Specificity of autoantibodies may be difficult to determine precisely but they sometimes show Rh specificity. Once the presence of an alloantibody has been excluded or defined, blood of the same Rh genotype as the patient should be used for transfusion. Frequently, no truly compatible donor blood can be found on cross-matching, in which case, in the absence of alloantibodies, the least incompatible units should be transfused.[46]

C. *IN VIVO* COMPATIBILITY TESTING

Occasionally, it is impossible to find truly compatible blood using conventional cross-matching techniques. If transfusion is required in such a patient, and time permits, *in vivo* survival of a cohort of cells may be assessed prior to transfusion. The most widely used technique is to inject small volumes (0.5 to 1 ml) of radiolabeled red cells, ^{51}Cr being used most commonly (though ^{99m}Tc or double labeling with ^{99m}Tc and ^{111}In has also been used), and the survival of labeled cells 1 hour and 24 hours after infusion is then measured. Other workers recommend that a small aliquot of radiolabeled cells should be included in the full unit when it is transfused. Survival of these cells is a helpful indicator of shortened survival or delayed hemolytic transfusion reaction.[48,49]

Survival of transfused cells can also be measured using an enzyme-linked antiglobulin test.[50] This technique measures transfused red cells antigenically distinct from the recipient's red cells. It is useful if the decision to estimate red cell survival is made after transfusion, or when radioisotopes are unavailable, or their use contraindicated.

It is likely that all these techniques will be superseded by cellular assays or the use of flow cytometry, as the latter technique obviates the use of radioisotopes and has been shown to produce accurate results when studied in parallel with ^{51}Cr survival.[51]

V. FUTURE DEVELOPMENTS

Currently available antibody screening, identification, and compatibility testing procedures are prone to certain imperfections, and new techniques are continually being developed and evaluated in an effort to improve patient care. Some innovative laboratory techniques are described briefly.

Solid-phase antiglobulin test for antibody screening — Solid-phase antiglobulin testing methods are available for antibody screening from commercial companies based on a method of Plapp et al.[52] Capture™-R, manufactured by Immunocor Inc., uses red cell ghosts immobilized to the surfaces of microplate wells. Reactions are visualized by the addition of anti-IgG-sensitized indicator red cells. The system can be automated to include an agglutination reader or adapted for enzyme-linked immunosorbent assay (ELISA) methodology for interpretation of the antibody screen. Some variants of solid-phase antiglobulin tests utilize incubation of test red cells with serum and washing of the tests by conventional liquid-phase techniques, but the final reading stage uses a solid-phase method, with anti-IgG and anti-C3d coated onto the microplate wells. Sensitivity is enhanced in comparison with liquid-phase microtiter IAT, although the wash phase remains[53,54] with its inherent problems.

ID gel centrifugation system — An antibody screening and identification system marketed in the U.K. by DiaMed-GB Ltd. utilizes a Sephadex™ gel incorporated into microtubes based on the method of Lapierre et al.[55] The gels may be neutral or impregnated with anti-human globulin. Enzyme-treated and LISS-suspended reagent cells are added to the reaction chambers above the gel and test serum is then introduced. After incubation and centrifugation the tests are read, without the requirement for washing the antiglobulin tests. The no-wash IAT reduces the potential for errors due to poor wash techniques or to elution of weakly bound antibodies. This increases the sensitivity of the test system and reduces hands-on labor involvement. Results are stable within the gels for several days, allowing for improved control possibilities. The gel system can be incorporated into an automated technique with image analysis of the results.

Flow cytometry — Flow cytometry (FCM) measures cellular characteristics within an automated electronic device. It is capable of analyzing specific features of a cell as it moves in front of stationary sensors. Its ability to assay quickly a large number of cells eliminates the risk of sampling error and reproducibility is excellent. The facility to detect and accurately quantitate minor red cell populations offers an excellent tool to the serologist for *in vivo* compatibility testing and the detection and quantitation of feto-maternal hemorrhage. It is also useful for demonstrating red blood cell chimerism and mosaicism. FCM can also be used to assess red blood cell antigen-site density, thereby detecting variant red blood cells. D antigen site density assay using FCM has confirmed variation in D antigen expression demonstrating strongest expression in R_2R_2 cells and easily differentiating between weak D (D^u) and D-negative cells.[56] Detection and quantitation of red cell antigen sites can also be useful for paternity and family studies. FCM can also be used to measure and quantify red cell-bound IgG in patients with warm autoimmune hemolytic anemia.

DNA analysis and transfusion medicine — In common with many other branches of medicine, the practical application of molecular biological techniques is leading to new insights and understanding. An improved understanding of the molecular basis of ABO polymorphism has also developed due to the use of cDNA probes and identification of specific restriction enzyme cleavage sites. Using these techniques, it is likely that DNA analysis will help to identify how ABO expression is manifest, and this should also help to elucidate the ways in which blood group chimeras, mosaics, and other anomalies occur and will increase the ability to use ABO groupings in linkage studies and forensic investigations.[57] Similar studies regarding the isolation and sequencing of genes coding for Rh proteins have been reported[58] and it is likely that by using these molecular techniques the structural basis of the common Rh phenotypes will soon be more fully understood.

VI. QUALITY ASSURANCE

Quality assurance is an essential aspect of good laboratory practice and it is the responsibility of all staff to ensure that quality is constantly monitored and maintained. There are several key factors.

1. Training — Laboratory personnel need to be trained correctly in order that individuals undertaking the performance of serologic tests can reach an agreed standard of proficiency in both practical and theoretical concerns relating to laboratory practice. "Training" should also encompass the realization that educational update requirements need to be met in order to continue the training process and ensure that the highest levels of expertise are maintained.

2. Standard operating procedures (SOP) — All staff must be aware that strict adherence to officially documented SOPs is necessary in order to achieve quality assurance of results. SOPs must be updated as appropriate, and new techniques must be evaluated and validated before being introduced, to ensure conformation with quality criteria.

3. Reporting — Accurate reporting of serologic results must be ensured, whether manually transcribed or electronically captured, with system checks incorporated to recognize anomalous results requiring further investigation. Reports of laboratory testing must be returned to the appropriate clinician rapidly in order to be of use for therapy or patient management. The results must, therefore, be clinically relevant, reliable, and reproducible, so that confidence in the laboratory results is ensured and the quality of health care continuously improved.

REFERENCES

1. **Landsteiner, K.,** Uber. Agglutinationserscheinungen normalen meuschlichen blutes, *Wien. Klin. Wochenschr.,* 14, 1132, 1901.
2. **Creite, A.,** Versuche uber die Wirkung des serumweisses nach injection in das blut, *Z. Rationelle Median,* 36, 195, 1869.
3. **Landois, L.,** *Die Transfusion des Blutes,* Vogel, Leipzig, 1875.
4. **Coombs, R. R. A., Mourant, A. E., and Race, R. R.,** Detection of weak and "incomplete" Rh agglutinins: a new test, *Lancet,* ii, 15, 1945.
5. **Issit, P. D.,** *Applied Blood Group Serology,* 3rd ed., Montgomery Scientific Publications, Miami, 1985.
6. **Salmon, C., Cartron, J. P., and Rouger, P. H.,** *The Human Blood Groups,* Masson Publishing USA, New York, 1984.
7. **Bird, G. W. G.,** Specific agglutinating activity for human red blood corpuscles in extracts of Dolichos biflorus, *Curr. Sci.,* 20, 198, 1951.
8. **Watkins, W. M.,** Biochemistry and genetics of ABO, Lewis and P blood group systems, in *Advances in Human Genetics,* Harris, H. and Hirschoruk, K., Eds., Plenum Press, New York, 1980.
9. **Petz, L. D. and Swisher, S. N., Eds.,** *Clinical Practice of Transfusion Medicine,* 2nd ed., Churchill Livingstone, New York, 1990.
10. **Hughes-Jones, N. C., Bloy, C., and Gorick, B. D.,** Evidence that the c, D and E epitopes of the human Rh blood group system are on separate polypeptide molecules, *Mol. Immunol.,* 25, 931, 1988.
11. **Cherif-Zahar, B., Bloy, C., Le Van Kim, C. et al.,** Molecular cloning and protein structure of a human blood group Rh polypeptide, *Proc. Nat. Acad. Sci. U.S.A.,* 87, 6234, 1990.

12. **Tippet, P.,** A speculative model for the Rh blood groups, *Ann. Hum. Genet.,* 50, 241, 1986.
13. **Moore, S. and Green, C.,** Identification of Rhesus polypeptide blood group ABH active-glycoprotein complexes in the human red cell membrane, *Biochem. J.,* 244, 735, 1987.
14. **Avent, N. D., Ridgewell, K., Mawby, W. J., Tanner, M. J. A., Anstee, D., and Kumpal, B. M.,** Protein sequence studies on Rh-related polypeptides suggest the presence of at least two groups of proteins which associate in the human red cell membrane, *Biochem. J.,* 256, 1043, 1988.
15. **Allen, F. H. and Tippett, P.,** A new Rh blood type which reveals the Rh antigen G, *Vox Sang.,* 3, 321, 1958.
16. **Tippett, P. and Sanger, R.,** Observations on subdivisions of the Rh antigen D, *Vox Sang.,* 7, 9, 1962.
17. **Tippett, P. and Sanger, R.,** Further observations on subdivisions of the Rh antigen D, *Arzliches Laboratorium,* 23, 47, 1977.
18. **Lomas, C., Tippett, P., Thompson, K. M., Melamed, M. D., and Hughes-Jones, N. C.,** Demonstration of seven epitopes on the Rh antigen D using human monoclonal anti-D antibodies and red cells from D categories, *Vox Sang.,* 57, 261, 1989.
19. **Clarke, C. A., Donohoe, W. T. A., McConnell, R. B., Woodrow, J. C., Finn, R., Krevaus, J. R., Kulke, W., Lehane, D., and Sheppard, P. H.,** Further experimental studies on the prevention of Rh haemolytic disease, *Br. Med. J.,* (i), 979, 1963.
20. **Hadley, T. J., Miller, L. H., and Haynes, J. D.,** Recognition of red cells by malaria and parasites: the role of erythrocyte binding proteins, *Transfus. Med. Rev. V,* 108, 1991.
21. **Fang, X., Kaslow, D. C., Adams, J. H. et al.,** Cloning of the Plasmodium vivax, Duffy receptor, *Mol. Biochem. Parasitol.,* 44, 125, 1991.
22. **Thompson, K., Barden, G., Sutherland, J., Beldon, I., and Melamed, M.,** Human monoclonal antibodies to human blood group antigens Kidd Jk^a and Jk^b, *Transfus. Med.,* 1, 91, 1991.
23. *Guidelines for the Blood Transfusion Services in the United Kingdom,* 3 volumes, joint publication of the U.K. Blood Transfusion Service and National Institute for Biological Standards and Control, 1989.
24. **Napier, J. A. F.,** The crossmatch, *Br. J. Haematol.,* 78, 1, 1991.
25. **Low, B. and Messeter, L.,** Antiglobulin test in low ionic strength solution for rapid antibody screening and crossmatching, *Vox Sang.,* 26, 53, 1974.
26. Guidelines for microplate techniques in liquid-phase blood grouping and antibody screening, *Clin. Lab. Haematol.,* 12, 437, 1990.
27. **Scott Marion, L.,** The principles and applications of solid-phase blood group serology, *Transfus. Med. Rev.,* V, 60, 1991.
28. **Engelfriet, C. P. and Ouwehand, W. H.,** ADCC and other cellular bioassays for predicting the clinical significance of red cell alloantibodies, in *Balliere's Clinical Haematology,* Vol. 3, No. 2, Contreras, M., Ed., Balliere Tindall, London, April 1990.
29. **Urbaniak, S. J., Greiss, M. A., Crawford, R. J., and Fergusson, M. J. C.,** Prediction of the outcome of Rhesus haemolytic disease of the newborn: additional information using an ADCC assay, *Vox Sang.,* 46, 323, 1984.
30. **Nance, S. J., Arndt, P., and Garraty, G.,** Predicting the clinical significance of red cell alloantibodies using a monocyte monolayer assay, *Transfusion,* 27, 449, 1987.
31. **Nance, S. J., Nelson, J. M., Arndt, P. A., Platt, L. D., and Garratty, G.,** Monocyte monolayer assay: an efficient noninvasive technique for predicting the severity of haemolytic disease of the newborn, *Am. J. Clin. Pathol.,* 92, 2283, 1989.
32. **Nance, S. J., Nelson, J., Horenstein, J., O'Neill, P., and Garratty, G.,** Predictive value of aminocentesis versus monocyte monolayer assays in pregnant women with Rh antibodies, *Transfusion,* 26 (Abstr.), 570, 1986.

33. **Hadley, A. G., Kumpel, B. M., Leader, D. A., Poole, G. D., and Fraser, I.,** Correlation of serological, quantitative and cell-mediated functional assays of maternal alloantibodies with the severity of haemolytic disease of the newborn, *Br. J. Haematol.*, 77, 221, 1991.
34. **Downing, I., Templeton, J. G., Mitchell, R., and Fraser, R. H.,** A chemiluminescence assay for erythrophagocytosis, *J. Biolumines c. Chemilumines c.*, 5, 243, 1990.
35. **Shwe, K. H., Love, E. M., Powell, S. B., Burgess, H. J., and Gunson, H. H.,** Evalution of anti-c quantitation and correlation with clinical outcome in sensitised pregnancies, Abstract BBTS Meeting, London, 1989.
36. **Nance, S. J. and Garratty, G.,** Correlates between in vivo haemolysis and the amount of RBC bound IgG measured by flow cytometry, *Blood*, 64, 88a, 1984.
37. **Petz, L. D. and Branch, D. R.,** Drug induced immune haemolytic anaemia, in *Immune Haemolytic Anaemias*, Chaplin, H., Jr., Ed., Churchill Livingstone, New York, 1985, 47.
38. **Branch, D. R. and Petz, L. D.,** A new reagent (ZAPP) having multiple applications in immunohaematology, *Am. J. Clin. Pathol.*, 78, 161, 1982.
39. **Edwards, J. M., Moulds, J. J., and Judd, W. J.,** Chloroquine dissociation of antigen-antibody complexes: a new technique for typing red blood cells with a positive direct antiglobulin test, *Transfusion*, 22, 59, 1982.
40. International Forum. Do you think that the crossmatch with donor red cells can be omitted when the serum of a patient has been tested for the presence of red cell alloantibodies with a cell panel?, *Vox Sang.*, 43, 151, 1982.
41. **Meyer, E. A. and Shulman, I. A.,** The sensitivity and specificity of the immediate-spin crossmatch, *Transfusion*, 29, 99, 1989.
42. **Grove Rasmussen, M.,** Routine compatibility testing, *Transfusion*, 4, 200, 1964.
43. Guidelines for compatibility testing in Hospital Blood Banks, in *Standard Haematology Practice*, Roberts, B., Ed., Blackwell Scientific, London, 1989.
44. **Schmidt, P. J., Ed.,** Standards for Blood Bank and Transfusion Services, 11th ed., American Association of Blood Banks, Arlington, VA, 1987.
45. **Laine, M. L. and Beattie, K. M.,** Frequency of alloantibodies accompanying autoantibodies, *Transfusion*, 25, 545, 1985.
46. **Walker, R. H., Kuban, D. J., Polesky, H. F., and Van der Hoeven, L. H.,** The 1980 comprehensive blood bank survey of the College of American Pathologists, *Am. J. Clin. Pathol.*, 78, 610, 1982.
47. **International Committee for Standardization in Haematology,** Recommended methods for radioisotope red cell survival studies, *Br. J. Haematol.*, 45, 659, 1980.
48. **Baldwin, M. L., Ness, P. M., Barrasso, C. et al.,** In vivo studies of the long term ^{51}Cr red cell survival of serologically incompatible red cell units, *Transfusion*, 25, 34, 1985.
49. **Davey, R. J.,** Long term ^{51}Cr survival of serologically incompatible red cell units, *Transfusion*, 25, 589, 1986.
50. **Kickler, T. S., Sith, B., Bell, W., Drew, H., Baldwin, M., and Ness, P. H.,** Estimation of transfused red cell survival using an enzyme-linked antiglobulin test, *Transfusion*, 25, 402, 1985.
51. **Nance, S. T. and Sinor, L. T.,** Applications of flow cytometry in blood transfusion science, in *Progress in Immunohaematology*, Moore, S. B., Ed., American Association of Blood Banks, Arlington, VA, 1988.
52. **Plapp, F. V., Sinor, L. T., Rachel, J. M., Beck, M. L., Coenen, W. M., and Bayer, W. I.,** A solid phase antibody screen, *Am. J. Clin. Pathol.*, 82, 719, 1984.
53. **Rachel, J. M., Sinor, L. T., Beck, M. L. et al.,** A solid-phase antiglobulin test, *Transfusion*, 25, 24, 1985.
54. **Ross, D. W. and Gordon, I.,** A solid-phase Coombs test for routine use, Poster presented at British Blood Transfusion Society Meeting, London, 1986.

55. **Lapierre, Y., Rigan, D., Adams, J., Josef, D., Merer, F., Gerber, S., and Drot, C.,** The gel test: a new way to detect red cell antigen-antibody reactions, *Transfusion,* 30, 109, 1990.
56. **Nicholson, G., Lawrence, A., Ala, F. A., and Bird, G. W. G.,** Semi-quantitative assay of D antigen site density by flow cytometric analysis, *Transfus. Med.,* 1, 87, 1991.
57. **Yamomoto, F., Clausen, H., White, T., Marken, J., and Hakomoni, C.,** Molecular genetic basis of the histo-blood group ABO system, *Nature,* 345, 229, 1990.
58. **Avent, N. D., Ridgewell, K., Tanner, M. J. A., and Anstee, D. J.,** cDNA Cloning of a 30 kD erythrocyte membrane protein associated with Rh (Rhesus) blood group antigen expression, *Biochem. J.,* 271, 821, 1990.

Chapter 10

AUTOMATION IN BLOOD GROUP SEROLOGY

W. Wagstaff and P. Davies

TABLE OF CONTENTS

ISBN 0-8493-4938-9

I. INTRODUCTION

The original concept that some form of mechanization could be used in blood group serology to reduce the laborious manual burden dates back to the mid-1960s. Since that time there have been many changes, both evolutionary and revolutionary, that have fundamentally altered the work patterns seen in blood grouping laboratories; perhaps the majority of work undertaken now is either partially or fully mechanized. It is not within the scope of this chapter to discuss or even enumerate all the various types of blood grouping systems available, although specific mention will be made of those which highlight a particular point of interest or of unique technology.

Areas to be covered are

1. The history of their development and introduction, highlighting specific changes which were important especially to the maintenance or improvement of quality aspects
2. The basic techniques employed and how these techniques have been improved and amended to overcome specific problems
3. The selection of reagents for use on the various types of equipment
4. A review of the way in which different systems are incorporated into existing laboratory work patterns

II. HISTORY AND DEVELOPMENT

In 1963, McNeil et al.[1] reported on preliminary investigations into the use of AutoAnalyser equipment for automatic blood grouping. This pioneering work was developed by Sturgeon and co-workers[2] in the same year, with the production of an automatic system for performing ABO grouping using continuous flow technology. The technique was quickly developed to include Rh typing and the use of continuous blotting paper to make a permanent record of the automated blood group reactions, these being interpreted by an experienced operator. This led to the release in 1965 of the AutoAnalyser BG system,[3] the first commercial blood grouping apparatus.

The original concept of Sturgeon was developed in the U.S. by Rosenfield and Haber in 1965[4] and in the U.K. in 1966 by Marsh et al.[5] to provide an automatic system very sensitive in the detection of irregular antibodies. The system was at least as sensitive as the traditional, manual two-stage enzyme technique for detecting anti-D. Lalezari,[6] in 1967, described an automated antibody detection system which did not incorporate enzyme, thus introducing an automated system that would reliably detect antibodies to the Duffy and MNS systems. The technique described involved the use of polybrene and low ionic media.

A fully automated blood grouping system using discrete rather than continuous flow analysis became commercially available in 1971,[7] the Kontron

Groupamatic 360 machine being based on the original concept of Matte.[8,9] This system was revolutionary not only in its use of discrete analysis but also in its unprecedented sampling rate of 300+ per hour, its use of a rudimentary type of positive sample identification and computerized data handling. Such sophistication, coupled with reliability and ease of use, was reflected in its high capital cost. A smaller version, the MG50, targeted at hospital blood banks, soon became available using the same technologies but different mechanics.

By the end of the 1970s the Groupamatic 360C represented the true state-of-the-art machine, offering not only routine ABO and Rh typing, but antibody detection, Rh phenotyping, Lewis typing, Kell typing, and microbiological testing for syphilis and HBsAg, along with true positive sample identification utilizing laser reading of barcoded labels.

By the late 1970s, Technicon had also introduced a revolutionary development of their BG system, again offering full red cell serology testing, positive sample identification and data processing, with a throughput of greater than 100 samples per hour.

During the 1980s, a great deal of attention was paid to the mechanization of conventional microplate grouping. The original idea of Bowley et al.[10] of using a microplate reader to detect and analyze hemagglutination reactions, has been greatly adapted and enlarged to encompass the long-awaited liquid handling systems, computer control, and positive sample identification. None of the systems using conventional microplates offers full automation because of the necessary manual intervention for the centrifugion and agitation stages.

In the mid-1980s, Kontron announced the successor to the Groupamatic 360, a machine coded as the G2000 which, while maintaining similar serological techniques, would offer greater mechanical and computer flexibility and reliability than the 360.

The Olympus PK7100[11] machine, while being based on microplates (albeit of an unconventional "amphitheater" design), is fully automated and may well be regarded as the state of the art in the late 1980s.

III. AUTOMATED TECHNIQUES

A. SINGLE-CHANNEL CONTINUOUS FLOW SYSTEMS

There are two basic techniques employed, either the bromelain-methyl cellulose system (BMC) of Sturgeon et al.[2] refined by Rosenfield and Haber[4] and Marsh et al.,[5] or the low ionic strength polybrene system (LISP) described by Lalezari.[6]

1. Antibody Screening

Both BMC and LISP share similar reaction manifolds — see Figure 1. A very high level of sensitivity can be obtained with correctly maintained and operated systems. The recording of results is based upon the potentiometric reading of a post-reaction hemolysate. There is no positive sample

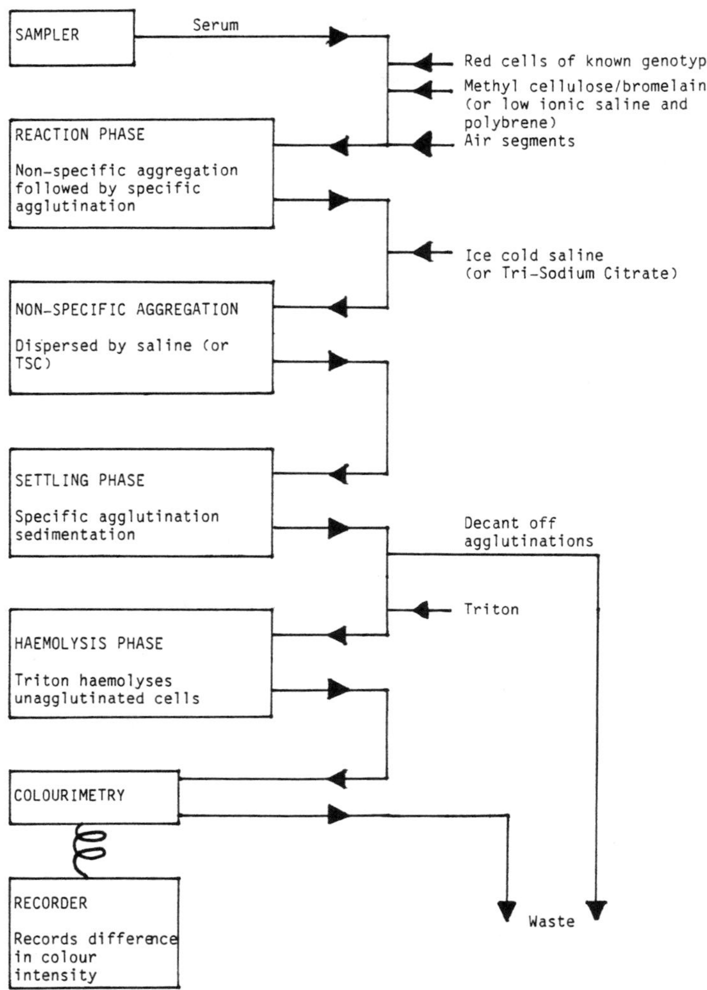

FIGURE 1. Schematic flow diagram of methyl cellulose/bromelain (or polybrene/low ionic saline) systems.

identification and therefore the identification of positive reactions may be difficult, often calling for repeating several potentially positive tests. As with all continuous flow technology, carry over may be a problem.

The BMC technique is probably the best technique, including manual ones, for detecting Rh antibodies, unfortunately being also the optimum technique for detecting anti-P_1, anti-Le^a, anti-Le^b, and anti-Bg^a. The very fact that these nonsignificant antibodies are detected at very low levels may cause problems when screening for clinically significant antibodies, therefore the reaction coil is often heated to 37°C to minimize the detection of cold antibodies. The use of an enzyme in the system limits the range of antibodies which may be detected. Obviously, antibodies to antigens which are denatured are not detected (e.g., Fy^a and M), and the system is unreliable for the detection of anti-Jk^a and Jk^b. While most anti-Kell are detected, a significant number give negative reactions by the technique.

The strength of the LISP system lies in its ability to detect the vast majority of irregular clinically significant antibodies; while it does not approach the sensitivity of the BMC technique with Rh antibodies, it certainly reacts well with anti-Fy^a, anti-Fy^b, anti-Jk^a, anti-Jk^b, anti-M, Anti-N, anti-S, anti-s, and many examples of anti-Kell. Occasionally, the LISP technique will fail to react with a clinically significant antibody which is easily demonstrable by manual technique; the most likely explanation of this would be the presence of polybrene antagonists in the patient's serum.

Most laboratories involved in large-scale antibody screening would not employ either of these techniques in isolation, but would use both techniques or one of them reinforced by the use of a manual antibody screen.

The selection of cells to be used for antibody screening may be problematic. Theoretically, nonpooled cells homozygous for the significant blood group antigens should be used. In reality, this is seldom possible and a compromise must be made. Often laboratories will use two-channel machines utilizing different cells in each channel. The use of pooled cells in a single channel will reduce sensitivity by up to 50%, depending upon the specificity of the antibody. Obviously, adequate control antisera must be used with each batch of samples tested.

The difficulty in selecting and obtaining screening cells in sufficiently large amounts, coupled with the requirement for a high level of operator skill, and the constant attention necessary means that these types of automated screening systems are only appropriate in laboratories dealing with a high antibody screening workload.

2. Antibody Identification

Antibodies may be identified using a similar system to that used for antibody detection, the best results being obtained using the LISP technique. Rather than testing unknown antisera against a single known cell, the test antiserum is tested against a panel of known cells. This technique is often used to assign specificity to antibodies which are detected by automated techniques but fail to react by traditional manual techniques. While the majority of these show no obvious specificity, some can be assigned specific activity. Although this minority often have Rh specificity, constant monitoring has usually shown them to be of no clinical importance.

3. Red Cell Phenotyping

Another system which relies on LISP technology is that of unknown red cells being tested against known antisera. This system is often used to confirm manually designated phenotypes. Rh phenotyping, MNSs, P_1, Lu^a, Le^a, Le^b, Fy^a, Fy^b, K, K, Jk^a, and Jk^b typing have all been successfully performed using this system. Many authorities would argue that Duffy and Kidd typing by this technique is more reliable than typing by manual techniques.

Very rare individuals may have a red cell defect which renders them unresponsive to polybrene, thus giving false-negative results by LISP techniques. Such red cells have apparent null-null phenotypes.

Antisera to be used should be carefully standardized and are often capable of still giving excellent reactions when massively diluted. Human polyclonal, animal polyclonal and monoclonal antibodies, together with lectins, have all been successfully used. Any antiserum which has been stored is capable of developing polybrene antagonistic activity, therefore all antisera used should be reevaluated at frequent intervals.

4. Antibody Quantitation

This technique is conventionally based on a BMC system and was originally described by Rosenfield.[4] The nature of the reaction demands that it be highly controlled in terms of reaction temperature, selection of test cells, and accurate reagent preparation. It was shown by Rosenfield that with such an AutoAnalyser system, colorimetric change in light transmission of the final hemolysate is directly proportional to antibody strength, over a specific range of antibody activity.

The technique is widely used to monitor anti-D levels during pregnancy in order to give a guideline to the clinical management necessary to limit the effects of hemolytic disease of the newborn. It is also used to assess the potency of anti-D donations which are to be used for the production of specific immunoglobulin. While mostly used to measure anti-D levels, the technique is now also used for the quantitation of other Rh antibodies.

5. Routine Blood Grouping Using Continuous Flow Technology

While the original Technicon BG15[3] machine may, with hindsight, seem a very rudimentary form of machine, it did indeed give most transfusion laboratories their first taste of automation. It was an excellent machine for confirming the blood groups of donations (the groups being first obtained from historical data or by manual grouping).

The serological technology of the BG15 was incorporated into the current Technicon AG16C, which is a fully computerized grouping machine offering positive sample identification. This type of machine is still used very successfully in many transfusion laboratories. The end point reactions are assessed potentiometrically, and computer analysis of these results allows the sample numbers, the ABO group, Rh type, and result of antibody screen to be directly printed out and/or fed directly to a host computer. The antibody screen has been greatly enhanced using both BMC and LISP technology to allow this machine to be used for the testing of both donor and patient samples.

The system is basically modular in design, which means that if one module fails it may be quickly and easily replaced to restore the system to serviceability. With the increasing importance and sophistication of computer control for these systems, it is often the availability, functionality, and reliability of the computer software which is the critical factor in the success of the system. A miniaturized continuous-flow system based largely on the AG16C has now been developed under the name of Compact.[12]

With continuous flow mechanisms there is no residual reaction which may be visually assessed to allow for a reinterpretation of any set of results. Thus the sample must be retested if even one essential channel gives an equivocal result.

Throughput for routine ABO grouping, Rh typing, and antibody screening of 100 samples per hour may be easily achieved. The rejection rate varies between 2 and 5% depending upon the testing protocol employed, about 1% of the samples initially tested commonly need to be passed for an alternative method of grouping.

B. BLOOD GROUPING USING DISCRETE AUTOMATED ANALYSIS

This type of mechanized analysis is based on the traditional manual methods of mixing cells and antiserum together in a well or tube, then observing the reaction. Various methods, mostly potentiometric, are employed to ascertain whether agglutination has occurred.

The first automated grouping system to employ discrete analysis was the Groupamatic 360. All Kontron machines use reusable discs which are made up of many specially constructed curvettes with concave transparent bases.

Diluted antisera together with enzyme-treated red cell dilutions are injected into the curvettes in precisely measured amounts using peristaltic pumps. Agglutination is encouraged by agitation and lateral centrifugation. An elaborate, carefully controlled sequence of agitation and rotation causes any agglutinated cells to move to the center of the curvette. The potentiometric detection system then measures the amount of cells present in both the center and periphery of the curvettes — see Figure 2.

Good light transmission of the periphery coupled with poor transmission at the center indicate a positive result. Equal transmission at center and periphery is indicative of a negative result. This system of dual reading means that empty cuvettes, over-strong red cell suspensions, and mixed-fixed agglutination reactions may be detected as being equivocal. In other single-site reading systems, such situations may well be subject to misleading interpretations.

The Kontron machines are under full computer control giving a print out of sample number, result of each channel, and an interpretation of the blood types, according to a programmed interpretation table. If the machine is not capable of analyzing the result of any channel, a trained technologist may

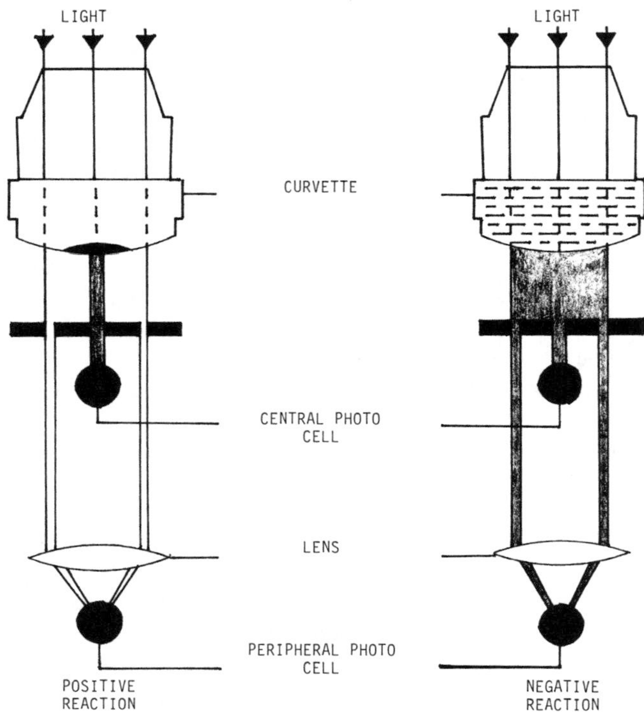

FIGURE 2. Cross-sectional diagram to show the reaction detection system of the Kontron Groupamatic.

visually inspect this channel and key in his interpretation, allowing the computer to reinterpret these edited results. The availability of on-line editing allows the rejection rate to be kept below 2%. The edited batch results are then automatically fed into a host computer.

A limitation of the Kontron blood grouping systems may well lie in the relative lack of sensitivity in the antibody screening systems employed. The incorporated enzymatic technique may well be sufficiently sensitive for testing blood donor samples, where the missing of a low-titer antibody in donor plasma will usually have no clinical sequelae, especially in a regime involving maximum usage of components. However, this may not be found acceptable in the testing of samples from patients.

Although attempts have been made to enhance antibody screening by modifying the technique, using trypsin-treated cells and polybrene, the modification significantly slows the sampling rate and is not fully reliable with all antibodies (especially Fy^a and Jk^a). Another alternative considered was the introduction of a washing stage, allowing indirect antihuman globulin tests to be performed. This system was also not viable because of the considerable reduction in throughput. At the moment it seems inevitable that if Kontron machines are to be used for testing patients, an alternative antibody screening technique must be considered.

C. MICROTITER PLATE-BASED SYSTEMS

Microplates were initially introduced into blood grouping serology as a convenient way of performing traditional manual grouping. Bowley was one of the first to attempt to read and interpret microplate grouping using a microplate reader developed for the reading of enzyme-linked immunosorbent assays (ELISA) coupled to a microcomputer.[10] The original systems were somewhat limited by the inflexibility of the computer software, the total lack of positive sample identification, and the unsophisticated reading system. This assessed the reaction in any well by a single reading, the difference between a positive and negative result being indicated by the presence or absence of red cells.

The original technique has been vastly improved by the introduction of more sophisticated, more flexible software, faster computers, and better reading techniques. The problem of sample identification has been overcome by the introduction of liquid handling systems, which are capable of dispensing both reagent and sample while reading a barcoded label on the sample tube. The introduction of such new technology has, of course, the drawback of developing the original concept of a cheap and easy-to-run system into a more complex and more expensive system. It has been suggested that the liquid handling stations of these systems could be easily reprogrammed to allow microbiological ELISA tests to be performed, thus the same equipment could be used both for performing routine red cell serology and for routine microbiological testing. The logistics of organizing such a system have not been considered in this chapter.

The modular approach allows a good deal of flexibility in the make up of a particular system. A simple system may be initially purchased with the view to expansion when resources allow. Two liquid handling systems may, for example, serve a single reader and reporting unit — see Figure 3.

Most of the current systems available are programmed only for ABO and Rh(D) typing. Modification may allow an enzyme antibody screen to be performed and Rh(C) and (E) typing of Rh(D) negative samples. There is a possibility of using microplate systems for large-scale antibody screening of antenatal and other patients, using an indirect antihuman globulin technique, though of course there would be considerable extra manual involvement in the washing stage. Even the most elaborate systems may require a great deal of user involvement in sample/plate barcode reading, centrifugation, and transfer of plate from one module to another.

The Olympus PK7100 is an automated grouping system based upon microplates, albeit very unconventional microplates. These avoid the necessity

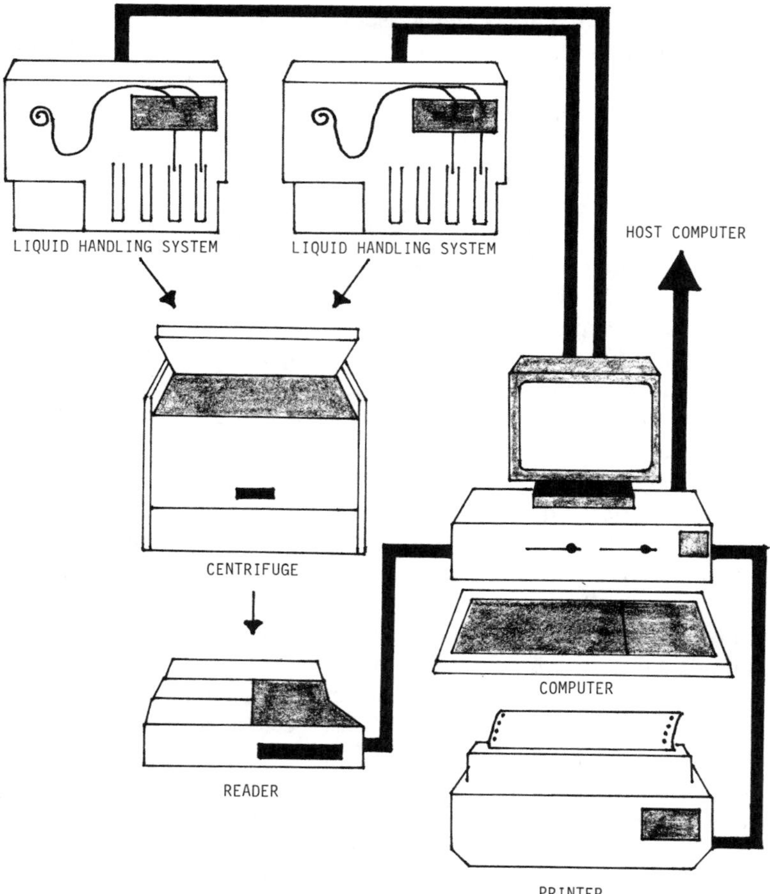

FIGURE 3. Diagrammatic representation of the modular approach of a microtiter-based system.

of centrifugation and agitation, thus allowing the PK7100 to be a fully mechanized blood grouping machine. The microplates are machined to give a V-shaped well with stepped rather than smooth sides, giving an amphitheater shape.

When cells and antisera are mixed together in this type of well, any agglutination settles out on the steps. Unagglutinated cells flow to the center of the well, forming a button of cells in the center at the point of the V. Thus a negative result shows cells only in the center, whereas a positive result will have cells evenly distributed throughout the base and sides of the well — see Figure 4.

Such a machine has cost a great deal to develop and this is reflected in the high capital cost. The use of more conventional microplates may enable

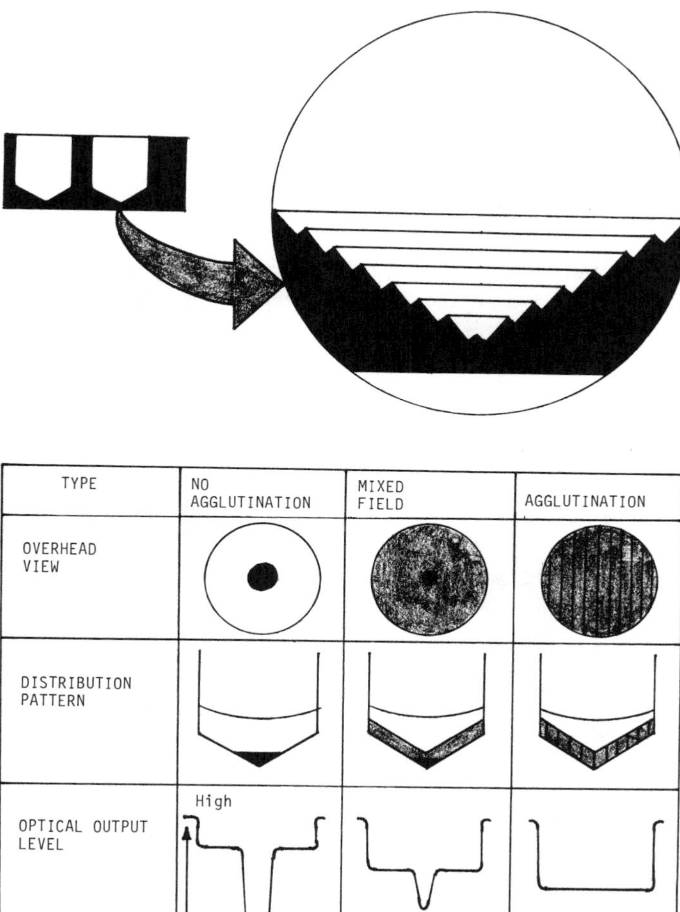

TYPE	NO AGGLUTINATION	MIXED FIELD	AGGLUTINATION
OVERHEAD VIEW			
DISTRIBUTION PATTERN			
OPTICAL OUTPUT LEVEL	High Low		
TRANSMISSION RATIO (CENT: PERIPHE)	LOW	MEDIUM	HIGH
RESULT	NEGATIVE (–)	DOUBTFUL	POSITIVE (+)

FIGURE 4. Cross-sectional view on Olympus microplate.

the machine to accommodate agglutination tests other than red cell serology, such as microbiological testing of blood samples, thus increasing its cost effectiveness.

Initial work with the Olympus system indicated that the proportion of positive results when screening blood donors for antibodies to red cell antigens was very high, perhaps falsely so. Modification of the antibody screen technique has reduced this number to comparability with other systems. The antibody screen is based on the use of enzymes and will not detect anti-Fy^a or MN antibodies reliably, therefore it is not a suitable stand-alone system for antibody screening of patients' samples.

In normal routine use, the Olympus PK7100 can test in excess of 300 samples per hour.

IV. SELECTION OF REAGENTS

The selection and standardization of reagents depend largely on which automated system is used and what the system is designed to achieve.

A. RED CELLS

Some laboratories may choose to perform reverse ABO grouping using A_1, A_2, and group B cells, although many laboratories have dispensed with the use of A_2 cells, thus reducing the rejection rate (many rejected groupings were due to the failure of anti-A to react well with A_2 reagent cells). For antibody screening, the selection of cells will depend largely on the technique used and the type of samples being tested.

In the case of blood donors, it is only useful to detect strong, clinically significant antibodies. Weaker Rh antibodies and the whole range of cold antibodies are usually considered to be of no significance from a transfusion point of view. Therefore the antibody screening technique employed may be relatively insensitive. The use of a single enzyme-treated cell (OR_1R_2K+) is adequate. Most grouping machines using this method will detect anti-D down to a level of 0.25 IU/ml. Of course, such a technique will not detect anti-Fy and Jk antibodies. Most authorities would suggest that the introduction of an extra test just to detect these antibodies is not cost effective. Some authorities would suggest that it is worthwhile selecting screening cells which are negative for the antigens that react with common cold antibodies (e.g., P_1), thus reducing the number of positive antibody screens which have to be confirmed and then identified. When screening patient samples, the situation is inevitably altered. The techniques employed must be capable of reliably detecting any significant antibody, therefore great care has to be exercised in the selection of screening cells appropriate to the choice of technique. It is clear that no single technique is optimum for detecting all types of antibodies, and that antibody detection is best done using cells homozygous for the major antigens. A good regime would be to use a continuous flow BMC technique against two separate cells (OR_1R_1K+ and OR_2R_2) in conjunction with a continuous flow LISP technique against cells selected mainly for their Duffy, Kidd, and MNS content. Some centers are now introducing antibody screening on microplates using both enzyme and antihuman globulin techniques. Problems have been encountered in developing an alternative automated or semiautomated reading system although solid-phase technology may well help to solve this problem.

B. ANTISERA

The selection and standardization of antisera suitable for use on automated systems has become somewhat of an art. Guidelines are available which indicate the minimum requirement for the standardization of such reagents. While techniques which use discrete analysis (especially microplate techniques) can easily be equated with traditional manual techniques with regard to standardization of sera, the techniques employing continuous flow analysis present fundamentally different problems.

It is acceptable that antisera to be used on automated grouping systems may be initially screened for unwanted antibodies by appropriate manual techniques. The selection of antibody dilution to be used must be based on testing on the appropriate equipment using the appropriate cells. Many antisera that work well by manual techniques perform badly on automated systems and vice versa. This may be seen most clearly in the case of some Duffy and Kidd antibodies which perform weakly by manual AHG technique but work superbly well at high dilution in continuous flow LISP techniques.

Antisera for use on automated grouping systems are invariably used at higher dilutions than in manual methods, thus leading to increased cost effectiveness. The selection and use of reagents that give complete agglutination of test cells may cause misleading results on an automated system; the aim is to produce several relatively small agglutinates as the typical positive result.

Often, monoclonal antibodies or lectins are used in automated grouping systems. The use of such reagents means that they do not require checking for extra, unwanted antibodies. Monoclonal antibodies, however, do seem to deteriorate relatively quickly, and so it is necessary to check them for sensitivity at frequent intervals. While guidelines may indicate how sensitivity testing should be performed on automated equipment, the actual level of sensitivity selected may be governed by the proposed use of the system. Thus reagent anti-D may be used much more economically if the desired result is the detection of ''normal'' D antigens, and not the vast range of variants, a criteria which is applicable to most patient testing. Similarly if anti-A,B is used only as a confirmatory reagent for anti-A and anti-B testing and no attempt is made to detect Ax, then it too may be used at a much higher dilution.

It is common practice in many laboratories to standardize a relatively large volume of antiserum then store it in frozen aliquots sufficient in size for a single day's use. Alternatively, some laboratories will make sufficient working reagents for several days, in which case there may be a danger of loss of sensitivity due to infection. This can be minimized by the incorporation of bacteriostatic agents and/or antibiotics, and the use of aseptic technique throughout. Guidelines for the production of reagents increasingly specify end-point sterilization of antisera, usually achieved by filtration.

In most automated systems, potentiators and enhancers such as albumin and methyl cellulose are used, these may well greatly increase the dilution factor at which the antisera may be employed. Similarly, the use of low ionic strength saline as a diluent has an enhancing effect, especially with Rh antibodies.

When an antiserum of a particular specificity has been used continually in one particular channel of a grouping machine, then traces will adhere to the coils, tubings, and wells of that channel, making the use of a serum with alternative specificity in that channel impossible without exceptionally thorough cleaning, or even replacement of all tubing, etc.

Most automated blood grouping systems are very dependent on the use of the enzyme, bromelain, to potentiate the agglutination reaction. The standardization of bromelain has been a cause of concern for some time. Some authorities would advocate the standardization of each batch by the use of a nonserological technique, (e.g., diazo-blue technique), while others would maintain that only serological standardization using known antisera and known red cells is permissible. Whichever line is followed, it must be acknowledged that inadequate storage or preparation technique may greatly affect the potency of the bromelain. Normally a stock solution is produced on a daily basis by dissolving a measured amount of bromelain in a fixed volume of saline or low ionic strength saline. The bromelain solution would appear to deteriorate very quickly.

V. HOW AUTOMATED SYSTEMS ARE INCORPORATED INTO LABORATORY SYSTEMS

Many transfusion centers use automated blood grouping systems as a method of confirming the ABO and Rh type of donations of blood, comparing the result with historical data. This approach means that the grouping system is essentially a quality control tool and many authorities suggest that the use of control samples are inappropriate, since virtually all the samples tested are of known group and may thus be regarded as controls. This pragmatic point of view may be short-sighted since all examples of all blood types will not be present in every run (e.g., Ax, D^u, etc.). On the other hand, the provision of a full range of controls in the volumes required for automated grouping may well prove difficult. If the system is used mainly for regrouping of donors, then the quality of the reagents used may be adjusted accordingly, which may produce significant financial savings.

Laboratories employing systems for the grouping of a significantly large proportion of first-time donors must be more stringent in their selection of reagents, and ensure that appropriate controls are used at frequent intervals. Even with the best reagents and good quality control procedures, it is essential that the results of a single analysis on a grouping machine are not accepted as definitive. There should always be a duplicate grouping, preferably using an alternative technology. If no alternative is available, then repeat grouping using different antisera should be performed on the same machine.

There is little doubt that the best available grouping system is still a manual one employing classical tube techniques, performed by an experienced operator. This may be regarded as an expensive alternative or even a waste of experienced human resources. If automated analysis is the only method employed, there is a real possibility of poorly expressed antigens being mistyped and this possibility must be taken into consideration. The issue of weak Ax blood as group O, for example, may be acceptable, depending upon financial constraints or the tradition of the testing laboratory. From a patient testing point of view, it may be of little practical importance whether a patient is Ax or O. If this is the case, then it may be preferable to make no attempt to identify weak antigens, thus erring on the side of clinical safety.

The accuracy and reliability of a blood grouping system is of little consequence if an adequate system of handling the results is not available. It is therefore highly desirable that automated systems that are under computer control be linked electronically with a host computer. The contribution to safety in transfusion made by electronic data-handling maneuvers such as computer-assisted labeling of packs and the widespread use of machine-readable labels cannot be overemphasized, but lies outside the scope of this chapter.

REFERENCES

1. **McNeil, C., Helmick, W. M., and Ferrari, A.,** A preliminary investigation into automated blood grouping, *Vox Sang.*, 8, 235, 1963.
2. **Sturgeon, P., Cedergren, B., and McQuiston, D.,** Automation of routine blood typing procedures, *Vox Sang.*, 8, 438, 1963.
3. Technicon Instruments Corporation, Research Park, Chauncey, New York.
4. **Rosenfield, R. E. and Haber, G. V.,** Proc. Technicon Symp. on Automation in Analytical Chemistry, New York, 1965.
5. **Marsh, W. L., Nichols, M., and Jenkins, W. J.,** Automated detection of blood group antibodies, *J. Med. Lab. Technol.*, 25, 335, 1968.
6. **Lalezari, P.,** A new method for detecting red blood cell antibodies, *Transfusion (Philadelphia)*, 8, 372, 1968.
7. Kontron International, Analytical Division, Head Office, Bernorstrasse-Snd 169, CH-8048, Zurich, Switzerland.
8. **Matte, C.,** Photométric précise des réactions d'agglutination sur plaques. Applications aux héamagglutinations, *Rev. Fr. Transfus.*, 6, 381, 1963.
9. **Matte, C.,** Détermination automatique des groupes sanguins. Réalisation d'un appareil expérimental, *Rev. Fr. Transfus.*, 12, 213, 1969.
10. **Bowley, A. R., Gordon, I., and Ross, D. W.,** Computer controlled automated reading of blood groups using microplates, *Med. Lab. Sci.*, 41, 19, 1984.
11. Olympus PK 7100, Olympus Optical Company (Europa), G. M. B. H., Postfact 104908, Wendenstrasse 14-16, 2000 Hamburg 1, West Germany.
12. Compact-10 Plus, Lep Scientific Limited, Sunrise Parkway, Linford Wood, Milton Keynes, MK14 6QF, U.K.

Chapter 11

PRODUCTION, CHARACTERIZATION, AND EVALUATION OF MONOCLONAL ANTIBODIES FOR BLOOD GROUPING

Douglas Voak, Lisbeth Messeter, J. R. Birch, and W. Ouwehand

TABLE OF CONTENTS

ISBN 0-8493-4938-9

I. INTRODUCTION

Monoclonal antibodies have now been produced to the red cell antigens A, A_1, B, A and B, H, I, M, N, Le^a, Le^b, P, P_1, LW, D, C, c, E, e, K, k, LKE, Lu^b, T, T_n, W^{rb}, MER2, Jk^a, and Jk^b, and to some complement and IgG determinents that are useful for the production of anti-human globulin reagents.

Selected stable cloned cell lines that produce high yields of useful monoclonal antibodies are now established for the production of blood grouping reagents as they provide unlimited quantitites of high-quality reagents at a price competitive to polyclonal reagents. They also have the ethical advantage of avoiding hyperimmunization of humans or animals.

This chapter reviews the principles of production, characterization, and evaluation of monoclonal antibodies for blood transfusion work. It explains how the various problems in the development of this technology were encountered and solved, and concentrates on the blood grouping reagents most important in routine blood transfusion work. For a detailed review of monoclonal antibodies useful in immunochemistry for the study of antigen structure and the distribution of blood group antigens in body tissues the readers are referred to the proceedings of the 2nd International Society of Blood Transfusion (ISBT) workshop on monoclonal antibodies against human red blood cells and related antigens.[1]

Safe blood transfusion practice requires the supply of thousands of liters of high-quality reagents for ABO and Rh(D) typing and antiglobulin reagents for antibody detection and identification.

Monoclonal antibodies for ABO and Rh(D) typing are now established in routine use.[2,3] Kohler and Milstein (1975)[4] first described the hybridoma technique for the production of monoclonal antibodies and the period of 1980 to 1984 saw the development of, and approval by the Food and Drug Administration (FDA) for, reagent sales in just four years.[2] This rapid replacement of polyclonal antisera was achieved because antisera produced by hyperimmunization of donors (the fact that they are polyclonal is irrelevant) is costly, involving the processing of larger numbers of separate small donations.

The success of monoclonal antibodies in routine blood transfusion work is such that they have now taken over 80% of the market for ABO and RhD typing reagents.

The main advantages of monoclonal antibodies are

- Freedom to use nonpurified antigens in immunization procedures
- Unlimited quantities of sera can be produced
- Identical antibody specificity in each batch (quantity produced may vary but it is easy to ensure quality control for reagent production)
- Free of contaminating antibodies
- Free of disease transmission, such as hepatitis
- Avoids the unethical repeated hyperimmunization of humans or animals

II. PRODUCTION OF HYBRIDOMAS

Monoclonal antibodies can be produced in different ways. In the original procedure as described by Kohler and Milstein,[4] splenic cells from hyperimmunized mice were fused with myeloma cells from other suitable mice strains, and a so-called mouse-mouse hybridoma was established. The sequence of events for the classical method of producing monoclonal antibodies has been described in detail by Galfre and Milstein[5] and Voak and Lennox[6] and is briefly summarized below (Figure 1).

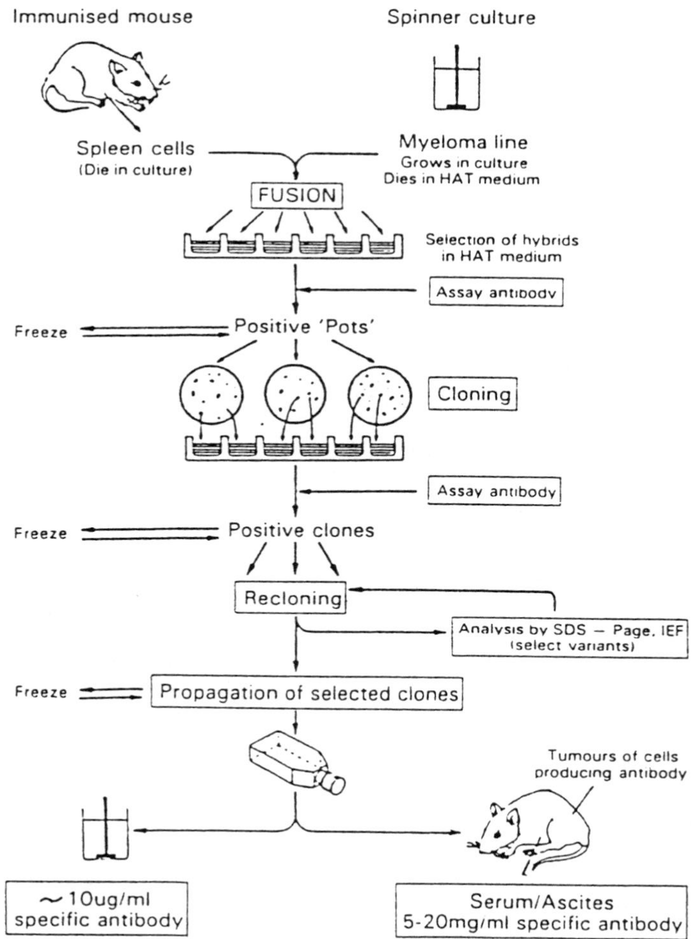

FIGURE 1. Sequence of events in the production of monoclonal antibodies. (From Galfre, G. and Milstein, C., *Meth. Enzymol.*, 73, 3, 1981. Reprinted with permission of Academic Press, New York.)

1. Immunization of a suitable animal (mostly mice). It is important to understand that an animal may make antibodies only if it lacks the determinants of the immunogen.
2. Fusion of the spleen cells from an immunized animal with suitable myeloma cells using polyethylene glycol (PEG). This is essential as antibody-forming cells from the spleen cannot be grown in culture — they die in just days. The production of a hybrid-myeloma combines the properties of myeloma cell immortality and high secretion with that of antibody production to provide an immortalized hybrid cell (when

cloned) that can provide unlimited quantities of antibody by tissue culture.

3. The hybridomas are selected from the myeloma cells by use of selective growth in HAT (Hypoxanthine, Aminopterin, Thymidine) medium which contains Aminopterin to kill off the myeloma cells that would otherwise overgrow the hybrid-meyloma cells.[7]
4. Useful antibody-secreting cell lines are selected by screening tests on supernatants with suitable indicator red cells.
5. The cell lines are cloned at least twice. This is essential to guarantee that the cell lines will not change in bulk culture.
6. Cell banks of cloned stable cell lines are stored in liquid nitrogen to guarantee supplies of the cell line that may be cultured or used in animals to produce ascitic fluid.
7. The isotype, heavy and light chain of the antibody may be determined.
8. Before use, the cell lines should be evaluated for freedom from mycoplasma infection. If infected, they may be cleaned by culture in appropriate antibiotics (e.g., Riboflaxin).

In addition to the classical mouse × mouse or rat × rat hybridomas, fusions have been performed with rat × mouse, and cell lines produced by two different species are called heterohybridomas.

III. IMPORTANCE OF A GOOD MYELOMA CELL LINE

The development of suitable myelomas was an important part of the technology. The first anti-A W61[8] gave poor agglutination with A_2B cells because the early NS1 myeloma produced its own K light chain (nonactive) that became incorporated into a high proportion of the IgM anti-A molecules (Figure 2), thus reducing their agglutinating efficiency with red cells of lower A site density (128,000). No reduction in reaction was seen with A_1 cells that have a much higher density of A sites.[9] This was called the HLK or mixed light chain phenomenon, as HLK hybrid myelomas make a variable mixture of three types of molecules (HL, HLK, and inactive HK, the last seen in IgG, but not IgM, multivalent antibodies). Subcloning the HLK W61 anti-A cell line produced a useful anti-A-secreting HL cell line.

However, the HLK phenomenon was overcome by using an improved myeloma cell line (NSO) which did not produce any unwanted heavy or light chains.[5] The use of NSO in fusions provides only HL (L or K) types, i.e., all the immunoglobulin is of spleen cell origin.

IV. ALTERNATIVE ROUTES TO MAKE ANTIBODY-PRODUCING CELL LINES

Human hybridomas have seen little use, since human-human cell lines are very unstable. A good human myeloma cell line has not yet been developed. Furthermore, the mouse system cannot make anti-D antibodies but

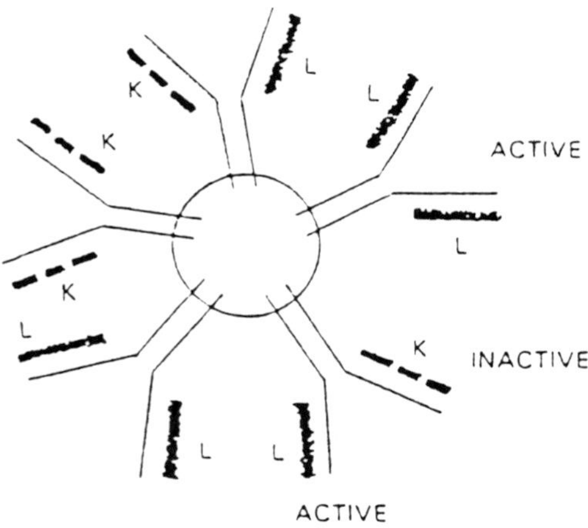

FIGURE 2. HLK antibodies: a mixture of K myeloma and L spleen light chains.

human antibody-secreting lymphocytes, stimulated by Epstein-Barr virus (EBV), have been used to make useful IgM and IgG monoclonal anti-D antibodies. Such cell lines need very careful cultivation to remain stable and improvements have been achieved by back-crossing human anti-D-secreting EBV cell lines to a mouse-human heteromyeloma[10] and most successfully to a mouse myeloma.[11]

Lowe et al. (1986) produced an interesting IgM anti-D (HD7) by direct fusion of anti-D-secreting B-lymphocytes from a recently boosted donor with a human lymphoblastoid line.[12] However, although interesting, as the anti-D misses Cat IV, the antibody yield was not high enough for commercial development.

Recently, new technologies in molecular biology have suggested that parts of monoclonal antibodies, perhaps as large as Fab, may be produced in bacteria, e.g., *Escherichia coli* (for a review see Reference 13). However, this technology is still in its early stages of development and it is not envisaged that it will replace conventional monoclonal antibody production techniques for several years. Nevertheless, it does offer fast screening procedures for rapid selection of high-affinity antibodies that can then be produced by conventional monoclonal tissue culture.

V. IMMUNIZATION AND ANTIGENS

If antibodies such as ABO, M, N, or complement are produced in mice or rats, an optimal protocol can be used for immunization and the spleen cells can be separated for fusion with a suitable myeloma cell line. This is clearly not possible for human cell lines, although strategies for *in vitro* immunization can be applied to enhance antibody production. Peripheral blood lymphocytes are generally used, as are lymphocytes which are isolated from lymph nodes.

In the case of production of antibody to blood group antigens obviously human red cells are most commonly used as antigens. One of the best monoclonal anti-A antibodies (MHO4) was accidentally made by Dr. Stux (personal communication) in Boston while attempting to make platelet antibodies; he did not even know the ABO group of the platelet donors used for the immunizations. In cases where the chemical structure of an antigen is known, natural or synthetic substances that carry this specific antigen have been useful. Thus, for the production of ABO antibodies, active human ovarian cyst material or synthetic blood group active haptens, coupled to a suitable carrier molecule, have been successfully used.

Since the selection and cloning procedure separates monoclonal antibodies from mixtures of antibodies, the immunizing antigens need not necessarily be highly purified before use. The ability to use impure antigens can be advantageous, since different specificities may be obtained by appropriate selection of a mixture of monoclonal antibodies obtained in the same immunization procedure.

VI. SELECTION OF HYBRIDOMAS

The antibodies from growing hybridomas are selected as soon as possible and the potential usefulness of the antibody is evaluated to ensure that any further work is undertaken only on antibodies meeting quality specification. In most casts, this testing is performed against selected test cells that may or may not be enzyme treated in order to detect IgG antibodies or simply to enhance sensitivity. Some laboratories may apply binding tests, usually enzyme-linked immunosorbent assay (ELISA) methods, where the microplates have been coated with the appropriate antigens. Those hybridomas that have been selected are cloned at least twice and then retested. This is, of course, tedious work as a successful immunization often gives rise to a large number of antibody-secreting hybridomas, but only a few prove useful after extensive testing. Those hybridomas that seem promising are then tested against a panel of selected cells to confirm specificity by at least saline and enzyme tests, and the potency and avidity are evaluated as described in the appropriate sections for the various specificities. It is now possible to determine the chemical specificity of ABO, H, I, P, and other antibodies by binding and inhibition assays using well-characterized structures.[14]

The isotype should be determined. When mice are immunized with human red cells or blood group active substances, antibodies are often IgM or IgG isotype, but IgA antibodies do occur.

Monoclonal antibodies from human cell lines are IgG or IgM, and the development of a saline test IgM monoclonal anti-D, C, c, E, e, D, Jk^a or

Jk^b is an important benefit for blood transfusion work; in particular, the production of large volumes of IgM anti-D has simplified D typing compared to that of ABO typing.

VII. CULTIVATION OF CELL LINES

Each cell line behaves in a characteristic way. Some cell lines are stable and do not easily switch isotypes. Cell lines for reagent purposes must be stable and must produce economic yields of antibody. A good cultivation procedure can often increase the antibody yield to several hundreds of milligrams per liter, but lower yields are much more common. Earlier hybridomas were often grown intraperitoneally in mice, since this was a rapid method of obtaining high antibody yields in ascitic fluid that are some 20- to 30-fold greater than achievable by tissue culture. However, production of ascitic fluid in mice is not to be encouraged for ethical reasons and to avoid the contaminants of ascitic fluids, the variable yields of small batches, and allergic reactions to mice in laboratory personnel.

Modern cultivation procedures with stable, suitable selected cell lines can be made highly cost effective. Depending on demand, the antibodies can be produced in roller-bottle systems for 20- to 60-liter scale or in 100- to 1,000-liter fermenters for bulk supply such as ABO and RhD reagents.

VIII. THE BULK PRODUCTION OF MONOCLONAL ANTIBODIES FOR BLOOD TYPING

The production of ABO blood typing reagents represented one of the first large-scale applications of monoclonal antibodies. New manufacturing methods were required to economically produce the required (kilogram) amounts. The choice was dictated by four key factors:

- *In vitro* cell culture can be scaled up by increasing the size of the culture vessel, allowing one to benefit from the economics of scale, especially with respect to labor and capital costs.
- This *in vitro* route avoids contamination of products with extraneous antibodies which may give false reactions.
- The process can be engineered to be highly reproducible.
- Human antibody-producing cells cannot be grown in mice but can be grown *in vitro*.

Many types of culture systems have been described for growing hybridoma cells. Birch et al. (1987)[15] opted to use large-scale suspension culture in bioreactors based on the airlift principle.

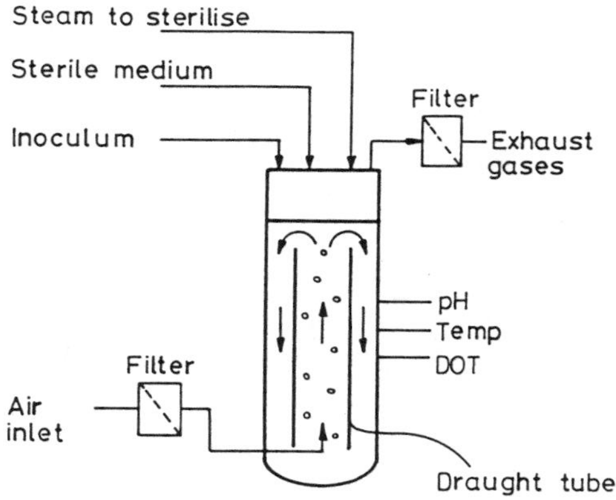

FIGURE 3. Principle of an airlift reactor.

IX. AIRLIFT REACTOR

Mixing in suspension culture reactors can be achieved either by mechanical stirring or by using the airlift principle. The airlift reactor was chosen because this is the simplest approach, doing away with the need for mechanical agitator systems and eliminating the possibility of microbial contamination through stirrer shaft seals. The principle of the airlift fermenter is shown in Figure 3. Air is injected into the base of the vessel to provide oxygen for cell growth and mixing of the culture. Mixing is aided by incorporating a draught tube or plate to separate "riser" and "downcomer" regions of the vessel. Efficient mixing is essential to ensure that cells are adequately supplied with nutrients and oxygen. Oxygen is poorly soluble in water and many cell culture systems are inefficient at supplying sufficient oxygen at high cell densities ($>10^6$/ml). In contrast, airlift fermenters have very good oxygen transfer characteristics which, unlike many systems, actually improve with increasing scale.[15]

ABO and RhD monoclonal antibodies used in the production of typing reagents are produced in reactors up to 1000-liter working volume. A photograph of a 1000-liter reactor is shown in Figure 4.

A. OPERATION OF AIRLIFT REACTORS

A large amount of engineering effort has been expended to ensure that sterility can be maintained during the production process. The stainless steel vessels with their associated vessels and pipework are sterilized by steam at high temperature and pressure. The culture medium is sterilized by filtration into the culture vessels and the gas mixtures used to aerate the culture are also sterilized by filtration.

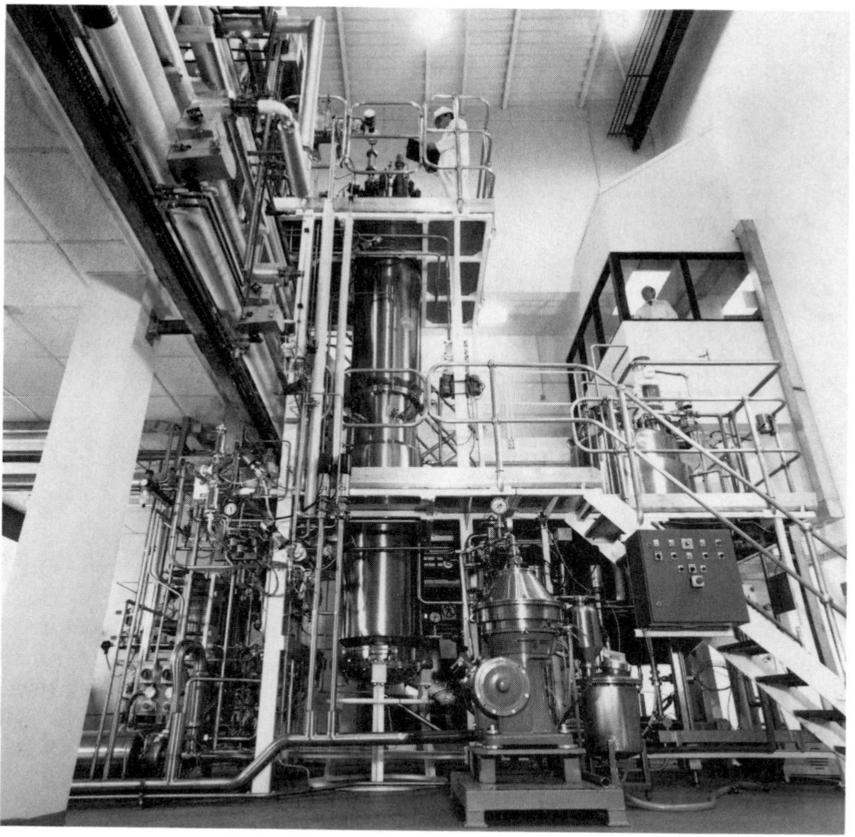

FIGURE 4. A 1000-liter airlift fermenter. (Courtesy of Celltech Ltd., Slough, England.)

The environment in the reactor has to be carefully controlled to ensure adequate growth and product synthesis. In particular, we routinely monitor and control pH, dissolved oxygen concentration, and temperature.

The pH is controlled by automatic injection of carbon dioxide into the culture vessel or by the addition of sodium hydroxide solutions. Dissolved oxygen is controlled by adjusting the rate of addition of air to the culture vessel. A heat exchanger is used to control the temperature of the vessel. Water at controlled temperature is pumped through jackets on the vessels.

A computer control system is used to achieve a high degree of automation. The control system provides automatic digital sequencing of valves and pumps (during sterilization, for example), control of key parameters, alarm monitoring, and provision of emergency action in the event of plant failure.

The bioreactors can be operated with proprietary culture media containing serum or with serum-free media. In practice, we find that virtually all hy-

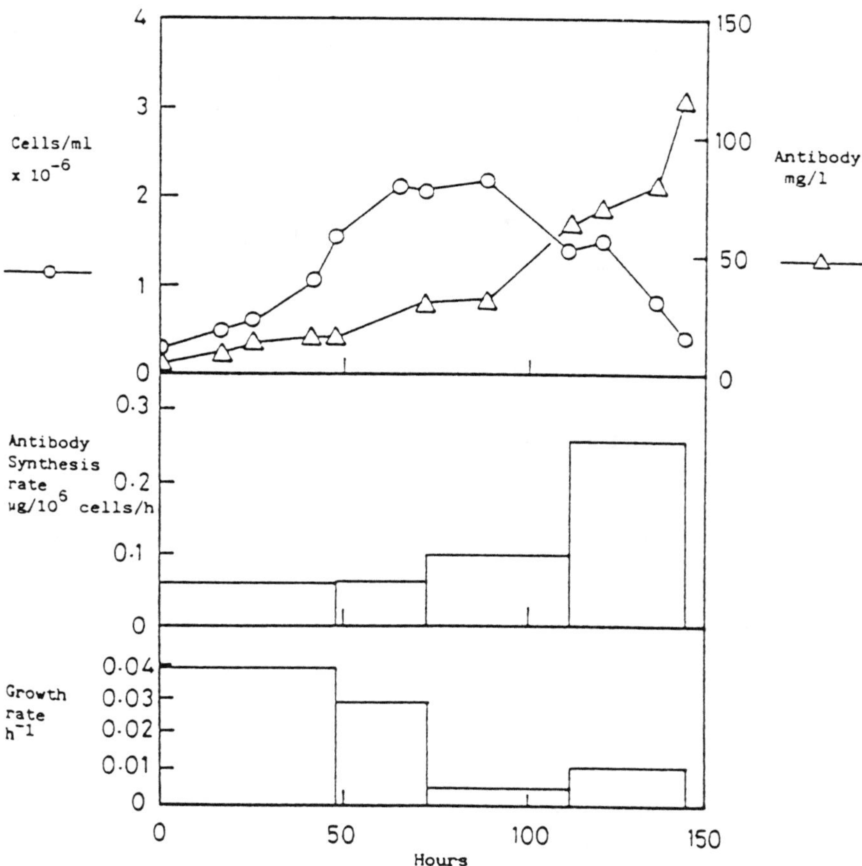

FIGURE 5. Antibody synthesis by a murine hybridoma. (Courtesy of Celltech Ltd.).

bridomas can be grown in serum-free media and that antibody yields are comparable with those seen in media supplemented with serum.

The operation of airlift fermenters has been described in more detail by Birch et al.[15]

B. PRODUCTION OF ANTIBODY

Growth and antibody (IgM) production by a murine hybridoma growing in an airlift reactor is shown in Figure 5. The production process is operated as a fed batch process. Small volumes of key nutrients and metabolites are fed to the vessel during the fermentations to increase antibody production.

It will be seen that a large proportion of the antibody is synthesized during the stationary and decline phase of the culture. The length of the production cycle varies between 140 and 400 hours (about 150 hours for the example given) and antibody levels reach 100 to 500 mg/l (115 mg/l for the cell line in Figure 4), depending on the cell line. The levels of antibody seen in the fermenters are typically two to three times higher than seen in roller culture systems that are suitable for small-scale production up to 60/l. This is a result of careful design of the culture medium and systematic process optimization.

C. PRODUCT RECOVERY

At the time of harvest, the culture broth in the reactor contains antibody in solution together with cells and cell debris. The latter are removed by continuous centrifugation. The clarified solution is then concentrated by tangential flow ultrafiltration to give a concentrate-containing antibody at a concentration of between 1 and 5 g/l. This concentrate is then processed further and formulated to produce a finished reagent.

X. PROBLEMS WITH MONOCLONAL ANTIBODIES

When producing monoclonal antibodies several problems are encountered. Many of these have been overcome when techniques have improved and knowledge increased. The problems relate to

- Stability of the antibody
- Specificity and potency
- Technical problems
- Blending of antibodies for optimal characteristics for slide and tube tests

Most laboratories have developed in-house tricks of the trade to enhance the properties of their antibodies. One problem, which in some instances has been difficult to overcome, is the antibody stability in storage at 4°C. This is generally most pronounced for antibodies of the IgM type; some lose considerable potency after only 6 to 18 months at 4°C, even if storage conditions are optimal. The IgM molecules of some anti-B antibodies may precipitate and give rise to turbid solutions that look as if they are infected. One anti-B, unstable at 4°C, showed remarkable stability at 37°C (personal communication, Hans Sonneborn), and yet, 37°C stability tests for 6 weeks are critical forced stability tests for other antibodies stable at 4°C.

There are several ways to improve stability, e.g., by adding "supportive" proteins such as bovine serum albumin at a level of from 1 to 7%. Another way is to control the pH of the solution to that optimum for the antibodies. (e.g., anti-M/N, discussed later). In some cases, none of these measures is successful and an otherwise useful antibody has to be discarded. Validation of stability by forced conditions — 4 to 6 weeks at 37°C, 1 hour at 56°C, and freezing and thawing 1 to 5 times — are the important parameters that should be included in the early evaluation of any new antibody. The later generations of monoclonal antibodies will replace earlier, less stable, less

TABLE 1
Examples of Monoclonal Antibodies to Red Cell Antigens (Literature)

Antibody specificity	Refs.	Antibody specificity	Refs.
A	8, 18, 22, 23	k	76
B	19, 21, 22	LW^a	57
A and B	21, 22, 24	T	77
H	66	T^n	Parsons (unpublished observations)
I	67		
Le^a	68, 69	MER 2	78
Le^b	22, 70	D	11, 38, 39
$P/P_1/P^k$	71	C	43, 79
LKE	72	c	43, 79
M	57, 59, 73	E	43, 79
N	56, 57	e	43, 79
Wr^b	74	Jk^a	80
K	75	Jk^b	80

potent, or less economic yield lines as part of the development of this technology. One interesting problem was observed with the IgM anti-C3d which was found to be lost during filtration as it combined with some standard filters;[16] a specific polysulfone filter has to be used with this material.

A serious problem seen with many monoclonal antibodies is the stickiness of the agglutinated red cells adhering to the test tube. This in turn makes reactions difficult to evaluate since vigorous shaking of the tubes will disperse the agglutinates. This problem is most apparent when diluted reagents are used, for example, in titration procedures. The dilution medium for monoclonal antibodies should therefore always contain protein, e.g., bovine serum albumin 1 to 7%. Several monoclonal antibodies are also dependent upon temperature and pH. When such antibodies are included in commercial reagents, this should be stated on the package insert to avoid false reactions upon inappropriate use.

A. USE IN ROUTINE SEROLOGICAL WORK

Monoclonal antibodies for routine blood group and anti-complement reagents were established in the early 1980s. The criteria for the specification for good-quality ABO, RhD, anti-C3d, and anti-IgG for bulk supply reagents is described in the appropriate sections. In addition there are now many other monoclonal antibodies to red cell antigens (Table 1).

However, before describing the characteristics of each of the main types of reagent, it is worthwhile dealing with the important principles of how the ABO, RhD typing, and antiglobulin reagents should be evaluated prior to use in routine work.

XI. STANDARDIZATION AND APPROVAL OF NEW REAGENTS

The consensus of opinion at the recent International Workshop "Reagents for the 1990s" of the ICSH/ISBT/FDA* and representatives of reagent manufacturers supported the policy proposed by Hoppe and Voak that:[17]

1. Field trials should commence only after manufacturers have established that their reagent achieves satisfactory performance by

   (*a*) Potency equal to or greater than the reference preparation
   (*b*) Its specificity (it should include a panel of useful rare cell types)
   (*c*) Being assessed in-house or by contract by a minimum of 300 tests
   (*d*) Having developed the recommended method(s)

2. For ABO and RhD typing reagents, the field trials must include the following:

   (*a*) 3000 to 5000 tests (generally at least 10% minimum negative or positive) must be done by manual and or microplate tests with additional automated tests of 5 days testing of samples
   (*b*) Additional manual tests must be done with 100 of each of the following:

Pregnant women	Cord samples
43-Day stored donor units	Frozen cells
Clotted samples	Anti-coagulated samples
Disease groups	Ethnic groups
Old people	

   (*c*) They must be held at three test sites with two reagent lots (one a production batch and blind coded)
   (*d*) Samples must represent the patient population with the various types of samples shown in 2 (*b*).
   (*e*) Samples must be run by parallel testing (anti-human globulin [AHG]) or comparison on the same samples (ABO and D) against an appropriate control reagent
   (*f*) Discrepancies must be studied by experts, and samples must be stored for reference
   (*g*) All methods/specimens must be covered by the package insert
   (*h*) Documentation must be accurate and comply with standards of good manufacturing practice

* International Committee for Standards in Haematology/International Society for Blood Transfusion/Food and Drug Administration

TABLE 2
Classification of Grades of Agglutination

Symbol	Score	Agglutinates
C	12	One clump
+ + +	10	Several large clumps
+ +	8	Smaller clumps
+	5	Granules
(+)	3	Small granules
W	1	Microscopic only
O	0	Negative

3. Changing an antibody in a reagent blend constitutes a new product, but the reagent may be approved on less than a full field trial if good reasons and data are provided to justify and validate the change
4. Stability data must be provided for the shelf life of the product for storage at 4°C, for example, 1 to 2 years with a provisional expiry date of 1 year, subject to extension when further data supplied
5. It was also considered that a product stored for 6 months at 4°C should be assessed for specificity using a panel of weak and strong reactors, in addition to stability tests

The evaluation of reagents for avidity and potency should be performed by experienced serologists using standard techniques and a defined scoring system to record the various grades of agglutination (Table 2).

The consensus of opinion at the Reagents for the Nineties workshop was that spin tube tests, incubated for 5 minutes, provide a reasonable time for uniform comparison of reagents. Standardization of centrifuge force and time is also important, and the various acceptable speeds and times that are adequate to sediment a cell button for sensitivity without causing excessive adherence of the cell button to the tube are

Relative centrifugal force (RCF)	100–110	200–220	500	1000
Time (seconds)	60	25–30	15–18	12–15

It was interesting to note that the use of 1000 RCF for 20 seconds was regarded as excessive by all participants at the workshop, and this widely used excessive spin force is recognized as causing reduced sensitivity due to the need to shake the cell tube to free the cell buttons from the tube.

XII. ANTIBODIES AGAINST ABO ANTIGENS

In 1980, the first monoclonal blood group antibody used in blood grouping — an anti-A — was described.[18] During the following few years, anti-Bs and anti-A + Bs were produced.[19–24] The antibodies were raised in mice and human red cells and natural or synthetic blood group active substances were usually used for immunization of the animals. Most of these antibodies are of the IgM type and, hence, good agglutinators; but also strongly agglutinating IgA and even IgG antibodies do exist. The first of these antibodies was of nearly the same quality as currently available polyclonal antibodies, or only slightly better. Very soon, superior reagents occurred and were commercialized. These anti-A antibodies could be formulated to detect even very weak variants, and thus made anti-A + B obsolete. In 1987, the International Society of Blood Transfusion arranged a workshop on monoclonal antibodies.[25] Many of the available ABO antibodies were tested in a number of laboratories worldwide and it was concluded that some of these antibodies, either alone or blended with other suitable monoclonal antibodies, were excellent reagents, and superior to polyclonal antibodies. At that time, no satisfactory single anti-A + B was in existence, but such antibodies have been produced lately, and the possibility of using a single antibody for this purpose was clearly shown in the Second International Workshop on Monoclonal Antibodies.[1]

These antibodies opened up a new vista of research into antigenic structure. Many of these antibodies have been extensively characterized in binding and inhibition assays and their fine specificity determined. The A and B hapten can occur on different chain types on the red cell.[14,26] A_1 and A_2 red cells differ both quantitatively and qualitatively. Both phenotypes contain A type 2 structure. A_1 red cells, in addition, also contain A type 3 and 4;[27] however, these structures do not occur on A_2 cells.

XIII. SPECIFICATION OF ABO REAGENTS

Selected mouse monoclonal anti-A, anti-B, and anti-A + B (A_1B) antibodies, often as optimal blends, exceed FDA requirements[28] and are excellent ABO typing reagents. These IgM antibody reagents should contain ethylene diamine tetracetate (EDTA) (0.1 *M*) at pH 7.01 to 7.03 to prevent hemolysis of red cells in the presence of fresh serum.[6]

The minimum specification for slide avidity tests with serum- or plasma-suspended cells and potency tube titration titers are shown in Table 3. Titrations of reagents under evaluation should always be performed in parallel to reference preparations. The FDA reference preparations are only available to licensed manufacturers or international standards organizations; however, FDA licensed reagents exceed the FDA minimum reference preparations and may be used until International Reference Preparations are completed. (They are currently under development by the Joint Working Party of the ICSH/ISBT on Blood Group Reagents.)

TABLE 3
Minimum Potency Specification of Monoclonal ABO Reagents

	FDA slide tests			
Reagent	**Avidity (seconds)**	**Intensity (clump size)**[a]	**Spin-tube titer after 5 minutes**[a]	**Negative controls**[a]
Anti-A[b]	10	$+++/A_2B$	$128/A_1$ $32/A_2B$	B and O
Anti-B	10	C/A_1B	128/B $64/A_1B$	A_1 and O
Anti-A,B[a]	10	C/A_2+B	$64/A_2$ 64/B	O

[a] Red cells.
[b] Should detect stronger examples of A_x.

It is most important to assess the reagents with several red cell types, as follows:

- Anti-A with A_1(1), A_2B(3), B(2), and O(2)
- Anti-B with B(1), A_1B(3), A_1(2), and O(2)
- Anti-A,B(A+B) with B(2), A_2(2), A_1(1), and O(2) and several examples of A_3, A_x and weak B variants (the latter are important if the population contains people of Asiatic origins)

It is essential to use A_2B and A_1B red cells to assess anti-A and anti-B, respectively. The weak A of A_2B and the weaker B of A_1B represent the weakest, commonly encountered examples of these antigens in routine grouping. Several examples are used because of the variability of the A/B antigen strength. It is important to avoid strong A_2B bloods that occur frequently and are H-deficient variants of A_1B genotype. The selection of A_2B red cells that are H-positive with Ulex anti-H is the simplest way of avoiding the H-deficient A_1B types.[29]

All reagents must be free of false reactions by 5-minute slides and by tube tests as described in the package insert. It is also worthwhile to check for false positives with enzyme-treated cells if the reagents are likely to be used in enzyme-enhanced systems.

Most monoclonal anti-Bs used for reagents do not detect acquired B,[9,20,30] but one very interesting antibody reacts well with cells of the B acquired phenotype and this antibody is inhibited very well with the deacetylated A structure.[14,20]

TABLE 4
Saline Titers of Tissue Culture Supernatant Monoclonal Anti-A Reagents

	Anti-A reagents[a]			
3% cells saline RT[b]	3D3 neat	MHO4 neat	BS-63 neat	Group B serum commercial X (U.S.)
A_1	1024	1024	512	512
A_2	512	512	512	256
A_1B	512	512	512	512
A_2B	64	256	256	64
A_2B weak	4	256	256	8
A_3B	0	256	128	1
A_3	4	256	128	4
A_x	0	64	32	0

Note: Saline tests negative × B, O, A_m, and A_{end} red blood cells.

[a] Anti-As that see A_x may show weak B (A) reactions.
[b] RT, Room temperature.

The use of anti-A,B(A+B) reagents is now questionable as good monoclonal anti-A reagents can reliably detect weak subgroups of A as well as many FDA licensed anti-A_1B(A+B) reagents. However, if it is mandatory to use anti-A,B for blood grouping, selected monoclonal antibodies — either as blends of anti-A + anti-B or as blends of cross-reacting anti-A,B with anti-A or anti-B, or more recently, single anti-AB reagents,[31] are more potent than most polyclonal reagents. These potent anti-AB antibodies have been shown to bind to a common part of the A and B antigen, which can be located terminally or at an internal portion of the antigen.[14]

Examples of the tube potency titers of various monoclonal anti-As and anti-Bs are shown in Tables 4 and 5.

Some superior anti-A monoclonals, for example MHO4 and BS 63, detect many examples of A_x and because they are so potent, they can also detect traces of A on the B cells of people with high levels of galactosyl transferase that show some cross reactions[32] and make a little A on these B cells. This phenomenon is called the B(A) (''funny B'').[33–35] The opposite phenomenon, called the A_1(B) (''funny A''), has been seen with only one superior monoclonal anti-B (BS 85).[36] The occurrence of B on A cells occurs only on adult A_1, not on A_2 or cord A cells and the transferase levels of the donors are not elevated.[37]

The main characteristics of the B(A) and A_1(B) phenomenon are

1. The B transferases make a little A (mostly in Blacks) in 0.2 to 0.8% of Bs. The A transferases make a little B in 1.41% of As

TABLE 5
Saline Titers of Tissue Culture Supernatant Monoclonal Anti-B Reagents

3% cells saline RT[a]	Anti-B reagents				
	NB1/19	3B4	5A5	BS-85	Group A serum commercial X (U.S.)
A_1B	256	64	256	256	64
A_2B	512	128	512	512	64
B	512	128	512	512	128
B cord	256	64	256	256	64
B weak[b]	0	32	64	32	64
A_1	0	0	0	0	0
O	0	0	0	0	0

[a] RT, Room temperature.
[b] Similar results obtained with 25 additional sub-groups of B.

2. The B(A) and A_1(B) reactions are very fragile, found in spin-tube tests and enzyme-enhanced microplate tests; the reactions are enhanced by albumin and protease enzymes
3. They are specifically inhibited: the B(A) reaction is inhibited by A saliva and the A_1(B) reaction by B saliva
4. Both phenomenon occur at high concentrations of antibody and are prevented by dilution of the antibody

These powerful anti-A and anti-B antibodies are used, blended with other less avid anti-A or anti-B antibodies, respectively, to optimize slide test reactions, and the use of the superior reagents at a dilution to avoid B(A) or A_1(B) reactions is an extra quality control step in ABO reagent production that was not needed with polyclonal reagents.

The ability to dilute the superior anti-A/anti-B is an obvious economic advantage in reagent production and these reagents also offer very economic ABO typing in automated systems such as the 16C Technicon in which they give reliable results at dilutions of 1 in 10 or more.

XIV. ANTIBODIES TO Rh ANTIGENS

A. ANTI-D ANTIBODIES

Monoclonal IgM and IgG anti-D antibodies have been prepared.[38–41] For reviews see References 42 and 43.

The major breakthrough in this area has been the large-scale supply of potent, stable, IgM monoclonal anti-Ds. This was first achieved by Thompson et al.,[11] using cell lines derived by back-crossing human anti-D-secreting

EBV-treated lymphocytes to mouse myelomas. These cell lines MAD-2, FOM 1, and the later lines, e.g., of BS 226 (Sonneborn Biotest) and BAC-9 (CNTS), grow well in tissue culture to give antibody supernatants with saline titers of 128 to 1024 × R_1r cells (by 5-minute spin-tube tests). Reagents made from these anti-Ds enable D typing to be performed by simple saline tube or slide tests and they work equally well at room temperature or 37°C; selected reagents are excellent for use in microplate or automated systems.

However, monoclonal anti-Ds are directed at various epitopes of the D mosaic and thus show limited specificity,[2,12,43–45] as shown by the examples in Table 6 with rare types of red cells from D categories (D-positive with anti-D in their serum) and D variants (D-positives with missing epitopes but no anti-D) and with weak D (D^u) types.

A simple solution to overcome the deficiency of IgM monoclonal anti-Ds with category/variants and the lack of sensitivity for weak D was to blend a high-titer (128 to 256 × R_1r) IgM anti-D with just sufficient IgG polyclonal anti-D to give reliable second-phase indirect antiglobulin tests (IAT) with the reagents, as shown in Table 7.

This type of IgM and IgG blend is now widely used commercially. These reagents are used in simple saline tests for the detection of normal D types and the negative tests converted to IAT only in manual donor blood testing and in babies' blood samples of Rh-negative mothers, unless the detection of weak D is mandatory in patient blood tests (e.g., as in Germany).

However, extensive testing with the IgM monoclonal anti-D (MAD-2) has revealed a low incidence of five strong D variants in 13,000 antenatal patients that were negative with MAD-2, but strongly positive with other IgM monoclonal anti-Ds and polyclonal reagents as shown by the examples HOW and Pol in Table 6.[13] We think it is possible that new D variants may continue to be discovered with each new monoclonal anti-D used in extensive routine work and we must accept that we are on a learning curve in terms of D epitope structure, as some of the D variants do not fit the patterns established for D categories. For recent reviews, see Thompson and Hughes-Jones[42] and Tippett and Moore;[43] there are at least seven epitopes of D and possible overlaps between these epitopes which may give rise to many D variants as seen by monoclonal IgM and IgG anti-Ds.

B. D TYPING WITHOUT INDIRECT ANTIGLOBULIN TESTS FOR WEAK D

Another approach to D typing, based on the streamlining of workloads and reducing costs, was presented by Van Rhenen and Overbeeke,[46] who discontinued the use of the IAT for weak D (D^u) on the grounds that Schmidt et al.[47] had demonstrated that weak D (D^U) was not immunogenic.

However, one example of primary and two examples of secondary immunizations were seen in the initial trial over 2 years, and they therefore developed a quality control protocol by which anti-Ds for donor blood testing

TABLE 6
Limited Specificity of Monoclonal Anti-Ds with D Category and D Variant Red Cells

	D Category Red Cells								D Variants[a]	
	III	IV	IV	V	V	VI	VI	VII	HOW	Pol
				Anti-Ds IgM (Saline)						
HD 7	+ + +	O	O	+ + +	+ + +	O	O	+	N/T	N/T
MAD-2	+ + +	C	C	+	O	O	O	+	O	O
BS 226	C	C	C	C	C	O	O	C	C	C
FOM-1	C	C	C	O	O	O	O	+	C	O
BAC-9	C	C	C	C	C	O	O	+ + +	O	C
				IgG(Alb)						
BS 221	C	+ + +	+ + +	C	C	+ +	O	+ + +	N/T	N/T
Polyclonal commerical	C	C	C	C	C	+ +	+ + +	+ + +	C	C

[a] Two of five examples found in screening 13,000 antenatal blood samples with MAD-2.

TABLE 7
Examples of a Monoclonal IgM and Polyclonal IgG Anti-D Blend for Saline D Typing and IAT Second Phase Weak D (D^u) Test

Spin-Tube Tests with 3% RBC in Saline[a]

	Normal D				Weak D			
	R_1R_1	**R_1R_2**	**R_1r**	**Cat.VI**	**R^u_1r**	**R^u_1r**	**R^u_2r**	**rr**
Blend								
MAD-2 Saline	C	C	C	O	O	O	+	O
IAT				+ + +	+ + +	+ + +	+ + +	O

[a] RBC, Red blood cells.

are evaluated against a cell panel of D variants and weak Ds, against which a reagent is required to give at least a 1+ grade of reaction by manual spin tube tests with at least 70% of the cell panel. The Central Laboratory of the Dutch Red Cross Blood Transfusion Service in Amsterdam (CLB) developed a potentiated IgM monoclonal anti-D and an enzyme test IgG polyclonal anti-D, with a recommendation that this combination of anti-D reagents, and not just monoclonal anti-D reagents, should be used to assess D in donor bloods by simple one-step direct tests. At the present time, 14 of the 22 donor testing laboratories have discontinued the IAT for weak D (D^u) and no further immunizations of Rh(D)-negative patients by weak D have been reported since adoption of the quality control procedure.

We certainly agree that sensitive automated donor blood testing by appropriately selected and standardized potentiated anti-D reagents can be achieved without the use of IAT for weak D (D^u).[48] However, the use of manual or microplate D typing tests for donor D typing is subject to individual worker skills, especially at the reading stage of the test. Weak D tests at the 1+ or even 2+ level of reaction are often very fragile and easily destroyed by over-agitation of tests (tubes and microplates).

Reactions of monoclonal and polyclonal anti-Ds with the weak D (D^u) red cells from the donor (3–41) that caused primary immunization in the Dutch trial are shown in Tables 8 and 9. Several problems were revealed by direct tests for weak D:

1. The red cells of 3–41 gave very fragile reactions of + to +/+ + with the IgM monoclonal anti-Ds that could detect this "immunogenic" weak D (D^u). Thus, staff training to guarantee detection of this weak D would be difficult to achieve with manual tests.
2. An IgM + polyclonal IgG blend detected the weak D (D_u) in the short 5-minute test, but was negative after a longer (15 minute) incubation test, as presumably the IgG anti-D had blocked the IgM anti-D reaction.

TABLE 8
Detection of an Immunogenic Weak D (3–41) by Direct Tests — Saline

Monoclonal IgM Anti-D	Spin-tube tests × 2% RBC in saline[a]					
	Weak D 3–41	R_1r	rr	Weak D 3–41	R_1r	rr
MAD-2 (BPL)	–	C	–	–	C	–
BS 226 (Biotest)	+/++	C	–	++	C	–
4319-1 (CLB)	++	C	–	+/++	C	–
BAC-9 (CNTS)	+/++	C	–	+/++	C	–
JAP RED X (Tokyo) (IgG Coupled Anti-IgG)	–	+++/C	–	–	C	–
(Blend IgM + IgG)	+/++	C	–	– (Blocked)	C	–
Incubation	5 Minutes at RT[b]			15 Minutes at 37°C		

[a] RBC, Red blood cells.
[b] RT, Room temperature.

TABLE 9
Detection of Immunogenic Weak D (3–41) by Direct Tests

	Spin-tube tests (15 minutes, 37°C) × 2% RBC[a]					
	RBC in serum			RBC in serum		
	Weak D 3–41	R_1r	rr	Weak D 3–41	R_1r	rr
Polyclonal	**Undiluted**			**1 + 5 Dilution[b]**		
Ortho	–	+++	–	+/++	C	–
Biotest	–	+++	–	+++	C	–
Diluent control	–	–	–	–	–	–

Note: Fragile agglutination × weak D 3–41.

[a] RBC, Red blood cells.
[b] Negative × 3–41 RBC in saline.

This type of observation has been seen many times (personal communication, J. Case [Gamma] and D. Davies [Ortho]).

3. Conventional polyclonal IgG anti-Ds did not detect 3–41 red cells with saline suspended cells or serum suspended cells, but if diluted to 1 + 5 with manufacturer's reagent diluent they would detect the cells only if the cells were suspended in serum. These reagents are not standardized

TABLE 10
Detection of Weak D (D^u) Types by Enhanced IgM Monoclonal Anti-Ds

Spin-Tube Tests (5 Minutes, Room Temperature) with 3% RBC in Saline[a]

	Anti-D reagents			
	BS 226 Not enhanced	**BS 226 Dextran**	**CLB 4319–1 Enhanced**	**Diluent control**
Weak D(D^u)				
1	+ +	+ + +	+ + +	O
2	+ +	+ +	+ +	O
3	+ +	+ +	+ +	O
4	+/+ +	+	W	O
5	+	+ +	O	O
6	O	O	+	O
7	O	+/+ +	O	O
8	O	+/+ +	O	O
9	O	+	O	O
10	W	+ +	+/+ +	O
Controls				
R_1r	C	C	C	O
rr	O	O	O	O

[a] RBC, Red blood cells.

to detect weak D by direct tests. They prozone with weak D as they contain a large amount of IgG anti-D (33 to 35 IU/ml) to enable them to work well with normal D by slide as well as by tube tests, but they are excellent for detection of weak D by IAT.

Furthermore, it must be remembered that product liability is only borne by manufacturers if their product is used as directed by the instructions on the packet insert.

C. DETECTION OF WEAK D BY POTENTIATED IgM MONOCLONAL ANTI-Ds

Some selected IgM monoclonal anti-Ds, for example, BS 226 from Hans Sonneborn, Biotest, are able to detect approximately 50% of the total 0.7% of East Anglian donors that are weak D. However, potentiation of the reagent by Dextran or albumin can increase the sensitivity to detect 80% of weak Ds by manual spin-tube tests. Table 10 lists some weak Ds found negative by one of the polyclonal IgG anti-Ds on our 16C Technicon machine. They have been tested with BS 226 and the potentiated CLB anti-Ds. The important points are that potentiation can increase the strength of the reaction, e.g., + may increase to + + and some negatives become + to + +, but different reagents show heterogeneity, e.g., weak Ds 7, 8, and 9 are detected by BS 226 but not 4319, whereas 4319 detects weak Ds 6 and 10 that are missed by BS 226.

Certainly, reagent developments are being made that can detect many examples of weak D by direct tests and reagent blends may further improve reagent ability to see D variants and different epitope variations in weak D.

A further important point is the effect of IgM anti-D concentration on detection of weak D. Our 16C Technicon, using BS 226 at a dilution of 1 in 40, with an enhanced enzyme (Bromelain) methyl cellulose system, detected all but one D^u and two Cat VI red cells in nearly 10,000 donor sample tests. By increasing the anti-D concentration to 1 in 25, our 16C Technicon detected the difficult D^u donor's cells, but the reagent did not recognize Cat VI which was detected by a selected enhanced polyclonal IgG anti-D reagent.

D. QUALITY ASSURANCE OF ANTI-D REAGENTS

The blend of IgM + polyclonal (or monoclonal) IgG anti-D requires an IgM anti-D titer of 128 or more by 5-minute tube tests with R_1r (pool of 4) red cells, and the quantity of IgG anti-D in the blend must be controlled to ensure it does not cause prozone (blocking) of the IgM anti-D reaction with the weakest common D-type R_1r cells after extended incubation tests, as recommended by the package insert.

The blending of IgG with IgM anti-D does reduce their ability to detect weak D (less D sites) in direct tests due to prozone (blocking) by the IgG anti-D. This type of reagent is designed to be used by IAT for detection of weak D (D^u) or variants not detectable by the IgM component anti-D(s).

XV. FUTURE DEVELOPMENTS

A. STANDARDS

The International Joint Working Party of the ICSH/ISBT for Standardization of Blood Group Reagents and Methods is preparing (1) an IgM monoclonal minimum potency standard with a titer of 64 to 128 $\times$ R_1r cells for use by manufacturers, and (2) a panel of D variants, D category, and weak D (D^u) red cells that are propertly evaluated for the assessment of anti-Ds for use in reagents. This will extend the work of Van Rhenen and Overbeeke[46] and include detailed serology with a panel of monoclonal anti-Ds and determination of the number of D sites with selected IgG monoclonal anti-Ds; e.g., the immunogenic cell 3–41 was found by Gorrick and Ouwehand to have only 500 D sites when studied with the Fog 1 IgG anti-D.[17]

B. REAGENTS

The present use of IgG polyclonal anti-D from hyperimmunized human volunteers guarantees a large supply of cheap polyclonal anti-D for reagent work. However, IgG anti-Ds that detect Cat VI and the other D variant types and weak Ds have been described by Kumpbell et al.[41] and they do have the monoclonal advantages of being reproducible for subsequent batches of reagents. In addition, IgG monoclonal anti-D(s), used at low concentrations with IgM anti-D blended reagents, offer the advantage of only needing one to two washes for the IAT for D^u.

C. OTHER Rh ANTIBODIES C, c, E, AND e FOR REAGENT USE

Since the second ISBT Workshop,[43] excellent IgM saline tests, anti-C, c, E, and e reagents have been developed and our recent trial of the reagents demonstrated that the anti-C and anti-E are better than conventional reagents for slide, spin-tube, microplate or automated tests.[42] The anti-c and anti-e were not quite so good, but they were generally better than the conventional reagents run in parallel with the 750 tube and 250 slide tests used in a clinical trial for Ortho Diagnostics.

D. ANTI-HUMAN GLOBULIN (AHG) REAGENTS WITH MONOCLONAL COMPONENTS

1. Monoclonal Anti-IgG

Conventional rabbit anti-IgG is easy to produce and has an excellent performance with a stability far in excess of a reagent shelf life of 2 years at 4°C. However, Downie et al.[49] did try to produce an anti-IgG blend for reagent use but it was not quite equal to the performance of rabbit anti-IgG, and it was noted that reaction with weak anti-Fy^a-sensitized red cells was the main limiting factor. However, in 1990 an anti-IgG (205), prepared by Drs. Lemieux and Broly, submitted in the anti-IgG workshop at the Lund symposium, was found to equal the performance of the ISBT/ICSH reference preparations R3P and RIIIM*.[50,51] Furthermore, Gamma Biologicals announced in the Washington Reagents for the 1990s workshop that they had applied to license a polyspecific AHG with a single monoclonal anti-IgG component (not 205).

2. Sequence of Tests to Evaluate Monoclonal Anti-IgG

These are based on the protocol of the ICSH/ISBT working party on antiglobulin reagents,[45,52] using the ICSH/ISBT reference antiglobulin reagents R3P and RIIIM. The sequence described below is designed to select useful antibodies and to minimize work by the rejection of unsuitable antibodies at each test sequence:

1. Samples should be tested with weak anti-Fy^a-sensitized red cells.
2. The anti-IgG should have a maximum potency titer with strongly IgG anti-D-sensitized red cells that is not less than that of R3P (the minimum potency AHG reagent).
3. The anti-IgG(s) should be tested by checkerboard titrations with weak anti-D-, anti-Kell-, and anti-Fy^a-sensitized red cells and they should

* Available from M. Overbeeke, CLB, Amsterdam.

TABLE 11
Selection of Useful Anti-IgGs

Anti-IgG Checkerboard Titrations with Anti-Fy^a

		Anti-Fy^a Sensitized Cells								
		N	**2**	**4**	**8**		**N**	**2**	**4**	**8**
R3P*	N	+ +	+ +	+	(+)	205 ($^1/_4$)	+ +/+ + +	+ +	+ +	+
	2	+ +	+	(+)	w		+ +/+ + +	+ +	+ +	(+)
	4	+	+	(+)	w		+ +	+ +	+	w
	8	(+)	w	–	–		+	+	(+)	–
198 (1/300)	N	+	+	+ +	+ +	207 (N)	+	+/+ +	+ +	+ +
	2	(+)	+	+ +	+ +		–	+	+ +	+
	4	–	w	+	+		–	w	(+)	+
	8	–	–	w	+		–	–	w	w

Dilutions to avoid prozones — Fail anti-D potency

* RIIIM similar.

have a performance close to that of the reference preparation(s) (R3P and RIIIM), e.g., the comparable performance of anti-IgG 205 to R3P is shown (Table 11) with anti-Fy^a-sensitized cells. The anti-IgGs 198 and 207 were not useful as single anti-IgGs for reagent work as their dilution to avoid prozones caused them to fail the maximum potency titer requirement, although that does not exclude them from possible use in blends of anti-IgG antibodies.

4. There should be no false positives against saline-suspended and protease enzyme-treated A_1, B, and O red cells.
5. Tests for prozones with weakly sensitized red cells should be carried out. The anti-IgG should not cause more prozone in time-delay tests than RIIIM (maximum potency ICSH/ISBT reference AHG reagents) as shown by the example of 205 in Table 12.
6. A high-potency anti-IgG equal to RIIIM offers considerable resistance to neutralization of residual serum from inadequately washed tests, as sometimes occurs with cell washing machines.[45] It is, therefore, useful to show that the anti-IgG is at least as resistant as R3P by inhibition tests with serum at a 1 in 3000 level with weak anti-D, anti-Kell, and anti-Fy^a.[45]
7. A useful additional test is to perform a slide avidity test with strong anti-D-sensitized cells.[50,51] The anti-IgG should agglutinate the sensitized cells as rapidly as the reference reagent, e.g., in about 5 to 10 seconds. In the case of anti-IgG (205), it was noted that a dilution of 1 + 3 had a considerably slower avidity time of greater than 4 minutes, although the freshly made reagent was satisfactory in tube tests with well-washed sensitized red cells.

TABLE 12
Prozone Tests of Anti-IgG with Weak Sensitized Red Cells

2 Vols Anti-IgG + Washed Sensitized RBC

Anti-IgG	Time delay before spin (minutes) 0	1	2	5	Sensitized RBC
RIIIM	+	+	$+^{w}$	0	Anti-D
205 (neat)	+	+	$+^{w}$	0	
RIIIM	+/++	+	$+^{w}$	0	Anti-Fy[a]
205 (neat)	+/++	+/++	$+^{w}$	0	
			Prozones		

8. The anti-IgG should detect at least the IgG1, IgG2, and IgG3 subclasses and ideally should also detect IgG4.[53]
9. Approval for reagent use requires: stability data for its shelf life at 4°C, preferably supported by data for 3 months at room temperature (25°C) and 6 weeks at 37°C; and extended tests with a wide range of weak antibodies of many specificities, especially after extended storage (e.g., 12 months) at 4°C.

Note that Anti-IgG neat supernatant 205(IgM) showed a failure to detect some antibodies after a 1-year storage at 4°C that gave clear 1+ reactions with our routine AHG reagent (CBT 24/4). Thus, it is essential to select a stable anti-IgG, and the economics dictate that this should be an IgM anti-IgG. However, a blend of two or three IgG anti-IgGs may prove to be more stable, although perhaps more expensive, reagents.

E. MONOCLONAL ANTI-COMPLEMENT (ANTI-C3c AND ANTI-C3d) FOR AHG

Conventional anti-C3c/C3d is costly to make and often contains a mixture of antibodies that varies considerably in production from batch to batch. The control of clean anti-C3d is complicated by the delicate balance between adequate anti-C3d potency and the occurrence of "false" positives with the C3d levels on normal red cells, especially as C3d uptake is increased when red cells are incubated in fresh serum, as in compatibility tests. Thus, some AHG reagents were assessed as clean with just-washed red cells by the old FDA false-positive test, but, nevertheless, gave false positives in routine work when the red cells were incubated in fresh serum.

The Joint Working Party on AHG Reagents of the ICSH/ISBT revised the false-positive test for AHG to include tests with fresh compatible serum as described below, and this procedure has also been adopted by the FDA.

TABLE 13
Three Types of AHG Free of "False" Positives in Crossmatch Tests

Various types of anti-C3 blended with rabbit serum anti-IgG	Spin-tube titers × EC3bi or EC3d indicator RBC			
	Immediate (15–30 second) tests			5-Minute delay[a]
	C3c	C3g	C3d	C3d
Conventional (rabbit) — C3c-C3d, e.g., R3P[b]	16	0	<1	4–8
Monoclonal — C3c-C3d e.g., RIIIM	64	0	2 increased	8
Monoclonal — C3d (BRIC 8) no C3c	0	0	32	32

[a] 5-Minute tests are essential to measure low levels of anti-C3d.
[b] May also contain some anti-C4c (titer 2–4) e.g., R3P.

TABLE 14
Complement-Coated Red Cells to Identify Anti-C3/C4 Specificities

	Indicator red cells				
	EiC3b/C4b	TRYP/EiC3b/C4b	EC3 ("EC3b")	EC4	TRYP EC4
C3 Fragments	c+ g+ d+	c− g− d+	a+ c+ d+ g−	None	None
C4 Fragments	c+ d+	c− d+	None	c+ d+	c− d+
Anti-C3c	+	−	+	−	−
Anti-C3g	+	−	−	−	−
Anti-C3d	+	+	+	−	−
Anti-C4c	+	−	−	+	−
Anti-C4d	+	+	−	+	+

Note: Antibodies must be negative with untreated and trypsin-treated non-sensitized cells.

The use of selected monoclonal anti-C3c(s) blended with anti-C3d(s) can produce a simulated polyclonal anti-C3c + anti-C3d blend as shown by the example of RIIIM which is the ICSH/ISBT reference AHG with monoclonal anti-complement components. Alternatively, selected IgM anti-C3ds such as BRIC-8[16,45,52] can provide a very potent anti-complement without the need to use anti-C3c, and they are as free of false positives as the reference AHG reagents R3P and RIIIM.

The titers of examples of three types of anti-complement in widespread use are shown in Table 13.

F. THE EVALUATION OF MONOCLONAL ANTI-COMPLEMENTS

The specificity pattern of antibodies to C3 and C4 components are easily determined by the use of C3- and C4-coated red cells prepared by low ionic methods, as shown in Table 14. These procedures have been reviewed by Voak et al.[45] and Engelfriet et al.[54] as a result of studies by a joint working party of the ISBT/ICSH on the standardization of anti-human globulin reagents. For detailed examples, see the workshop report on anti-complement from the 1989 Lund meeting.[50,51]

A recommended sequence of tests is as follows:

1. Exclude anti-C4 antibodies by tests with EC4/EC4d.
2. This enables the anti-C3 antibodies to be assessed by titration with EiC3b/C4 to find the potency titer* dilution equivalent to that of the reference reagent RIIIM. (The C3d component of RIIIM exceeds the minimum potency FDA reference preparation.)
3. Check the antibody at dilutions for possible reagent use for freedom from false positives. This is achieved by simulated crossmatch tests with fresh ABO-compatible sera against old stored red cells (21 to 30 days) from CPD-A1 donor pack segment lines, as they represent the worst scenario for C3d uptake.
4. Monoclonal anti-complement found satisfactory against low ionic indicator EiC3c/C3d should then be assessed against antibody-bound complement tests. This is important especially for anti-C3c(s) as some have been found to fail with EAJk^a or EALe^a. It should be noted that the "EC3b" low ionic system of Fruitstone[55] is, in fact, whole C3 and has C3a, C3c, and C3d, and is negative with anti-C3g and free from C4 components.[45] This system is useful in the characterization of anti-C3g as its C3g is concealed. However, some IgM anti-C3ds, e.g., BRIC-8 do not work reliably with this EC3 system, although they work well with EiC3b/C4 and the latter reflects the C3 state of *in vitro* bound complement that presents C3c, C3g, and C3d.

Recent claims at the Washington Reagents Workshop[17] (Pennec, 1990) that 3 of 400 donor bloods showed C3d polymorphism and were negative with some anti-C3ds deserves further evaluation, but may reflect quantitative and not qualitative variation.

G. OTHER MONOCLONAL, ANTIBODY BLOOD TYPING REAGENTS

Conventional anti-M and anti-N reagents are difficult to make and give very poor reproducibility batch to batch. Therefore, it was not surprising that monoclonal anti-M and anti-N antibodies were among the first blood group monoclonals to find application in routine work.

Each monoclonal anti-M and anti-N needs to be assessed for its optimum pH as their optimum activity and specificity are very pH dependent.[56–60]

* *Note:* The upper limit of anti-complement for potency is restricted only by freedom from false positives; e.g., BRIC-8 anti-C3d is clean but far more potent than conventional anti-C3d or the anti-C3d component in RIIIM.

TABLE 15
A Specific Monoclonal Anti-M (BS 57)

Spin-Tube Titers (Room Temperature at pH 8.0)

	Saline	Trypsin destroyed	Chymotrypsin enhanced
3% RBC			
MM	16,000	0	64,000
MN	16,000	0	64,000
$M^{v}N$	16,000	0	64,000
$M^{c}N$	0	0	0
Control			
NNSs	0	0	0

Position 1		**Position 5**
M Serine	M^{c}	Glycine
N Leucine		Glutamic acid

Monoclonal anti-N antibodies, like all anti-N antibodies, cross-react with the N-like antigen called ''N'', which is on Glycophorin B and is not a product of the N gene.

Fortunately, ''N'' occurs at a lower site density than that of the N gene in heterozygotes. Thus, it is relatively easy to make monoclonal anti-N reagents ''specific'' for agglutination by a given method, by selecting the dilution at which they fail to detect ''N'' of MM red cells, but have an adequate reaction with MN red cells. It is important to use S + MM red cells for the negative control in selecting the ''specific'' anti-N dilution, because these red cells have 30% more ''N'' than ss MM red cells.[61–63]

Some monoclonal anti-M reagents may not be cross-reactive with N, but the M antigen is the product of only the M gene. Thus, it is possible to have specific monoclonal anti-M antibodies that do not react at all with the N or ''N''-like antigens, e.g., BS-57 as shown in Table 15. However, BS-57 does not detect the variant M^{c} because, presumably, glycine is an important part of the M determinant recognized by BS-57 and it is replaced by glutamic acid in M^{c}.[64] However, this is a useful discrepancy and M^{c} is easily recognized if the second anti-M reagent is selected to ensure it is reactive with M^{c}.

Anti-Le^{a} and anti-L^{b} monoclonal reagents[22,65] have been used routinely for several years and should be evaluated as with conventional reagents, including an A_1 Le^{b} cell to demonstrate if an anti-Le^{b} requires a high H status for adequate reactions, as is typical of most reagents.

Recently, excellent IgM monoclonal anti-Jk^{a} and anti-Jk^{b} reagents have been described by Thompson and Hughes-Jones,[80] and these reagents have simplified an IAT typing test to a simple direct test.

Monoclonal antibodies are playing an increasingly important role in routine blood grouping and research. For reviews of recent research applications of monoclonal antibodies studied extensively at ISBT international workshops, the readers are referred to the works edited by Rouger and Salmon[25] and Messeter and Johnson.[1] These studies clearly demonstrate that selected monoclonal antibodies are excellent research probes for studying the fine immunochemical structure of many antigens and their distribution in body tissues.

REFERENCES

1. **Messeter, L. and Johnson, U., Eds.,** Proceedings of the 2nd ISBT Workshop on monoclonal antibodies against human red blood cells and related antigens. Lund, Sweden, *J. Immunogenet.,* 17, 213, 1990.
2. **Voak, D.,** Monoclonal antibodies in blood grouping, *Biotest Bull.,* 3, 177, 1988.
3. **Voak, D.,** Monoclonal antibodies as blood grouping reagents, in *Bailliere's Clinical Haematology,* Vol. 3, No. 2, Contreras, M., Bailliere Tindall, Harcourt, Brace, Jovanovich, London, 1990, 219.
4. **Kohler, G. and Milstein, C.,** Continuous cultures of fused cells secreting antibody of predefined specificity, *Nature,* 256, 495, 1975.
5. **Galfre, G. and Milstein, C.,** Preparation of monoclonal antibodies, strategies and procedures, *Meth. Enzymol.,* 73, 3, 1981.
6. **Voak, D. and Lennox, E.,** Principles of monoclonal antibodies in blood transfusion work, *Biotest Bull.,* 4, 281, 1983.
7. **Littlefield, J. W.,** Selection of hybrids from matings of fibroblasts in vitro and their presumed recombinants, *Science,* 145, 709, 1964.
8. **Barnstable, E. J., Bodmer, W. F., Brown, G. et al.,** Production of monoclonal antibodies to group A erythrocytes, HLA and other human cell surface antigens: new tools for genetic analysis, *Cell,* 14, 9, 1978.
9. **Voak, D., Lennox, E., Sachs, S., Milstein, C., and Darnborough, J.,** Monoclonal anti-A and anti-B development as cost-effective reagents, *Med. Lab. Sci.,* 39, 109, 1982.
10. **Bron, D., Feinberg, M. B., Nelson, N. H. T., and Kaplan, H. S.,** Production of human monoclonal IgG antibodies against Rhesus (d) antigen, *Proc. Natl. Acad. Sci. U.S.A.,* 81, 3214, 1984.
11. **Thompson, K. M., Melamed, M. D., Eagle, K. et al.,** Production of human monoclonal IgG and IgM antibodies with anti-D Rhesus specificity using heterohybridomas, *Immunology,* 58, 157, 1986.
12. **Lowe, A. D., Green, S. M., Voak, D. et al.,** A human-human monoclonal anti-D by direct fusion with a lymphoblasted line, *Vox Sang.,* 51, 212, 1986.
13. **Winter, G. and Milstein, C.,** Man-made antibodies, *Nature,* 349, 293, 1991.
14. **Oriol, R., Samuelsson, B. E., and Messeter, L.,** ABO antibodies serological behaviour and immuno-chemical characterization, *J. Immunogenet.,* 17, 279, 1990.
15. **Birch, J. R., Lambert, K., Thompson, P. W., Kenney, A. C., and Wood, L. R.,** in *Large Scale Culture Technology,* Lydersen, K., Ed., Carl Hanser, Verlag, Berlin, 1987, 1.
16. **Holt, P. D. J., Donaldson, C., Judson, P. A. et al.,** NBTS BRIC-8. A monoclonal anti-C3d antibody, *Transfusion (Philadelphia),* 25, 267, 1986.

17. Reagents for the 90's, Convenors A. Hoppe and D. Voak, 1st International Meeting of the International Society of Blood Transfusion/International Committee for Standards in Haematology/Food and Drug Administration and Reagent Manufacturers, Washington, D.C., Nov. 7–9, 1990; Immunohaematology, 7, 57, 1991.
18. **Voak, D., Sachs, S., Alderson, T., Takei, F., Lennox, E., Jarvis, J., Milstein, C., and Darnborough, J.,** Monoclonal anti-A from a hybrid myeloma: evaluation as a blood grouping reagent, *Vox Sang.*, 39, 13, 1980.
19. **Sachs, S. and Lennox, E.,** Monoclonal anti-B as a new source of blood typing reagents, *Vox Sang.*, 40, 99, 1981.
20. **Salmon, Ch., Rouger, Ph., Doimel, Ch., Edelman, L., and Bach, J. F.,** ABH subgroups and variants. Use of monoclonal antibodies, *Biotest Bull.*, 4, 300, 1983.
21. **Voak, D., Lowe, A. D., and Lennox, E.,** Monoclonal antibodies: ABO serology, *Biotest Bull.*, 4, 291, 1983.
22. **Messeter, L., Brodin, T., Chester, M. A. et al.,** Mouse monoclonal antibodies with anti-A, anti-B and anti-A,B specificities: some superior to human polyclonal ABO reagents, *Vox Sang.*, 46, 185, 1984.
23. **Lowe, A. D., Lennox, E., and Voak, D.,** A new monoclonal anti-A culture supernatant with the performance of hyperimmune human reagents, *Vox Sang.*, 46, 29, 1984.
24. **Moore, S., Chirnside, A., Micklem, L. R. et al.,** A mouse monoclonal antibody with anti-A(B) specificity with agglutinates Ax cells, *Vox Sang.*, 47, 427, 1984.
25. **Rouger, Ph. and Salmon, Ch., Eds.,** Monoclonal antibodies against human red blood cell and related antigens, Proc. 1st International Society of Blood Transfusion Workshop on Monoclonal Antibodies, Paris, Sept., 1987.
26. **Clausen, H. and Hakomori, S. I.,** ABH and related histo-blood group antigens; immunochemical differences in carrier isotopes and their distributions, *Vox Sang.*, 56, 1, 1989.
27. **Clausen, H., Levery, S. B., Nudelman, E., Tsuchiua, S., Hakomori, S. I. et al.,** Repetitive A epitope (type 3 chain A) defined by blood group A, specific monoclonal antibody 1H-1: chemical basis of qualitative A, and A2 distinction, *Proc. Natl. Acad. Sci. U.S.A.*, 82, 1199, 1985.
28. **Hoppe, A. H.,** Considerations in the Selection of Reagents, American Association of Blood Banks, Washington, D.C., 1979, Appendix 1, p. 15.
29. **Voak, D., Lodge, T. W., Stapleton, R. R., Fogg, H., and Roberts, H. E.,** The incidence of H deficient A2 and A2B bloods and family studies on the AH/ABH status of an Aint and some new variant blood types, *Vox Sang.*, 19, 73, 1970.
30. **Monro, A. C., Inglis, G., Blue, A., Sheridan, R., and Mitchell, R.,** An evaluation of mouse monoclonal anti-A and anti-B as routine blood grouping reagents, *Med. Lab. Sci.*, 39, 123, 1982.
31. **Broly, H.,** Second International Society of Blood Transfusion Workshop on Monoclonal Antibodies against Human Red Blood Cells and Related Antigens, Lund, Sweden, April, 1990.
32. **Greenwell, P., Yates, A. D., and Watkins, W. M.,** Blood group A synthesising activity of the blood group B gene specified 3-galactosyl transferase, in *Glyconjugates,* Schaur, R., Boer, P., Buddecke, E., and Kramer, M. F., Eds., Vliegenthart and Wiegendt, Stuttgart, 1979, 268.
33. **Beck, M. L., Hardman, J. T., and Henry, R.,** Reactivity of a licensed murine monoclonal anti-A reagent with group B cells, *Transfusion,* 26, 572, 1986.
34. **Treacy, M. and Stroup, M.,** Proceedings of a scientific forum on blood grouping anti-A (murine monoclonal blend) Bioclone, Sept., 1986, Raritan, NJ, Ortho Diagnostics DS, 1987, p. 1.
35. **Goldstein, J., Lenny, L., Davies, D., and Voak, D.,** Further evidence for the presence of A antigen on group B erythrocytes through the use of specific exoglycosidases, *Vox Sang.*, 57, 142, 1989.

36. **Sonneborn, H. H. and Voak, D.,** Monoclonal Antibodies Detect Overlapping Specificities of A and B Glycosyl Transferases, Abstr. (postep) Congr. of Int. Soc. Haematol. Milan, 1988.
37. **Voak, D., Sonneborn, H., and Yates, A.,** The detection of traces of B on A1 cells by a monoclonal anti-B: characteristics of the B(A) phenomenon, *Transfusion Med.*, 2, 119, 1992.
38. **Doyle, A., Jones, T. J., Bidwell, J. L., and Bradley, B. A.,** In vitro development of human monoclonal antibody secreting plasmacytomas, *Hum. Immunol.*, 13, 199, 1985.
39. **Crawford, D. H., Barlow, M. J., Harrison, J. F., Winger, L., and Huehns, E. R.,** Production of human antibody to Rhesus D antigen, *Lancet,* 1, 386, 1983.
40. **Goosens, D., Champonier, F., Rouger, P., and Salmon, C.,** Human monoclonal antibodies against blood group antigens. Preparation of a series of stable EBV immortalised clones producing high levels of antibody of different isotype and specificities, *J. Immunol. Meth.*, 101, 193, 1987.
41. **Kumpel, B. M., Poole, G. D., and Bradley, B. A.,** Human monoclonal anti-D antibodies. Their production, serology, quantitation and potential use as blood grouping reagents, *Br. J. Haematol.*, 71, 125, 1989.
42. **Thompson, K. M. and Hughes-Jones, N. C.,** Production and characterization of monoclonal anti-Rh, in *Bailliere's Clinical Haematology,* Vol. 3, No. 2, Contreras, M., Ed., Bailliere Tindall, Harcourt, Brace, Jovanovich, London, 1990.
43. **Tippett, P. and Moore, S.,** Monoclonal antibodies against Rh and Rh-related antigens, *J. Immunogenet.*, 17, 309, 1990.
44. **Lomas, C., Tippett, P., Thompson, K. M., Melamed, M. D., and Hughes-Jones, N. C.,** Demonstration of seven epitopes on the Rh antigen D using human monoclonal anti-D antibodies and red cells from D categories, *Vox Sang.*, 57, 261, 1989.
45. **Voak, D., Downie, D. M., Moore, B. P. L., and Engelfriet, C. P.,** Anti-human globulin reagent specification: the European and ISBT/ICSH view, *Biotest Bull.*, 1, 7, 1986.
46. **Van Rhenen, D. J. and Overbeeke, M. A. M.,** Quality of anti-D sera by a panel of donor red cells with weak reacting D antigens and with partial D antigens by the Federation of Netherlands Red Cross Blood Banks, *Vox Sang.*, 57, 273, 1989.
47. **Schmidt, P. J., Morrison, E. G., and Schol, J.,** The antigenicity of the Rh (Du) blood factor, *Blood,* 20, 196, 1962.
48. **Contreras, M. and Knight, R. C.,** The Rh-negative donor, *Clin. Lab. Haematol.*, 11, 317, 1989.
49. **Downie, D. M., Voak, D., Jarvis, J., Waldmann, H., and Spitz, M.,** The use of monoclonal antibodies to human IgG in blood transfusion serology, *Biotest Bull.*, 4, 348, 1983.
50. **Voak, D. and Nilsson, U.,** Report of studies on monoclonal anti-IgG antibodies. Second ISBT Workshop on Monoclonal Antibodies, *J. Immunogenet.*, 17, 331, 1990.
51. **Voak, D. and Nilsson, U.,** Report of studies on monoclonal antibodies to complement components. Second ISBT Workshop on Monoclonal Antibodies, *J. Immunogenet.*, 17, 337, 1990.
52. **Engelfriet, C. P. and Voak, D.,** International reference polyspecific anti-human globulin reagents, *Vox Sang.*, 53, 241, 1987.
53. **Frame, T., Bot, A., Vlug, A., and Eijk, R.,** Subclass and epitope specificities of monoclonal anti-IgG antibodies, Second International Workshop on Monoclonal Antibodies to Red Cell Antigens and Related Determinants, Lund, Sweden, 1–4 April, 1990.
54. **Engelfriet, C. P., Overbeeke, M. A. M., and Voak, D.,** The antiglobulin test (Coombs test) and the red cell, in *Progress in Transfusion Medicine,* Vol. 2, Cash, J., Ed., Churchill Livingstone, Edinburgh, 1987, 74.
55. **Fruitstone, M. J.,** C3b sensitised erythrocytes, *Transfusion (Philadelphia),* 18, 125, 1978.
56. **Fraser, R. H., Munro, A. C., Williamson, A. R., Barrie, E. K., Hamilton, E. A., and Mitchell, R.,** Mouse monoclonal anti-N, *J. Immunol.*, 9, 295, 1982.

57. **Sonneborn, H. H., Uthemann, H., Munro, A. C., Bruce, M., Fraser, R. H., and Inglis, G.,** Reactivity of monoclonal antibodies directed against blood group antigens M and N, *Dev. Biol. Stand.,* 57, 61, 1984.
58. **Sonneborn, H. H. and Ernst, M.,** Further characterisation and standardisation of mouse monoclonal antibodies reacting with M/N blood group antigens, *Dev. Biol. Stand.,* 67, 97, 1987.
59. **Nichols, M. E., Rosenfield, R. E., and Rubinstein, P.,** Two blood group M epitopes disclosed by monoclonal antibodies, *Vox Sang.,* 49, 134, 1985.
60. **Rubocki, R. and Milgrom, F.,** Reactions of murine monoclonal antibodies to blood group MN antigens, *Vox Sang.,* 51, 217, 1986.
61. **Voak, D., Davies, D., Sonneborn, H. et al.,** The application of monoclonal antibodies for the detection of genetic markers of human red cells, in *Advances in Forensic Haematogenetics,* Vol. 2, Mayer, W. R., Ed., Springer-Verlag, Berlin, 1988, 268.
62. **Voak, D., Downie, D. M., Moore, B. P. L. et al.,** Replicate tests for the detection and correction of errors in anti-human globulin (AHG) tests: optimum conditions and quality control, *Haematologia,* 21(1), 3, 1988.
63. **Anstee, D. J. and Lisowska, E.,** Monoclonal antibodies against glycophorins and other glycoproteins, *J. Immunogenet.,* 17, 301, 1990.
64. **Dahr, W., Uhlenbruck, G., Jansen, E., and Schmalish, R.,** Different N-terminal amino acids in the MN glycoprotein free MN and NN erythrocytes, *Hum. Genet.,* 35, 335, 1977.
65. **Fraser, R. H.,** (Abstract) British Blood Transfusion Society Conference, Manchester, September, 1984.
66. **Salmon, Ch., Rouger, Ph., Doinel, Ch., Edelman, L., and Bach, J. F.,** ABH subgroups and variants. Use of monoclonal antibodies, *Biotest. Bull.,* 4, 300, 1983.
67. **Feizi, T.,** Demonstration by monoclonal antibodies that carbohydrate structures of glycoproteins and glycolipids are oncodevelopmental antigens, *Nature,* 314, 53, 1985.
68. **Fraser, R. H., Allen, E. K., Inglis, G., Munro, A. C., Mackie, A. C., and Mitchell, R.,** Production and immunochemical characterization of mouse monoclonal antibodies to human Le^a blood group structures, *Exp. Clin. Immunogenet.,* 1, 145, 1984.
69. **Young, W. W., Johnson, H. S., and Tamura, Y.,** Characterization of monoclonal antibodies against the human Le^b blood group antigen, *J. Biol. Chem.,* 256, 13223, 1983.
70. **Fraser, R. H., Mackie, A., Inglis, G., Murphy, M. T., and Mitchell, R.,** Characterization of anti-glyco conjugate monoclonal antibodies, *Rev. Fr. Transfus. Immuno-Haematol.,* 30(5), 633, 1987.
71. **Von dem Borne, A. E. G., Bos, M. J. E., Joustra-Mass, N., Tromp, J. F., Van Wijingaarden-du-bois, R., and Tetteroo, P. A. T.,** A murine monoclonal IgM antibody specific for bleed group P antigen (globoside), *Br. J. Haematol.,* 63, 35, 1986.
72. **Tippett, P., Andrews, P. W., Knowles, B. B., Salter, D., and Goodfellow, P. N.,** Red cell antigens P (Globoside) and Luke: identification by monoclonal antibodies defining the murine state specific embryonic antigens -3 and -4 (SSEA-3 and SSEA-4), *Vox Sang.,* 51, 53, 1986.
73. **Fraser, R. H., Ingils, G., Mackie, A., Munroe, A. C., Allan, E. K., Mitchell, R., Sonneborn, H. H., and Uthemann, H.,** Mouse monoclonal antibodies reacting with M blood group related antigens, *Transfusion,* 25, 261, 1985.
74. **Anstee, D. J. and Edwards, P. A. W.,** Monoclonal antibodies to human erythrocytes, *Eur. J. Immunol.,* 12, 228, 1982.
75. **Parsons, S. F., Judson, P. A., and Anstee, D. J.,** BRIC-18: monoclonal antibody with a specificity related to the kell blood group system, *J. Immunogenet.,* 9, 377, 1982.
76. **Sonneborne, H. H., Uthemann, H., and Pfeffer, A.,** Monoclonal antibody specific for human blood group k (Cellano), *Biotest. Bull.,* 1, 328, 1983.
77. **Rahman, R. A. F. and Longnecker, B. M.,** A monoclonal antibody specific for the Tomsen-Freidenreich cryptic T antigen, *J. Biol. Chem.,* 129, 2021, 1982.

78. **Daniels, G. L., Tippett, P., Palmer, D. K., Miller, Y. E., Geyer, D., and Jones, C.,** MER2, a red cell polymorphism defined by monoclonal antibodies, *Vox Sang.*, 52, 107, 1987.
79. **Thompson, K., Barden, G., Sutherland, J., Beldon, I., and Melamid, M.,** Human monoclonal antibodies to human blood group antigens Kidd Jk^a and Jk^b, *Transfus. Med.*, 9, 91, 1991.
80. **Thompson, K., Barden, G., Sutherland, J., Beldon, I., and Melamid, M.,** Human monoclonal antibodies to C, c, E and G antigens of the Rh system, *Immunology,* 71, 323, 1990.

Chapter 12

MICROPLATE BLOOD GROUPING TECHNIQUES

Marion L. Scott

TABLE OF CONTENTS

ISBN 0-8493-4938-9

I. INTRODUCTION

Over the last twenty years there have been various trends in the development of blood grouping techniques. Due to revolutionary developments in biotechnology, polyclonal human-based reagents for ABO and D grouping have been able to be replaced by monoclonal reagents, giving better performance in terms of increased reaction strength, shorter incubation times, and lot-to-lot consistency. The introduction of the use of low ionic strength solutions has also improved the sensitivity and speed of tests. Tile techniques have been almost completely superseded by tube techniques; currently many laboratories are adopting microplate techniques.

The 96-well microplate format was first used in viral serological investigations[1] and has since been adopted as a convenient, efficient means of handling batches of immunodiagnostic tests in many disciplines. Wegman and Smithies[2] described the application of this format to blood grouping tests in 1966, detailing a technique using V-well microplates and 0.03% red cell suspensions for saline, enzyme, and antiglobulin methods. Subsequent publications[3–5] confirmed the versatility of this format for blood grouping tests, which could be used with a wide range of volumes and concentrations of reagents in U- and V-well plates. In 1984, two groups of workers[6,7] described the automated interpretation of ABO and Rh grouping tests in microplates.

All of these workers used liquid-phase techniques, based on hemagglutination as the endpoint. In 1978, Rosenfield and co-workers[8] proposed the use of novel solid-phase techniques in microplates, where a positive reaction was no longer signaled by agglutination, but by hemadsorption, possibly convertible to a color reaction. His ideas were developed by several groups of workers,[9–14] and now the exciting new developments of solid-phase microplate techniques are starting to be used routinely. The use of this type of system opens up totally new possibilities for microplate blood grouping methodology.

The motives driving these changes are to improve the accuracy and efficiency of blood grouping tests and to offer a fast, reliable service at a low cost. In recent times, difficulty in the recruitment of staff and competition for funds has increased this motivation. Every laboratory is looking for ways to deal with their workload in the most staff-time- and cost-effective manner. Many laboratories who have adopted microplate methods (liquid or solid phase) have done so not just because it is the "latest up-to-date technology", but rather of necessity as the only way they can cope with a high workload, poor funding, and short staffing.

This chapter details the various ways in which microplate technology is being used in blood group serology, and indicates advantages and disadvantages of each technique. Consideration is given to the quality assurance required for the introduction of this type of technology into a laboratory.

II. LIQUID-PHASE TECHNIQUES

A. RANGE OF TESTS

Microplates are being used in liquid-phase techniques for ABO and Rh(D) typing, antibody screening, crossmatching, and rare phenotype screening. The type of techniques being used are basically very similar to tube techniques, with some modifications to take account of the use of a plastic container for the reaction mixture, the lower total volume of the wells compared to tubes, and adaptation to enable automated reading of test results using some type of through-plate spectrophotometer/nephelometer. The microplate is effectively being used as a convenient block of 96 small test tubes. Techniques are based on direct agglutination for ABO and Rh(D) typing (sometimes with potentiators) and antiglobulin and enzyme tests for antibody detection. As with tube techniques, there is much variation between laboratories in the precise method used.

B. PROBLEMS ASSOCIATED WITH THE USE OF PLASTIC

Problems associated with the use of plastic rather than glass are those of nonspecific protein absorption to the plastic, sometimes causing monolayering of red cells, and static charges, making the dispensing of reagents difficult. Incorporation of a nonionic detergent such as Tween 20 into blood grouping reagents prevents many of the monolayering problems, as does pretreatment of plates with the detergent and/or proteins such as albumin or casein. Static charge reduction may be achieved by simply prewashing plates in water, or standing the plates on a damp tissue.

C. READING METHODS

The method of reading the results in microplates varies between workers. Most tests consist of incubation of reactants followed by centrifugation and then manual or machine assessment of the degree of hemagglutination. Care must be taken with the centrifugation of microplates to ensure an even *g* force across the plate. This is achieved by ensuring free movement of swing-out plate carriers and using a centrifuge with a large radius. Agglutination may be assessed by resuspension or streaming. For resuspension, the contents of the wells are mixed using a mechanical rotary shaker at a defined speed for a defined length of time. Again, care must be taken to ensure that all wells are subjected to the same amount of agitation — in fact, this is easier to achieve with the mechanical mixing of a microplate than the manual resuspension of tests in a series of test tubes! The degree of agglutination is assessed as for a tube technique. If an automated through-plate spectrophotometer is being used, it may be desirable to potentiate reactions, such that differentiation between positive and negative results is easier. Various workers have developed the use of cocktails of combinations of proteolytic enzymes, protamine sulfate, and low-ionic-strength saline (LISS) for the suspension of red cells to facilitate machine reading of ABO and Rh(D) typing plates. With improvements in typing reagents and developments in machine reading, the use of these types of potentiators is often no longer necessary.

Agglutination may also be assessed by streaming, where the plate is held at a defined angle to the horizontal for a defined length of time and the movement of the cell button observed and assessed by eye. In a negative reaction, the cells all stream freely downwards in one line, whereas positive agglutinated cells will move down in one clump. This method of reading is more sensitive than resuspension, and is used by some workers for antibody detection where the agglutination may be weak. However, this type of reading method cannot be used in automated readers and interpretation is subjective.

Different types of automated through-plate readers are now available for assessing agglutination reactions in microplate wells. A general purpose, unmodified, single light beam enzyme-linked immunosorbent assay (ELISA) reader can be used if the plate and the reader are tilted, such that agglutinated cells fall out of the path of the light beam. Alternatively, dedicated single light beam machines can be used flat, when the light beam has been offset to pass through the well outside the area occupied by agglutinated cells. Newer machines take many readings across each well to build up a pattern of readings to assess the degree of agglutination. The increasing availability of sophisticated image analysis technology at affordable prices means that this type of reader may take over as the best automated means of assessing agglutination reactions.

D. TYPES OF PLATES

In general, U-well plates are used for resuspension techniques, using 1 to 3% red cell suspensions. For streaming techniques it may be preferable to use V-well plates and a lower concentration of red cells — typically 0.5 to 1% to obtain optimum sensitivity.Other considerations in the selection of microplates for liquid-phase techniques should be the type of plastic and the supplier. Plates giving a low binding of protein should be used — *not* those sold for ELISA and other solid-phase techniques. In general, this means using nonactivated polystyrene plates. The molding quality of the plates is important, particularly if an automated reader is to be used, and it is important to buy from a manufacturer with good quality assurance.

E. REAGENT STANDARDIZATION

Reagents standardized for use in tube techniques need to be restandardized for microplate use. Generally, microplate techniques are more sensitive, so dilution and greater economy of reagents may be achievable. Reactions should always be assessed with strong and weak phenotype cells when considering dilution of a reagent. Also, greater sensitivity may reveal contaminant specificities in a reagent that were not detectable by tube technique. Some monoclonal antibodies which work well in glass tubes may give an unacceptable degree of monolayering in a microplate due to their stickiness to plastic. Addition of dyes to reagents should be considered as it facilitates checking whether or not a particular reagent has been added to a microplate well — this is difficult to assess by eye in inner wells.

F. DRIED MICROPLATES

Dried microplates with reagents for ABO and Rh(D) typing already dispensed in the wells are available from a few manufacturers.[15–16] These provide a microplate typing system in a kit form which can be very useful, for example, to small units operating in remote locations. They have been proposed as a simple, appropriate means of bedside confirmatory testing of ABO and Rh group.[16]

G. ANTIGLOBULIN METHODS

Most laboratories find it relatively easy to adopt microplate techniques for ABO and Rh(D) typing. However, many laboratories have experienced difficulties in adapting antiglobulin antibody screening techniques to a microplate system. Extending the number of washes prior to antihuman globulin (AHG) reagent addition is normally necessary when adapting a tube technique to a microplate. The full well volume of a microplate is five to ten times less than a tube, such that the washing efficiency of each step is lower. Adsorption of IgG to the plastic during the incubation stages may cause monolayering and neutralization of AHG — blocking plates prior to use may be essential. Standardization of AHG reagents for microplate use is essential, as prozones may occur in microplates at dilutions of anti-IgG suitable for use in tubes. These types of problems with the liquid-phase antiglobulin test in microplates have led several laboratories to investigate the use of a solid-phase antiglobulin test, described below.

H. QUALITY ASSURANCE

Detailed proposals for the quality assurance of liquid-phase microplate techniques are given in the U.K. "Guidelines for Microplate Techniques in Liquid-Phase Blood Grouping and Antibody Screening".[17] Since few manufacturers issue instructions for use of their reagents in a microplate technique, it is up to the user to carry out sufficient testing to ensure that the performance of the reagents they are using is adequate in their microplate technique.

I. ADVANTAGES OF USING MICROPLATES

Overall, the advantages of using microplates for liquid-phase blood group serology are the increased sensitivity of reactions, the concomitant possible economies with reagents, the speed and ease of use of the plates, and the availability of a large range of automated and semiautomated equipment for handling all phases of tests in a microplate format. At the simplest level, use of multichannel pipettes allows simultaneous addition of reagent to 8 or 12 tests at a time by one worker. At higher levels, fully automated plate dispensers, washers, incubators, shakers, and readers are available, with stacking systems to take many plates. Robotic systems are available to sample from tubes into microplates. The modular nature of the automation means that automated microplate systems have considerable advantages over continuous flow automated systems — if one part of the system fails, that operation can be performed by hand until corrected, leaving the rest of the system fully functional. The sample identity integrity provided by bar coding on sample tubes, microplates, and computer storage and analysis of results is invaluable in a busy modern laboratory.

J. DISADVANTAGES OF USING MICROPLATES

The disadvantages of using microplates for liquid-phase blood group serology are that tests must, by nature of the format of the plate, be batched. This may not be appropriate for the working practices of all laboratories, or in certain situations where, for example, a single emergency grouping or antibody screen is required. However, microplate wells are now available as strips of wells rather than whole plates, so that small batches of tests can be run in microwell strips, using the same methodology as for using a whole plate. Some retraining of staff and purchase of new equipment is required in a laboratory switching from tubes to microplates. However, these initial costs are normally rapidly offset by the increased productivity achieved using a microplate system.

III. SOLID-PHASE TECHNIQUES

A. GENERAL PRINCIPLES

In a solid-phase microplate assay, one of the components of the test system is immobilized on the plastic surface of the microplate well prior to starting the test. The immobilized component serves to capture specific components from the test solution, allowing simple separation from the other elements of the reaction mixture and measurement. Solid-phase microplate methods have been developed for all the blood grouping tests, encompassing red cell typing, antibody screening, and crossmatching. Solid-phase microplate tests retain all the advantages of the liquid-phase microplate systems while achieving higher sensitivity, ease of use, and automation.

B. SOLID-PHASE CELL TYPING

The principles of this system are shown in Figure 1. Partially purified monoclonal blood group specific antibody is coated onto the microplate under carefully controlled and optimized conditions. This can either be achieved by direct coating of antibody onto the plate[10,13] (as shown in Figure 1), or specific capture of antibody onto a plate precoated with the appropriate type of red cell.[18] Excess antibody is washed away. At this stage the coated plate can be

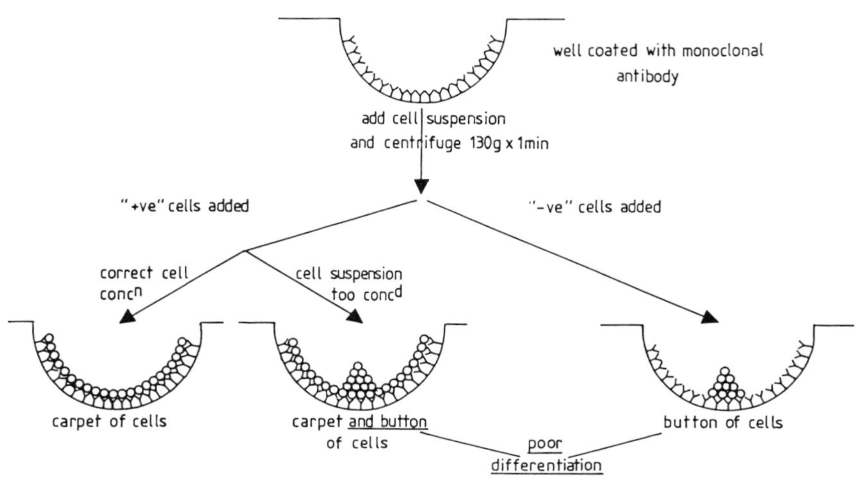

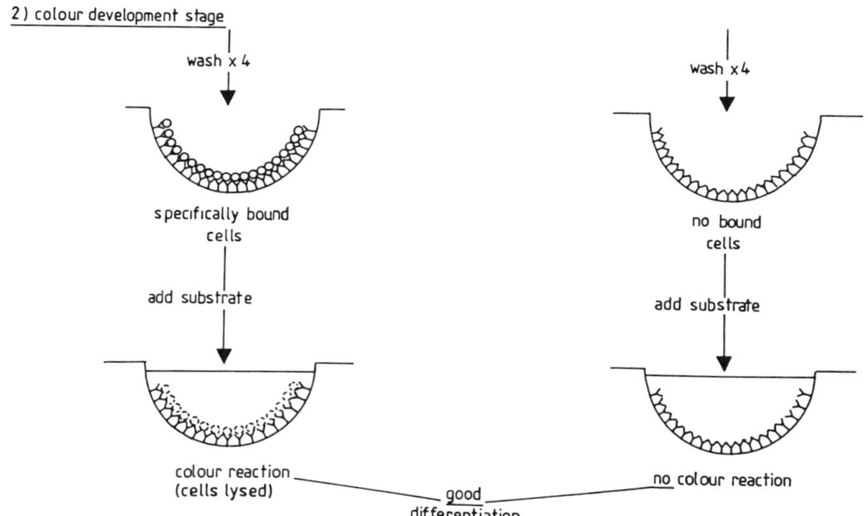

FIGURE 1. Schematic diagram of solid-phase cell grouping.

dried and stored. Coated plates are stable for up to two years at 4°C. To use, the test red cell suspension is added to the plate and the plate centrifuged. Positive red cells adhere to the antibody and form a carpet of cells around the well. Negative red cells button in the bottom of the well. At this stage the plate can be read by eye or using a through-plate reader. To aid visual or machine reading, the plate can be washed to remove nonadherent red cells.

If chromogenic peroxidase substrate is then added, the potent hemoglobin peroxidase of the adherent positive cells will cause rapid color development. The use of this washing and color development stage makes the test more robust and less liable to reading errors caused by the use of too concentrated a cell suspension (leading to the presence of a button of cells in a positive as well as a negative test well) or over-centrifugation (leading to partial collapse of the carpet monolayer).

The advantages of this type of system over the equivalent liquid-phase microplate test are the sensitivity achieved and the use of a reading system not dependent on hemagglutination. Visual reading of red cell monolayers is easier and more objective for an inexperienced worker than resuspension of cells and assessment of the degree of agglutination. The availability of the washing and color development stages render this system very suitable for easy automation using a simple single light beam through-plate reader. The advantages of using prepared plates are the same as for dried liquid-phase plates. The solid-phase system can be prepared on microwell strips, if required, for use in situations where batching of tests to fill a whole microplate is not appropriate. A system based on the same principles has recently been described using smaller 72-well Terasaki plates.[18]

C. SOLID-PHASE ANTIBODY SCREENING

It is in this area of solid-phase tests that the main advantages of solid-phase techniques are to be realized, due to the technical problems of reproducibly performing sensitive liquid-phase microplate antiglobulin tests. The use of solid-phase methods obviates many of the problems inherent in liquid-phase tests. There are two main types of solid-phase antibody detection methods in current use. In the first type, reagent red cells, red cell stroma, or blood group antigens are immobilized on the solid phase. In the second type, components of the antiglobulin detection system are immobilized on the solid phase. I shall refer to these second types of assays as solid-phase antiglobulin tests — see below.

The principles of the first type of system are shown in Figure 2. Red cell membranes or ghosts are immobilized onto the plastic by first coating the plate with poly-L-lysine to render the surface strongly positively charged. The red cells then stay bound on the plastic by charge interaction. (Alternatively cells may be bound onto the plastic specifically by precoating the plastic with a red cell-specific lectin or antibody, or other suitable chemical treatment.) At this stage, if ghosts have been used, the plate can be dried and stored. Test serum is added to the coated plate, incubated, and the plate washed to remove free immunoglobulin. It is at this stage that the technique has considerable advantages over a liquid-phase technique, as no centrifugation and resuspension of the red cells is involved — washing is achieved by simply filling the well with wash fluid and emptying it. The number of red cells used is considerably less than in a liquid-phase test — only a monolayer is

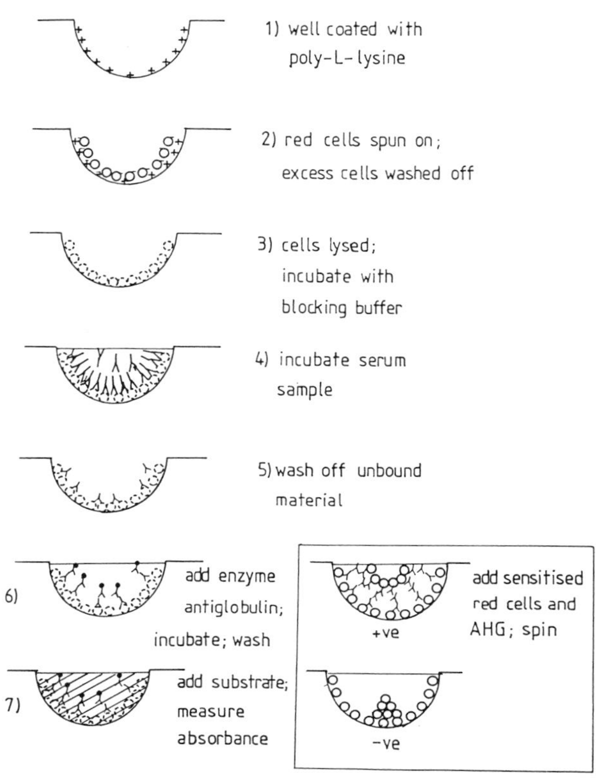

FIGURE 2. Schematic diagram of solid-phase antibody screening.

present, so that the washing efficiency and the ratio of antibody to antigen are high.

Detection of bound antibody may be achieved by several different methods. An enzyme-conjugated antiglobulin reagent can be used, followed by washing, color development, and reading in a through-plate spectrophotometer. Alternatively, a red cell indicator system can be used. Indicator red cells are prepared by sensitizing Rh(D)-positive red cells to a standard level with IgG anti-D. Sensitization to a standard level is most easily achieved using a monoclonal anti-D. Addition of antiglobulin reagent at a standardized dilution produces indicator red cells that are coated with antiglobulin reagent, but are not agglutinated. When these cells are added to the microplate wells and the plate spun, the antiglobulin reagent will bind the indicator red cells to any IgG bound on the solid-phase red cell monolayer. The appearance of a positive reaction is thus a monolayer of adherent cells compared to a button of cells in a negative reaction.

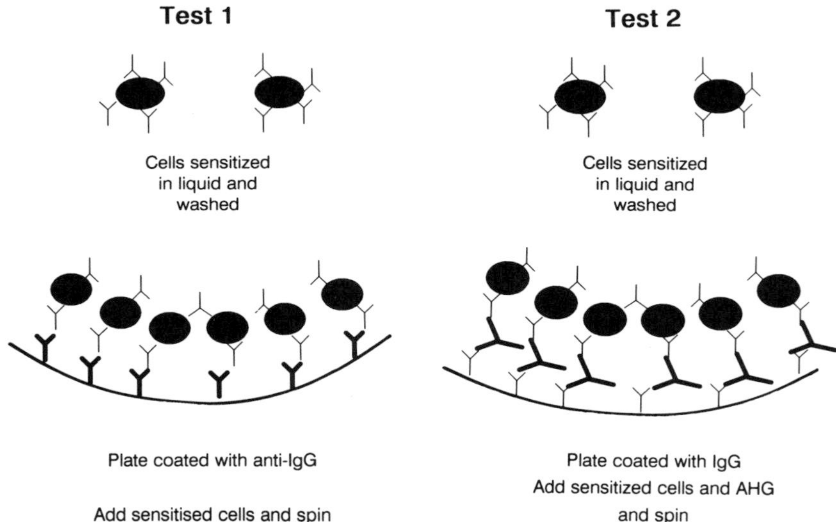

FIGURE 3. Schematic diagrams of three versions of the solid-phase antiglobulin test. The antiglobulin reagent is shown in bold type.

This type of system with a red cell indicator has been very successfully developed and marketed by Immucor (Georgia) as their Capture R system. Microwells are available as either whole plates, or strips of eight wells. The system has high sensitivity and good freedom from false-positive reactions when compared to a conventional liquid-phase antiglobulin test. Again, the use of a reading system not dependent on hemagglutination has considerable advantages. Visual reading of red cell monolayers is easier and more objective for an inexperienced worker than resuspension of often weakly agglutinated cells and assessment of the degree of agglutination. If dried ghosts are used in this system it has considerable logistic advantages in the production, standardization, and use of screening cells. After selection of a good screening cell panel, many solid-phase plates or strips of wells can be prepared and dried from this panel and used over several years. The lifetime of selected screening cells is thus greatly extended. The possibilities of preparing dried plates or strips for antibody identification are also opened up by this technology.

D. SOLID-PHASE ANTIGLOBULIN TESTS

Several variants of solid-phase antiglobulin tests (in which components of the AHG detection phase are immobilized on the plastic) are in current use. The principles are shown in Figure 3. In all these tests, the test red cells are incubated with the serum sample and washed in liquid phase. They do not, therefore, have the same advantages in terms of ease and efficiency of

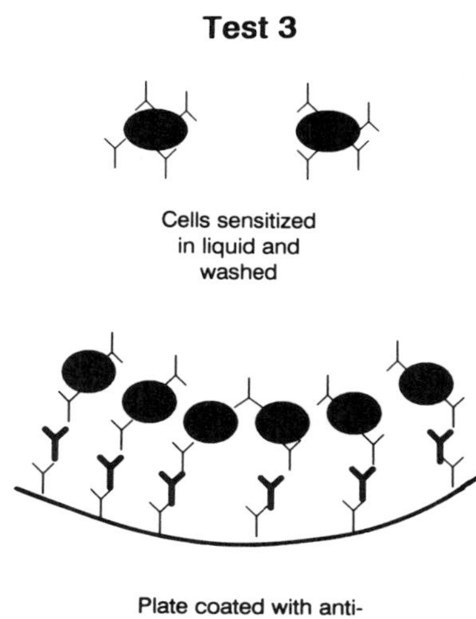

FIGURE 3 (continued).

washing that the first type of method has. The solid-phase part of the test is purely designed to convert the reading method from hemagglutination to solid-phase adherence.

In one variant,[9] the plastic well is coated with anti-IgG and, in some cases, anti-C3d. Addition of washed sensitized or unsensitized cells and centrifugation results in a carpet forming with sensitized cells due to adherence of the IgG to the solid-phase anti-IgG, or a button with unsensitized cells.

In another variant,[19,20] the plastic well is coated with normal IgG, usually by using a dilution of group AB serum. Washed sensitized or unsensitized cells are added with conventional liquid AHG reagent and the plate centrifuged. Sensitized cells form a carpet around the well due to the AHG reagent bridging between IgG on the sensitized cells and IgG coated on the plastic. Unsensitized cells button in the bottom of the well.

In another variant, the plastic well is coated with anti-antiglobulin reagent (e.g., anti-rabbit IgG if the antiglobulin reagent was raised in rabbits). Washed sensitized or unsensitized cells are added with conventional liquid AHG reagent and the plate centrifuged. Sensitized cells form a carpet around the well as they have bound components of the antiglobulin reagent which are in turn bound by the anti-antiglobulin reagent coating the well. Unsensitized cells button in the bottom of the well. A system based on this type of methodology is available commercially from Biotest (Frankfurt, Germany) as their SolidScreen system.

These three variants of solid-phase antiglobulin tests all offer a more sensitive test system than the liquid-phase antiglobulin test with the use of a reading system not dependent on subjective interpretation of hemagglutination. Visual reading of red cell monolayers is easier and more objective for an inexperienced worker than resuspension of often weakly agglutinated cells and assessment of the degree of agglutination. All of these types of tests can be converted to a color reaction by washing the plate and adding chromogenic peroxidase substrate, as for red cell typing.

E. QUALITY ASSURANCE OF SOLID-PHASE METHODS

Solid-phase blood grouping methods are still in a period of active research and development. It is difficult to generalize on suitable methods for quality assurance at this stage.

Quality assurance of solid-phase cell typing must be undertaken by different means to those used for liquid-phase techniques. It is not possible to perform comparative potency titrations of blood grouping reagents in this type of technique, as the grouping reagent antibody must be coated onto the well at optimum concentration. Assurance of adequate performance can only be achieved by testing the solid-phase system with panels of weak-phenotype red cells. This should be carried out to validate the performance of a solid-phase grouping method in comparison to existing laboratory procedures prior to adopting the solid-phase technique. It should also be carried out as preacceptance testing of new batches of coated plates, and weak-phenotype red cells should be routinely included as daily or batch controls.

Any proposed solid-phase antibody detection system should be tested in parallel with current tube techniques with a dilution series of at least three weak (titers of 8 to 16 in conventional LISS spin-tube AHG techniques) nonsaline reactive sera (to include anti-D, anti-Kell, and anti-Fy^{a}). The sensitivity of detection of the solid-phase system should at least equal that of the liquid-phase tube technique, using a validated AHG reagent. Preacceptance testing using such sera should be carried out when a new batch number kit is used, or on new batches of coated plates and new batches of antiglobulin reagent. Daily or batch controls should include samples known to contain strong, weak, and no antibody (inert AB serum).

IV. CONCLUSIONS

Microplate technology has much to offer to blood grouping techniques. Use of microplates as more convenient containers than tubes for liquid-phase agglutination-based tests has opened up the world of modular semi- and fully automated systems to the blood group serologist, with considerable savings in staff time and increased efficiency in the laboratory.

Use of microplates as plastic supports for solid-phase-based assays has introduced totally new concepts into blood grouping techniques, with a move away from hemagglutination as an endpoint. The higher sensitivity of such test methods, coupled with the ease of use and availability and automation will make this the technology of the future.

REFERENCES

1. **Sever, J. L.,** Application of a microtechnique to viral serological investigations, *J. Immunol.,* 88, 320, 1962.
2. **Wegmann, T. G. and Smithies, O.,** A simple haemagglutination system requiring small amounts of red cells and antibodies, *Transfusion,* 6, 67, 1966.
3. **Crawford, M. N., Gottman, F. E., and Gottman, C. A.,** Microplate system for routine use in blood bank laboratories, *Transfusion,* 10, 258, 1970.
4. **Warlow, A. and Tills, D.,** Micromethods in blood group serology, *Vox Sang.,* 35, 354, 1978.
5. **Parker, J. L., Marcoux, D. A., Hafleigh, E. B., and Grumet, F. C.,** Modified microtiter tray method for blood typing, *Transfusion,* 18, 417, 1978.
6. **Bowley, A. R., Gordon, I., and Ross, D. W.,** Computer controlled automated reading of blood groups using microplates, *Med. Lab. Sci.,* 41, 19, 1984.
7. **Severns, M. L., Schoeppner, S. L., Cozart, M. J., Friedman, L. I., and Schanfield, M. S.,** Automated determination of ABO/Rh in microplates, *Vox Sang.,* 47, 293, 1984.
8. **Rosenfield, R. E., Kochwa, S., and Kaczera, Z.,** Solid-phase serology for the study of human erythrocyte antigen-antibody reactions, in *Proc. XII Congress of Int. Soc. Haematol. and XV Congress of Int. Soc. Blood Transfusion,* Karger, Basel, Switzerland, 1978, 27.
9. **Moore, H. H. and Conradie, J. D.,** Solid-phase indirect anti-human globulin test for identification of red blood cell antibodies in human sera, *Transfusion,* 22, 540, 1982.
10. **Sinor, L. T., Rachel, J. M., Beck, M. L. et al.,** Solid-phase ABO grouping and Rh typing, *Transfusion,* 25, 21, 1984.
11. **Plapp, F. V., Sinor, L. T., Rachel, J. M. et al.,** A solid-phase antibody screen, *Am. J. Clin. Pathol.,* 82, 719, 1984.
12. **Lee, H., Canavaggio, M., Germain, C. et al.,** The production and standardisation of monoclonal antibodies as ABO blood typing reagents: their application in a microelisa system, *Proc. 18th Congress Int. Soc. Blood Transfusion,* Karger, Basel, Switzerland, 1984.
13. **Scott, M. L. and Phillips, P. K.,** Development of a solid-phase microplate system for ABO and D grouping, Poster presented at British Blood Transfusion Soc. Annual Meeting, Oxford, 1985.
14. **Sharon, R., Duke-Cohan, J. S., and Galili, U.,** Determination of ABO blood group zygosity by an antiglobulin rosetting technique and cell based enzyme immunoassay, *Vox Sang.,* 50, 245, 1986.
15. **Hazenberg, C. A. M., Mulder, M. B., and Beelen, J. M.,** A comparison of precoated microplates with manual tube techniques for routine blood group typing, *Labmedica,* June/July, 1988, p. 43.
16. **Blakeley, D., Tolliday, B., Colaco, C., and Roser, B.,** Dry instant blood typing plate for bedside use, *Lancet,* 336, 854, 1990.
17. British Society for Haematology and British Blood Transfusion Society, Guidelines for microplate techniques in liquid-phase blood grouping and antibody screening, *Clin. Lab. Haematol.,* 12, 437, 1990.
18. **Sinor, L. T., Stone, D. L., Rolih, S. D., and Eatz, R. A.,** RBC typing by solid-phase red cell adherence in 72-well terasaki plates, *Abstracts of Int. Soc. Blood Transfusion Congress,* AABB, Arlington, VA, 1990.
19. **Ross, D. W. and Gordon, I.,** A solid-phase Coombs test for routine use, Poster presented at British Blood Transfusion Society Annual Meeting, London, 1986.
20. **Rachel, J. M., Sinor, L. T., Beck, M. L. et al.,** A solid-phase antiglobulin test, *Transfusion,* 25, 24, 1985.

Chapter 13

PRETRANSFUSION COMPATIBILITY ASSURANCE: PAST AND PRESENT

Bahman Habibi

TABLE OF CONTENTS

ISBN 0-8493-4938-9

I. DEFINITION

Pretransfusion compatibility assurance (PCA) consists of policies and procedures aimed at the prevention of immediate or secondary hemolytic transfusion reactions. This terminology, designed to convey the broad sense of this major field of transfusion medicine, is proposed in preference to those currently used, such as pretransfusion or compatibility testing, since these terms tend to restrict the subject to its ''testing'' and laboratory facets. The same criticism applies to ''crossmatch'' which is inappropriate per se, since, for several decades now, the routine practice has been not to ''cross'' the major match with the minor, the recipient's serum vs. donor's cells test remaining the only component of this originally bidirectional procedure.

II. BACKGROUND

The evolution of the concept of PCA has both fostered and followed the development of applied immunohematology since the discovery and recognition of the role of ABO groups in blood transfusion at the dawn of the 20th century (Figure 1) (see References 1 and 2 for review). The pioneer approach to PCA consisted of ABO blood typing and/or the mixture of donor and recipient's whole blood at room temperature. The First World War fostered the development of whole blood transfusions and witnessed the emergence of the group O ''universal donor'' approach, questioning, to some extent, the usefulness of pretransfusion testing in settings where such donors were available.

During the 1940s, coincidental with the recognition of Rh blood groups, the need was appreciated to detect ''incomplete'' antibodies. The advent of agglutination-enhancing methods using albumin, proteases, and antiglobulin thus introduced a major refinement in the laboratory implementation of the PCA. Over the next two decades, the major and minor match gained common acceptance. Coincidental with the discovery of new transfusion- or pregnancy-induced alloantibodies and with the recognition of new blood group systems, screening tests for irregular antibodies in recipients were introduced and panels of reagent red blood cells were made available both by blood centers and the

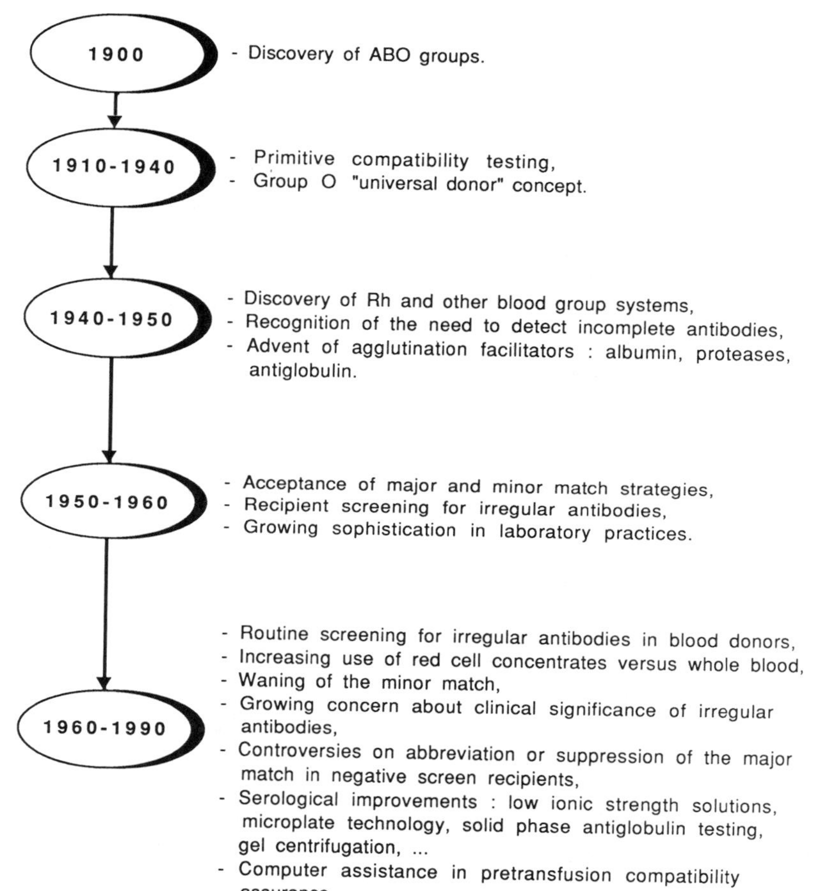

FIGURE 1. Development and refinements of pretransfusion compatibility assurance.

industry. During this period, the fear of ‘‘missing’’ an antibody and the quest for perfection in serological compatibility played a leading role in the choice of PCA strategies. This trend resulted in progressive sophistication of procedures and caused an increase in the work-load, costs, and outdating, a longer delay in the release of blood units, and, consequently, an increase in the number of unsatisfied clinicians.

Since the 1970s, laboratory practices have been more critically assessed in a search for reasonable simplification and this has resulted in the progressive implementation of some radical changes in blood centers.

1. Systematic screening for irregular antibodies in donors’ plasma has become routine in most countries with developed transfusion services,

thereby discarding from direct therapeutic use whole blood or plasma units containing clinically significant antibodies.

2. The so-called ''minor crossmatch'' has ceased to be required in parallel with the growing use of red cell concentrates rather than whole blood. However, in many countries, the medical jargon is still paradoxically continuing to use the prefix ''cross-'' almost irremediably stuck to the popular ''major crossmatch'' which, as stated earlier, is but a one-side test!
3. Major concern has been focused on the clinical significance of irregular antibodies, thus deliberately ignoring others, especially the cold-reacting ones.[3]
4. In countries where the major match was a regulatory requirement for the implementation of PCA, the very usefulness of the antiglobulin phase of the match or even of the entire procedure has been strongly questioned in settings where recipients have a negative antibody screen. This is mainly for time-saving and cost-containment reasons.[1,2,4–6]
5. The use of low ionic strength solutions[7–9] has become almost standard practice for suspension of red blood cells. The procedure enhances the indirect antiglobulin test, replaces albumin, shortens the incubation time of the compatibility testing, and consequently results in the delivery of blood to patients in a more rapid and effective way.
6. Besides the breakthrough represented by the use of low ionic strength solutions, the laboratory techniques used to implement PCA have achieved a wide range of improvements. In recent years, they have evolved from test tubes into microplates and from the classical liquid phase into solid-phase[10] and gel-centrifugation[11] technologies which are more elegant, easier to handle, and of equivalent if not higher sensitivity.
7. Finally, automation, bar codes, computers, and data processing have radically changed many areas of blood banking activities. These include not only administration of the blood bank, processing and labeling of donated blood, but also maintenance of patients' records, transfusion laboratory practice, and release of blood, all of which are integral components of the PCA.

III. BASIC CONSIDERATIONS

To implement PCA in a given blood center, the choice of operating strategy is mainly based on environmental issues such as the number of patients and the geographic area to be served, the blood usage profile of the health care facility, the blood inventory issues such as supply, demand, and outdating figures, the availability of qualified personnel, the degree of effective implementation of standard operating procedures, the reliability of the donor-recipient identification system, the extent to which transfusionists get themselves involved in the management of patients, and, finally, the discipline and collaboration with clinicians and nurses which is most instrumental in obtaining reliable scientific information regarding adverse reactions and efficacy of blood transfusion in general.

Given the number and complexity of the above variables no single and universally applicable recipe could be recommended in implementing PCA. The best approach is the global quality assurance in the blood center, in the hospital ward, and within the blood center — the bedside communication system. It would be, therefore, the duty of medical directors of transfusion services to determine the most appropriate technical and strategic choices to be adapted to their specific environment while considering the following basic reflections.

A. STAFF TRAINING AND QUALIFICATION

Whatever the strategy, the universally stressed prerequisites are the training and qualification of the staff, and the establishment of standard operating procedures covering blood grouping, screening for clinically significant antibodies, record keeping, and communication of immunologic data.

B. PREVENTION OF ABO INCOMPATIBILITY

Even in the 1980s, over three quarters of the severe hemolytic transfusion accidents are caused by ABO incompatibility. From 1976 through 1985 the United States Food and Drug Administration received reports of 158 fatalities due to acute posttransfusion hemolysis. ABO incompatibility was by far the most common cause (131/158) and accounted for 37% of all the transfusion-associated fatalities reported.[12]

The above figures reflect only a fraction of the reality. Nonfatal, clinically unrecognized, or deliberately unrevealed ABO incompatible transfusions seem to be much more frequent; this is particularly so since, in most countries, there is no mandatory reporting mechanism to allow objective assessment and monitoring of this transfusion morbidity.

Since by far the most common causes of ABO incompatibility are identification errors and poor operational practices, the prevention of such errors both at the transfusion service and at the bedside must remain a major and permanent concern.

C. PREVENTION OF NON-ABO INCOMPATIBILITIES

Undetected or improperly identified irregular antibodies represent the second major cause of hemolytic transfusion reactions.[13] Clinically significant alloantibodies are currently found in approximately 1 to 4% of prospective transfusion recipients. Their incidence, characteristics, and diversity must be borne in mind when setting up procedures designed to prevent their harmful effects on transfused patients. Such antibodies are encountered either in patients without obvious exposure to foreign antigens (''naturally occurring'' antibodies) or in individuals with a prior history of blood transfusion or pregnancy (''immune'' antibodies).

TABLE 1
Irregular Antibodies Found in Routine Screening of 106,939 Blood Donors

Anti-D ± C ± E	118	Anti-P_1	223
Anti-E	17	Anti-Le^A	84
Anti-c	6	Anti-Le^B ± Le^A	82
Anti-C	2	Anti-H	43
Anti-C^W	2	Anti-M	3
Anti-e	1	Anti-N	1
Anti-K	5	Anti-Lu^A	1

Note: Donors from the National Blood Transfusion Center, Paris; incidence: 0.55%.

TABLE 2
Some Naturally Occurring and Pregnancy-Induced Alloantibodies Capable of Causing Hemolytic Transfusion Reactions on the First Transfusion

Frequent	Anti-Lewis, -P_1, -Wr^A, anti-''private''
Rare	Anti-H, -Tj^A, -K, -P, Rh29, -Rh17, -Lan, -U, -K^U, -Kp^B, -Fy^3, -Jk^3, -Ve^A, -Sc_1, Duclos

''Naturally occurring'' antibodies and those resulting from pregnancy are seen in healthy untransfused people who are prospective blood recipients in trauma centers and surgery and maternity wards. Table 1 shows the incidence of these antibodies in a population of healthy blood donors, and, by extension, among these people as patients. Obviously, the absence of a transfusion history offers little protection and the use of type-specific blood without antibody screening, even in these apparently low-risk populations, could cause hemolytic reactions. Table 2 shows some naturally occurring or pregnancy-induced alloantibodies that also may be detected at the time of the first transfusion of the patient. Many of these antibodies are capable of causing hemolytic transfusion reactions.

''Immune'' antibodies occur predominantly in women and in previously transfused patients. Table 3 shows their incidence in the author's laboratory where 488,618 pretransfusion screening tests had been performed over a period of 10 years. Of these, 15,215 individuals were found positive, 6,326 of whom had alloantibodies of the immune type and the remaining 8,889 had autoagglutinins or naturally occurring alloantibodies. The distribution of the latter is but slightly predominant in women (female to male ratio 1.26) whereas in the former category 73% of immunized patients were women (female to male ratio 2.66). Obviously, antibody frequency figures vary according to countries, ethnic groups, and techniques. They form the scientific background

TABLE 3
Incidence of "Immune" and "Naturally Occurring" Antibodies in Patients Screened in Anticipation of Transfusion

"Immune" antibodies			"Naturally occurring" antibodies		
Specificity	No. Patients	Female/male ratio	Specificity	No. Patients	Female/male ratio
Anti-D	2133	3.77	Auto-agglutinins	3743	1.28
Anti-C(Rh-neg.)	648	2.66	Anti-Le^a	1776	1.17
Anti-E(Rh-neg.)	212	2.02	Anti-P	1288	1.38
Anti-E(Rh-pos.)	1006	1.73	Anti-Le^b	749	1.17
Anti-K	778	2.48	Anti-Le^a + Le^b	694	1.26
Anti-c	367	2.63	Anti-H+I	382	1.31
Anti-Fy^a	220	2.54	Anti-M	157	1.34
Anti-C(Rh-pos.)	82	1.82	Anti-N	31	0.93
Anti-Jk^a	78	2.39	Anti-Lu^a	69	1.22
Anti-S	69	1.65			
Anti-Jk^b	49	2.76			
Anti-e	48	2.20			
Anti-Fy^b	13	12			
Anti-s	8	1			
Rare or unidentified antibodies	615				
Total (mean)	6326	(2.66)	Total (mean)	8889	(1.26)

Note: From the National Blood Transfusion Center, Paris.

for the choice of laboratory techniques and operational policies aimed at the prevention of transfusion incompatibilities.

D. LACK OF STRICT CORRELATION BETWEEN *IN VITRO* AND *IN VIVO* COMPATIBILITIES

High-titer, low-avidity antibodies such as Ch^a, Rg^a, Cs^a, Kn^a and most cold-reacting naturally occurring antibodies such as anti-H, anti-Lewis, anti-M, anti-I, anti-Pl, fail to cause significant *in vivo* destruction of serologically incompatible red cells. Conversely, in rare circumstances, especially in multiply transfused patients, transfused red cells have a poor *in vivo* survival despite serologic compatibility with the recipient's serum.[14–16] It should be remembered, as warned about several decades ago by pioneer transfusionists,[15,17] that we have still no universal *in vitro* technique for the detection of all clinically significant antibodies. Despite their increasing maturation, our *in vitro* tests do not infallibly reflect *in vivo* compatibility or incompatibility between donor and recipient. The reasonable choice is therefore a compromise between possible and feasible. This compromise will, however, have to be adapted to environmental conditions and keep abreast of scientific and technical progress.

E. IMMUNOLOGIC COMPATIBILITY AND OTHER VARIABLES OF RED CELL VIABILITY

Aside from any immunologic considerations, the current standards hold that a blood unit may be infused into a recipient even if 70% of the transfused red cells are destroyed in the first 24 hours (the widely accepted threshold for the calculation of storage periods of 21 and 35 days). The contrast is obviously striking between the enthusiastic sophistication of screening methods aimed at the detection of all antibodies in *occasional* patients and this institutionally tolerated up to 30% destruction of transfused red cells in *all* recipients. Organized efforts leading to improving this threshold would have a greater impact in terms of patient care than those that advocate increasing sophistication of laboratory tests to detect some debatable immunological incompatibility.

IV. IMPLEMENTATION

As shown in Figure 2, two main strategies are currently implemented for transfusion of red cells or whole blood. The process is obviously complex and involves multiple practices and individuals geographically dispersed in the blood center (donor processing laboratory, recipient processing laboratory, blood delivery unit), in the hospital ward (operating rooms, physicians, nurses), and within the blood center (bedside-communication system). This section will focus on the specific steps and practices which support PCA strategies.

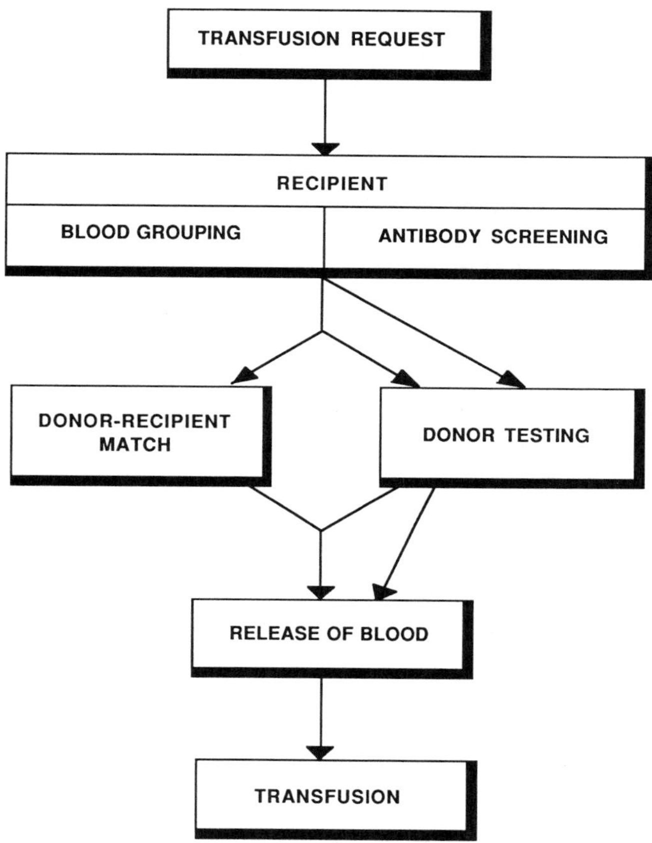

FIGURE 2. Current strategies for transfusion of red cells or whole blood.

A. TRANSFUSION REQUEST

Specimen collection for pretransfusion testing must be more exacting than for other clinical laboratory tests, although the same principles basically apply to all. Blood specimens must be labeled at the bedside immediately after collection: data must show first and last names, identification number, and date of collection. Positive identification of the patient is essential. In addition to consulting the patient's identification information on the chart or attached to the bed or to the patient's body (e.g., wristband or identification discs), conscious patients should be asked to give at least their first and last names and birth date. Accompanying request forms must be meticulously filled in (sex, last name, first name, date of birth, identification number) and dated and signed by the responsible physician or nurse. Additional information such as diagnosis, transfusion history, previous pregnancies, or already identified antibodies may be helpful both in problem solving and in selecting the most appropriate blood product.

Computer transmitted or telephoned requests should comply with strict preestablished procedures and any improvisation by the hospital or the laboratory staff should be prohibited.

In an emergency, when the patient's identity is unknown, a temporary wristband with an emergency identification number should be used and later cross-referenced with the patient's definitive identification markers.

Blood specimens should optimally be drawn into two stoppered tubes, one containing citrate or ethylene diamine tetraacetate (EDTA), for red cell typing, the other without anticoagulant for antibody screening. If the blood is collected from an infusion line, the tubing should be flushed with saline and the first few milliliters of blood withdrawn should be discarded.

Antibody screening and major match must be performed on samples collected within 3 days of the scheduled transfusions when the patient has been pregnant or transfused within the preceding 3 months or if the history is uncertain or unavailable. It seems appropriate to generalize the above arbitrary 3-day limit to all specimens used for pretransfusion testing to avoid problems that might occur because of record-keeping errors or inaccurate history.[18]

Before a specimen is processed a qualified member of the staff must confirm that identity information on the request form and on the label are identical. A new specimen must be obtained in case of doubt or discrepancy.

B. RECIPIENT BLOOD GROUPING

ABO type must be determined by both red cells and serum grouping using anti-A, anti-B, and anti-AB reagents for the former, and group A, B and, optionally, A_2 test cells for the latter. Any discrepancy between the results or any serological problems must be resolved before entering the data in the patient's records and a temporary decision must be taken in case of emergency regarding the appropriate group of the blood to be transfused.

The serum of infants less than 2 to 6 months of age contains little or no anti-A or anti-B except that transferred from the mother. If it is an established policy within the transfusion service to deliver cards to blood recipients, no such document should be issued until the age of 1 or 2 years when the red cell antigens and serum antibodies have matured into their definitive adult picture.

The RhO(D) type must be determined by a rapid and reliable method using potent anti-D serum capable of recognizing regular and high-grade D weak antigens. Provided the reagent and the technique used meet this requirement, further testing for D^u antigen by the indirect antiglobulin technique on apparently D-negative patients is not required. An exception is made for the apparently D-negative neonates born to D-negative mothers, since the discovery of a D^u type baby would lead to the mother being given immunoprophylaxis although the chance of such a neonate causing Rh sensitization of its mother is probably remote.[19]

The use of an adequate control for each D typing is mandatory for recipients. Agglutination of red cells by the antiserum diluent alone makes D typing impossible to interpret. One may thus avoid false typing of D-negative patients as D-positive and their consequent transfusion with D-positive blood.

ABO and D typing should optimally be carried out by two technicians working independently and, whenever possible, using two lots of reagents. It is also sound practice to require similarity between the results of two different specimens before definitive entry in the patient's records and before type-specific blood is issued for transfusion.

Patient's records must be checked for previous results of blood typing. Any discrepancy might imply a clerical or technical error which must be resolved before further proceeding. The same must apply to antibody screening since, as will be discussed below, previously identified antibodies may become undetectable over time[20] but nevertheless hemolytically active *in vivo,* especially if boosted by transfusion of incompatible red cells, leading thereby to delayed hemolytic transfusion reactions.

C. RECIPIENT ANTIBODY SCREENING

Detection of clinically significant antibodies is the aim of this step of the PCA strategy. Clinically significant antibodies are those known to have caused immediate or delayed hemolytic transfusion reactions or hemolytic disease of the newborn.

The choice of the antibody detection and identification techniques depends on several variables: size and workload of the laboratory, clinical situations to be covered, proportion of emergency cases to be supported, and the technical staff and financial capacity of the blood bank. Many techniques and substances have been developed to enhance red cell antibody reactions: indirect antiglobulin test, proteases, bovine albumin, methylcellulose, polyethylene glycol, Polybrene, low ionic strength solutions, etc., but no single technique available today can detect all possible irregular antibodies. The use of more than one technique may therefore be advisable. Moreover, new scientific achievements may result in modification of previously established policies. Continuous flow hemagglutination, low ionic strength solution techniques, solid-phase antiglobulin testing, and gel centrifugation are examples of this evolution and emphasize the need for each laboratory director to adapt his/her techniques with common sense and objectivity, bearing in mind that *in vivo* and *in vitro* characteristics of antibodies are not always closely correlated. An example of a reasonable choice for routine practice in nonautomated laboratories would be the use of two manual techniques: indirect antiglobulin testing at 37°C, using an antiglobulin reagent with good anti-IgG and anti-complement activities, and a papain test at 37°C. The low ionic polycation test[8,9] and the manual polybrene test[21–24] are rapid but sensitive methods and may be recommended as routine, especially when a prompt response is needed.

Apart from the technique itself, the reliability of antibody screening depends on the reagents and other technical parameters. The reagent red cells used should consist of two to five selected samples expressing as many blood group antigens with clinically significant antibodies as possible. It is currently required in the U.S. that the following 18 antigens be present on the red cells: D, C, E, c, e, M, N, S, s, Pl, Le^a, Le^b, K, k, Fy^a, Fy^b, Jk^a, and Jk^b.[25] It is not exceptional that weak and yet significant antibodies remain undetected by reagent red cells bearing single-dose antigens.[26–28] It is therefore advisable that at least one of the screening samples has a double-dose homozygous expression of at least D, c, Jk^a, Jk^b, Fy^a, and Fy^b antigens, which are most commonly implicated in such settings.

Pooling of reagent red cell samples decreases the sensitivity of antibody screening; most authors therefore agree not to consider it as a recommended practice.

The serum to cell ratio affects the sensitivity of the reaction: the higher the ratio, the higher, to some extent, the detection rate of weak antibodies. The optimum serum to cell ratio should therefore be determined by each laboratory for each technique.

Agglutination and/or hemolysis, which are the visible endpoints of red cell-antibody reactions, should be read in an accurate and consistent way by all personnel in the laboratory according to standard operating procedures covering details such as tilting to dislodge cells from the bottom of the tube, the use of reading devices (concave mirror, microscope), and grading of reactions, etc.

Discrepant opinions have been expressed regarding the need for the anti-complement component of antiglobulin reagents[1,2,29] which, compared to anti-IgG only reagents, has the disadvantage of picking up more insignificant antibodies and the advantage of detecting some examples of complement-fixing antibodies such as anti-Jk^a, anti-Fy^a, or anti-K.[26,30]

Including a direct antiglobulin test or autocontrol as part of routine antibody screening is costly, time consuming, and of limited value.[31] There is consensus agreement that the test should only be performed when investigating a suspected hemolytic transfusion reaction or a drug-induced or autoimmune hemolytic anemia; in situations where all screening red cell samples are positive; and in testing a neonate exposed to materno-fetal red cell incompatibility.

A negative antibody screen becomes invalid with time and must be repeated even after a few days, because intervening immunologic events such as pregnancies and transfusions unknown to the physician may change the patient's immunohematologic status. In patients receiving a series of transfusions within a short period of time, most authorities are of the opinion that the antibody screening should be repeated at least every 2 or 3 days.

D. DONOR TESTING

ABO and Rh(D) typing require the same attention as for recipient blood typing. Blood bags must only be labeled after two sets of ABO and D typing have been completed or after having confirmed the agreement between the results of a single set of tests performed on the donation with the donor's previous records. After labeling of the blood bag a final red cell typing performed on a tubing segment attached to the bag must validate the ABO blood type and the label must be signed by the staff member having performed the final check.

Provided the anti-D reagent and the technique used are capable of recognizing high-grade D weak antigens, D^u testing of apparently D-negative donor units by indirect antiglobulin test may not seem to be warranted. However, the D^u testing of such units is still required in some countries whereas, in others, it is replaced by C and E testing, the blood unit being labeled Rh(D)-negative only if both C and E antigens are absent from the red cells.

Antigens other than A, B, and D, commonly involved in red cell alloimmunization (see Table 3) should be tested for in a selected population of donors, preferably of group O or A, in order to support transfusion of patients either with irregular antibodies or at high risk of being immunized by such antigens.

If group O whole blood is to be used for recipients of other blood groups, a screening test for "immune" anti-A or anti-B should be done, using a standard technique easily applicable to routine blood processing. Although such techniques are not unanimously defined, they include: hemolysis of A_1 or B red blood cells (RBC) in the presence of human complement, titers over 64, failure of inhibition by group-specific substances, or failure of inactivation by dithiothreitol treatment. Units of whole blood or plasma defined as containing dangerous levels of anti-A or anti-B should bear a label recommending their use exclusively in recipients of the same ABO group.

Screening of serum for irregular antibodies should be against one or two selected RBC samples by a rapid and simple technique shown to detect those antibodies active at 37°C. Apart from its usefulness in providing potential sources of blood grouping reagents, this screening is especially recommended in testing whole blood and plasma used in neonatal transfusions, where the injection of such antibodies may cause destruction of the patient's own RBC. Donors should be informed about the presence of irregular antibodies and be given appropriate recommendations in case they might need blood transfusions themselves; their plasma should be used for nontransfusion purposes.

Every measure should be taken to ensure correct labeling of blood units and blood components. Details and definition of these measures vary according to the blood facility and represent one of the principal responsibilities of the medical director.

E. DONOR-RECIPIENT MAJOR MATCH

The procedure, which, as mentioned previously, is still inappropriately referred to in the professional jargon as a "major crossmatch", consists of testing the recipient serum against donor red cells using the same serological techniques as for antibody screening. The test aims at detecting incompatibility between the patient and red cell units which have already been selected for transfusion on the basis of patient blood typing and antibody screening. Two main reasons have classically supported the major match as part of the PCA: first, detection of an ABO incompatibility inadvertently escaped from the previously described control barriers, and second, detection of clinically significant antibodies against red cell antigens absent from the antibody screening cells while present on the donor cells.

During the late 1970s and 1980s in the U.S., mainly for time and labor savings in the laboratory and for cost-containment reasons, it was advocated that, for patients with a negative antibody screen, the antiglobulin phase of the major match could be dropped with reasonable safety and replaced by an abbreviated immediate spin match for ABO incompatibility[32–35] (see also References 1, 2, 4, and 5 for review).

This concept, which was first introduced in the U.S. as early as 1964,[36] gained progressively broader audience and was possibly further fostered by the fact that in several western European blood centers, this strategy had been successfully implemented for years.[37] Although, as a consequence of this trend, the antiglobulin phase of the match was made optional in negatively screened patients in 1984 by the FDA and the American Association of Blood Banks,[38] surveys by the College of American Pathologists showed that, in 1987, less than 15% of the U.S. laboratories had actually dropped the test.[39]

The reluctance to abbreviate the major match is substantiated by reports showing the possibility of an incompatible donor-recipient match despite a negative antibody screen.[14,40]

Garratty,[5] reviewing data from four large American hospitals, found that 65 antibodies of potential clinical significance were detected by the major match and not by the screening method in 1.1 million compatibility tests, yielding an incidence of one potential antibody per 17,000 compatibility tests, if the antiglobulin phase of the match was not performed.

Another study, quoted by Shulman,[41] revealed 11 antibodies to low-frequency antigens (Di^a, Wr^a, Kp^a, f, Lu^a), and unidentified, during a 2-year period where 10,600 screening and 4,500 major match tests had been performed.

In order to estimate the clinical magnitude of these *in vitro* incompatibilities, Shulman reviewed the incidence of hemolytic transfusion reactions from 20 American hospitals performing approximately 1,300,000 abbreviated major matches. Five patients who had negative antibody screening and abbreviated match tests had experienced overt hemolytic transfusion reactions due to antibodies (anti-Jk^a, anti-Wr^a, anti-C, anti-c, and anti-Kp^a) that had been missed by the antibody screen.[41]

On the other hand, the practical value of the wisdom-dictated half-measure represented by the immediate-spin room-temperature match has been questioned on practical grounds since: (1) compatible immediate-spin matches were documented between A_2 or A_2B donor units and O or B recipients[42–46] although one should be cautious not to overestimate the magnitude of the problem;[47,48] (2) false-positive reactions are much more common than true positive ones mainly due to rouleaux and cold-reacting antibodies;[49] and (3) the calculated cost savings compared to the nonabbreviated match was negligible.[50]

The above considerations have led several authors to advocate complete demise of the major match and its replacement by an appropriate compatibility testing algorithm including duplicate ABO testing of donor and recipient blood and a manual clerical check to ensure ABO compatibility.[51–54] The actual implementation of such a strategy has reportedly caused no ABO incompatible transfusion over a 20-month period where 6,043 patients received 14,618 units of red cell products without a major match.[41,52]

In practical terms, the numerous scientific and environmental uncertainties and variables referred to earlier (Section III), on the one hand, and the preceding discussion on the other hand, show how difficult it is to recommend a universally applicable compatibility testing strategy. As indicated in Figure 2, two algorithms are currently implemented in developed blood centers in the world: the short one referred to as "type and screen" includes recipient blood grouping and antibody screening followed, if all tests are negative, by the release of blood without further laboratory testing. The long one, referred to as "type, screen, and match", includes recipient blood typing and antibody screening followed by a full or abbreviated major match before release of blood. Table 4 is a comparative summary of key issues related to each strategy. It is up to the blood center medical director to choose the most appropriate policy, taking into account local conditions.

1. Type and Screen

An example of this policy is outlined by the algorithm currently used in the author's center:

1. Upon admission to the hospital, patients susceptible to or immediately requiring blood transfusion, are "typed and screened". Blood typing is performed using microplate techniques and two different batches of anti-A, anti-B, anti-AB, and anti-D, as well as A_1, A_2, and B reagent red cells, by two independent technicians. Except in emergency, blood transfusion is authorized only after a second typing on a new blood sample and the results are filed in a computer. Upon request, blood units are released after a manual or computer check of the donor-recipient compatibility.

TABLE 4
Comparison of Type and Screen vs. Type, Screen, and Match

Type and screen (TS)	Type, screen, and match (TSM)
1. Communication simplified. The clinician needs only request TS before transfusion. The inconvenience is the definition of suitable timing for TS in relation to multiple transfusions.	1. Patient serum tested against every blood unit transfused. Reasonably safe procedure to detect incompatibility due to irregular antibodies.
2. Avoids sequestration of blood units for identified patients. Decrease in cost and workload. Outdating better controlled.	2. With units set up for individual patients, major risk of ABO incompatibility avoided, provided bedside identification is reliable. Heavier cost and workload. May lead to outdating of matched units not used by patient.
3. Permits detection of weak antibodies that require double-dose antigens.	3. Rarely, weak antibodies requiring double-dose antigens may be missed.
4. Requires suitable reagent red cells.	4. Identification of an antibody is required.
5. Misses antibodies against low-frequency or ''private'' antigens.	5. Antibodies to low-frequency or ''private'' donor antigens are detected.
6. Identification of an antibody quickly carried out at convenient time.	
7. Decreases blood bank control at clinical end. May dangerously restrict blood bank involvement to simple execution of serological tests and delivery of blood on demand.	6. Contributes to maintaining medical role of blood bank and facilitates its active participation in hemotherapy of patients.

2. Antibody screening is carried out using the following techniques:

   - A polybrene two-channel autoanalyzer system with two different reagent red cells
   - A manual microplate papain technique with two different reagent red cells
   - A gel-centrifugation technique including a polyspecific antiglobulin and two different reagent red cells
   - A low-ionic-strength saline (LISS)-antiglobulin or solid-phase antiglobulin technique including an anti-IgG antiglobulin with three different reagent red cells

   The antibody screening is thus performed using three technical approaches (autoanalyzer polybrene, papain, and Coombs) and at least six different reagent red cells selected to express, in a homozygous state, the antigens D, c, Jk^a, Jk^b, Fy^a, and Fy^b; in a homo- or heterozygous state, the antigens C, E, e, K, M, N, S, s, P_1, Le^a, Le^b, and, if possible, some low-frequency antigens such as C^w and Kp^a.

3. If the screen is negative, ABO, D-compatible blood is released. If not, antibody identification is initiated using the technique(s) in which the antibody reacts and a 10 (or more)-sample panel of reagent red cells.
4. If the positive screen is found to be related to autoagglutinins or cold-reacting natural antibodies such as anti-H (in group A_1 or A_1B patients), anti-P_1, anti-Lewis, anti-Lu^a, anti-M, or anti-N, no major match is performed and phenotypically compatible blood units, respectively A_1, A_2B, P_2, Lewis(−), Lu(a−), M−, N−, are released after the final manual or computer check of the patient-unit compatibility.
5. If the positive screen is found to be related to a warm-reacting alloantibody such as anti-D, -C, -E, -c, -K, -k, -Fy, -Jk, -S, -s, or -Lu^b, phenotyped blood is selected and matched with the patient's serum in the technique(s) in which the antibody was found to be reactive. The rationale behind the major match in this setting is that (1) a patient immunized to such antigens could be at higher risk of developing other alloantibodies which might be missed by the antibody screen, and (2) the major match would represent a double check of the red cell phenotype of the selected blood unit for the index antigen.
6. If the specificity of a warm-reacting alloantibody cannot be established, a major match is performed with ABO, D-compatible units before the release of blood.
7. Immediately before transfusion, the ABO groups of the patient and of the blood unit are checked at the bedside by the clinician, anesthesiologist, or under their responsibility by a trained nurse, and blood is transfused if no problem has been encountered.

2. Type, Screen, and Match

If the choice is the long compatibility testing algorithm, it is of paramount importance to take all possible measures to prevent outdating, unnecessary matching, and waste of resources while ensuring an efficient supply of blood in emergency cases.

The demand for "standby" matched blood in elective surgery should be restricted to those procedures in which a critical review of the records has shown a real need for transfusion. A realistic maximum blood order schedule should be discussed, implemented, and periodically revised by the blood center director and the surgical team.[55]

A tested mechanism should be provided to issue blood with virtually no waste of time in life-threatening emergency situations. For example, ABO and D-compatible or group O, D-negative units could be released immediately while starting or completing antibody screening and match. In the case of serologically established incompatibility, transfusion should be stopped or prevented by telephone, the unit should be replaced by serocompatible blood, and physicians of both patient and blood center should be immediately notified.

F. RELEASE OF BLOOD

The release of blood is a major step in the PCA policy and should be controlled by well-trained staff.

Pertinent information should be registered in the blood center records: identification and blood group of the patient, identification number and blood groups of the donors, date and hour of the release, and name of the person issuing the blood.

A tag or label should be securely attached to the blood unit indicating, at least, the recipient's last and first names, as well as the blood unit's donor identification number. Furthermore, the blood unit should be checked for its expiration date and for abnormal appearance: color, leaking, clotting, etc.

In some countries a patient blood card bearing ABO and D groups and, if applicable, special typing and antibody information, may be forwarded together with the blood order. Such cards can be very useful when it is necessary to identify blood donors of a certain type, or as a warning in patients with a rare blood type or an important blood group antibody, thus saving time and effort in serologic testing. However, because of the possibility of transcription errors and of the recording of inaccurate serologic data, blood group cards should be issued only by laboratories of advanced capability. Otherwise, they may be misleading or even dangerous. Blood group cards should never be accepted in lieu of appropriate pretransfusion testing of either recipients or donors.

G. TRANSFUSION OF BLOOD

Before blood that has been grouped and matched for a patient is actually transfused, one or, preferably, two trained persons should check the information on the blood container against that on the patient or his chart to verify that the blood is indeed prepared and intended for that person and is compatible. A further useful step is to have the person who verified the blood sign a statement on a transfusion form.

In some countries, a bedside confirmation of the recipient and donor blood types is carried out. However, the procedure may provide false security if performed by relatively untrained individuals using reagents of uncertain potency. Bedside blood grouping in no way substitutes for careful verification of patient and donor identification and match.

Observation of the patient during and after blood transfusion is another task to be accomplished by nurses. Any abnormal sign and evidence of poor tolerance of blood is cause to stop the transfusion promptly and inform the patient's physician and the blood bank.

Evaluation of the efficacy of transfused red cells must be an integral part of the transfusion procedure and be documented by means of the patient's hemoglobin rise and its duration, taking into account the amount of RBC transfused, the patient's blood and plasma volume, the degree of marrow regeneration, and the bleeding status. Active observation and follow-up of patients is necessary to identify and study mechanisms of ineffective transfusions and to prevent them whenever possible.

H. WARD-LABORATORY COORDINATION

The operating procedures and communication between hospital wards and the transfusion service are critical for the immunologic safety of blood transfusions and must be formulated and reviewed by the hospital transfusion committee. This committee, including the blood bank director and appropriate representatives of hospital administration, physicians, anesthesiologists, and nurses, is a formal focus of review and evaluation, criticism, decision, and control of the various aspects of blood transfusion activity in the hospital. Policies to be described in the following section must be explained and adopted by this representative committee, which should eventually issue instructions to all hospital medical, technical, and administrative staff involved in transfusion activities. Obviously, the efficacy of such a committee is proportional to the interest and energy devoted to it by its members, and the support its decisions receive from clinical and administrative authorities in the hospital.

I. PRETRANSFUSION COMPATIBILITY ASSURANCE IN SPECIAL SITUATIONS

1. Emergency Transfusions

Maintenance of blood volume in bleeding patients pending pretransfusion tests is the most vital emergency measure to be taken, using crystalloid solutions, colloids, plasma, or albumin. It must be stressed that, in capable laboratories, blood grouping and compatibility testing may be accomplished in 20 to 45 minutes, depending on the techniques used, if no serological problem arises.

In each case, the clinician must evaluate the anticipated benefits against the hazards of transfusing a patient with group O Rh-negative or -positive or type-specific blood before the completion of antibody screening and compatibility testing. To justify such transfusions, they must be considered life saving.

In patients known to have an irregular antibody, phenotyped units negative for the corresponding antigen may be delivered in emergency situations while compatibility testing is being completed, or serologically compatible blood may be given before the appropriate phenotyping has been performed.

2. ABO Nonspecific Transfusions

Although the basic rule of ABO compatibility is that one must not give blood having antigens against which the recipient has antibody, it is possible to give transfusions of O blood to A or B recipients and A or B blood to AB recipients. However, such transfusions should consist of red cell concentrates rather than whole blood, to avoid infusing large amounts of plasma containing antibodies against the recipient's A or B antigens.

In patients massively transfused with type-nonspecific whole blood or plasma, the change back to type-specific blood is based on the presence or absence of anti-A or anti-B in the recipient's plasma. The simple rule is therefore to require *in vitro* compatibility between the patient's serum and donor's red cells at the time of transfusion.

3. Transfusion of D-Positive Blood to D-Negative Recipients

This may be considered in emergencies for male patients and older women when D-negative units are unavailable. Every effort should be made to avoid such transfusions in young girls and women of childbearing age. In any case, not only should one make sure that the patient is not already immunized against the D antigen, but also the possible appearance of anti-D should be checked for in the patient's serum over the next few months.

4. High-Frequency Antibodies and Autoantibodies

The presence in the patient's serum of an antibody reacting equally with all RBC samples in the panel, or in the blood units to be transfused, may indicate one of two possible situations, depending on the reactivity of the patient's own red cells and serum in the ''auto-control''.

If the auto-control is negative, the antibody is probably recognizing a high-frequency or ''public'' antigen. Identification of such antibodies may sometimes be easy, e.g., anti-H, but often it requires availability of rare antigen-negative red cell samples to identify the specificity. Reference laboratories have to be consulted and transfusion postponed pending preparation of compatible blood units from regional, national, or international banks of frozen rare blood.

The patient's family should also be tested in the search for like phenotypes. Whenever possible, such individuals must be encouraged to donate blood regularly, which will be preserved, frozen, and be available for the family's needs as well as for unrelated, rare, people having the same phenotype.

If the auto-control is positive, an autoantibody is presumably present, and serologically compatible blood may be impossible to identify. Direct antiglobulin and elution tests may help to characterize the autoantibody and the practical approach to blood transfusion should be considered as follows:

- Red cell transfusions should be considered only in patients with clinically threatening signs of anemic hypoxia, and not in those with well-tolerated anemia.
- Autoantibodies are generally directed against high-frequency or public antigens, so *in vivo* incompatibility can hardly be avoided. But this does not cause shock and acute renal failure, although it leads to destruction of transfused RBC at a rate that is difficult to predict.
- Patients with a past history of transfusions and of overt transfusion reactions must be submitted to careful screening for alloantibodies which are usually masked by autoantibodies and are potentially more harmful.

If initial serological findings suggest an IgM autoantibody (complement-type direct antiglobulin test, saline-active antibody, activity at 22°C, etc.), inactivation of the serum by dithiothreitol may eliminate the IgM and allow IgG alloantibodies to be identified.

If initial results suggest an IgG autoantibody (IgG-type direct antiglobulin test, antibody optimally reacting at 37°C or at the second phase of the indirect antiglobulin test using an anti-IgG antiglobulin, etc.), one may resort to comparative titration of serum against RBC with selected phenotypes or to repeated absorptions of serum on autologous red cells or on red cell samples from known donors lacking antigens such as K, c, E, Fy^a, or JK^a, which are commonly involved in posttransfusion alloimmunization.

5. Transfusion in the Neonatal Period

Labeling of blood specimens from the newborn requires extreme care in order to avoid errors of identification, which occur more easily in maternity hospitals where the baby has still no formally established civil identity.

Laboratory testing for anemic or icteric babies should systematically include ABO and Rh grouping and a direct antiglobulin test on the baby's blood. In addition, an antibody screen should be done on the mother's serum if not performed shortly before delivery. Some anemic conditions may thus be easily diagnosed, and transfusion errors avoided.

Red cells to be transfused in the neonatal period must be compatible with the mother's serum with respect to ABO and other blood group antigens. Blood group antibodies in the newborn are mostly IgG and come from the mother. Transfusion of A blood to an A child born to an O mother may cause hemolytic anemia and hyperbilirubinemia, because the A antigen site density of transfused adult red cells is higher than the newborn's own antigenically immature cells. Also, group O Rh-negative blood should by no means be considered a panacea. Abuse of this type of blood, without appropriate pre-transfusion testing, not only deprives other patients, but it may also be detrimental to mother and baby if the former has irregular antibodies to red cell antigens other than D.

Compatibility between transfused plasma and a newborn's red cells is another prerequisite, either within the ABO group, with special emphasis on immune anti-A or anti-B in donor plasma, or with respect to other blood group systems.

6. Prevention of Alloimmunization

According to a survey conducted in Paris,[56] new cases of D immunization showed a 36% decrease from 1970 through 1979, due to the prophylactic use of anti-D immunoglobulin, whereas the number of pregnant women carrying other antibodies, mainly anti-c, -E, and -K showed an increase from 17 to 92 cases over the same period. Of these women, 80% had a history of transfusions in contrast to about 10% of pregnant women in general. Because hemolytic disease of the newborn may result from anti-c and anti-K, in particular, it has been argued that girls or women should not be transfused with E, c, and K antigens if they lack them on their own red cells. However, this practice could lead to complex inventory problems as well as more costly pretransfusion testing, and the concept has not yet received unanimous acceptance.

Injection of anti-D immune globulin within the 72 hours following inadvertent or intentional transfusion of Rh-positive blood or cellular blood components to Rh-negative recipients, especially young women, may also be recommended. A dose of 10 to 20 μg of anti-D immune globulin per milliliter of transfused red cells forms a reasonable basis for calculation of the amount required, which may of course be enormous. The use of Rh immune globulin in these circumstances should be guided by common sense and clinical judgment, particularly if large amounts of Rh-positive blood were transfused. Age, sex, clinical status, availability of intravenous vs. intramuscular anti-D immunoglobulin, the possibility of partially extracting transfused Rh-positive red cells by exchange transfusion using Rh-negative blood prior to administration of anti-D immunoglobulin and the time elapsed since transfusion are the main factors to be considered in the management of such cases.

Whenever possible, autologous transfusions in elective surgery should be encouraged, considering, but not unduly exaggerating, the risks of alloimmunization and of disease transmission from homologous transfusions.

Preventive measures against immunization are of secondary concern compared to the basic organizational measures described in the preceding sections for the prevention of incompatible transfusions in patients with preexisting immune, naturally occurring, regular, or irregular antibodies.

V. CONCLUSIONS

Risk-benefit and cost-benefit issues have, over the past two decades, opened the scope of interest in compatibility testing, which was once restricted to bench workers, to other blood banking components such as management and hospital transfusion committees. Despite considerable progress, much work has to be done to improve our understanding of the numerous variables participating in immune red cell destruction and to enhance the predictive values of our *in vitro* compatibility tests. Evaluation and documentation of the efficacy of red cell transfusions should not be regarded as an investigational added burden, but as an integral part of standard operating procedures. Personal involvement of clinicians in this evaluation is a key element to achieve better policies of pretransfusion compatibility assurance.

REFERENCES

1. **Oberman, H. A.,** The crossmatch: past, present and future, in *A Seminar on Immune Mediated Cell Destruction,* American Association of Blood Banks, Arlington, VA, 1981, 29.
2. **Oberman, H. A.,** The crossmatch. A brief historical perspective, *Transfusion,* 21, 654, 1981.
3. **Giblett, E. R.,** Blood group alloantibodies: an assessment of some laboratory practices, *Transfusion,* 17, 199, 1977.
4. **Garratty, G.,** The role of compatibility tests. Report of a meeting sponsored by the Bureau of Biologics for the Blood Products Advisory Committee, *Transfusion,* 22, 169, 1982.
5. **Garratty, G.,** Abbreviated pretransfusion testing, *Transfusion,* 26, 217, 1986.
6. **Masouredis, S. P.,** Pretransfusion tests and compatibility: questions of safety and efficacy, *Blood,* 59, 873, 1982.
7. **Low, B. and Messeter, L.,** Antiglobulin test in low ionic strength salt solution for rapid antibody screening and crossmatching, *Vox Sang.,* 26, 53, 1974.
8. **Rosenfield, R. E., Shaikh, S. H., Innella, F., Kaczera, Z., and Kochwa, S.,** Augmentation of hemagglutination by low ionic conditions, *Transfusion,* 19, 499, 1979.
9. **Ahn, J. H., Rosenfield, R. E., and Kochwa, S.,** Low ionic antiglobulin tests, *Transfusion,* 27, 125, 1987.
10. **Plapp, F. V., Sinor, L. T., and Rachel, J. M.,** A solid phase antibody screen, *Am. J. Clin. Pathol.,* 82, 719, 1984.
11. **Gerber, H., Lapierre, Y., and Hitzler, W.,** Gel centrifugation test: a comparative study of a new method in red blood cell serology, in *Transfusion in Europe,* Castelli, D., Genetet, B., Habibi, B., and Nydegger, U., Eds., Arnette, Paris, 1990, 343.
12. **Sazama, K.,** Report of 355 transfusion-associated deaths: 1976 through 1985, *Transfusion,* 30, 583, 1990.
13. **Habibi, B.,** Immunologic Safety in Blood Transfusion, Guide No. 8, International Society of Blood Transfusion, ISBT Publications, Paris, 1984.
14. **Mintz, P. D., Haines, A. L., and Sullivan, M. F.,** Incompatible cross match following non reactive antibody detection test, *Transfusion,* 22, 107, 1982.
15. **Mollison, P. L., Engelfriet, C. P., and Contreras, M.,** *Blood Transfusion in Clinical Medicine,* 9th ed., Blackwell Scientific, Oxford, 1989.
16. **Davey, R. J., Gustafson, M., and Holland, P. V.,** Accelerated immune red cell destruction in the absence of serologically detectable alloantibodies, *Transfusion,* 20, 348, 1979.
17. **Rosenfield, R. E.,** Compatibility tests: an appraisal, *Med. Clin. North Am.,* 50, 1643, 1966.
18. American Association of Blood Banks, Technical Manual, 10th ed., Arlington, VA, 1989, 269.
19. **Schmidt, P. J., Morrison, E. G., and Stohl, J.,** The antigenicity of the RhO (D^u) blood factor, *Blood,* 20, 196, 1962.
20. **Ramsey, G. and Larson, P.,** Loss of red cell alloantibodies over time, *Transfusion,* 28, 162, 1988.
21. **Lalezari, P. and Jiang, A. F.,** The manual polybrene test: a simple and rapid procedure for detection of red cell antibodies, *Transfusion,* 20, 206, 1980.
22. **Lown, J. A. G., Johnson, W., and Ivey, J. G.,** Eighteen months' experience with a manual polybrene crossmatch in a large hospital transfusion laboratory, *Vox Sang.,* 55, 229, 1988.
23. **Fisher, G. A.,** Use of the manual polybrene test in the routine hospital laboratory, *Transfusion,* 23, 151, 1983.

24. **Ferrer, Z., Wright, J., Moore, B. P. L., and Freedman, J.,** Comparison of a modified manual hexademethrine bromide (polybrene) and a low ionic-strength solution antibody detection technique, *Transfusion,* 25, 145, 1985.
25. Code of Federal Regulations Title 21, parts 600 to 799, Revised as of April 1, 1988, Subparts 606 and 660, U.S. Government Printing Office, Washington, D.C.
26. **Habibi, B.,** unpublished observations.
27. **Shulman, I. A., Nelson, J. M., Okamoto, M., and Malone, S. A.,** The dependence of anti-Jk[a] detection on screening cell zygosity, *Lab. Med.,* 16, 602, 1985.
28. **Shulman, I. A., Yaowasiriwatt, M., Saxena, S., and Nelson, J. M.,** Influence of reagent red cell zygosity on anti-Fy[a] detection, *Lab. Med.,* 20, 37, 1989.
29. **Garratty, G. and Petz, L. D.,** The significance of red cell bound complement components in development of standards and quality assurance for the anti-complement components of antiglobulin sera, *Transfusion,* 16, 297, 1976.
30. **Howard, J. E., Winn, L. C., Gottlieb, C. E., Grumet, F. C., Garratty, G., and Petz, L. D.,** Clinical significance of the anti-complement component of antiglobulin antisera, *Transfusion,* 22, 269, 1982.
31. **Judd, W. J., Barnes, B. A., Steiner, E. A., Oberman, H. A., Averill, D. B., and Butch, S. H.,** The evaluation of a positive direct antiglobulin test (autocontrol) in pretransfusion testing revisited, *Transfusion,* 26, 220, 1986.
32. **Boral, L. I. and Henry, J. B.,** The type of screen: a safe alternative and supplement in selected surgical procedures, *Transfusion,* 17, 163, 1977.
33. **Oberman, H. A., Barner, B. A., and Friedman, B. A.,** The risk of abbreviating the major crossmatch in urgent or massive transfusion, *Transfusion,* 18, 137, 1978.
34. **Lee, K. and Lachance, V.,** Type and screen for elective surgery. Results of one year's experience in a small community hospital, *Transfusion,* 20, 324, 1980.
35. **Huang, S. T., Lir, J., Floyd, D. M., and Cole, G. W.,** Type and hold system for better blood utilisation, *Transfusion,* 20, 725, 1980.
36. **Grove-Rasmussen, M.,** Routine compatibility testing. Standards of the AABB as applied to compatibility tests, *Transfusion,* 4, 200, 1964.
37. **Heisto, H.,** Pretransfusion blood group serology. Limited value of the antiglobulin phase of the crossmatch when a careful screening test for unexpected antibodies is performed, *Transfusion,* 19, 761, 1979.
38. American Association of Blood Banks, Standards for Blood Banks and Transfusion Services, 11th ed., Arlington, VA, 1984.
39. **Harrison, C. R. and Set, J. D.,** Comprehensive Blood Bank 1987 Survey, College of American Pathologists, Skokie, IL, 1987.
40. **Oberman, H. A., Barnes, B. A., and Steiner, E. A.,** Role of the crossmatch in testing for serologic incompatibility, *Transfusion,* 22, 12, 1982.
41. **Shulman, I. A.,** Controversies in red blood cell compatibility testing, in *Immune Destruction of Red Blood Cells,* Nance, S. J., Eds., American Association of Blood Banks, Arlington, VA, 1989, 171.
42. **Berry-Dortch, S., Woodside, C. H., and Boral, L. I.,** Limitations of the immediate spin crossmatch when used for detecting ABO incompatibility, *Transfusion,* 25, 176, 1985.
43. **Shulman, I. A.,** ABO incompatibility missed by saline immediate spin compatibility testing, *Transfusion,* 21, 469, 1981.
44. **Shulman, I. A., Nelson, J. M., Tai Lam, H., and Meyer, E.,** Unreliability of the immediate-spin crossmatch to detect ABO incompatibility, *Transfusion,* 25, 589, 1985.
45. **Sererat, S., Beatty, J., Schifano, J. V., and Lau, P.,** Why not antiglobulin compatibility testing?, *Transfusion,* 25, 589, 1985.
46. **Judd, W. J., Steiner, E. A., O'Donnell, D. B., and Oberman, H. A.,** Discrepancies in reverse ABO typing due to prozone. How safe is the immediate-spin crossmatch?, *Transfusion,* 28, 334, 1988.

47. **Park, H.,** Limitation of the immediate-spin crossmatch, *Transfusion,* 25, 588, 1985.
48. **Pohl, B. A.,** Immediate-spin crossmatch: how serious are the problems?, *Transfusion,* 25, 588, 1985.
49. **Meyer, E. A. and Shulman, I. A.,** The sensitivity and specificity of the immediate-spin crossmatch, *Transfusion,* 29, 99, 1989.
50. **Shulman, I. A., Nelson, J. M., Kent, D. R., Jacobs, V. L., Nakayama, R. K., and Malone, S. A.,** Experience with a cost effective crossmatch protocol, *JAMA,* 254, 93, 1985.
51. **Suoboda, R.,** Passing the crossmatch by screening antibodies, *Lab. World,* 32, 26, 1981.
52. **Soloway, H. B., McClanslin, M., and Belliveau, R. R.,** Is the routine crossmatch obsolete?, *Med. Lab. Observ.,* 20, 27, 1988.
53. **Shulman, I. A. and Kent, D.,** Safety in transfusion practice. Is it safe to eliminate the major crossmatch for selected patients?, *Arch. Pathol. Lab. Med.,* 43, 270, 1989.
54. **Baumgarten, R. K.,** Elimination of the crossmatch, *Transfusion,* 27, 445, 1987.
55. **Friedman, B. A., Oberman, H. A., Chadwick, A. R., and Kingdon, K. L.,** The maximum surgical blood order schedule and surgical blood use in the United States, *Transfusion,* 16, 380, 1976.
56. **Pinon, F., Cregut, R., and Brossard, Y.,** Immunisation érythrocytaire chez la femme enceinte, *Rev. Franc. Transfus. Immunohematol.,* 24, 483, 1981.

Chapter 14

EXTERNAL QUALITY ASSESSMENT OF BLOOD GROUPING ANTIBODY SCREENING, AND CROSSMATCH PROCEDURES WITHIN THE UNITED KINGDOM*

Peter K. Phillips

TABLE OF CONTENTS

* The views expressed are not necessarily those of the members of the Steering Committee or the Scheme Organiser of the U.K. National External Quality Assessment Scheme for blood group serology.

ISBN 0-8493-4938-9

I. INTRODUCTION

In the U.K. clinical laboratories exist within the public (state) and private sectors. There is no licensing of reagents or techniques, and no accreditation of laboratories, although the U.K. Association of Independent Hospital Pathology Laboratories, the Association of Clinical Pathologists, the Royal College of Pathologists, and the Institute of Medical Laboratory Sciences support the principle of accreditation based on good laboratory practices and active participation in external schemes that assess the performance of the laboratory.

The United Kingdom National External Quality Assessment Scheme (U.K. NEQAS) for blood group serology is but one of the several schemes which cover the range of pathology specialities. Currently, the others are autoimmune serology, blood coagulation, clinical chemistry, clinical cytogenetics, cytopathology, drug assay, hematology, histopathology, hormones, immunochemistry, medical microbiology, trace elements, and tissue (HLA) typing. Details of these schemes may be obtained from Department of Health, Room 416B, Eileen House, 80 Newington Causeway, London, SE1 6EF.

All laboratories should have a rigorous, documented mechanism of assuring the quality of their work, that is from the collection of the specimen through to the receipt of the results by the originator of the request. The performance of routine and on-call staff should be assessed regularly by the replicate testing of materials the identity of which is unknown to the tester and, preferably, is included within a batch of routine specimens. U.K. NEQAS cannot replace this local quality assurance. Its aim is to obtain a "snapshot" of the performance of U.K. clinical laboratories by distributing a common test material and comparing the results of each laboratory against the consensus result. This gives the laboratories an opportunity to compare their performance against that of their peers and assists in the evaluation of different procedures, equipment, material, and personnel between participating laboratories.

Participation in the U.K. NEQAS is on a voluntary basis. U.K. public and private sector laboratories are encouraged to participate in all relevant schemes by professional bodies, the Department of Health, and the Association of Independent Pathology Laboratories. The clinical laboratories of the U.K. armed forces also participate, whether based within the U.K. or overseas. In addition, membership of the schemes is open to commercial manufacturers of appropriate instruments, reagents, or therapeutic products supplied within the U.K. There are a small number of non-U.K. participants in most schemes, either on a reciprocal basis between the organizing laboratories of national schemes or where the number of laboratories within a country is too small to support a viable scheme of their own.

Participating laboratories are identified by a laboratory code known only to the participant and the scheme Organizer. The blood group serology scheme is unusual in having regional advisers, usually within the regional transfusion centers. In certain of the U.K. regions, by unanimous agreement, participants have made their identity available to their regional adviser. Within the blood group serology scheme, the laboratory code comprises a five-digit number comprising a two-digit regional code, a two-digit laboratory number unique to that region, and a one-digit check number (modulus 11), which is mathematically derived from the other four and is used to detect an incorrect laboratory code either through error by the participant or by the data-entry operator.

In order to provide the safeguards necessary for the operation of external assessment schemes, within the U.K. there is a system of interacting committees to segregate the key functions: the operation of the schemes, the acceptance of criteria for satisfactory performance, and the monitoring of the activity of the schemes.[7]

A. OPERATION OF THE SCHEMES

Each scheme has a scheme Organizer who is appointed by the U.K. Department of Health. The Organizer is a senior member of the appropriate profession with acknowledged skills in the particular speciality of the scheme. The scheme Organizer is responsible for the direction of the scheme and the nature of its exercises. Many schemes have a scheme Manager who, as agent of the Organizer, undertakes the day-to-day functions of the scheme and may provide central laboratory facilities that are available to a succession of scheme organizers.

The scheme Organizer is supported and is advised on the overall operation of the scheme by a steering committee of technical and clinical advisers together with a representative of the U.K. Department of Health. The steering committee is chaired by an independent expert and considers, for example, the frequency of distribution of exercise material, the methods of analysis to be performed, and the presentation of data to participants. The steering committee is not concerned with the performance of individual participants, except where this might indicate a failure in operation of the scheme.

The scheme Organizers and Chairmen of the steering committees report to the Advisory Committee on Assessment of Laboratory Standards (ACALS) of the U.K. Department of Health. ACALS is an interdisciplinary body with the members sitting in their own right, not as the representative of any professional body or organization. Its role is to ensure that the various schemes set similar standards and to promote the exchange of ideas among the schemes.

B. CRITERIA FOR SATISFACTORY PERFORMANCE

Each scheme is monitored by one of three U.K. National Quality Assurance Advisory Panels: Chemical Pathology, Hematology, or Medical Microbiology. These panels are responsible for maintaining satisfactory standards of analytic work undertaken in U.K. private or public sector laboratories for the detection, diagnosis, or management of disease in humans. Members of the Panels are nominated by a professional body or are co-opted. It is these Panels that determine, in conjunction with the scheme Organizers, the criteria for acceptable performance in the U.K. schemes. Participants with a performance deemed to be unsatisfactory by the defined criteria are referred by the scheme Organizer to the Panel without disclosure of the participant's identity. If the Panel decides to intervene, a letter is forwarded to the participant by the scheme Organizer offering assistance and advice, and seeking details on the measures that have been taken by the participant to improve their performance. The participant may reply to the Panel disclosing their identity or reply anonymously via the scheme Organizer. If the participant's performance remains unsatisfactory, the identity of the participant is disclosed to the Panel for further direct communications.

C. MONITORING THE ACTIVITY OF THE SCHEMES

The Advisory Panels are accountable to the Joint Working Group on Quality Assurance, which consists of representatives from various professional bodies. This Group has no access to information on individual participants or to communications between an Advisory Panel and an individual participant. The role of the group is primarily to consider the develoment of quality assurance practices within the U.K., that is to monitor the activity of the Advisory Panels and their relationship with the professions, scheme Organizers and other Panels, and to consider any new quality assurance activities within existing or additional areas of laboratory practice.

II. EXERCISE FORMAT

Participants may register to participate in the ABO and Rh(D) grouping, antibody screen, or crossmatch components of the exercise. In addition, those participants registering for antibody screen may register to participate in the antibody identification component of the exercise.

Until the end of 1989, U.K. NEQAS (blood group serology) exercises were either to assess ABO and Rh(D) grouping with antibody screen or crossmatch procedures. In order to assess the complete group, screen, and crossmatch procedure, U.K. NEQAS (blood group serology) exercises now comprise up to a maximum of five "patient" paired red cell-serum samples and up to a maximum of three "donor" red cell samples. The "donor" samples are not labeled with their ABO or Rh(D) group and participants are not required to group these "donor" samples. For the purpose of the NEQAS exercise, participants are to assume that the "donor" samples are nominally ABO, Rh(D), and antigen compatible with each "patient" sample, even though the "patients" may be of different ABO or Rh(D) status from each other and atypical (allo) antibody may be present. This arrangement permits exercises to be distributed that assess the ability to detect ABO or Rh(D) incompatibilities.

At dispatch, the red cell samples are some 10 to 14 days post-donation. Results are to be returned to the organizing laboratory within two weeks from dispatch. Participants are asked to use only the techniques that they undertake routinely for non-urgent investigations, although future exercises may assess urgent investigations. A direct antiglobulin test on the "patient" red cell sample is to be undertaken if this is routine practice or is indicated by the reaction of the "patient" red cell sample with the serological controls for the grouping reagents. Participants are to interpret their serological results, that is, state the ABO, Rh(D), and atypical antibody status of the "patient" samples and, for each combination of "patient" serum and "donor" red cell samples, to state whether compatible or incompatible.

Previously, participants were not required to interpret the results of the crossmatch or of the antibody screen. Any positive result recorded for a particular crossmatch was interpreted by the organizing laboratory as indicating an incompatibility. Similarly, any positive result for a particular antibody screen investigation was interpreted as the detection of atypical antibody. It was noted that participants tended to record weak positive results, particularly with enzyme techniques, perhaps to avoid the error penalty of failing to detect a true incompatibility or the true presence of atypical antibody, particularly since the failure to observe a true compatibility was not defined as an error. In practice, false-positive reactions that delay the provision of blood are not acceptable. For this reason, participants now are asked to interpret their results and a missed compatibility has been defined as a minor error.

The record form distributed with the exercise permits the recording of results for the following techniques.

- ABO Grouping
  ''Patient'' red cells with
    anti-A
    anti-B
    anti-A,B
    anti-A_1
  ''Patient'' serum with
    A_1 red cells
    A red cells
    A_2 red cells
    B red cells
    O red cells

- Auto control
  The ''patient'' red cell sample tested with the corresponding ''patient'' serum sample.

- D Grouping
  Potentiated anti-D (with its reagent control). This is defined as an anti-D reagent comprising IgG antibody and macromolecules, or albumin in excess of some 50 g/l, to enable the direct agglutination of Rh(D)-positive red cells. Since such reagents can cause agglutination of Rh(D)-negative cells coated with IgG, a reagent control prepared to the same formulation but with no anti-D activity is normally available from the manufacturer to ensure the validity of the results.

  Saline anti-D, that is, a reagent comprising IgM anti-D, or chemically modified IgG anti-D, which affects the direct agglutination of Rh(D)-positive red cells.

Albumin anti-D (with its reagent control), that is, an IgG anti-D reagent standardized for use with albumin, typically by displacement of the supernate test medium following the incubation of serum and cell suspension.

Enzyme anti-D (with its reagent control), that is, an IgG anti-D reagent standardized for use with an enzyme preparation.

Antiglobulin anti-D (with its reagent control), that is, an IgG anti-D reagent standardized for use in an antiglobulin technique.

- Direct antiglobulin test
  Using polyspecific anti-human globulin or anti-IgG with separate anti-C_3d.

- Antibody screen
  Using any of the techniques described in the crossmatch section below.

- Antibody identification
  The identity of the atypical antibody detected.

- Crossmatch of a ''patient'' serum with a ''donor'' red cell sample
  Direct agglutination test, in a low or normal ionic strength medium incubated at a temperature of less than 30°C.

  Direct agglutination test, in a low or normal ionic strength medium incubated at a temperature of 30 to 37°C.

  Enzyme test, that is, a test *not* using an antiglobulin reagent, employing an enzyme either to pretreat the red cell sample or included as a reagent with red cells and serum in the same tube.

  Albumin test, that is, a test *not* using an antiglobulin reagent, employing albumin either to displace or replace the supernate test medium after a period of incubation.

  Antiglobulin test, that is, any test using an antiglobulin reagent.

  Any other test, that is, any test not included in the above, for example, a polybrene technique but without the involvement of an antiglobulin reagent.

The results from microplate or automated procedures are entered under the heading corresponding to the particular technique used, that is, an enzyme test performed in a microplate would be entered under the enzyme heading.

III. THE "CORRECT" RESULT

Prior to Exercise 1989E3, the "correct" result for the exercise was determined from ten participants selected from regional transfusion centers, district hospitals, and teaching hospitals, and included the organizing laboratory. A selection criterion for these participants was the use of all the techniques represented on the result form, with the possible exception of the "any other test" category of techniques. For a given investigation and technique, if eight or more of these participants agreed on the nature (positive or negative) of the result then that result was deemed to be correct. If the "correct" result was positive, its grade of reaction was the average of these participants obtaining a positive result. If between two and eight of these participants agreed on the nature of the result for a given investigation and technique, then either a positive or negative result from the participants was acceptable as "correct".

Over a period of time, some of the participants whose results contributed to the "correct" results either ceased to undertake all the techniques or undertook them specifically for the exercise. Either case resulted in an unsatisfactory basis for the determination of the "correct" result; the former diminished the number of laboratories on which the "consensus" result for a given technique and assessment was determined, the latter resulted in participants who routinely employed less frequently used techniques, being assessed against a "correct" result determined from a select, small number of participants who undertook that technique specifically for the exercise. For these reasons, the "correct" result for a given technique and investigation is now determined as the consensus from all U.K. participants who undertake that technique and investigation. For subgroups of A, the "correct" subgroup is determined from those participants undertaking subgrouping. If more than 80% of U.K. participants agree on the nature of the result then that result is deemed correct. If less than ten U.K. laboratories perform a given technique for an investigation, the "correct" result for that technique is not determinable. Analysis of several exercises has shown that the average grade of reaction for a given technique and investigation, determined from all U.K. participants using that technique, did not differ markedly from the result determined using the ten select participants except, as beneficial measure, that the incidence of equivocal "correct" results was diminished.

If 80% or less of the U.K. participants agree on the nature of the result, then the results of those who had made no errors in the previous eight exercises are considered. If more than 80% of these better-performing agree on the result, then it is deemed to be correct.

IV. EXERCISE MATERIAL

Donations of plasma and of red cell units are obtained from the U.K. Regional Transfusion Centres. The donations have been tested and found negative for hepatitis B surface antigen and HIV antibody. The plasma is defibrinated by the addition of thrombin and calcium, heated to destroy residual fibrinogen, filtered through a 0.2-μm filter and aseptically dispensed into vials which then are sealed with rubber closures and aluminum "flip-top" caps. After labeling, the vials are stored frozen until the exercise material is packaged. These "serum" samples contain no preservative. The red cell units are washed and resuspended in a sterile, modified Alsever's solution containing antibiotics and dispensed into vials.

The red cell and serum samples are packaged into rigid polystyrene boxes, which are placed into stout envelopes together with the documentation for the exercise and dispatched within the U.K. by first class mail. Packages for non-U.K. participants are dispatched by registered air mail using the Non-Infectious Perishable Biological Substances service and carry a customs declaration stating that the contents are of negligible commercial value. All packages are indicated to contain pathological specimens and the temperature of storage on arrival. In addition, the packages are indicated as containing NEQAS materials in order to be externally differentiated from clinical specimens at the receiving laboratory. In general, the addressee is the technologist in routine charge of the laboratory. This avoids the delays that can occur if the addressee is the pathologist in charge of the laboratory, particularly since the pathologist may not be located permanently at the site of the participating laboratory.

With the numerous specimen containers and labels in routine use within the U.K., it is inevitable that exercise material will be presented in containers distinct from those in use within the participant's laboratory. For manufacturing convenience, the material is presented in nominal 5-ml, rubber-stoppered, glass vials with a "flip-off" aluminum seal. The "patient" serum sample is defibrinated plasma and therefore hypertonic, hyperionic, and of a lower protein concentration than true serum. Currently, defibrination is performed by the addition of calcium ions and bovine thrombin, removal of the compressed fibrin clot, and filtration. Heating to 50°C for 20 minutes is necessary to destroy residual fibrinogen which otherwise would convert slowly to fibrin on storage. However, this heating induces a degree of polymerization of IgG protein which appears to be responsible for the "stickiness" of the "patient" sera, sometimes the subject of comments by participants who use microplate techniques. More effective methods of defibrination are being investigated that would obviate the necessity for heating. "Patient" sera do not contain serologically active components of complement and are probably anti-complementary to some extent. "Patient" sera do not contain antibodies that are dependent upon complement fixation for their detection. However,

TABLE 1
Grading System Used for U.K. NEQAS Exercises

Grade	Appearance
5	Cell button remains in one macroscopically visible clump
4	Cell button dislodges into several macroscopically visible clumps
3	Cell button dislodges into many small macroscopically visible clumps
2	Cell button dislodges into finely granular, but definite, small, macroscopically visible clumps
1	Cell button dislodges up to fine granules that are microscopically visible only
0	Negative result

the absence of active complement components has been said to be an explanation for the incidence of undetected ABO incompatibilities in some exercises. Similarly, the formulation of the ''patient'' red cell and ''donor'' red cell samples has been criticized, but the formulation is very similar to that of many red cell screening and identification panels distributed widely within the U.K., for use without washing in normal ionic strength test procedures.

The preferred presentation of the ''patient'' sample would appear to be a clotted specimen for those participants using traditional, manual methods of testing and an anti-coagulated specimen for participants with automated systems. Although it would be possible to distribute contrived anti-coagulated whole blood ''patient'' samples, probably there would be insufficient residual material for distribution to those participants using manual methods of delivery. In addition, there are logistical difficulties involved in distributing at one time, two different presentations of the same exercise material. Furthermore, the provision of separate ''patient'' red cells and serum samples does increase the flexibility of the organizing laboratory to distribute a wide range of materials without unintentionally distributing a patient's sample with an autoantibody to some minor red cell antigen system, particularly since the actual red cell units to be used for an exercise are not received by the organizing laboratory until one week before dispatch.

Both the layout of the record form and the scoring system have generated some comment from participants. Before the introduction of the Scheme, the scoring system used within the U.K. varied widely between participants. Although many participants have changed their routine scoring system to that of the Scheme, some participants translate their own scoring system before entry of the results onto the record form and a few participants continue to forward results using their own scoring system for translation by the organizing laboratory. Table 1 indicates the scoring system in use for the Scheme. In principle, it would be possible for participants to register their own record forms and scoring system with the organizing laboratory, who would hold that format on computer. Participants could forward their results using their own forms and at the point of entering the data onto the computer, the participant's form would be displayed for data entry and the results arranged electronically into the required internal format for analysis. This approach may be used in the future but is expected to be demanding in computer data storage and electronic processing requirements.

The documentation enclosed with the exercise material comprises:

- A questionnaire on the particular reagents and techniques to be used in that exercise
- A memorandum containing various information such as cautionary statements, from where replacement material can be obtained in the case of breakages, and the definition of errors for the Scheme
- Instructions for the exercise, including the scoring system to be used
- A two-part carbonless record form
- A self-adhesive label addressed to the organizing laboratory for returning one copy of the completed result form together with the questionnaire
- The detailed report on the previous exercise

In addition, a copy of the detailed report on the previous exercise is sent to the pathologist in charge of the laboratory.

V. CLASSIFICATION OF ERRORS

Errors are defined as:

- For U.K. participants, the failure to return results before the closing data of the exercise without a valid reason. Being too busy to undertake the exercise is not a valid reason for nonparticipation.
- For participants registered to participate in the crossmatch component of the exercise, the failure to detect a true incompatibility between a "patient" serum and a "donor" red cell sample. The failure to observe a true compatibility is a minor error, although the Steering Committee has forwarded to the Advisory Panel the recommendation this should be an error.
- For participants registered to undertake the grouping component of the exercise, the incorrect ABO grouping (excluding subgroups of A) or Rh(D) grouping, including the identification of a Rh(D)-negative sample as D^u. The identification of a Rh(D)-positive sample as D^u is a minor error. The incorrect identification of the subgroup of A is a minor error. This is, a group A_2 red cell sample identified as group A is not an error but identified as group A_1 is a minor error.
- For participants registered to undertake the antibody screen component in the exercise, the failure to detect, or the false detection of, atypical (allo) antibody in a "patient" serum sample.
- For participants registered to undertake the antibody identification component, the failure to identify, or fully identify, the atypical antibodies correctly detected in the screening procedure.
- Minor errors do not contribute to the definition of poor performance.

TABLE 2
Distribution of the Number of Crossmatches and Group with Antibody Screens Undertaken Within the U.K., as Determined by Questionnaire

No. of crossmatches undertaken per week[a]	% Participants[b]	No. of group with antibody screens undertaken per week[c]	% Participants[d]
≤10	13	≤50	24
11–50	35	51–100	14
51–100	27	101–150	14
101–150	9	150–200	9
151–200	5	201–250	9
201–500	3	251–300	6
>500	1	301–400	8
No answer	7	>401	9
		No answer	7

[a] Exercise 89/2.
[b] Total number of participants returning questionnaires: 378.
[c] Exercise 89#3.
[d] Total number of participants returning questionnaires: 403.

VI. POOR PERFORMANCE

Poor performance by a participant is defined as the occurrence of one or more errors in an exercise. Two or more poor performances within a series of four consecutive exercises result in the classification as a Persistent Poor Performer. Details of such performances are reviewed by the scheme Organizer for referral to the Advisory Panel. Participants with poor performance and particularly those with persistent poor performance are encouraged to seek assistance.

VII. PARTICIPANTS

In 1989, 501 participants were registered to undertake the crossmatch component of the exercise, 508 to undertake the ABO and Rh(D) grouping component, 504 to undertake the antibody screen component, and 386 to undertake the identification of atypical antibodies detected in the screening procedure. 75 participants were from the private sector. Excluding participants from the overseas laboratories of the U.K. armed forces, there were 16 non-U.K. participants.

Table 2 shows the distribution of the number of crossmatches and of groups with antibody screening per week within the laboratories of the participants, as reported in returned questionnaires.

Within the U.K., most (95%, Exercise 89E3) participants perform manual serological tests, manually dispensing the reagents and reading the results by

TABLE 3
Use of Microplate Techniques Within the U.K. (Exercise 89/A)

Procedure	% Participants[a]
ABO Grouping	33
Rh(D) Grouping	32
Antibody screen	
By enzyme	19
By antiglobulin	9
Crossmatching	
By enzyme	1
By antiglobulin	3
Predispensed plates used	
Stored at 4°C	4
Stored frozen	7
Solid-phase microplate technology used	1

[a] Percentage of participants returning questionnaires.

eye (75%, Exercise 89E3). Automated dispensing and automated observation of test results is undertaken primarily for ABO and Rh(D) grouping, essentially using microplate techniques. Table 3 shows the use of microplate techniques within the U.K.

VIII. COMPUTING FACILITIES

The computing facilities at the organizing laboratory comprise an IBM® clone personal computer operating under MS-DOS®, with 640-Kbyte memory, 20-Mbyte hard disk, 720-Kbyte 3.5-inch diskette drive, 360-Kbyte diskette drive, and a 132-column printer. These facilities are duplicated to provide a reverse facility. Bespoke computer programs are written by an experienced serologist within the organizing laboratory and compiled to assembler language (Turbo Pascal®, Borland). The use of a serologist with proven programming skills has proved more successful than the use of a professional programmer whose understanding of serology and serological practices is limited.

The organizing laboratory is registered as a data user under the U.K. Data Protection Act, 1984, which exists to prevent the misuse of data stored electronically. The organizing laboratory holds personal information provided by the participants in the form of exercise results, questionnaire responses, and names with addresses of the pathologists and technologists in charge of the participating laboratories. On request, a participant is entitled to view their personal information.

The various computer programs are selected from a menu of options accessible when the computer is switched on. These programs are used to maintain the registration details, print address labels, enter the serological results and questionnaire responses, analyze the serological performance, maintain the participants' cumulative performance file, and print out the participants' initial reports.

IX. ANALYSIS OF RESULTS AND REPORTING TO PARTICIPANTS

On receipt by the organizing laboratory, the participants' results are scrutinized for obvious errors. Instances of an incomplete or missing laboratory code number often can be resolved by reference to the postal frank or the originator's address, which may appear on the envelope. Participants who make an error in their serological investigations are informed by telephone without revealing the nature of the error or the correctness of any other results. Further exercise material is dispatched for repeat testing although the initial results stand as a record of the participant's achievement in that exercise. The serological results are entered twice onto the computer in order to detect random errors of entry by the keyboard operator. All the data for an exercise exist on removable diskette. This arrangement avoids the computer's fixed disk from becoming cluttered with data from successive exercises, while preserving the exercise's data in an electronic form for any future use.

The keyboard entry on the exercise data involves a great deal of time and effort. The ideal solution would be for the participants to send electronically their results and questionnaire responses direct to a receiving computer at the organizing laboratory. Unfortunately, the large majority of participants do not have the necessary computer facilities. As a less satisfactory solution, computer programs have been written to enable those participants with IBM®-compatible computers to enter their data onto a diskette for mailing to the organizing laboratory. Although maintaining lists of those participants requiring the variously sized diskettes and mailing diskettes is an additional task, this is outweighed by the benefits of receiving data in an electronically readable form, although measures to prevent the transfer of computer viruses have to be implemented.

Any erroneous result arising from the operation of the scheme is corrected; for example the provision of an incorrect or invalid sample, or the incorrect entry of results into the computer. An erroneous result arising from the participant's action remain as their record of achievement, for example, a missed incompatible crossmatch or a transcription error. However, in the analysis to determine the performance within the U.K. or in the calculation of the "correct" result for the exercise, the results of participants with obvious transcription or transposition errors are excluded in order that the data are more representative of the true U.K. serological performance.

Following the analysis of each participant's result against the "correct" result, a report is produced for each participant which reproduces their own results along with the corresponding "correct" result. Any errors of false-

TABLE 4
An Example of the Use of the Chi-Square Test in 2-by-2 Tables

Serum to red cell concentration	Antiglobulin reaction: False negative	Antiglobulin reaction: Correct positive	Totals
Less than or equal to 20:1	20	76	96
Greater than 20:1	35	278	313
Totals	55	354	409

Note: Number of participants with a false-negative, correct positive antiglobulin reaction in the detection of antibodies, vs. the serum to red cell concentration ratio [(100 × volume of serum added)/(volume of red cell suspension added × percentage cell suspension)]. Percentage of participants with false-negative antiglobulin reactions using: (1) serum to red cell concentration ratio of less than or equal to 20:1 — 20/96 (21%); (2) serum to red cell concentration ratio of greater than 20:1 — 35/313 (11%). Chi-square = 5.08 for 1 degree of freedom, $0.01 < 2P < 0.05$.

positive or false-negative reactions incurred by the participant are indicated on the report together with the distribution of errors incurred by all U.K. participants. The report is printed in duplicate; one copy is addressed to the pathologist, the other to the technologist in charge of the laboratory, and is distributed within two weeks of the closing date of the exercise.

The analysis of performance vs. technique is undertaken by bespoke programs after electronically transferring the serological performance and questionnaire data into a database (RBase®, Microrim). The particular database was chosen for the ease with which a technologist unskilled in computer languages can extract information from the database using a prompt facility which guides the user through the sequence of keyboard entries required to extract certain information, for example, the number of participants with a false-negative antiglobulin test in the antibody screen of "patient" 3 and who use a low ionic strength saline (LISS) addition technique.

The data from the analysis of performance with the technique is arranged in the form of a 2-by-2 table (see Table 4). The statistical significance of the analysis is obtained from a Chi-squared test with Yates' correction, or occasionally by Fisher's exact analysis.[1] The analysis compares the deviation of the observed frequencies of occurrence with those expected and determines the probability that the observed distribution of results was obtained by chance alone. If the nature of any difference in the frequency of occurrence is not known or cannot be predicted from prior knowledge, the statistical test should be interpreted as a two-tailed test, otherwise a one-tailed test can be used

TABLE 5
Percentage of Participants Routinely Using a Given Reagent for ABO and Rh(D) Grouping

Year	ABO Cell grouping				ABO Serum (reverse) grouping				
	Anti-A	Anti-B	Anti-A,B	Anti-A_1	A1 cells	A cells	A2 cells	B cells	O cells
1985	99	100	91	23	83	21	35	99	62
1986	100	100	90	20	84	18	38	99	58
1987	nd	nd	nd	nd	nd	nd	nd	nd	nd
1988	100	100	87	19	81	20	38	98	55
1989	100	100	88	17	83	19	36	98	53

Direct Antiglobulin Test

Year	Auto	PolySp.AHG[a]	anti-IgG	anti-C3d
1985	67	78	15	14
1986	63	79	9	9
1987	nd	nd	nd	nd
1988	59	63	5	5
1989	54	60	4	5

[a] PolySp., polyspecific; nd, not determined.

TABLE 5 (continued)
Percentage of Participants Routinely Using a Given Reagent for ABO and Rh(D) Grouping

Rh (D) Grouping

Year	Potentiated[b]	Control	Saline[b]	Albumin[b]	Control	Enzyme[b]	Control	AGH[b]	Control
1985	38	27	31	57	43	27	19	18	15
1986	36	27	33	55	40	25	15	17	11
1987	nd	nd	nd	nd	nd	nd	nd	nd	nd
1988	37	25	62	34	25	20	12	13	10
1989	35	24	67	30	20	18	11	6	4

Additional Grouping Procedures	1985	1986	1988	1989
Anti-A_1 only for A_1/A_2 differentiation	19	19	17	14
AHG Anti-D only for samples observed to be Rh(D)-negative	48	39	34	27

[b] See Section II for definition of reagents. nd, Not determined.

which is more powerful in revealing a true statistical difference. However even with such *a priori* evidence, two-tailed interpretations are used in the analyses of NEQAS data in order to err on the side of caution. The relationship between the Chi-square statistic and the two-tailed probability (2P) that the observed distribution of results has arisen by chance, depends on a factor termed the number of degrees of freedom. Suffice it to say that for these 2-by-2 tables, the number of degrees of freedom is one. The two-tailed probability of the observed distribution of results occurring by chance is determined by reference to statistical tables,[6] with entry at one degree of freedom and the Chi-square statistic.

In general, a two-tailed probability of less than 5% that the observed results have been obtained by chance alone is accepted as indicating statistical significance, that is with the 2-by-2 tables, that the frequency of occurrence of the two factors is different; a factor other than chance alone has contributed to the distribution of results. In the evaluation of performance with technique, it is important to be aware that multiple analyses of the same set of data eventually will produce a statistically significant result by chance with the probability of this occurrence increasing with the number of multiple analyses. With such analyses, it is unwise to accept a probability in the range of 5% to 1% as an indication of statistical significance, at least without *a priori* evidence to support that conclusion. In any instance, any statistical significance should be supportable by a logical explanation of the inferred conclusion. For example, analysis of the data shown in Table 4 indicates that the observed distribution of results has arisen by chance with a two-tailed probability (2P) in the range 5% to 1%. Since it is known that the detection of antibody in the antiglobulin test is dependent on the serum to red cell concentration ratio,[9] it could be concluded that the exercise data illustrate a dependency of the frequency of false-negative to correct positive antiglobulin reactions in the detection of antibodies, on the serum to red cell concentration ratio.

X. CHANGES IN SEROLOGICAL METHODS

With ABO grouping (see Table 5) there has been a slight reduction in the use of anti-A,B, of group O cells, and of anti-A_1. With Rh(D) grouping, there has been a marked reduction in the use of albumin displacement, enzyme and antiglobulin anti-D blood grouping reagents with a concomitant increase in saline anti-D blood grouping reagents due to the availability of monoclonal IgM anti-D reagents — the reagent of choice for tests on patient material. The reduction in the use of antiglobulin anti-D blood grouping reagent may be in response to a letter circulated by the scheme Organizer which indicated the high incidence of true Rh(D)-negative samples being grouped as Rh(D)-positive because of false-positive antiglobulin reactions. However, it should be noted that 27% of participants continue to use an antiglobulin anti-D blood

TABLE 6
Percentage of Participants Routinely Using a Given Technique for Antibody Screen

Year	Technique: Direct agglutination <30°C	Direct agglutination ≥30°C	Enzyme	Albumin	Antiglobulin	Other
1983	76	38	83	31	96	nd
1984	72	36	83	25	96	nd
1985	70	31	80	22	94	nd
1986	64	30	78	18	94	nd
1987	nd	nd	nd	nd	nd	nd
1988	56	28	79	12	96	5
1989	50	28	80	19	98	3

Note: nd, Not determined.

TABLE 7
Percentage of Participants Routinely Using a Given Technique for Crossmatching

Year	Technique: Direct agglutination <30°C	Direct agglutination ≥30°C	Enzyme	Albumin	Antiglobulin	Other
1981	99	71	61	68	100	nd
1982	99	68	66	60	100	nd
1983	97	68	66	56	100	nd
1984	94	66	67	49	100	nd
1985	93	65	66	45	100	nd
1986	91	63	65	40	100	nd
1987	nd	nd	nd	nd	nd	nd
1988	82	63	58	29	100	4
1989	78	65	55	25	100	3

Note: nd, Not determined.

grouping reagent with samples found to be Rh(D)-negative in initial testing with other types of blood grouping reagents.

In antibody screening procedures (see Table 6) and crossmatching techniques (see Table 7) direct agglutination tests at a temperature less than 30°C and albumin tests have declined in use. It is to be noted that the majority of direct agglutination tests are performed at temperatures less than 30°C, predominantly at room temperature.

There are many combinations of techniques in routine use. Some participants used anti-A_1 only to differentiate red cell samples found to be group

TABLE 8
Most Frequently Used Serological Techniques; Group, Screen, and Crossmatch

Sample	Technique	1985[a]	1986[a]	1988[a]	1989[a]
Non-group A sample	Anti-A + anti-B + anti-A,B	69	72	71	73
Group A sample	Anti-A + anti-B + anti-A,B	53	56	58	60
Non-group A sample	A_1 + B cells		25	25	28
	A_1 + A_2 + B + O cells	25			
Group A sample	A_1 + B cells		25	25	27
	A_1 + A_2 + B + O cells	25			
Rh(D)-Positive sample	Saline anti-D			20	27
	Albumin anti-D	21	20		
Rh(D)-Negative sample	Saline anti-D			12	19
	Albumin anti-D + antiglobulin anti-D	14	12		
Positive antibody screen	Enzyme + antiglobulin				31
	Direct (<30°C) + enzyme + antiglobulin	28	29	27	
Negative antibody screen	Enzyme + antiglobulin				24
	Direct (<30°C) + enzyme + antiglobulin	28	29	27	
Incompatible crossmatch	Direct (<30°C) + direct (≥30°C) + enzyme + antiglobulin	23	23	20	19
Compatible crossmatch	Direct (<30°C) + direct (≥30°C) + enzyme + antiglobulin	21	23	20	19

[a] Percentage of participants.

A; other participants use an antiglobulin anti-D blood grouping reagent only on red cell samples shown to be negative with other types of anti-D blood grouping reagents. Table 8 shows the percentage of participants using the most popular technique for group and screen and crossmatch procedures over the period 1985 to 1989.

A. VARIATIONS IN ANTIGLOBULIN TECHNIQUES

Table 9 shows the variants of the antiglobulin test used over the period 1980 to 1989. Tile techniques are those in which, after incubation with the test serum and subsequent washing, the test red cells are deposited on a tile or slide and mixed with the antiglobulin reagent. This technique continued in use over the 1980s despite antiglobulin reagents being formulated for use only with tube techniques since, in general, it is difficult to produce an

TABLE 9
Use of a Given Antiglobulin Crossmatch Technique, Expressed as a Percentage of Participants Using Antiglobulin Techniques

Antiglobulin technique[a]	Year								
	1980	1982	1983	1984	1985	1986	1987	1988	1989
Tile technique	18	10	5	5	nd	4	nd	2	0
Tube technique									
NIS[b]	75	50	49	40	nd	29	nd	22	18
LIS-Suspension[c]	25	43	43	52	nd	62	nd	73	76
LIS-Addition[d]	nd	7	4	6	nd	8	nd	7	5
Albumin-AGT[e]	19	11	7	6	nd	6	nd	nd	5

Note: nd, Not determined.

[a] Usage averaged over all exercises for that year.
[b] A normal ionic strength solution is used to suspend the test cells.
[c] A low ionic strength solution is used to suspend the test cells.
[d] A reaction mixture is used comprising test cells in a normal ionic strength medium, test serum and a low ionic strength medium added as a separate component.
[e] A reaction mixture is used comprising test cells in a normal ionic strength medium, test serum and bovine serum albumin added as a separate component.

antiglobulin reagent at an optimal dilution for both rapid tube and tile techniques. Antiglobulin reagents prepared for rapid tube methods have a much higher concentration of anti-IgG which tends to cause prozones if used for tile techniques, particularly with antibodies of low potency.

Normal ionic strength techniques have declined at the gain of low ionic strength techniques, probably because of the shorter incubation period that the latter technique offers. Albumin-antiglobulin techniques, where bovine albumin is included with the cell/serum mixture, have decreased in usage but continue to be used by a small proportion of participants despite the fact that the increased sensitivity shown originally with this technique[18] has been demonstrated to be due to the low ionic strength formulation of the particular albumin used in that study (Voak, personal communication). A 1989 review of the antiglobulin reagents available within the U.K. did not reveal any reagents where this technique was recommended by the manufacturer.

A small proportion of participants use a low ionic strength addition technique where the reaction mixture comprises test cells suspended in a normal ionic strength medium, serum and a low ionic strength medium added as a separate component.

Currently, 62% of participants use an antiglobulin reagent manufactured within the public sector; the remainder use a commercial product.

TABLE 10
Use of a Given Enzyme Technique in Antibody Screening Procedures, Expressed as a Percentage of Participants Using Enzyme Techniques

Enzyme technique	1983-D	1984-C	1988-A	1989E3
One-stage layer	19	18	11	11
One-stage mix	42	44	22	18
One-stage delay	nd	nd	nd	5
One-stage inhibitor	nd	nd	nd	1
Two stage	40	39	68	66

Note: nd, Not determined.

B. VARIATIONS IN ENZYME TECHNIQUES

In general, enzyme procedures are either one stage or two stage. In the former, enzyme, red cells and test serum are present together within the same tube. In the latter, the red cells are incubated with the enzyme and are washed for subsequent treatment with the test serum. One-stage procedures can be subdivided into:

- One-stage layer — where test serum is overlaid with the enzyme preparation which in turn is overlaid with the red cell suspension; it is important that a narrow tube (about 6 × 50 mm) is used to maintain the stratification of the reactants so that the red cells gravitate through the enzyme into the serum
- One-stage mix — where test serum, enzyme, and red cells are mixed and incubated
- One-stage inhibitor — where red cells are incubated with the enzyme preparation, following which an enzyme inhibitor is added, followed by the test serum, and the mixture is briefly incubated.
- One-stage delay — where red cells are incubated with the enzyme preparation, following which the test serum is added and the mixture briefly incubated.

The enzyme most frequently used is papain which is used by 80% of those participants using an enzyme technique. Bromelain and ficin are used by 17% and 3%, respectively, of such participants (Exercise 1983-D, 1984-D, 1988-A, 1989E3). These proportions have remained virtually constant over the 1980s. Some 60% of participants using papain (70% for users of bromelain) prepare their own reagent or it is prepared by the regional transfusion center; the remainder use a commercial product. 80% of participants use an enzyme technique for antibody screen. Table 10 shows the variations in enzyme techniques used.

TABLE 11
Use of a Given Enzyme Technique in Crossmatch Procedures, Expressed as a Percentage of Participants Using Enzyme Techniques

Enzyme technique	1982/3	1984/2	1989/2A
One-stage layer	26	24	30
One-stage mix	59	53	37
One-stage delay	nd	nd	12
One-stage inhibitor	nd	nd	1
Two stage	14	21	21

Note: nd, Not determined.

Over the period 1983 to 1989, there has been a decrease in the use of one-stage enzyme procedures for antibody screen procedures with a corresponding increase in two-stage procedures where the test cells are pretreated with the enzyme reagent, washed free of enzyme, and subsequently used in tests with the serum.

One-stage enzyme methods, especially one-stage mix, continue to be used in antibody screening procedures. There is no justification for a one-stage mix technique in antibody screening where there should be adequate time to pretreat the two or three screening red cell samples, if an enzyme test is required.

In crossmatch techniques, two-stage enzyme methods are less frequently used, probably because of the number of donor red cell samples that would need to be treated. 55% of participants use an enzyme procedure for the crossmatch. Table 11 shows the variations in enzyme techniques used.

XI. THE USE OF SENSITIVITY AND REACTIVITY CONTROLS

A. ANTIGLOBULIN TESTS

Some 70 to 80% of participants state the use of a control to assure adequate sensitivity of the antiglobulin test, that is, they use an antiserum of known specificity and potency in parallel with the tests being performed. Eighty to ninety per cent of participants state that they add red cells, sensitized with IgG antibody, to each test with a negative result to assure adequate reactivity of the anti-IgG component of the antiglobulin reagent present within the tube.

In exercises 1989/2 and 1989-A, involving the detection of anti-D samples at 0.3 and 0.1 International Units per milliliter (IU/ml) in the crossmatch using R_1r and R_1R_1 red cell samples and in the antibody screen, there was no association of the ability to detect antibody with the use of a sensitivity

TABLE 12
Relationship Between the Use of an Antiserum Sensitivity Control and the Ability to Detect Anti-D in the Antiglobulin Test[a]

Sensitivity control	Number of false-negative antiglobulin test results	Number of correct positive antiglobulin test results
Used	317[b]	1227
Not used	154[c]	559

[a] Anti-D 0.3 and 0.1 IU/ml in the crossmatch using R_1r and R_1R_1, red cells and in the antibody screen. Exercises 1989-A, 1989/2.
[b] Incidence of false-negative antiglobulin test result: sensitivity control used, 21%.
[c] Incidence of false-negative antiglobulin test result: sensitivity control not used, 22%.

Chi^2 test, $2P < 0.05$, not statistically significant.

TABLE 13
Relationship Between Use of IgG-Sensitized Control Red Cells and the Ability to Detect Anti-D in the Antiglobulin Test[a]

IgG-Sensitized red cells	Number of false-negative antiglobulin test results	Number of correct positive antiglobulin test results
Used	384[b]	1435
Not used	87[c]	353

[a] Anti-D 0.3 and 0.1 IU/ml in the crossmatch using R_1r and R_1R_1 red cells and in the antibody screen. Exercises 1989-A, 1989/2.
[b] Incidence of false-negative antiglobulin test result: IgG-sensitized control cells used, 21%.
[c] Incidence of false-negative antiglobulin test result: IgG-sensitized control cells not used, 20%.

Chi^2 test, $2P < 0.05$, not statistically significant.

antiserum control or with the use of IgG-sensitized control red cells (see Tables 12 and 13).

The failure to observe a statistically significant relationship between the detection of antibody with the use of sensitivity and reactivity controls is disappointing. It may have been that the sensitivity controls used by the participants were too potent or that the IgG-sensitized control cells were too heavily sensitized to detect the inhibitory effect of any residual serum. Sensitized control cells will not detect false-negative tests due to mishandling of the agglutinates by the worker, particularly when dislodging the red cell button from the bottom of the tube prior to observation.

Antiglobulin reagents formulated for use in immediate spin-tube techniques that are made to U.S., or similar, specifications contain higher concentrations of anti-IgG than previous generations of reagents, particularly those for use in slide techniques. Strongly IgG-sensitized control cells will produce a clear reaction with immediate spin-tube antiglobulin reagents that have been partially neutralized to an extent that weak antibodies are not detected that would have been detected by the fully active antiglobulin reagent. Ideally, IgG-sensitized control cells should effect a weak macroscopic reaction to demonstrate adequate reactivity of the anti-IgG component. However, in practice, many users will avoid using weakly IgG-sensitized control cells because inevitable technical variation would result in an impractical proportion of their tests being repeated because of macroscopically negative results with the weakly IgG-sensitized cells. In addition, the ability of IgG antibody of low equilibrium constant to transfer rapidly from the sensitized control cells to the test cells where these have the same antigen but present in greater quantity, and for the IgG antibody to elute from the sensitized cells on storage after preparation, can limit the usefulness of weak, IgG-sensitized control cells.[18]

Consideration of the value of sensitivity and reactivity controls should not be in isolation from other internal quality assurance procedures. Staff and cell washing systems should be regularly assessed by performing blind, replicate testing of known inert and weak antibodies. The detection of the latter is particularly dependent upon the method used to dislodge the red cells from the bottom of the tube, following centrifugation after the addition of the antiglobulin reagent. Current cell washing systems are capable of blockage in wash spigots or of a nonuniform distribution of wash material which can cause the failure of the antiglobulin test in one particular tube of the washing system. The addition of weak IgG-sensitized control cells to each tube with a negative result would detect such failures, whereas the sensitivity antiserum control would not — unless it happened to be situated at that particular tube location. Perhaps the use of IgG-sensitized control cells will remain until cell washing systems are available which assure the efficacy of the washing process at each location within the cell washer.

B. ENZYME TESTS

Some 90% of participants state the use of a serological control to assure adequate sensitivity of the enzyme test, for example anti-C + D or soybean extract. In exercise 1989E3, those participants who used a serological sensitivity control had a significantly lower incidence of false-negative enzyme

TABLE 14
Relationship Between the Use of a Serological Sensitivity Control and the Ability to Detect Anti-D 0.3 IU/ml in the Antibody Screen, Using Enzyme Tests: Exercise 89E3

Incidence of false negative enzyme test result: serological sensitivity control used, 22/290 (8%)
Incidence of false negative enzyme test result: serological sensitivity control not used, 10/55 (18%)

$\text{Chi}^2 = 4.97$ for 1 degree of freedom, $0.01 < 2P < 0.05$.

test results in the detection of anti-D 0.3 IU/ml in the antibody screen (see Table 14).

XII. THE DETECTION OF ANTI-D AT 0.3 AND 0.1 INTERNATIONAL UNITS PER MILLILITER

Anti-D diluted to 0.3 and 0.1 IU/ml has been issued periodically as exercise material. Tables 15 and 16 show the detection rate of the anti-D 0.3 and 0.1 IU/ml in the crossmatch and antibody screen procedures. Thes anti-D antisera are prepared by dilution in group-compatible plasma of a pool of anti-D antisera which has been quantitated by a continuous flow automated system by several laboratories within the U.K. A new pool was produced for use from 1985 onwards.

The U.K. guidelines for compatibility testing in hospital blood banks[19] state that anti-D 0.3 IU/ml should be readily detectable in the antiglobulin test. The antiglobulin test is consistently more sensitive in the detection of anti-D antibodies present in exercise material than the enzyme or albumin techniques. It is seen that, in general, with respect to the crossmatch against R_1r or R_1R_1 test red cells, some 95% of participants are able to detect anti-D 0.3 IU/ml using the antiglobulin test, the corresponding figure for albumin and enzyme techniques being 72 and 65%, respectively. For anti-D 0.1 IU/ml, it is seen that the detection rate in the crossmatch is 73% (antiglobulin), 38% (albumin), and 47% (enzyme).

The better performance of the enzyme technique in antibody screening is probably due to the greater use of two-stage enzyme tests than in crossmatch procedures. Two-stage tests are where washed, enzyme-treated screening red cells are prepared for subsequent use; enzyme, test cells, and serum are not together in the same tube.

XIII. THE PERFORMANCE OF VARIOUS ANTIGLOBULIN TECHNIQUES

Variants of the antiglobulin technique having different sensitivities, in general, will be revealed only by the use of antibody specificities of low

TABLE 15A
Detection Rate of Anti-D 0.3 IU/ml in the Crossmatch

Exercise	Against	Detection rate[a]		
		Enzyme	Albumin	Antiglobulin
1981–4	R_1R_1 Cells	66	70	93
	R_1r Cells	66	68	90
1982–1	R_1r Cells	51	66	88
	R_2r Cells	66	76	94
1983–2	R_1R_1 Cells	68	83	98
	R_1r Cells	72	85	98
1983–4	R_1R_1 Cells	54	88	98
	R_1R Cells	57	80	97
1984–3	R_1R_1 Cells	52	83	98
1985–3	R_1R_1 Cells	79	86	99
	R_1r Cells	82	76	96
1989–2	R_1R_1 Cells	84	61	96
	R_1r Cells	40	40	93
1989E3	R_1r Cells	66	51	93
Average detection rate		65	72	95

[a] Participants detecting antibody by the technique, as a percentage of those using that technique.

TABLE 15B
Detection Rate of Anti-D 0.3 IU/ml in the Antibody Screen

Exercise	Detection rate[a]		
	Enzyme	Albumin	Antiglobulin
1983–B	74	82	95
1985–A	89	76	99
1988–A	93	74	100
1989E3	89	59	99
Average detection rate	86	73	98

[a] Participants detecting antibody by the technique, as a percentage of those using that technique.

potency. Furthermore, the association of a particular variation with a poor sensitivity may be observed only with certain antibody specificities or only with some examples of that antibody specificity.

A. THE EFFECT OF GLASS VS. PLASTIC TUBES

The use of plastic tubes in the antiglobulin test has been shown in three exercises to be associated with a lower detection rate, or with a weaker reaction grade. This is probably due to the greater degree of agitation that is required

TABLE 16A
Detection Rate of Anti-D 0.1 IU/ml in the Crossmatch

Exercise	Against	Detection rate[a]		
		Enzyme	Albumin	Antiglobulin
1983–4	R_1R_1 Cells	28	54	84
	R_1r Cells	32	62	84
1985–3	R_1R_1 Cells	64	nd	88
	R_1r Cells	63	nd	71
1989–2	R_1R_1 Cells	55	24	59
	R_1r Cells	42	12	52
Average detection rate		47	38	73

[a] Participants detecting antibody by the technique, as a percentage of those using the technique; nd, not determined.

TABLE 16B
Detection Rate of Anti-D 0.1 IU/ml in the Antibody Screen

Exercise	Detection rate[a]		
	Enzyme	Albumin	Antiglobulin
1985–C	66	65	82
1989–A	81	56	90
Average detection rate	74	61	86

[a] Participants detecting antibody by the technique, as a percentage of those using that technique.

to dislodge the cell button from the tube following centrifugation prior to reading of the result. In addition, the electrostatic charge on plastic tubes is known to cause a variation in the delivery from a Pasteur pipette held close to the mouth of the tube.[10]

The poorer performance of the antiglobulin test in plastic tubes has been reported by other workers.[2] In Exercise 1989/2, glass tubes were used by 50% of participants (see Table 17).

B. THE EFFECT OF LOW IONIC STRENGTH ADDITION VS. SUSPENSION

The conventional low ionic strength technique uses red cells washed and suspended in a low ionic strength medium — this is termed low ionic strength *suspension*. For certain investigations, this would necessitate the same red cell sample being prepared as a normal ionic strength and as a low ionic strength suspension. Therefore, some participants add a differently formulated

TABLE 17
The Effect of Glass vs. Plastic Tubes in the Antiglobulin Test

Exercise 1986–3: detection of anti-Jk^a in the antibody screen
Detection rate using glass tubes, 51/129 (40%)
Detection rate using plastic tubes, 54/202 (27%)
$Chi^2 = 5.38$ for 1 degree of freedom, $0.01 < 2P < 0.05$
Exercise 1988/2: detection of anti-K in the crossmatch using Kk red cells
Occurrence of grade 1 or 2 reactions using glass tubes, 6/164 (4%)
Occurrence of grade 1 or 2 reactions using plastic tubes, 27/220 (12%)
$Chi^2 = 7.81$ for 1 degree of freedom, $0.005 < 2P < 0.01$
Exercise 1989/2: detection of incompatibilities due to anti-D and anti-Fy^a using R_1R_1, R_1r, and Fy(a + b +) red cells
All incompatibilities detected using glass tubes, 108/187 (58%)
All incompatibilities detected using plastic tubes, 86/189 (46%)
$Chi^2 = 5.17$ for 1 degree of freedom, $0.01 < 2P < 0.05$

TABLE 18
The Effect of Low Ionic Strength in the Antiglobulin Technique — Addition vs. Suspension

Exercise 1989/1	
False-negative antiglobulin reactions — low ionic strength (addition)	7/30 (23%)
False-negative antiglobulin reactions — low ionic strength (suspension)	29/299 (10%)
$Chi^2 = 3.90$ for 1 degree of freedom, $0.01 < 2P < 0.05$	

low ionic strength medium as a separate component of a reaction mixture which comprises serum, red cells suspended in normal ionic strength medium, and the low ionic strength medium — this is termed low ionic strength *addition*.

The use of low ionic strength addition has been associated with a greater incidence of false-negative antiglobulin reactions (see Table 18). This may be due to the addition of the low ionic strength medium, which, although not affecting the serum to red cell concentration ratio, will dilute the reactants, changing the position and rate of attainment of equilibrium.

C. THE EFFECT OF SERUM TO RED CELL RATIO

The serum to red cell ratio is defined as:

$$\frac{(\text{volume of serum added} \times 100)}{(\text{volume of red cell suspension added}) \times (\text{percentage red cell suspension})}$$

and ignores the effect of any other added material. For a technique comprising 2 volumes of serum mixed with 1 volume of 3% red cell suspension, the serum to red cell concentration ratio would be 67:1. Using a 10% cell suspension by the same technique would result in a 20:1 ratio.

TABLE 19
The Effect of Serum to Red Cell Concentration Ratio on the Detection of Antibody in the Antiglobulin Test

Anti-K vs. Kk cells: Exercise 1986–3	
Detection rate, serum to red cell concentration ratio ≤20:1	59/81 (73%)
Detection rate, serum to red cell concentration ratio >20:1	203/241 (84%)
$Chi^2 = 4.47$ for 1 degree of freedom, $0.01 < 2P < 0.05$	
Anti-K (different sample from above) vs. Kk cells: Exercise 1986–3	
Detection rate, serum to red cell concentration ratio ≤20:1	19/67 (28%)
Detection rate, serum to red cell concentration ratio >20:1	78/155 (50%)
$Chi^2 = 8.30$ for 1 degree of freedom, $0.001 < 2P < 0.05$	
Anti-Fy^a vs. Fy(a + b +): Exercise 1986–3	
Detection rate, serum to red cell concentration ratio ≤20:1	3/7 (43%)
Detection rate, serum to red cell concentration ratio >20:1	206/211 (98%)
$Chi^2 = 38.45$ for 1 degree of freedom, $2P < 0.001$	
False-negative antiglobulin reactions in the detection of antibodies (anti-E, K, Fy^a, and c): Exercise 1989/1	
Detection rate, serum to red cell concentration ratio ≤20:1	76/96 (79%)
Detection rate, serum to red cell concentration ratio >20:1	278/313 (89%)
$Chi^2 = 5.08$ for 1 degree of freedom, $0.01 < 2P < 0.05$	
False-negative antiglobulin reactions in the detection of anti-D 0.1 IU/ml: Exercise 1989/A	
Detection rate, serum to red cell concentration ratio ≤20:1	49/67 (73%)
Detection rate, serum to red cell concentration ratio >20:1	278/321 (87%)
$Chi^2 = 6.61$ for 1 degree of freedom, $0.01 < 2P < 0.05$	

The greater the serum to red cell concentration ratio for a given antibody/antigen, the more antibody will be bound at equilibrium. Serum to red cell concentration ratios of 20:1 or less have been associated with a lower detection rate of antibodies in the antiglobulin test (see Table 19).

Most (92%) of the participants (Exercise 1989-2) do not use any method of assuring the red cell suspension other than by eye. It is known that experienced serologists can differ sixfold in the concentration of the red cell suspension prepared to a nominal concentration, and that a drop from a single Pasteur pipette can differ by up to 2.6-fold.[4,10] The serum to red cell concentration ratios used for the analysis in this section were determined from details of the techniques as reported by the participants' questionnaires returned to the organizing laboratory; the actual ratios may have been different.

D. TUBE OR TILE ANTIGLOBULIN TEST

As detailed in Section X.A, it has been the practice of some participants to remove the red cells from the tube after washing following the incubation phase of the antiglobulin test, onto a slide or tile for mixing with the antiglobulin reagent. The use of tile antiglobulin technique has been associated with the poorer detection of antibodies in the antiglobulin test (see Table 20).

It is probable that the participants using a tile technique were using antiglobulin reagents characterized only for a tube technique, since a review

TABLE 20
Tube vs. Tile Antiglobulin Technique

Anti-Fy^a vs. Fy(a + b +): Exercise 1986–3	
Detection rate using tile techniques	10/13 (77%)
Detection rate using tube techniques	307/318 (97%)
Chi^2 = 7.52 for 1 degree of freedom, $0.005 < 2P < 0.01$	
Anti-Jk^a vs. Jk(a + b+): Exercise 1986–3	
Detection rate using tile techniques	0/13 (0%)
Detection rate using tube techniques	105/318 (33%)
Chi^2 = 4.86 for 1 degree of freedom, $0.01 < 2P < 0.05$	

TABLE 21
Normal vs. Low Ionic Strength Antiglobulin Technique

Anti-K vs. Kk red cells: Exercise 86–3	
Detection rate using normal ionic strength techniques	83/93 (89%)
Detection rate using low ionic strength techniques	176/229 (77%)
Chi^2 = 5.69 for 1 degree of freedom, $0.01 < 2P < 0.05$	
Anti-Jk^a vs. (Jka + b) red cells: Exercise 1986–3	
Detection rate using normal ionic strength techniques	19/93 (20%)
Detection rate using low ionic strength techniques	85/229 (37%)
Chi^2 = 7.68 for 1 degree of freedom, $0.005 < 2P < 0.05$	
Anti-K vs. Kk red cells: Exercise 1986–3	
Detection rate using normal ionic strength techniques	72/93 (77%)
Detection rate using low ionic strength techniques	99/229 (43%)
Chi^2 = 29.68 for 1 degree of freedom, $2P < 0.001$	

of the antiglobulin reagents available within the U.K. at that time did not reveal any reagent for which a tile technique was recommended.

E. NORMAL VS. LOW IONIC STRENGTH TECHNIQUES

For antisera issued in these exercises, low ionic strength techniques have a greater detection rate than normal ionic strength techniques, with the exception of anti-K antisera (see Table 21).

Anti-K is the non-complement-fixing antibody specificity often referenced as a specificity being poorly detected by low ionic strength techniques.[11] It is known that the detection of blood group antibodies is dependent on the serum to red cell concentration ratio (see Section XIII.C above). The "conventional" low ionic strength technique of 1 volume of 3% red cells suspended in a low ionic strength medium to 1 volume of serum effects a serum to red cell concentration ratio of 33:1, compared with the "conventional" normal ionic strength technique of 1 volume of 3% red cells suspended in a normal ionic strength medium to 2 volumes of serum, which effects a 67:1 ratio. A technique which increases the serum to red cell concentration ratio of low ionic strength (suspension) tests while preserving the ionic strength of the incubation mix is 2 volumes of 1.5% red cell suspended in a low ionic medium added to 2 volumes of serum.[20] This effects at 67:1 serum to red cell ratio,

TABLE 22
Macroscopic Observation vs. Macro- with Microscopic Observation in the Antiglobulin Technique

Exercise 1988/1: ABO and anti-K incompatibilities	
Incidence of at least one false-negative antiglobulin test, macroscopic observation only	7/82 (9%)
Incidence of at least one false-negative antiglobulin test, macroscopic and microscopic observation	10/335 (3%)
$Chi^2 = 3.87$ for 1 degree of freedom, $0.01 < 2P < 0.05$	
Exercise 1989/2: Anti-D vs. R_1r red cells	
Detection of anti-D at 0.1 IU/ml, macroscopic observation only	24/177 (14%)
Detection of anti-D at 0.1 IU/ml, macroscopic and microscopic observation	170/199 (85%)
$Chi^2 = 190.87$ for 1 degree of freedom, $2P < 0.001$	

and presents the same number of red cells to the antiglobulin reagent as the "conventional" 1 volume of 3% red cells to 1 volume of serum. Such a technique appears to detect examples of anti-K antibody with a greater assurance than the "conventional" low ionic strength (suspension) technique.[8,19]

F. METHOD OF READING

Using a magnifying mirror or lens or microscope to determine the result of the antiglobulin tests that are negative on macroscopic observation is associated with a greater detection rate than macroscopic observation alone (see Table 22).

The increased sensitivity of microscopic observation will be revealed with the use of antibodies of low potency. Exercise 1988/1 involved the detection of incompatibilities due to anti-A with A_2B and A_2 red cell samples and to anti-K with Kk red cell samples. The statistical significance for the detection of the anti-D at 0.1 International Units per ml clearly illustrates the increased sensitivity of microscopic observation of tests that are negative on macroscopic observation.

G. EFFECT OF INCUBATION PERIOD IN THE LOW IONIC STRENGTH ANTIGLOBULIN TEST

The low ionic strength technique is recommended to have an incubation period of 15 minutes or greater.[21] It has been observed that participants using an incubation period of more than 15 minutes have a greater detection rate than those using 15 minutes or less. It is not known whether participants prewarmed their test materials (see Table 23).

TABLE 23
Exercise 1988/1: Low Ionic Strength Antiglobulin Technique[a]

Detection rate of all antibodies using an incubation period of 15 minutes or less	74/82 (90%)
Detection rate of all antibodies using an incubation period of greater than 15 minutes	177/181 (98%)
$Chi^2 = 5.75$ for 1 degree of freedom, $0.01 < 2P < 0.05$	

[a] Compatibility testing involving anti-A with A_2 and A_2B red cells and anti-K with Kk red cells.

XIV. THE USE OF THE MANUFACTURER'S RECOMMENDED METHODS OF USE FOR THE ANTIGLOBULIN TEST

The antiglobulin technique, as reported by questionnaire, of those participants using the most frequently used antiglobulin reagent within the U.K. was assessed for compliance with the manufacturer's recommended methods of use. The conditions of centrifugation after the addition of the antiglobulin reagent were excluded from the analysis since the manufacturer permitted the use of other suitable combinations of relative centrifugal force and time.

In Exercise 1986-D, 9 (10%) of the 93 participants using this reagent by a low ionic strength technique, used the manufacturer's recommended method. None (0%) of the 36 participants using the reagent by a normal ionic strength technique used the manufacturer's recommended method. In Exercise 1988/1, the corresponding figures were 2/123 (2%) and 2/40 (5%).

The manufacturer's recommended method of use for the normal ionic strength method was: 2 volumes of serum to 1 volume of 3% red cells in phosphate-buffered saline or saline, mix, and incubate for 60 minutes at 37°C. Wash at least three times in phosphate-buffered saline. Add two volumes of antiglobulin reagent, centrifuge, and observe for agglutination, macro- and microscopically. For the low ionic strength method, the recommended method was: 1 volume of serum to 1 volume of 3% red cells in low ionic strength medium, mix, and incubate for 15 minutes at 37°C and proceed as with the normal ionic strength technique.

The majority of the differences from the manufacturer's recommended techniques were in two areas: the serum to red cell ratio and the period of incubation (see Tables 24 and 25).

The methods of use recommended by the manufacturer of any reagent are those by which the reagent has been characterized for potency, specificity, and, for a slide technique, avidity. If the recommended methods are not suited to the practices of a laboratory, then an alternative product which is recommended for the desired method should be sought. Alternatively, the user may fully characterize the reagent for the desired method of use. However, the

TABLE 24
Exercise 1988/1: Use of Manufacturer's Recommended Antiglobulin Technique — the Period of Incubation

Normal ionic strength technique		Low ionic strength technique	
Incubation period (min)	% Participants using the reagent	Incubation period (min)	% Participants using the reagent
15	6	10	3
20	13	15[a]	30
30	12	20	38
35	0	25	3
40	4	30	16
45	17	31–60	10
50	2	>60	1
60[a]	42		
>60	3		

[a] Recommended incubation period.

TABLE 25
Exercise 1988/1: Use of Manufacturer's Recommended Antiglobulin Technique — the Serum to Red Cell Concentration Ratio

Serum to red cell concentration ratio	Normal ionic strength technique[a]	Low ionic strength technique[a]
≤10:1	1	1
>10:1 to ≤20:1	12	20
>20:1 to <30:1	2	12
>30:1 to <40:1[b]	25	43
>40:1 to <50:1	14	14
>50:1 to <60:1	2	0
>60:1 to <70:1[c]	18	7
>70:1 to <80:1	10	0
>80:1	15	2

[a] Percentage of participants using the reagent.
[b] Ratio of the recommended low ionic strength technique is 33:1.
[c] Ratio of the recommended normal ionic strength technique is 67:1.

TABLE 26
The Detection Rate[a] of Anti-D Using One- and Two-Stage Enzyme Techniques

Technique	1989/2[b]	1989E3[c]
Two stage	129/164 (79%)	216/226 (96%)
One-stage mix	136/291 (47%)	37/75 (49%)
One-stage layer	170/236 (72%)	25/39 (64%)
One-stage delay	84/96 (88%)	14/16 (88%)
One-stage inhibitor	4/4 (100%)	2/2 (100%)

[a] (Number of positive results)/(expected number of positive results).
[b] Anti-D 0.3 and 0.1 IU/ml vs. R_1r and R_1R_1 red cells — crossmatch procedure.
[c] Anti-D 0.3 IU/ml vs. R_1r red cells — crossmatch procedure.

user should be aware that liability for the correct performance of the reagent by a method not included in the manufacturer's package insert, will be with the user.

XV. THE PERFORMANCE OF VARIOUS ENZYME TECHNIQUES

Section X.B detailed the usage of various enzyme procedures. Table 26 shows the detection rate of anti-D using these procedures. The number of participants using the one-stage inhibitor technique[15] is too small to enable conclusions to be drawn. The one-stage mix is particularly insensitive, yet is the most frequently used one-stage technique. The detection rate using the one-stage mix is significantly different from that using the one-stage delay ($Chi^2 = 47.25$ for 1 degree of freedom, $2P < 0.001$). Many participants using a one-stage mix technique in crossmatch procedures who wish to use an enzyme technique should be able to use a one-stage delay technique,[12] after validation with their particular enzyme preparation. The poor performance of the one-stage mix technique has been attributed to the digestion by the enzyme of antibody immunoglobulin and serum albumin.[14]

XVI. THE CONSEQUENCES WITHIN THE U.K. OF USING AN ANTIGLOBULIN TEST ALONE IN CROSSMATCH AND ANTIBODY SCREEN PROCEDURES

Exercise 1989-2 included anti-D 0.1 IU/ml, anti-D 0.3 IU/ml, and three group O "donor" red cell samples of presumptive Rh genotypes, R_1R_1, R_1r, and rr. The result of the antiglobulin and enzyme tests for the two anti-D antisera are summarized in Table 27.

TABLE 27
Distribution of Antiglobulin and Enzyme Test Results[a]

Antiserum	Grade of reaction[b]	Antiglobulin test, red cells		Enzyme test, red cells	
		R_1R_1	R_1r	R_1R_1	R_1r
Anti-D 0.1 IU/ml	0	182	214	108	138
	1	93	101	25	23
	2	107	87	42	27
	3	50	33	43	36
	4	10	6	20	14
	5	2	2	3	2
Anti-D 0.3 IU/ml	0	17	30	38	60
	1	42	60	27	36
	2	100	136	41	41
	3	178	134	61	52
	4	91	65	57	36
	5	16	18	17	15

[a] Number of participants having a stated grade of reaction for a given test.

[b] Grade 0, negative reaction; grade 1, agglutination visible microscopically only; grades 2 to 5, weak to maximum agglutination, macroscopically visible.

In this exercise, there were 3486 antiglobulin tests with compatible serum-red cell combinations, of which 63 tests were falsely positive, and 1914 enzyme tests with compatible serum-red cell combinations, of which 33 were falsely positive.

The relationship between the test result obtained and the correct result can be written as:

Test result	Correct result: Positive	Correct result: Negative
Positive	a	b
Negative	c	d

where a is the number of correctly positive test results; b is the number of falsely positive test results; c is the number of falsely negative test results; and d is the number of correctly negative test results.

The following can be defined for the test:

- *Sensitivity*, the number of correctly positive test results expressed as a proportion of the results that should be positive, that is, $a/(a + c)$
- *Specificity*, the number of correctly negative test results expressed as a proportion of the results that should be negative, that is, $d/(b + d)$
- *False-positive rate,* the number of falsely positive test results expressed as a proportion of all positive test results, that is, $b/(a + b)$

- *False-negative rate,* the number of falsely negative tests results expressed as a proportion of all negative test results, that is, c/(c + d)

It should be noted that the false-positive and false-negative rates depend on the proportion of tests that should be positive or negative in the sera subjected to test; if all the sera ought to have positive test results, there can be no false-positive result.

The sensitivity and specificity of the enzyme and antiglobulin test can be calculated from the exercise data as:

	Anti-D antiserum			
	0.1 IU/ml Red cell sample		**0.3 IU/ml Red cell sample**	
Parameter	**R_1r**	**R_1R_1**	**R_1r**	**R_1R_1**
Antiglobulin test				
Sensitivity	0.517	0.590	0.932	0.962
Specificity	0.982	0.982	0.982	0.982
Enzyme test				
Sensitivity	0.425	0.552	0.740	0.842
Specificity	0.983	0.983	0.983	0.983

The greater sensitivity of the antiglobulin test compared to the enzyme is apparent, as is the greater sensitivity with the use of a R_1R_1 compared to a R_1r red cell sample.

Given a batch of test antiserum in which a proportion "P" contains an antibody that is detectable by the antiglobulin test, then the false-positive and false-negative rates of the test can be determined from the following equations:

$$\text{False-negative rate} = \frac{P(I - S)}{F(I - P) + P(I - S)}$$

$$\text{False-positive rate} = \frac{(I - F)(I - P)}{(S \times P) + (I - F)(I - P)}$$

where S and F are the sensitivity and specificity, respectively, for the particular antibody-red cell sample test.

For a given proportion of anti-D antisera in a batch of sera tested using a R_1R_1 red cell sample, the false-positive and false-negative rates can be calculated as shown in Table 28A for the antiglobulin test, and in Table 28B for the enzyme test, using the calculated sensitivities and specificities.

Using R_1R_1 red cells and with anti-D at 0.3 IU/ml present in 1% of test sera, a false-negative antiglobulin test is expected in 4 of 10,000 tests. If the antiglobulin test were the only test used to detect the antibody in the crossmatch or antibody screen procedure, this figure would be the number of missed incompatibilities or false-negative antibody screens, assuming 1% of the test

TABLE 28A
Proportion of False-Negative and False-Positive Antiglobulin Test Results Expected in a Batch of Sera Tested with R_1R_1 Red Cells

Proportion of anti-D antisera in a batch of test sera	Anti-D antiserum 0.1 IU/ml False-positive tests	Anti-D antiserum 0.1 IU/ml False-negative tests	Anti-D antiserum 0.3 IU/ml False-positive tests	Anti-D antiserum 0.3 IU/ml False-negative tests
0.999 (99.9%)	0.0000	0.9976	0.0000	0.9748
0.99	0.0003	0.9764	0.0002	0.7930
0.9	0.0034	0.7898	0.0021	0.2583
0.7	0.0129	0.4935	0.0080	0.0828
0.5	0.0296	0.2945	0.0184	0.0373
0.3	0.0665	0.1518	0.0418	0.0163
0.1	0.2154	0.0443	0.1441	0.0043
0.01	0.7513	0.0042	0.6494	0.0004
0.001 (0.1%)	0.9682	0.0004	0.9492	0.0000

TABLE 28B
Proportion of False-Negative and False-Positive Enzyme Test Results Expected in a Batch of Sera Tested with R_1R_1 Red cells

Proportion of anti-D antisera in a batch of test sera	Anti-D antiserum 0.1 IU/ml False-positive tests	Anti-D antiserum 0.1 IU/ml False-negative tests	Anti-D antiserum 0.3 IU/ml False-positive tests	Anti-D antiserum 0.3 IU/ml False-negative tests
0.999 (99.9%)	0.0000	0.9978	0.0000	0.9938
0.99	0.0003	0.9783	0.0002	0.9409
0.9	0.0034	0.8040	0.0022	0.5913
0.7	0.0130	0.5154	0.0086	0.2727
0.5	0.0299	0.3131	0.0198	0.1385
0.3	0.0670	0.1634	0.0450	0.0644
0.1	0.2170	0.0482	0.1538	0.0175
0.01	0.7530	0.0046	0.6665	0.0016
0.001 (0.1%)	0.9685	0.0005	0.9528	0.0002

sera to contain anti-D at 0.3 IU/ml and the use of R_1R_1 red cells (or other antibodies and red cell samples having the equivalent sensitivity in the test). The use of an enzyme test in conjunction with the antiglobulin test would reduce the incidence of missed incompatibility or false-negative antibody screen from 4 in 10,000 to 6.4 in 100,000,000 — assuming that the antibody were detectable in the enzyme test with a sensitivity equivalent to anti-D at 0.3 IU/ml with R_1R_1 red cells; that the performance of the two techniques were independent; and that a positive enzyme test reaction with a negative antiglobulin test reaction would result in further investigation.

In the seven U.K. NEQAS exercises over the period 1988 to 1989, if participants had used the antiglobulin test alone, there would have been 608

TABLE 29
Performance of the Antiglobulin Test Alone and Antiglobulin with Enzyme Test in U.K. NEQAS Exercises Over the Period 1988 to 1989

		No. of participants who *would* have failed to detect the antibody using	
Exercise	Antibody-red cell sample	Antiglobulin test alone	Antiglobulin and enzyme test together
1988–1	Anti-A vs. A_2	1/429	0/429
	Anti-A vs. A_2B	15/427	2/427
	Anti-K vs. Kk	4/428	2/428
	Anti-B vs. A_2B	0/428	
	Anti-A,B vs. A_2	0/428	
	Anti-A,B vs. A_2B	0/428	
1988–2	Anti-B vs. B	0/440	
	Anti-K vs. Kk	2/440	1/440
	Anti-A vs. A_2	5/439	0/439
	Anti-A vs. A_2	1/439	0/439
	Anti-K vs. Kk	7/439	4/439
	Anti-A vs. A_2	1/439	0/439
	Anti-K vs. Kk	3/439	0/439
1988–A	Anti-D 0.3 IU/ml (screen)	2/419	0/419
	Anti-D 0.3 IU/ml (screen)	1/419	0/419
	Anti-K vs. Kk	0/438	
	Anti-E vs. R_2R_2	15/439	1/439
1989–1	Anti-Fy^a vs. Fg(a + b −)	52/439	52/439
	Anti-c vs. R_2R_2	0/439	
	Anti-D 0.1 IU/ml vs. R_1R_1	182/444	81/444
	Anti-D 0.1 IU/ml vs. R_1r	214/443	123/443
1989–2	Anti-D 0.3 IU/ml vs. R_1R_1	17/447	2/447
	Anti-D 0.3 IU/ml vs. R_1r	30/443	8/443
	Anti-K vs. Kk	3/444	1/444
	Anti-Fy^a vs. Fy(a + b −)	5/444	5/444
1989E3	Anti-Fy^a vs. Fy(a + b −)	5/444	5/444
	Anti-D 0.3 IU/ml (screen)	5/427	1/427
	Anti-D 0.3 IU/ml vs. R_1r	32/428	10/428
	Anti-Fy^a vs. Fy(a + b −)	4/423	4/423
	Anti-Fy^a vs. Fy(a + b −)	10/428	10/428
1989–A	Anti-D 0.1 IU/ml (screen)	57/431	13/431
	Anti-D 0.1 IU/ml (screen)	56/431	13/431
	Anti-Fy^a (screen)	13/431	13/431

Note: Total number of participants who would have failed to detect antibodies in 1988 to 1989 using an antiglobulin test alone: crossmatch procedure, 608; antibody screen procedure, 134; total, 742. Total number of participants who would have failed to detect antibodies in 1988 to 1989 using both an antiglobulin and enzyme test: crossmatch procedure, 311; antibody screen procedure, 40; total 351.

missed incompatible crossmatches and 134 false-negative antibody screenings. With the use of the antiglobulin and enzyme tests, these figures would be reduced to 311 and 40 respectively (see Table 29). The greater fall observed in false-negative antibody screening results compared to missed incompatibilities with the use of both antiglobulin and enzyme tests is probably a reflection of the greater use of the more sensitive two-stage enzyme test, rather than one-stage tests, in antibody screening procedures.

The number of U.K. participants undertaking only an antiglobulin tests has increased slowly from 0% in 1984 to 4% in 1989 for crossmatching, and from 5% in 1985 to 8% in 1989 for antibody screen procedures. An analysis of these laboratories has shown a better performance than in the U.K. as a whole. Presumably, such laboratories have a well-controlled, assured antiglobulin test procedure covering all aspects of the test: staff, reagent, equipment, and technique. A laboratory seeking to restrict antibody screen and crossmatch procedures to the antiglobulin test may justify its introduction by referring to performance of those laboratories already using only the antiglobulin test. From the analysis of the antiglobulin test over the U.K. as a whole, this would appear to be unwise — at least without introducing the additional factors present in those better-performing laboratories which make their antiglobulin procedure an effective test.

XVII. CONCLUDING COMMENTS

The aim of U.K. NEQAS is to assist laboratories to attain an adequate degree of performance. By indicating techniques that are associated with poor performance, it is hoped that participants — particularly those at the lower end of the performance spectrum — will review their practices. The philosophy of any external scheme must be one of education, not punition. External quality assessment schemes cannot be more than an adjunct to a laboratory's own internal quality procedures. Nevertheless, external schemes are the way in which a laboratory can demonstrate its ability against that of its peers, to the people dependent on its services.

The performance of participants depends on the nature of the exercise material. ABO and Rh(D) grouping appears satisfactory, at least serologically; almost all the grouping errors in the exercises are due to transcription of results or transposition of the exercise material. To some extent this may be because the U.K. NEQAS result form and samples are not as used by that participating laboratory. However, the importance of clerical error in transfusion laboratories should not be underestimated, particularly with respect to ABO errors.[13,16]

Performance in the antibody screen depends on the potency of the particular antibody and on the antigen profile of the screening cells used. A point for concern is the introduction of group and screen policies followed by an "immediate-spin" crossmatch where alloantibody has not been detected in the antibody screen using an antiblobulin test. The concern is not so much the policy, although it is known that the immediate-spin crossmatch does not detect all ABO incompatibilities,[2,5,17] particularly between group B patients and group A_2B donor blood. The concern is more with a lack of specification within the U.K. for the screening cells used in antibody screen procedures. Antibodies such as anti-Fy^a, anti-Jk^a, anti-Jk^b, anti-S, anti-s, and anti-Fy^b do often require a homozygous expression of the corresponding antigen for their ready detection. In a recent exercise (1990E1), 41 participants failed to detect anti-S in the antibody screen but detected this antibody in the crossmatch using SS red cells. Anti-Jk^a, not detected by an antibody screen using Jk(a + b+) red cells, has resulted in a severe delayed hemolytic transfusion reaction although the antibody was readily detected in the original sample when tested with Jk(a + b −) red cells (A. Black, personal communication).

It is felt that there is scope for improvement in the performance of the antiglobulin test within the U.K. The use of plastic tubes, inappropriate serum to red cell concentration ratio, nonobservance of the manufacturer's method of use, and the use of Pasteur pipettes with low ionic strength antiglobulin procedures should receive corrective attention. Where the manufacturer's recommended method of use is not followed, in countries with Product Liability legislation, users should be aware that liability for the correct performance of the reagent will rest with them, not the manufacturer.

The low ionic strength formulation commonly used[10] when mixed with an equal volume of serum has an ionic strength equivalent to 0.09 *M* NaCl, ignoring the effect of ionized buffer salts. Variation in delivery from a Pasteur pipette will be reflected in variation in the ionic strength of the incubated mix. False-positive reactions due to the binding of complement components at too low an ionic strength are unlikely. Much more likely, are false-negative reactions due to too high an ionic strength resulting in insufficient antibody-antigen reaction within the incubation period. The delivery of Pasteur pipettes is variable,[4] particularly with the use of plastic tubes,[10] where the electrostatic charge influences the size of the drop. In addition, plastic tubes tend to retain liquid on their sides and the cell button is more difficult to dislodge following centrifugation prior to reading of the test. With low ionic strength tests, particularly with plastic tubes, a pipette having a fixed volume of delivery should be used.[10]

The serum to red cell concentration ratio is a major factor in determining the sensitivity of tests; 92% of participants prepare red cell suspensions for use by eye alone, without reference to any comparator. The variability in preparation of cell suspension is marked[4] and will be reflected in the serum to red cell concentration ratio, as will variations in delivery from a Pasteur pipette. Serological reactions are biochemical reactions and are influenced by factors such as temperature, pH, ionic strength, and the ratio of reactants. It does appear that the antiglobulin test is more demanding in the preparation of red cell suspensions than can be assured by eye alone and in the delivery of reagents than can be obtained using a Pasteur pipette. A few laboratories assure the red cell suspension using a colorimeter which determines the concentration of red cells within a Pasteur pipette held in a light path; however, this device is not widely available (Inverness Blood Transfusion Centre, Scotland). The majority of participants use a Pasteur pipette for the low ionic strength antiglobulin test (86%, Exercise 1989/1).

The general performance of enzyme tests is not satisfactory, primarily because of the continued use of one-stage mix, both in antibody screen and crossmatch procedures. Where an enzyme test is required, there is little or no reason why a two-stage enzyme test cannot be used for antibody screen and a one-stage delay for crossmatch procedures where an enzyme test is required and the number of donor units to be tested makes the use of two-stage enzyme tests impracticable. The one-stage mix enzyme test is not worth the effort of undertaking in antibody screen or crossmatch procedures. Despite exercise reports demonstrating the poor performance of one-stage mix procedures, they continue to be used by 37% of participants using an enzyme technique for crossmatch and by 18% of participants using an enzyme technique for antibody screening, enzyme techniques being used by 55% of participants in crossmatch and by 80% of participants in antibody screen procedures.

The use of an antiglobulin anti-D grouping technique continues. This is used by 6% of participants with all test samples and by an additional 27% of participants on samples found to be negative with other anti-D grouping procedures. This situation probably reflects confusion whether the D^u status should be determined for patient samples and the absence of a policy on this issue. Users of antiglobulin anti-D grouping reagents should be aware that the specificity of the antiglobulin test result is not 100% (Exercise 1989-2, see Section XVI).

Adequate performance in clinical laboratories depends on a combination of factors, including suitable equipment, appropriate procedures and reagents, and trained, motivated, assured staff, operating within a framework of quality management. There is a loop of activity: information passing from the participants to the U.K. NEQAS organizing laboratory in the form of serological and questionnaire exercise data, and from the organizing laboratory to the participants in the form of analyses in which the reasons for poor performance are reported. The final part of this loop is for the appropriate staff in participating laboratories to review their practices and performance against that of their peers and to introduce changes where these are indicated; time will tell whether U.K. NEQAS has been successful in its aim.

ACKNOWLEDGMENT

U.K. National External Quality Assessment Scheme (NEQAS) (blood group serology) is supported by a grant from the U.K. Health Ministries.

REFERENCES

1. **Bailey, N. T. J.,** *Statistical Methods in Biology,* The English Universities Press, London, 1959, 58.
2. **Berry-Dortch, S., Woodside, C. H., and Boral, L. I.,** Limitations of the immediate-spin crossmatch when used for detecting ABO incompatibility, *Transfusion,* 25, 176, 1985.
3. **Black, D. and Kay, J.,** Influence of tube type on the antiglobulin test, *Med. Lab. Sci.,* 43, 169, 1986.
4. **Greendyke, R. M., Wormer, J. L., and Banzhaf, J.,** Quality Assurance in the blood bank, *Transfusion,* 71, 286, 1979.
5. **Judd, W. J., Steiner, E. A., O'Donnell, D. B., and Oderman, H. A.,** Discrepancies in reverse ABO typing due to prozone. How safe is the immediate-spin crossmatch?, *Transfusion,* 28, 334, 1988.
6. **Lentner, C., E.,** *Scientific Tables,* Vol. 2, Ciba-Geigy, Basel, 1982, 34.
7. **Lewis, S. M. and Jennings, R. D.,** United Kingdom External Quality Assessment Schemes. Background and terms of reference, Department of Health, London, 1989.
8. **Merry, A. H., Thomson, E. E., Lagar, J., Howell, P., Voak, D., Downie, M., and Stratton, F.,** Quantitation of antibody binding to erythrocytes in LISS, *Vox Sang.,* 47, 125, 1984.
9. **Mollison, P. L., Engelfriet, C. P., and Contreras, M.,** *Blood Transfusion in Clinical Medicine,* 8th ed., Blackwell Scientific, Lond, 1987, 481.
10. **Moore, H. C. and Mollison, P. L.,** Use of a low-ionic-strength medium in manual tests for antibody detection, *Transfusion,* 16, 291, 1976.
11. **Molthan, L. and Strohm, P.,** Haemolytic transfusion reaction due to anti-Kell undetectable in low-ionic-strength solution, *Am. J. Clin. Pathol.,* 4, 629, 1981.
12. **Odel, W. R., Roxby, D. J., Ryall, R. G., and Seshadli, R. S.,** A LISS spin enzyme method for the detection of red cell antibodies and its use in routine antibody screen procedures, *Transfusion,* 23, 373, 1983.
13. **Sazama, K.,** Transfusion-associated fatalities reported to the FDA between 1976 and 1985, Presented at a Conference of the American Society of Clinical Pathologists, March, 1988; quoted by Schmidt, P. J., The algorithm and the crossmatch, *Transfusion,* 29, 95, 1989.
14. **Scott, M. L., Voak, D., and Downie, D. M.,** Optimum enzyme activity and a new technique for antibody detection: an explanation for the poor performance of the one-stage mix technique, *Med. Lab. Sci.,* 45, 7, 1988.
15. **Scott, M. L. and Phillips, P. K.,** Sensitive two-stage papain technique without cell washing, *Vox Sang.,* 52, 67, 1987.
16. **Shulman, I. R. and Kent, D.,** Safety in transfusion practice — is it safe to eliminate the major crossmatch for selected patients?, *Arch. Pathol. Lab. Med.,* 113, 270, 1989.
17. **Shulman, I. A., Nelson, J. M., Lam, H. T., and Meyer, E.,** Unreliability of the immediate-spin crossmatch to detect ABO incompatibility (letter), *Transfusion,* 25, 589, 1987.
18. **Stroup, M. and Maclroy, M.,** Evaluation of the albumin antiglobulin technique in antibody detection, *Transfusion,* 5, 184, 1965.
19. **Voak, D., Downie, D., Haigh, T., and Cook, N.,** Improved antiglobulin tests to detect difficult antibodies: detection of anti-Kell by LISS, *Med. Lab. Sci.,* 39, 363, 1982.
20. **Voak, D., Downie, D. M., Moore, B. P. L., Ford, D. S., Englefriet, C. P., and Case, J.,** QC of anti-human globulin tests: use of replicate tests to improve performance, *Biotest Bull.,* 1, 41, 1986.
21. **Waters, A. H.,** Guidelines for compatibility testing in hospital blood banks, *Clin. Lab. Haematol.,* 9, 333, 1987.

Chapter 15

TISSUE TYPING AND THE USE OF MONOCLONAL ANTIBODIES TO HLA ANTIGENS

R. J. T. Hancock

TABLE OF CONTENTS

ISBN 0-8493-4938-9

I. INTRODUCTION

"Tissue typing" is a term commonly used to describe the identification of the HLA antigens expressed by particular individuals or cells. This has routinely been done by testing the reactivities of viable cells against panels of alloantisera to HLA specificities in microcytotoxicity assays (e.g., References 67 and 79). The antisera are commonly obtained from women immunized in the course of pregnancy by paternally derived foreign HLA antigens expressed by the fetus, though antisera produced in other ways, e.g., by planned immunization of volunteers, have also been used. More recently the use of monoclonal antibodies to polymorphic HLA determinants has been introduced and in addition, monoclonal antibodies to nonpolymorphic "framework" determinants have provided valuable reagents for the analysis of HLA molecules.[7,70]

This chapter will briefly review some of the recent developments in the production, analysis, and use of monoclonal antibodies to HLA antigens, relate them to the increased understanding of the structure and biological functions of HLA molecules, and indicate how monoclonal antibodies may make further contributions in the future. It will concentrate on antibodies to polymorphic determinants expressed at the cell surface, though monoclonal antibodies can contribute in other ways.[66,82,84,95]

II. HLA ANTIGENS — STRUCTURE AND FUNCTION

The HLA (human leukocyte series A) antigens are an exceptionally polymorphic group of glycoproteins detectable at the cell surface. They can be divided into two groups, the class I molecules (including HLA-A, B, and C), detectable on the majority of nucleated cells and the class II molecules (including HLA-DR, DP, and DQ) which show a more restricted distribution. The specificities recognized in 1989[9] are listed in Table 1A. These molecules are of great medical interest because of their relevance to histocompatibility i.e., in matching donor and recipient in organ transplantation[16] and because of the associations of particular HLA antigens and diseases.[39]

The biological reasons for the enormous polymorphism shown by these molecules, which is also found in comparable molecules, encoded by comparable clusters of genes (the so-called major histocompatibility complex, or MHC, antigens) in other species, were obscure until the discovery of the phenomenon of MHC restriction provided an attractive hypothesis. It was found that the T lymphocytes of the immune system recognized foreign antigen in the context of MHC antigens and could not recognize it if it was presented in the context of an inappropriate MHC antigen. Very briefly,[42,61,69] T lymphocytes expressing a particular glycoprotein marker (CD8) (which included cytotoxic T cells capable of killing virus-infected targets) were restricted by class I and T lymphocytes, expressing another glycoprotein marker,

CD4, which included regulatory T cells with a ''helper'' function, were restricted by class II antigens. The capacity to recognize antigen in this ''restricted'' manner was acquired in the thymus. The discovery of restriction suggested that the existence of polymorphism at the MHC locus could confer an advantage on a population by making it more difficult for a microorganism to evade immune surveillance by ''molecular mimicry'' of a particular HLA antigen. Restriction could also be related to the immunogenicity of MHC molecules; MHC polymorphisms were recognized as ''foreign'' because they resembled self-MHC + foreign (e.g., microbial) antigen (see Reference 23). Some of the more recent advances in understanding of the structure and function of HLA molecules are listed below.

No attempt will be made to discuss the mechanisms which determine whether antigens are restricted by class I or class II; the reader is referred to other recent articles (e.g., References 42, 61, and 69).

A. CLASS I

Class I MHC antigens, which can be detected on most nucleated cells, are bimolecular complexes of a glycosylated 44-kDa heavy chain tightly but noncovalently bound to the 11.6-kDa β_2-microglobulin (Figure 1). It is the genes for the heavy chains which are located in the MHC on chromosome 6 (see Figure 2) while the gene for the β_2-microglobulin is located on chromosome 15.[24] Though ''nonclassical'' class I genes are capable of expression,[40,49] most of the information on the structure of class I molecules is based on investigations of the A, B, and C MHC loci and their products and it is these products, which are polymorphic, which are of most interest to tissue typists. The heavy chains have three extracellular domains (α_1, α_2, and α_3), a transmembrane portion, and a cytoplasmic domain (Figure 1). The extracellular domains of the heavy chain contain two disulfide loops (Figure 1) and the amino acid sequence of the α_3 domain shows highly significant homology with immunoglobulin constant regions as does β_2-microglobulin.[78]

The crystallographic structures of two HLA class I molecules, A2 and Aw68, have been recently determined[10,11,22] and, together with the large amount of information now available on the sequences of MHC genes, have shed considerable light on the mechanisms by which MHC molecules regulate immune responses. The crystallographic investigations showed that carboxy-terminal parts of both the α_1 and α_2 domains of the class I heavy chains are coiled in an α-helical conformation while the amino-terminal regions are arranged in flattened β-pleated sheets. The two α-helical parts form the sides of a groove and the flattened β-pleated sheets its floor. The crystallographic investigations also showed the presence within this groove of ill-defined material which, it was suggested, represented a mixture of bound peptides. Since there was already evidence that cytotoxic T cells could recognize peptides in the context of MHC, e.g., that target cells pulsed with synthetic influenza virus peptides became sensitized to killing by flu-specific cytotoxic T cells (see Reference 91 for review), it was rational to propose that peptides

TABLE 1A
List of Recognized HLA Specifities[9]

A	B	C	D	DR	DQ	DP
A1	B5	Cw1	Dw1	DR1	DQw1	DPw1
A2	B7	Cw2	Dw2	DR2	DQw2	DPw2
A3	B8	Cw3	Dw3	DR3	DQw3	DPw3
A9	B12	Cw4	Dw4	DR4	DQw4	DPw4
A10	B13	Cw5	Dw5	DR5	DQw5(w1)	DPw5
A11	B14	Cw6	Dw6	DRw6	DQw6(w1)	DPw6
Aw19	B15	Cw7	Dw7	DR7	DQw7(w3)	
A23(9)	B16	Cw8	Dw8	DRw8	DQw8(w3)	
A24(9)	B17	Cw9(w3)	Dw9	DR9	DQw9(w3)	
A25(10)	B18	Cw10(w3)	Dw10	DRw10		
A26(10)	B21	Cw11	Dw11(w7)	DRw11(5)		
A28	Bw22		Dw12	DRw12(5)		
A29(w19)	B27		Dw13	DRw13(w6)		
A30(w19)	B35		Dw14	DRw14(w6)		
A31(w19)	B37		Dw15	DRw15(2)		
A32(w19)	B38(16)		Dw16	DRw16(2)		
Aw33(w19)	B39(16)		Dw17(w7)	DRw17(3)		
Aw34(10)	B40		Dw18(w6)	DRw18(3)		
Aw36	Bw41		Dw19(w6)			
Aw43	Bw42		Dw20	DRw52		
Aw66(10)	B44(12)		Dw21			
Aw68(28)	B45(12)		Dw22	DRw53		
Aw69(28)	Bw46		Dw23			
Aw74(w19)	Bw47		Dw24			
	Bw48		Dw25			
	B49(21)		Dw26			
	Bw50(21)					
	B51(5)					
	Bw52(5)					
	Bw53					
	Bw54(w22)					
	Bw55(w22)					
	Bw56(w22)					
	Bw57(17)					
	Bw58(17)					
	Bw59					
	Bw60(40)					
	Bw61(40)					
	Bw62(15)					
	Bw63(15)					
	Bw64(14)					
	Bw65(14)					
	Bw67					
	Bw70					
	Bw71(w70)					
	Bw72(w70)					

TABLE 1A (continued)
List of Recognized HLA Specifities[9]

A	B	C	D	DR	DQ	DP
	Bw73					
	Bw75(15)					
	Bw76(15)					
	Bw77(15)					
	Bw4					
	Bw6					

Note: Where specificities are splits of a broader one, the broad specificity is listed in parentheses. Every HLA-B locus molecule has either the Bw4 or Bw6 epitope. In addition HLA-Aw24 and HLA-A32 have the Bw4 epitope and HLA-Cw3 is cross-reactive with Bw6. The B-locus specificities associated with Bw4 and Bw6 are as follows: Bw4: B5, B13, B17, B27, B37, B38(16), B44(12), Bw47, B49(21), B51(5), Bw52(5), Bw53, Bw57(17), Bw58(17), Bw59, Bw63(15), Bw77(15); Bw6: B7, B8, B14, B18, Bw22, B35, B39(16), B40, Bw41, Bw42, B45(12), Bw46, Bw48, Bw50(21), Bw54(w22), Bw55(w22), Bw56(w22), Bw60(40), Bw61(40), Bw62(15), Bw64(14), Bw65(14), Bw67, Bw70, Bw71(w70), Bw72(w70), Bw73, Bw75(15), Bw76(15). The DR specificities associated with DRw52 and DRw53 are as follows: DRw52: DR3, DR5, DRw6, DRw8, DRw11(5), DRw12(5), DRw13(w6), DRw14(w6), DRw17(3), DRw18(3); DRw53: DR4, DR7, DR9.

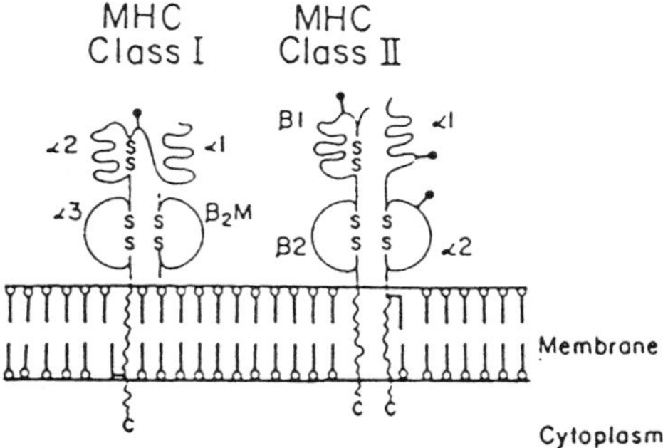

FIGURE 1. Class I and class II MHC antigens. S-S indicates disulfide bonds between cysteine residues. C, Carboxy terminus; ↑ , carbohydrate side chains. (After Korman et al., Reference 53.)

bound in the cleft of the MHC class I molecule acted as targets for class I restricted CD8-positive cytotoxic T lymphocytes. The structure of the class I heavy chain is shown in Figure 3 and the interaction with T lymphocytes summarized, in cartoon form, in Figure 4. The latter cartoon also gives a model for the mechanism of restriction of cytotoxic CD8-positive lymphocytes by class I, i.e., that the CD8 molecule binds specifically to class I, more specifically to the α_3 domain.[81]

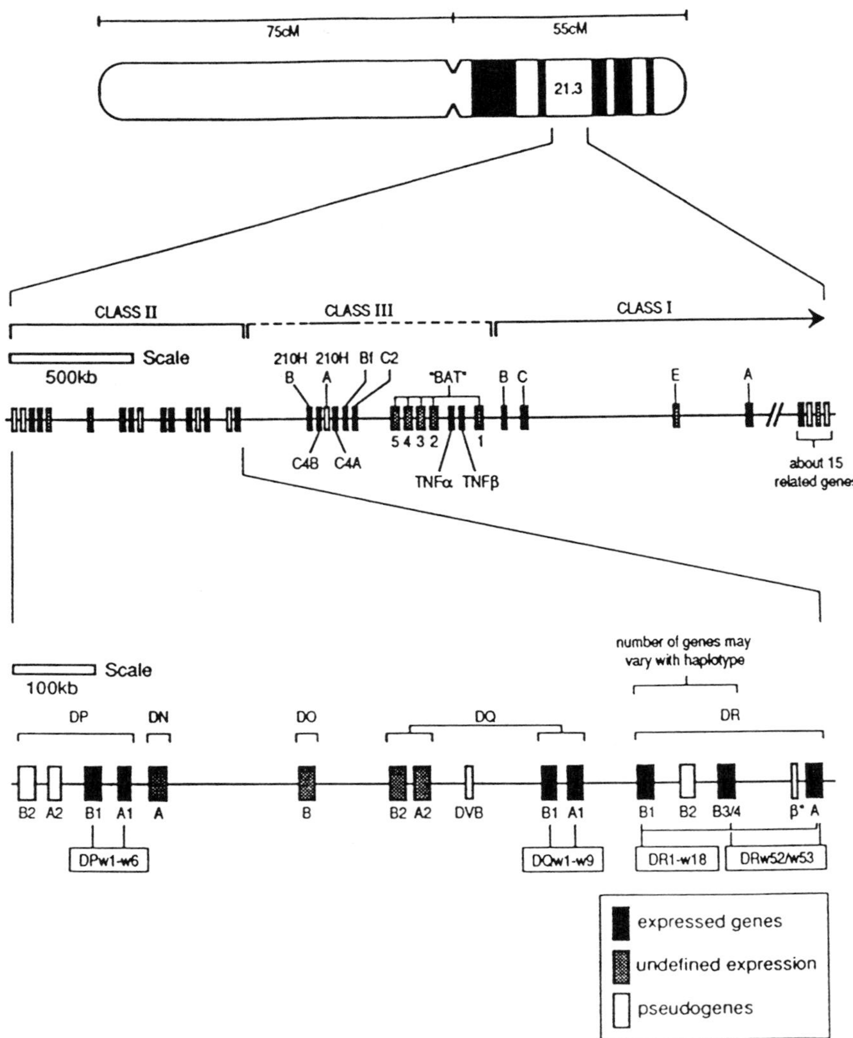

FIGURE 2. Arrangement of HLA genes on chromosome 6. The molecular characteristics of the products of the class I and class II genes are listed in Table 1B. The so-called class III genes (for tumor necrosis factor, TNF; "HLA-B-associated transcript" genes, BAT; 21 hydroxylase, 210H; and complement components, C2, C4, Bf) are localized on the map, but are not dealt with in the course of this chapter. (From figure provided by Dr. J. Bidwell.)

This three-dimensional model also allowed the localization of residues which had been identified as critical for the formation of selected alloantigenic determinants by comparisons of the sequences of class I antigens with their reactivities with particular monoclonal antibodies or cytotoxic T cells. Most

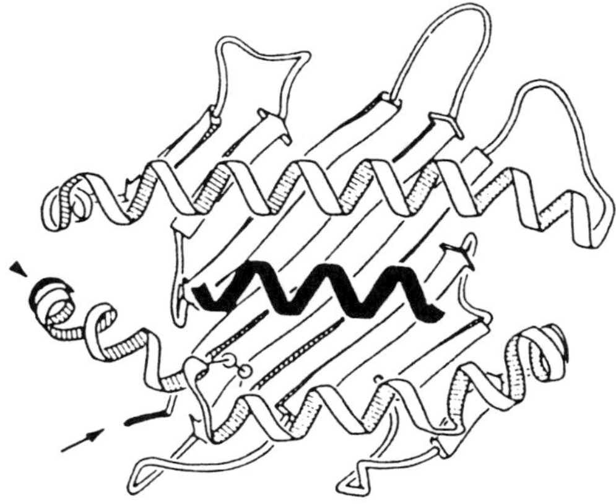

FIGURE 3. Model of class I, showing the peptide-binding groove. α-Helices shown as helical ribbons; β-strands as broad arrows. Amino terminus of α_1 domain shown by black arrow and carboxy terminus of α_2 by arrowhead. Darkened helix represents bound peptide. (From Parham, P. et al., in *Immunobiology of HLA,* Vol. 2, Dupont, B., Ed., Springer-Verlag, Berlin, 1989, 10. With permission.)

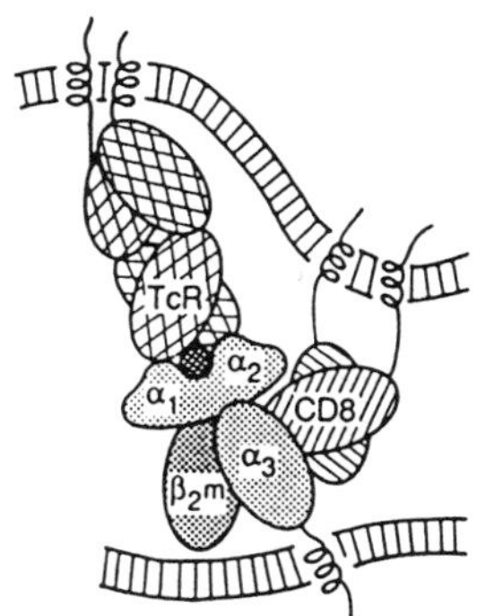

FIGURE 4. Interaction of peptide + class I with T cell receptor. Figure also shows interaction of CD8 with class I. (From Parham, P., *Nature,* 342, 617, 1989. With permission.)

of the sequences critical for reactions with monoclonal antibodies were found on the α-helices with at least one residue in each epitope solvent exposed and apparently accessible to direct recognition by antibody. However, substitutions need not necessarily alter binding at the same site and examples of substitutions which apparently alter antibody binding elsewhere have been reported,[92] and not all alloantigenic class I determinants can be correlated with particular sequences.[93]

Plotting the residues critically involved in recognition by T cells provided a rather different picture. Though some of these variant residues were potentially directly accessible to the T-cell receptor, i.e., their side chains faced "up" (using the convention that the diagram of the class I molecule shown in Figure 3 is a view from "above"), the majority pointed into the groove, suggesting that alloreactivity may involve the recognition by the T cell of a complex between allo-HLA and peptide, whether derived from class I or some other molecule. There is other evidence that peptide binding may be involved in alloantigen formation.[37,72]

The initial reports[10,11] were supported by subsequent evidence[73] that the majority of the polymorphic residues in class I molecules which showed high variability were in positions in the α-helices of the α_1 and α_2 domains where their side chains either pointed "up" and were potentially able to interact with the T-cell receptor or into the groove, where they could interact with peptide. All these data were consistent with the view that class I polymorphisms altered the "self"-antigens which would be recognized by the T-cell receptor in association with foreign peptides or the capacity of the MHC molecules to bind and present polypeptides. They, therefore, very specifically related MHC polymorphism to the capacity to develop immune responses to foreign antigens and illuminated the mechanisms of allorecognition.

Sequence information also provides insights into the ways in which individual loci may be related to one another. The sequences investigated show evidence of locus-specific character, including both the location of polymorphic positions and ways in which small sequences are arranged. This can be interpreted as evidence that genetic exchange between alleles of the same loci has been a more important mechanism in the generation of HLA-A, -B, and -C diversity than genetic exchange between alleles at different loci.[73,75] There is, however, also evidence of some genetic exchange (gene conversion) between alleles at different loci.[75] Extensive sharing of polymorphisms between chimpanzee and human A, B, and C MHC loci has been interpreted as evidence that much of the current polymorphism originated before the emergence of *Homo sapiens*.[75]

B. CLASS II

Class II antigens are found on a more limited range of cells than class I. These include B lymphocytes, activated T lymphocytes, dendritic cells, and cells of the macrophage myeloid series. Unlike class I, the class II antigens were originally defined by cellular reactions, i.e., the capacity of class II disparate cells to stimulate T-cell proliferation. Subsequently, serological determinants which correlated with the T-cell-defined determinants were delineated. Like class I, they are glycoprotein dimers of a heavy (α) and light (β) chain (see Figure 1), but unlike class I the genes for both chains are located in the MHC complex (see Figure 2). Most of the information currently available relates to three families of class II molecules,[9] DP, DQ, and DR

TABLE 1B
Names for Class I and Class II Genes in the HLA Region

Name	Previous equivalents	Molecular characteristics
HLA-A	—	Class I α chain
HLA-B	—	Class I α chain
HLA-C	—	Class I α chain
HLA-E	E, "6.2"	Associated with class I 6.2 kb *Hind*III fragment
HLA-F	F, "5.4"	Associated with class I 5.4 kb *Hind*III fragment
HLA-G	G, "6.0"	Associated with class I 6.0 kb *Hind*III fragment
HLA-DRA	DRα	DR α chain
HLA-DRB1	DRβ1, DR1B	DR β1 chain determining specificities DR1, DR3, DR4, DR5, etc.
HLA-DRB2	DRβII	Pseudogene with DR-β-like sequences
HLA-DRB3	DRβIII, DR3B	DR β3 chain determining DRw52 and Dw24, Dw25, Dw26 specificities
HLA-DRB4	DRβIV, DR4B	DR β4 chain determining DRw53
HLA-DRB5	DRβIII	DR β5 chain found in DR2 haplotypes
HLA-DQA1	DQα1, DQ1A	DQ α chain as expressed
HLA-DQB1	DQβ1, DQ1B	DQ β chain as expressed
HLA-DQA2	DXα, DQ2A	DQ α-chain-related sequence, not known to be expressed
HLA-DQB2	DXβ, DQ2B	DQ β-chain-related sequence, not known to be expressed
HLA-DOB	DOβ	DOβ chain
HLA-DNA	DZα, DOα	DN α chain
HLA-DPA1	DPα1, DP1A	DP α chain as expressed
HLA-DPB1	DPβ1, DP1B	DP β chain as expressed
HLA-DPA2	DPα2, DP2A	DP α-chain-related pseudogene
HLA-DPB2	DPβ2, DP2B	DP β-chain-related pseudogene

Note: After report by World Health Organization Nomenclature Committee (Reference 8). The class I genes for HLA-F and HLA-G, which are not named in Figure 2 map telomeric to HLA-A (Reference 49).

(see Figure 2). In DP molecules the β-chain is polymorphic while the α-chain is less so.[2] In DQ, both α- and β-chains show significant polymorphism. In most genotypes the DR specificity (DR1, DR3, etc., see Table 1A) is coded for by the genes at the DRB1 locus and the "supertypic" DRw52 and w53 specificities are coded for by genes at the DRB3 and DRB4 loci, respectively (see Table 1B). However, in DR2 the gene at the B5 is the more polymorphic and both the B1 and B5 loci apparently code for DR2 determinants.[45] The number of DRB genes varies between genotypes.

Both light and heavy chains of class II molecules have four domains, two extracellular (see Figure 1), and the extracellular domains of the α- and β-chains contain, respectively, one and two disulfide loops. The membrane-proximal extracellular domains (α_2 and β_2) show homology with immunoglobulin while the membrane-distal domains show lower but significant homology with class I α_1 and α_2 domains.

TABLE 2
Association of DR and Dw Specificities

HLA alleles[a]	HLA-DR specificities	HLA-D-associated (T-cell-defined) specificities
DRB1*0101	DR1	Dw1
DRB1*0102	DR1	Dw20
DRB1*0103	DR'BR'	Dw'BON'
DRB1*1501	DRw15(2)	Dw2
DRB1*1502	DRw15(2)	Dw12
DRB1*1601	DRw16(2)	Dw21
DRB1*1602	DRw16(2)	Dw22
DRB1*0301	DRw17(3)	Dw3
DRB1*0302	DRw18(3)	Dw'RSH'
DRB1*0401	DR4	Dw4
DRB1*0402	DR4	Dw10
DRB1*0403	DR4	Dw13
DRB1*0404	DR4	Dw14
DRB1*0405	DR4	Dw15
DRB1*0406	DR4	Dw'KT2'
DRB1*0407	DR4	Dw13
DRB1*0408	DR4	Dw14
DRB1*1101	DRw11(5)	Dw5
DRB1*1102	DRw11(5)	Dw'JVM'
DRB1*1103	DRw11(5)	—
DRB1*1104	DRw11(5)	Dw'FS'
DRB1*1201	DRw12(5)	Dw'DB6'
DRB1*1301	DRw13(w6)	Dw18
DRB1*1302	DRw13(w6)	Dw19
DRB1*1303	DRw13(w6)	Dw'HAG'
DRB1*1401	DRw14(w6)	Dw9
DRB1*1402	DRw14(w6)	Dw16
DRB1*0701	DR7	Dw17
DRB1*0702	DR7	Dw'DB1'
DRB1*0801	DRw8	Dw8.1
DRB1*0802	DRw8	Dw8.2
DRB1*0803	DRw8	Dw8.3
DRB1*0901	DR9	Dw23
DRB1*1001	DRw10	—
DRB3*0101	DRw52a	Dw24
DRB3*0201	DRw52b	Dw25
DRB3*0202	DRw52b	Dw25
DRB3*0301	DRw52c	Dw26
DRB4*0101	DRw53	Dw4, Dw10, Dw13, Dw14, Dw15, Dw17, Dw23

TABLE 2 (continued)
Association of DR and Dw Specificities

HLA alleles[a]	HLA-DR specificities	HLA-D-associated (T-cell-defined) specificities
DRB5*0101	DRw15(2)	Dw2
DRB5*0102	DRw15(2)	Dw12
DRB5*0201	DRw16(2)	Dw21
DRB5*0202	DRw16(2)	Dw22

[a] This table summarizes the T-cell-defined Dw type usually, though not necessarily always, associated with a particular allele. Alleles are named according to the World Health Organization Nomenclature Committee report, August, 1989.[8] The first part of the name indicates the locus, the second the most closely associated specificity.

A three-dimensional structure for class I molecules based on the crystallographic structure of class I has been proposed[12] in which α-helically coiled parts of the α_1 and α_2 domains form the sides and β-pleated sheets the floor of a peptide-binding cleft. In this model, as in that for class I, residues shown to be critically involved in the formation of epitopes recognized by monoclonal antibodies to polymorphic determinants are solvent accessible, while residues critically involved in recognition by T cells (including those associated with allorecognition) include residues which would be directly accessible to the T cell and others which would be expected to affect peptide binding. This model provides a mechanism for class II-restricted T-cell recognition of antigens and, since mutations in the class II molecule are expected to alter the binding of peptides or the antigenic context in which they are recognized, is consistent with earlier work mapping ''immune response'' genes to the class II region of the MHC.[44] The model also suggests that alloreactivity can involve the recognition of peptide plus allo-HLA and there is experimental evidence consistent with this (e.g., see References 19, 58, and 64).

As in the case of class I molecules, sequence information also provides insights into the way in which individual genes and loci may be related to one another (see, e.g., References 25 and 26).

There has been (see, e.g., References 1, 43, and 86) debate about the relative contributions of various class II epitopes to the stimulation of T lymphocytes in primary cultures, though it is agreed that determinants coded for by the DR and DQ class II determinants can stimulate substantial proliferation in primary mixed lymphocyte cultures[1] and that DP disparity is more readily demonstrated in secondary cultures.[76] The associations of Dw types, determined by proliferative responses in primary mixed lymphocyte cultures, with individual DR alleles are listed in Table 2.

III. MONOCLONAL ANTIBODIES TO HLA ANTIGENS

Sera from women immunized by pregnancy have been a major source of antibodies for the analysis of HLA antigens. These sera are mixtures of antibodies and may require absorption before use for tissue typing or the analysis of antigenic cross-reactivity. Individual sera are available in only limited quantities and the necessity for continual serum screening involves significant costs. The development of techniques for the production of monoclonal antibodies offered the hope that it would be possible to produce monospecific reagents in essentially unlimited quantities. Some of the work on production, screening, and analysis of monoclonal anti-HLA antibodies is briefly reviewed below, with particular emphasis on more recent developments.

A. PRODUCTION OF RODENT MONOCLONAL ANTIBODIES TO HLA ANTIGENS

These techniques are well established[21] and will not be described in detail. The essentials are that lymphocytes from an immunized animal (usually a mouse) are fused to a tumor cell line, the antibodies produced by these hybrid cells analyzed, and selected hybridomas plated out at limiting dilutions to produce monoclonal antibody-producing colonies.

Animals have been immunized with a variety of preparations, including purified HLA antigens,[7,30] whole cells, and mouse cells transfected with human genes and expressing HLA antigens.[38,96] More recently, it has been possible to use transgenic mice which have had HLA genes introduced into their genomes.[28] The specificities of the antibodies produced are discussed in a subsequent section.

B. PRODUCTION OF HUMAN MONOCLONAL ANTIBODIES TO HLA ANTIGENS

The production of human monoclonal antibodies in general has lagged behind the production of mouse monoclonal antibodies, partly because of the lack of generally accepted appropriate fusion partners. Nevertheless, in 1986, several groups reported the *in vitro* production of human monoclonal antibodies to HLA antigens, two to public determinants on class II[20,54] (one following a preliminary report in 1985[41]), one to HLA-DQw2,[77] and one with specificity for HLA-DR5.[29] Since then, a series of human monoclonal antibodies to HLA antigens have been reported,[31,33–35,50–52,53,57,66,97] most of them from a relatively small number of centers. In general, they have been produced by obtaining cells from individuals immunized *in vivo* by mechanisms including pregnancy (e.g., Reference 34) and planned immunization (e.g., Reference 77) and infecting the B cells with Epstein-Barr virus (EBV) to produce antibody-secreting B-cell lines. These are "cloned" and/or fused to an appropriate cell line. Fusion partners include both mouse (e.g., Reference 31) and human (e.g., Reference 35) lines. Although relatively straightforward in principle, the procedures are often difficult to put into practice. EBV-immortalized antibody-producing B-cell lines are frequently difficult to clone and/or cease antibody production. Various procedures have been used to address these problems, including the use of medium "conditioned" by growing B-cell lines,[29] cloning cells in soft agar,[56] and, as an alternative to cloning by limiting dilution, the "picking" of clusters of cells with a finely drawn pipette and their transfer to individual wells.[27] It is a little hard to compare the efficacies of the different protocols at this stage, particularly since it is possible that the B-cell lines to which they are being applied are heterogeneous and evolving populations. It is a not uncommon finding that a protocol which is helpful with a cell line fairly soon after its production is less effective after the cell line has been grown for a longer period. The capacity of the cell line to produce or respond to growth factors may alter with time. Differences between the B-cell lines may also contribute to the differences in the usefulness of particular fusion partners observed by different laboratories, as may other factors.[85] However, bearing in mind the above caveats, it seems worth pointing out that a high proportion of the publications describing human monoclonal antibodies to HLA antigens utilize the technique of "cluster picking".

C. SCREENING AND ANALYSIS

The screening procedures applied in the production of monoclonal antibodies are determined by the objectives of the program. Where the aim is to provide a class-specific antibody (e.g., anti-HLA class II), supernatants can be screened initially against a target expressing class II (e.g., a B-cell line) and a target which does not express class II (e.g., MOLT4). Where the objective is to produce antibodies to polymorphic HLA determinants, supernatants can be screened against a panel of target cells, some of which would be expected to react with the antibody and some of which would not. Decisions also have to be made on whether the screening is to be confined to a particular type of assay (e.g., cytotoxicity) or combinations (e.g., cytotoxicity and enzyme-linked immunosorbent assay [ELISA]) and again, this is related to the overall aim of the program. Since the quantities of antibody available at the early stages of monoclonal antibody production are limited, it is desirable to use assays which use small quantitites of antibody. The standard microcytotoxicity assay[79] uses only one microliter of antibody and solid-phase ELISA assays which utilize microELISA readers[18,32] in which the antigen (usually glutaraldehyde-fixed cells) is attached to the bases of wells of Terasaki tissue-typing plates and use only 5 μl of supernatant. Other binding assays which use small quantities of antibody have also been reported.[50] It is sometimes useful to carry out a prescreen for the presence of immunoglobulin.[32]

Once selected antibodies have been grown up in larger volumes, more extensive analyses can be applied to them. It is possible to analyze cytotoxic antibodies against panels of lymphocytes using standard microcytotoxicity procedures provided the following points are borne in mind.

(1) It cannot be emphasized too strongly that some batches of complement which are satisfactory for the analysis of alloantisera produce sporadic "extra" cytotoxicity when used with monoclonal antibodies. A simple explanation for this phenomenon is that the sera used as complement sources (usually obtained from rabbits) also contain cytotoxic xenoantibodies i.e., "anti-species" antibodies. When they are used with whole human serum the activity of these xenoantibodies is blocked by reactions with similar antigens on serum proteins. When they are used with monoclonal antibodies suspended in tissue culture medium + fetal calf serum, this blocking effect is absent and sporadic cytotoxicity of target cells results. This problem can be avoided by screening complement batches for the absence of cytotoxicity against cells suspended in tissue culture medium + fetal calf serum and rejecting inappropriate batches. Alternatively, it may be possible to block this cytotoxicity by adding human serum to the monoclonal antibody. This may not be appropriate for all monoclonal antibodies, and there have been recommendations that human serum should not be used in medium for their dilution, but it is clearly effective with some (K. Gelsthorpe and V. Joysey, personal communication).

(2) The antibodies have to be used at an appropriate dilution. It is possible to produce monoclonal antibodies at very high titers, but if they are added to tissue-typing plates in this concentrated form it is very easy for them to be carried over to contaminate reagents in surrounding wells. Conversely if they are diluted too much, the antibody apparently sometimes sticks to the plastic of the container, leading to lack of reactivity. However these are addressable problems and by diluting the antibodies to an appropriate dilution in a fairly protein-rich medium such as Medium 199 + 20% fetal calf serum, and taking appropriate precautions to prevent carryover, it is possible to use them on the same plates as alloantisera (e.g., see References 17 and 46). Some workers place a well containing tissue culture medium next to the monoclonal antibody well as a control for carryover. Alternatively, the wells containing the monoclonal antibody can be at the edge of the plate so that these are the last wells to have cells or complement added.

The above procedures are satisfactory for the analysis of cytotoxic antibodies with readily recognized specificities, but where the antibodies are not cytotoxic, or where the specificity is not readily recognizable, alternative/additional procedures may be used. The antibodies can be tested in binding assays against larger panels of cells to determine their specificity and the results of both binding and cytotoxicity assays can be supplemented by various blocking procedures, e.g., determining the inhibitory effects of preincubating the targets with antibodies of known specificity.[30,50,51,55] Although assays of this type need to be interpreted cautiously and critically, since blocking may result from steric hindrance rather than a genuine competition for the same molecule,[71] they can provide useful information with monoclonal antibodies just as they have with sera.[4,87] Alternatively, it is possible to purify antigens from the cells either electrophoretically[90] (e.g., Reference 97) or by binding monoclonal antibodies to HLA determinants (e.g., see Reference 50). A further approach is to test their reactivity against cells transfected with HLA genes and expressing single products.[5,38,97]

D. SEROLOGICAL SPECIFICITIES AND ANTIGENIC CROSS-REACTIVITIES DEFINED BY MONOCLONAL ANTIBODIES

It is clear that some serological specificities previously defined by allo-antisera can be identified by monoclonal antibodies. It is not possible to give an unqualified list of these specificities because different protocols and laboratories may produce different conclusions. However, a guide to progress in the area can be obtained from the reports of the International Histocompatibility Workshops, which have analyzed increasing numbers of these reagents,[47,68] and also by consulting the register of monoclonal antibodies maintained by Colombani et al.[17] In a recent report,[17] monoclonal antibodies submitted to the 10th International Histocompatibility Workshop were compared with those in the register and the results are summarized in Table 3 (A and B). Approximately one third of HLA specificities could be recognized by monoclonal antibodies, the overwhelming majority of them derived from mice. The use of monoclonal antibodies as tissue-typing reagents is clearly possible. The development of further reagents of this type requires (1) the existence of single antigenic determinants/epitopes unique to individual HLA antigens or groups of antigens and (2) the production of cells immunized by these epitopes in sufficient numbers to make their immortalization and cloning practical. Some guidance on the likely existence of such epitopes can be obtained by comparing the sequences of different HLA molecules, mapping the residues which distinguish individual antigens on the three-dimensional structure,[65,74] and relating them to the reactivities with existing serological reagents. Using this approach, it has, for instance, been concluded that the production of a single specific anti-A2 monoclonal antibody is unlikely and that the A2 specificity is defined by a combination of antibodies to different A2 epitopes.[74]

The efficacies of the various procedures to increase the frequency of antibodies to polymorphic epitopes remain to be fully evaluated. The use of different mouse strains may be helpful.[80] Immunizing mice with mouse cells transfected with human HLA genes and expressing HLA antigens can produce informative reagents (see, e.g., Reference 38 and 96) and the production of hybrid mouse/human class II molecules[63] offers the possibility of immunizing

TABLE 3A
Summary of Monoclonal Antibodies to HLA Class I Specificities

HLA	Number in WS[a]	Number in Register	HLA	Number in WS[a]	Number in Register
A2	2	6	B7	0	1
A2 + A28	13	22	B7 (+ B27 + Bw22 + B40 +)[b]	6	17[c]
A2 + Aw69	2	7	B27	1	5[d]
A3	5	8	B27 + Bw47	1	2
A3 + A11	1	4	B8	4	4
A9	2	3	B8 (+ B14 + B16 + B18 +)[b]	1	4
A10	2	2	B13	4	8
A25	0	1[c]	Bw4 (+ A23 + A24 + A32)[b]	4	8
A25 + A32	2	5	Bw6	2	9
A29	1	7	A2 + B17	0	2
A30 + 31	1	1	A2 + B16	0	1
A31	1	1	Aw19 + B7 +	0	2
Cw1 + Cw3	0	1	A32 + B27	0	2

[a] 10th International Histocompatibility Workshop.
[b] Specificities in parentheses are those generally associated with the main specificity.
[c] Includes one human MoAb.
[d] Includes two human MoAbs.

From Colombani, J. et al., *Tissue Antigens*, 34, 97, 1989. With permission.

mice with molecules with a more limited number of human determinants. However, what is being examined is the response of the mouse's immune system to human HLA antigens, and immunization of mice with transfectant cells has also produced antibodies which were apparently directed to a framework determinant or which showed cross reactions other than those usually defined by human alloantisera.[88] Immunizing normal mice with cells from transgenic mice expressing HLA antigens[48] is subject to the same caveat. The use, as ''responders'', of transgenic mice expressing HLA antigens could, however, be expected to address some of these problems since the mice would be expected to be tolerant to the HLA antigens which they express and immunizations between transgenic mice expressing different HLA antigens have allowed the production of monoclonal antibodies to polymorphic determinants.[28] It should not be expected that this approach will be entirely without problems, since the expression of a particular human HLA antigen by a transgenic mouse does not necessarily lead to complete tolerance to that antigen.[3]

The use of human cells for the production of monoclonal antibodies may be expected to be helpful since one would not expect the production of the ''anti-species'' antibodies produced by mice. However, though specific typing reagents[31,51,52] and human monoclonal antibodies recognizing cross-reactivities similar to those previously identified by alloantisera have been produced,[97]

TABLE 3B
Summary of Monoclonal Antibodies to HLA Class II Specificities

HLA	Number in WS[a]	Number in Register
DR1 + DR4	2	5
DR2	0	2[b]
DR3	3	3
DR3 + DRw6	1	6
DR4	1	2
DR5	2	4[c]
DR7	4	4
Non-DR7	4	10
DRw52	6	25[b]
DRw53	1	5[b]
DQw1	9	25[b]
DQw2	3	4[b]
DQw3	7	11
DQw4(WA)	2	2
DQw7(TA10)	3	5
DQw6 + DQw8 + DQw9(2B3)	0	5[b]
DPw2 + DPw3 + DR5	0	1
DPw2 + DPw4	1	1

[a] 10th International Histocompatibility Workshop.
[b] Includes one human MoAb.
[c] Includes two human MoAbs.

From Colombani,, J. et al., *Tissue Antigens,* 34, 97, 1989. With permission.

many of the antibodies identify cross reactions which have not been commonly described with alloantisera.[33,55] It is not clear to what extent this is because monoclonal antibodies are particularly powerful tools for the identification of cross-reactivity and to what extent it reflects the use of EBV, which is a polyclonal activator[14] and may immortalize cells which make relatively little contribution to circulating serum antibody. Only further work will determine the degree to which the identification of cross reactivities by monoclonal antibodies will be followed by their identification in serum, as has happened in the past.[15,62] What is clear is that monoclonal antibodies identify determinants to which antibodies can be produced and may therefore be helpful in identifying polymorphisms which may affect graft survival and provide guidance on the production of further typing reagents, whether these polymorphisms are ultimately "typed" serologically or by molecular genetic techniques.[6,13,94]

Monoclonal antibodies may therefore have a role not only in current tissue typing but also in the development of further typing reagents in the future.

ACKNOWLEDGMENTS

I would like to thank Dr. Jeff Bidwell, Bristol, and Baillière Tindall Ltd. for permission to use the summary of knowledge on the molecular genetics of HLA loci in Figure 2; Munksgard International Publishers Ltd., Copenhagen, for permission to use material in Figure 1 (© 1985) and Table 3 (© 1989); and Springer-Verlag, Heidelberg, for permission to use material in Figure 3. Figure 4 is reprinted by permission from *Nature,* Vol. 342, pp. 617–692, © 1989, Macmillan Magazines Ltd.

In this chapter I have given my personal view of this subject. It should not be taken as the official position of any organization.

REFERENCES

1. **Bach, F. H. and Reinsmoen, N. L.,** The role of HLA-DR and HLA-DQ products in T lymphocyte activation and in contributing to 'Dw specificities', *Hum. Immunol.,* 16, 271, 1986.
2. **Bell, J. I., Todd, J. A., and McDevitt, H. O.,** Molecular structure of human class II antigens, in *Immunobiology of HLA,* Vol. 2, Dupont, B. Ed., Springer-Verlag, Berlin, 1989, 40.
3. **Bernhard, D. J., Ai-Xuan, T. L., Barbosa, J. A., Lacy, E., and Engelhard, V. H.,** Cytotoxic T lymphocytes from HLA-A2 transgenic mice specific for HLA-A2 expressed on human cells, *J. Exp. Med.,* 163, 1157, 1988.
4. **Bernoco, D., Bernoco, M., Ceppellini, R., Poulik, M. D., van Leeuwen, A., and van Rood, J. J.,** B-cell antigens of the HLA system: a simple serotyping technique based on non-cytotoxic anti-β_2 microglobulin reagents, *Tissue Antigens,* 8, 253, 1976.
5. **Biddison, W. E., Anderson, R. A., Cowan, E. P., Turner, R. V., Coligan, J. E., Hannestad, K., Hansen, T., and Maloy, W. L.,** Structural studies of an HLA-O3 alloantigenic epitope defined by a human hybridoma antibody, *Immunogenetics,* 30, 54, 1989.
6. **Bidwell, J. L., Bidwell, E. A., Savage, D. A., Middleton, D., Klouda, P. T., and Bradley, B. A.,** A DNA-RFLP typing system which positively identifies serologically well defined and ill defined HLA-DR and DQ alleles, including DRw10, *Transplantation,* 45, 640, 1988.
7. **Bodmer, J. G. and Bodmer, W. F.,** Monoclonal antibodies to HLA determinants, *Br. Med. Bull.,* 40, 267, 1984.
8. **Bodmer, J. G., Marsh, S. G., and Albert, E.,** Nomenclature for factors of the HLA system, 1989, *Immunol. Today,* 11, 3, 1990.
9. **Bodmer, W. F., Albert, E., Bodmer, J. G., Dupont, B., Mach, B., Mayr, W. R., Sasazuki, T., Schreuder, G. M. Th., Svejgaard, A., and Terasaki, P. I.,** Nomenclature for factors of the HLA system, 1987, in *Immunobiology of HLA,* Vol. 1, Dupont, B., Ed., Springer-Verlag, Berlin, 1989, 72.
10. **Bjorkman, P. J., Saper, M. A., Samraoui, B., Bennett, W. S., Strominger, J. L., and Wiley, D. C.,** Structure of the human class I histocompatibility antigen. HLA-A2, *Nature,* 329, 506, 1987.

11. **Bjorkman, P. J., Saper, M. A., Samraoui, B., Bennett, W. S., Strominger, J. L., and Wiley, D. C.,** The foreign antigen binding site and T cell recognition regions of class I histocompatibility antigens, *Nature,* 329, 512, 1987.
12. **Brown, J. H., Jardetzky, T., Saper, M. A., Samraoui, B., Bjorkman, P. J., and Wiley, D. C.,** A hypothetical model of the foreign antigen binding site of class II histocompatibility molecules, *Nature,* 332, 845, 1988.
13. **Bugawan, T. L., Horn, G. T., Long, C. M., Mickelson, E., Hansen, J. A., Ferrara, G. B., Angelini, G., and Erlich, H. A.,** Analysis of HLA-DP allelic sequence polymorphism using tne in vitro enzymatic DNA amplification of DP-α and DP-β loci, *J. Immunol.,* 141, 4024, 1988.
14. **Casali, P. and Notkins, A. L.,** Probing the human B-cell repertoire with EBV: polyreactive antibodies and $CD5^+$ B lymphocytes, *Annu. Rev. Immunol.,* 7, 513, 1989.
15. **Claas, F., Catelli-Visser, R., Schreuder, I., and van Rood, J.,** Alloantibodies to an antigenic determinant shared by HLA-A2 and -B17, *Tissue Antigens,* 19, 388, 1982.
16. Clinical transplantation, in *Immunobiology of HLA,* Vol. 2, Dupont, B., Ed., Springer-Verlag, Berlin, 1989, 515.
17. **Colombani, J., Lepage, V., Raffoux, C., and Colombani, M.,** HLA typing with monoclonal antibodies: evaluation of 356 HLA monoclonal antibodies including 181 studied during the 10th International Histocompatibility Workshop, *Tissue Antigens,* 34, 97, 1989.
18. **Durbin, H. and Bodmer, W. F.,** A sensitive micro-immunoassay using β-galactosidase/anti-β-galactosidase complexes, *J. Immunol. Meth.,* 97, 19, 1987.
19. **Eckels, D. E., Gorski, J., Rothbard, J., and Lamb, J. R.,** Peptide mediated modulation of T-cell allorecognition, *Proc. Natl. Acad. Sci. U.S.A.,* 85, 8191, 1988.
20. **Effros, R. B., Hulette, C. M., Ettenger, R., Dillard, L. C., Zeller, E., Duong, R., and Walford, R.,** A human-human hybridoma secreting anti-HLA class II antibody, *J. Immunol.,* 137, 1599, 1986.
21. **Fazekas de St Groth, S. and Scheidegger, D.,** Production of monoclonal antibodies: strategy and tactics, *J. Immunol. Meth.,* 35, 1, 1980.
22. **Garrett, T. P. J., Saper, M. A., Bjorkman, P. J., Strominger, J. L., and Wiley, D. C.,** Specificity pockets for the side chains of peptide antigens in HLA-Aw68, *Nature,* 342, 692, 1989.
23. **Gaston, J. S. H., Rickinson, A. B., and Epstein, M. A.,** Cross-reactivity of self-HLA-restricted Epstein-Barr virus-specific cytotoxic T-lymphocytes for allo-HLA determinants, *J. Exp. Med.,* 158, 1804, 1983.
24. **Goodfellow, P. N., Jones, E. A., van Heyningen, V., Solomon, E., Bobrow, M., Miggiano, V., and Bodmer, W. F.,** The β_2-microglobulin gene is on chromosome 15 and not in the HLA region, *Nature,* 254, 267,
25. **Gorski, J. and Mach, B.,** Polymorphism of Ia antigens: gene conversion between two DR β loci results in a new HLA-D/DR specificity, *Nature,* 322, 67, 1986.
26. **Gorski, J.,** HLA-DR β chain polymorphism-second domain polymorphism reflects evolutionary relatedness of alleles and may explain public serologic epitopes, *J. Immunol.,* 143, 329, 1989.
27. **Hammerling, U., Kosinski, S., Chua, R., and Livingston, P.,** Production of human monoclonal alloantibodies: considerations of an optimal strategy, *Perspect. Immunogenet. Histocompatibility,* 6, 61, 1984.
28. **Hammerling, G. J., Chamberlain, J. W., Dill, O., Yang, S. Y., Dupont, B., Khan, R., Chua, R., Weissman, S. M., and Hammerling, U.,** Self-tolerance to HLA focuses the response of immunized HLA-transgenic mice on production of antibody to precise polymorphic HLA alloantigens, *Proc. Natl. Acad. Sci. U.S.A.,* 87, 235, 1990.
29. **Hancock, R. J. T., Martin, A., Stinchcombe, V., Jones, T. J., Smythe, J., Laundy, G. J., and Bradley, B. A.,** In vitro production of anti-HLA-DR antibodies by human B-cell lines, *Tissue Antigens,* 28, 228, 1986.

30. **Hancock, R. J. T., Harvey, J., Evans, P. R., Hodges, E., Molnar, J., Martin, A., Lewis, L., Cohen, B., Laundy, G., MacIver, A. G., and Bradley, B. A.,** Expression of polymorphic B-cell antigens on human kidneys, *Tissue Antigens,* 31, 165, 1988.
31. **Hancock, R. J. T., Martin, A., Laundy, G. J., Smythe, J., Roberts, I., Cooke, H., Pera, S., Bowerman, P., and Bradley, B. A.,** Production of monoclonal human antibody to HLA-DR5(DRw11) by mouse/human heterohybridomas, *Hum. Immunol.,* 22, 135, 1988.
32. **Hancock, R. J. T., Yendle, J. E., and Bradley, B. A.,** MicroELISA assays of anti-HLA activity and isotype of human monoclonal antibodies, *Tissue Antigens,* 33, 437, 1989.
33. **Hancock, R. J. T., Martin, A., Jackson, D., Yousaf, K., Brady, C., Laundy, G. J., and Bradley, B. A.,** Production of monoclonal human antibody with unusual anti-HLA-B7 activity by mouse/human heterohybridomas, Proc. Fourth European Histocompatibility Conference, March, 1990.
34. **Hansen, T., Kolstad, A., Thorsby, E., and Hannestad, K.,** A human-human hybridoma producting cytotoxic antibody to HLA-B15, cross-reacting with B17, B15, B35 and B18, *Tissue Antigens,* 29, 246, 1987.
35. **Hansen, T., Kolstad, A., Mathisen, G., and Hannestad, K.,** A human-human hybridoma (Tr7E2) producing cytotoxic antibody to HLA-DQw1, *Hum. Immunol.,* 20, 307, 1987.
36. **Hansen, T. and Hannestad, K.,** Simple rosette assay for HLA-B27 typing of whole blood samples, *Tissue Antigens,* 30, 198, 1987.
37. **Heath, W. R., Hurd, M. E., Carbone, F. R., and Sherman, L. A.,** Peptide-dependent recognition of H-$2K^D$ by alloreactive cytotoxic T lymphocytes, *Nature,* 341, 749, 1989.
38. **Heyes, J., Austin, P., Bodmer, J., Bodmer, W., Madrigal, A., Mazzilli, M. C., and Trowsdale, J.,** Monoclonal antibodies to HLA-DP transfected mouse L cells, *Proc. Natl. Acad. Sci. U.S.A.,* 83, 3417, 1986.
39. HLA and disease association, in *Immunobiology of HLA,* Vol. 2, Dupont, B., Ed., Springer-Verlag, Berlin, 1989, 399.
40. **Holmes, N.,** New HLA class I molecules, *Immunol. Today,* 10, 52, 1989.
41. **Hulette, C. M., Effros, R. B., Dillard, L. C., and Walford, R. L.,** Production of a human monoclonal antibody to HLA by human-human hybridoma technology, *Am. J. Pathol.,* 121, 10, 1985.
42. **Janeway, C. A.,** The role of CD4 in T-cell activation: accessory molecule or co-receptor?, *Immunol. Today,* 10, 234, 1989.
43. **Jaraquemada, D., Navarette, C., Ollier, W., Awad, J., Okoye, J., and Festenstein, H.,** HLA-Dw specificity assignments are independent of HLA-DQ, HLA-DR and other class II specificities and define a biologically important segregant series which strongly activates a functionally distinct T cell subset, *Hum. Immunol.,* 16, 259, 1986.
44. **Kaufman, J. K., Auffray, C., Korman, A. J., Shackelford, D. A., and Strominger, J. L.,** The class II molecules of the human and murine major histocompatibility complex, *Cell,* 36, 1, 1984.
45. **Kawai, J., Ando, A., Sato, T., Nakatsuji, T., Tsuji, K., and Inoko, H.,** Analysis of gene structure and antigen determinants of DR2 antigens using DR gene transfer into mouse L cells, *J. Immunol.,* 142, 312, 1989.
46. **Kennedy, L. J., Bourel, D., Dejour, G., Fauchet, R., and Bodmer, J. G.,** A European workshop to investigate technical problems of using HLA monoclonal antibodies in microcytotoxicity assays, *Tissue Antigens,* 29, 43, 1987.
47. **Kennedy, L. J., Marsh, S. G. E., and Bodmer, J.,** Cytotoxic monoclonal antibodies, in *Immunobiology of HLA,* Vol. 1, Dupont, B., Ed., Springer-Verlag, Berlin, 1989, 301.
48. **Kievits, F., Wuffels, J., Lokhorst, W., Boerenkamp, W. J., and Ivanyi, P.,** HLA expression and function in single and double HLA-B27-transgenic mice, *Tissue Antigens,* 34, 50, 1989.

49. **Koller, B. H., Geraghty, D. E., DeMars, R., Duvick, L., Rich, S. S., and Orr, H. T.,** Chromosomal organization of the human major histocompatibility complex class I gene family, *J. Exp. Med.*, 169, 469, 1989.
50. **Kolstad, A., Hansen, T. Y., and Hannestad, K.,** A human-human hybridoma antibody (TrB12) defining subgroups of HLA-DQw1 and -DQw3, *Hum. Immunol.*, 20, 219, 1987.
51. **Kolstad, A., Hansen, T., and Hannestad, K.,** A cytotoxic human-human hybridoma antibody (TrH6) specific for HLA-DRw52, *Tissue Antigens*, 31, 90, 1988.
52. **Kolstad, A., Bratelie, A., and Hannestad, K.,** A cytotoxic human-human hybridoma antibody (TrC7) specific for HLA-A29, *Tissue Antigens*, 33, 546, 1989.
53. **Korman, A. J., Boss, J. M., Spies, T., Sorrentino, R., Okada, K., and Strominger, J.,** Genetic complexity and expression of human class II histocompatibility antigens, *Immunol. Rev.*, 85, 45, 1985.
54. **Kosinski, S., Hammerling, U., and Yang, S. Y.,** A human monoclonal antibody to an HLA-DRw53(MT3)-like epitope on Class II antigens, *Tissue Antigens*, 28, 150, 1986.
55. **Kosinski, S., Ferrara, G. B., Yang, S. Y., and Hammerling, U.,** A human monoclonal antibody against HLA-A25, *Tissue Antigens*, 29, 177, 1987.
56. **Kosinski, S. and Hammerling, U.,** A new cloning method for antibody-forming lymphoblastoid cells: increase in cloning efficiency by inclusion of human fibroblasts into semisolid agarose growth layer, *J. Immunol. Meth.*, 94, 201, 1986.
57. **Kosinski, S., Yang, S. Y., Pistillo, M. P., and Hammerling, U.,** A supertypic HLA Class II determinant shared by DR1 and DRw9, and crossreactive with DR2, defined by human monoclonal antibody, *Hum. Immunol.*, 21, 221, 1988.
58. **de Koster, H. S., Anderson, D. C., and Termijtelen, A.,** T-cells sensitised to synthetic HLA-DR3 peptide give evidence of continuous presentation of denatured HLA-DR3 molecule by HLA-DP, *J. Exp. Med.*, 169, 1191, 1989
59. **Krangel, M. S.,** Two forms of HLA class I molecules in human plasma, *Hum. Immunol.*, 20, 155, 1987.
60. **Lechler, R. I., Lombardi, G., Batchelor, R. J., Reinsmoen, N., and Bach, F. H.,** The molecular basis of alloreactivity, *Immunol. Today*, 11, 83, 1990.
61. **Long, E. O.,** Intracellular traffic and antigen processing, *Immunol. Today*, 10, 232, 1989.
62. **McMichael, A. J., Parham, P., Rust, N., and Brodsky, F.,** A monoclonal antibody that recognises an antigenic determinant shared by HLA-A2 and -B17, *Hum. Immunol.*, 1, 121, 1980.
63. **Maddox, J. F. and Bodmer, J. G.,** Hybrid human-mouse class II molecules: localisation of antibody binding sites, in *Immunobiology of HLA*, Dupont, B., Ed., Springer-Verlag, Berlin, 1989, 373.
64. **Marrack, P. and Kappler, J.,** T-cells can distinguish between allogeneic major histocompatibility complex products on different cell types, *Nature*, 332, 840, 1988.
65. **Marsh, S. G. E. and Bodmer, J. G.,** HLA-DR and -DQ epitopes and monoclonal antibody specificity, *Immunol. Today*, 10, 305, 1989.
66. **Mazzoleni, O., Longo, A., Angelini, G., Colonna, M., Tanigaki, N., Delfino, D., Pistillo, M. P. P., Kun, L., and Ferrara, G. B.,** Human monoclonal antibody MP8 detects a supertypic determinant encoded by DPB alleles DPB2.1, DPB3, DPB4.2, DPB8, DPB9, DPB10, and DPB 14, *Immunogenetics*, 30, 502, 1989.
67. **Ray, J. G., Ed.,** NIAID Manual of Tissue Typing Techniques, 1979–1980, Publ. No. 80-545, Department of Health, Education and Welfare, National Institutes of Health, 1979.
68. **Nelson, K., Bodmer, J., Martin, A., Navarette, C., and Strong, D. M.,** Micro EIA and monoclonal antibodies, in *Immunobiology of HLA*, Vol. 1, Dupont, B., Ed., Springer-Verlag, Berlin, 1989, 292.
69. **Nuchtern, J. G., Biddison, W. E., and Klausner, R. D.,** Class II MHC molecules can use the endogenous pathway of antigen presentation, *Nature*, 343, 74, 1990.

70. **Parham, P., Androlewicz, M. J., Brodsky, F. M., Holmes, N. J., and Ways, J. P.,** Monoclonal antibodies: purification, fragmentation and application to structural and functional studies of class I MHC antigens, *J. Immunol. Meth.*, 53, 133, 1982.
71. **Parham, P., Antonelli, P., Herzenberg, L. A., Kipps, T. J., Fuller, A., and Ward, F. E.,** Further studies on the epitopes of HLA-B7 defined by murine monoclonal antibodies, *Hum. Immunol.*, 15, 44, 1986.
72. **Parham, P., Clayberger, C., Zorn, S. L., Ludwig, D. S., Schoolnik, G. K., and Krensky, A. M.,** Inhibition of alloreactive cytotoxic T-lymphocytes by peptides from the α_2 domain of HLA-A2, *Nature*, 325, 625, 1987.
73. **Parham, P., Lomen, C. E., Lawlor, D. A., Ways, J. P., Holmes, N., Coppin, H. L., Salter, R. D., Wan, A. M., and Ennis, P. D.,** Nature of polymorphism in HLA-A, -B, and -C molecules, *Proc. Natl. Acad. Sci. U.S.A.*, 85, 4005, 1988.
74. **Parham, P., Lawlor, D. A., Salter, R. D., Lomen, C. E., Bjorkman, P. J., and Ennis, P. D.,** HLA-A,B,C: patterns of polymorphism in peptide-binding proteins, in *Immunobiology of HLA*, Vol. 2, Dupont, B., Ed., Springer-Verlag, Berlin, 1989, 10.
75. **Parham, P., Lawlor, D. A., Lomen, C. E., and Ennis, P. D.,** Diversity and diversification of HLA-A,B,C alleles, *J. Immunol.*, 142, 3937, 1989.
76. **Park, M. S., Takenouchi, T., Terasaki, P. I., Tonai, R., and Barbetti, A.,** HLA-DP region complexity by CDC, RFLP and cellular assays, in *Immunobiology of HLA*, Vol. 2, Dupont, B., Ed., Springer-Verlag, Berlin, 1989, 311.
77. **Pistillo, M. P., Hammerling, U., Dupont, B., and Ferrara, G. B.,** In vitro production of a human HLA alloantibody of restricted specificity (DQw2) via Epstein-Barr virus transformation, *Hum. Immunol.*, 15, 109, 1986.
78. **Ploegh, H. L., Orr, H. T., and Strominger, J. L.,** Major histocompatibility antigens: the human (HLA-A,B,C) and murine (H2-K, H2-D) class I molecules, *Cell*, 24, 287, 1981.
79. **Ray, T. R.,** Antibodies in HLA serology, in *Antibodies, a Practical Approach*, Vol. 2, Catty, D., Ed., IRL Press, Oxford, 1989.
80. **Sachs, J. A., Fernandez, N., Kurpisz, M., Okoye, R., Ogilvie, J., Awad, J., Labeta, A., and Festenstein, H.,** Serological biochemical and functional characterisation of three different HLA-DR monoclonal antibodies derived from C57B16 mice, *Tissue Antigens*, 28, 199, 1986.
81. **Salter, R. D., Norment, A. M., Chen, B. P., Clayberger, C., Krensky, A.M., Littman, D. R., and Parham, P.,** Polymorphism in the α_3 domain of HLA-A molecules affects binding to CD8, *Nature*, 338, 345, 1989.
82. **Sakaguchi, K., Ono, R., Tsujisaki, M., Richiardi, P., Carbonara, M. S., Park, R., Tonai, R., Terasaki, P. I., and Ferrone, S.,** Anti-HLA-B7, B27, Bw42, Bw54, Bw55, Bw56, Bw67, Bw73 monoclonal antibodies: specificity, idiotypes, and application for a double determinant immunoassay, *Hum. Immunol.*, 21, 193, 1988.
83. **Schroeijers, W. E. M., de Koster, H. A., van Rood, J. J., and Termijtelen, A.,** HLA-DRβIII and HLA-DP induce comparable proliferation in primary mixed lymphocyte culture, *Tissue Antigens*, 32, 145, 1988.
84. **Skornik, J. C.,** HLA-A2 epitopes recognized by alloantibodies from broadly sensitized patients, *Hum. Immunol.*, 18, 277, 1987.
85. **Shoenfeld, Y. and Zamir, R.,** The significance of HLA studies in human-human hybridomas, *Tissue Antigens*, 32, 209, 1988.
86. **Sterkers, G., Zeliszewski, D., Freidel, A. C., Gebuhrer, L., Betuel, L., and Levy, J. P.,** Both HLA-DR and HLA-DQ determinants contribute to HLA-Dw typing, *Hum. Immunol.*, 20, 233,1987.
87. **Taylor, C. J., Chapman, J. R., Fuggle, S. V., Ting, A., and Morris, P. J.,** A positive B cell crossmatch due to IgG anti-HLA-DQ antibody present at the time of transplantation in a successful renal allograft, *Tissue Antigens*, 30, 104, 1987.

88. **Thurau, S. G., Wildner, G., Kuon, W., Weiss, E. H., and Riethmuller, G.,** Expression and immunogenicity of HLA-B27 in high-transfection recipient P815: a new method to induce monoclonal antibodies directed against HLA-B27, *Tissue Antigens,* 33, 510, 1989.
89. **MacQueen, J. M., Ed.,** Tissue Typing Reference Manual, South-Eastern Organ Procurement Foundation, Richmond, VA, 1987.
90. **Towbin, H., Staehlin, T., and Gordon, J.,** Electrophoretic transfer of proteins from polyacrylamide gels to nitrocellulose sheets: procedure and some applications, *Proc. Natl. Acad. Sci. U.S.A.,* 76, 4350, 1979.
91. **Townsend, A. and Bodmer, H.,** Antigen recognition by class I-restricted T lymphocytes, *Annu. Rev. Immunol.,* 7, 601, 1989.
92. **Toubert, A., Raffoux, C., Boretto, J., Sire, J., Sodoyer, R., Thurau, S. T., Amor, B., Colombani, J., Lemonnier, F. A., and Jordan, B. R.,** Epitope mapping of HLA-B27 and HLA-B7 antigens by using intradomain recombinants, *J. Immunol.,* 141, 2503, 1988.
93. **Trapani, J. A., Mizuno, S., King, S. Y., and Dupont, B.,** Molecular mapping of a new public HLA class I epitope shared by all HLA-B and HLA-C antigens and defined by a monoclonal antibody, *Immunogenetics,* 29, 25, 1989.
94. **Uryun, N., Maeda, M., Tsuji, K., and Inoko, H.,** A simple rapid method for HLA-DRB and -DQB typing by digestion of PCR-amplified DNA with allele specific restriction endonucleases, *Tissue Antigens,* 35, 20, 1990.
95. **Vartdal, F., Gaudernack, G., Funderud, S., Bratlie, A., Lea, T., Ugelstad, J., and Thorsby, E.,** HLA class I and II typing using cells positively selected from blood by immunomagnetic isolation — a fast and reliable technique, *Tissue Antigens,* 28, 301, 1986.
96. **Viken, H. D., Gaudernack, G., and Thorsby, E.,** Characterisation of a monoclonal antibody recognising a polymorphic epitope mainly on HLA-DPw2 and DPw4 molecules, *Tissue Antigens,* 34, 250, 1989.
97. **Yendle, J. E., Bowerman, P. D., Yousaf, K., Roberts, I. M., Cohen, B., Barber, L., Lechler, R., Hancock, R. J. T., and Bradley, B. A.,** Production of a cytotoxic human monoclonal antibody with specificity for HLA-DR4 and DRw10 by cells derived from a highly sensitised kidney recipeint, *Hum. Immunol.,* 27, 167, 1990.

Chapter 16

DETECTION OF PLATELET, GRANULOCYTE, AND MONOCYTE ANTIBODIES

C. P. Engelfriet, R. W. A. M. Kuijpers, R. J. L. Klaassen, and A. E. G. Kr. von dem Borne

TABLE OF CONTENTS

ISBN 0-8493-4938-9

I. GENERAL PRINCIPLES

Techniques for the detection of platelet antibodies are based on different principles. The first methods that were developed depended on a secondary result of platelet-antibody interaction, such as agglutination, the activation of complement, or a disturbance of platelet function. Techniques based on the last principle suffered from the serious drawback that many nonimmunological factors may affect platelet function *in vitro* and such techniques are no longer used. Techniques based on complement activation often proved to be much less sensitive than techniques of a later generation and, in any case, most platelet antibodies are noncomplement-binding. The platelet agglutination test has the disadvantage that only IgM antibodies are detectable with it and, although in theory IgM antibodies of low affinity might be optimally detected in this test, it was shown to be less sensitive compared to later techniques for detecting known IgM antibodies.

The classical antiglobulin test, based on the agglutination of sensitized cells by antiglobulin serum, proved to be inapplicable because of the tendency of platelets to aggregate spontaneously, particularly after being washed. However, all the more successful techniques developed for platelet antibody detection are based on the antiglobulin principle in various ways: the radioimmunoassay,[1] the immunofluorescence test,[2] the enzyme-linked immunosorbent assay,[3] and the mixed red cell adherence assay.[4] Several varieties of these assays have been described in which binding of immunoglobulins to platelets is detected by antiglobulin reagents, either directly or indirectly (antiglobulin consumption, or two-stage assays) and either qualitatively or quantitatively.[5] A general problem in techniques based on the antiglobulin principle is the presence of Fc-receptors for IgG on platelets. This may cause binding of inert IgG and this interferes in several of the techniques.

More recently, methods have been developed to detect antibody binding to particular platelet membrane glycoproteins. Radioimmunoprecipitation and sodium dodecyl sulfate-polyacrylamide gel electrophoresis (SDS-PAGE) was one of the first of these methods.[6] A popular new method is the immunoblot (Western blot).[7] Also, assays have been developed using chemically purified glycoproteins or glycoproteins caught by monoclonal antibodies bound to a solid phase from whole platelet lysate.[8–10]

An interesting modification of the latter methods, the monoclonal antibody-specific immobilization of platelet antigens assay, or MAIPA, has recently been described by Kiefel et al.[11]

An example of each of the above techniques will be described and discussed in this chapter.

II. RADIOIMMUNOASSAY

In this technique, use is made of ^{125}I-labeled anti-immunoglobulin or -complement antibodies for detecting antibodies or complement bound to platelets. It was first described by Soulier et al.[1] and Mueller-Eckhardt et al.[12] A more recent version of the radioimmunoassay was described by LoBuglio et al.[13] In this assay monoclonal anti-human IgG is applied instead of a polyclonal reagent. The highly restricted antigenic specificity and the single binding affinity of the monoclonal reagent were considered to be of advantage with regard to the specificity of the assay. Another important step is centrifugation of the platelet suspension over Percoll to remove platelet fragments, which have been found to be an important source of nonspecifically bound anti-IgG.[14] It was found that, on the platelets of normal individuals, there are 169 $\pm$ 79 molecules of IgG per platelet, 10 to 100 times fewer than measured in assays in which polyclonal anti-IgG is used and in which no steps are undertaken to remove platelet fragments.

Another advantage is that the assay is quantitative, not only in measuring antibodies, but also for determining the number of antigens on the cell surface. Using this technique, the number of autoantibodies on the platelets of immune thrombocytopenia (ITP) patients was found to range from 790 to 13095 molecules.[13] A disadvantage of this radio immunoassay is that IgM and IgA antibodies, which quite often occur without IgG (particularly the former), are not detected.

A slightly modified assay, the monoclonal antibody radioimmunoassay (MARIA), in which a sucrose gradient is used to separate the platelets, has been adapted for the use of anti-IgG subclass and anti-IgM antibodies.[15] The assay is described in Addendum I. It was shown that this assay is somewhat more sensitive in the detection of platelet auto- and alloantibodies than the immunofluorescence test (see below).

III. IMMUNOFLUORESCENCE TEST

An immunofluorescence test using paraformaldehyde-treated platelets has been described.[2] The advantages of treatment with paraformaldehyde are a diminished uptake of aggregated Ig and immune complexes and swelling of platelets with expulsion of platelet-associated Ig.[16,17] In this technique, use is made of fluorescein-iso-thio-cyanate (FITC)-labeled antiglobulin reagents. Advantages of the technique are as follows: the fluorescence of individual platelets is assessed which circumvents the problem of cell fragments and anti-Ig and class- and subclass-specific reagents can be applied. The technique is, however, relatively insensitive. It was shown[15] that at least 1000 molecules of IgG must be bound to a platelet to produce a positive reaction. This number of antibodies is well above that capable of inducing platelet destruction (>450 as shown by results obtained in the MARIA).

The immunofluorescence test described by von dem Borne et al.[2] has been chosen as the standard technique by the Working Party on Platelet Serology of the International Society of Blood Transfusion and the International Committee of Standardization in Haematology. The test is now performed as a microassay and is described in Addendum II.

Another version of the immunofluorescence test was described by Schneider and Schnaidt.[18] This test is performed on Hamax glass slides with 60 rings to which freshly washed platelets firmly adhere. Nonspecific fluorescence is avoided by the use of F(ab′)2 fractions of antiglobulin reagents.

Fluorescence flow cytometry has also been applied in platelet serology to quantitate bound platelet alloantibodies[2] and to determine platelet-associated IgG in thrombocytopenia.[19,20] Using this technique, Dunstan and Simpsom[21] have shown that the number of A, B, and Le antigens per cell is much more variable than that of platelet-specific antigens, such as HPA-1a and 1b or HLA antigens.

IV. THE ENZYME-LINKED ANTIGLOBULIN TEST

The use of an enzyme (peroxidase)-labeled antiglobulin for detecting platelet antibodies was first described by Tate et al.,[3] using platelets in suspension. After incubation of sensitized platelets with enzyme-linked antiglobulin serum, substrate is added and the reaction product quantified. Since then, a number of enzyme-linked immunosorbent assays (ELISA) have been described for the measurement of platelet-associated IgG.[22–32] Intact platelets, platelet lysates, and platelet monolayers on slides or in microtiter plates were applied. Horai et al.[26] were the first to use a solid-phase technique in microtiter plates. The following enzymes have been applied: peroxidase, peroxidase/antiperoxidase complex, and alkaline phosphatase.

The results of most ELISA methods are semiquantitative, but quantitative methods have also been described. These methods have been made quantitative by quantitation and standardization of the numbers of platelets bound to the wells of microtiter trays and by the use of quantitated IgG standards.[33,34] In another technique, fixed numbers of intact platelets in suspension were sensitized and then coated onto the wells of microtiter plates and again calibration curves were applied.[11] A drawback in solid-phase ELISA is that some sera cause nonspecific binding to plastic. The ELISA used in our laboratory is described in Addendum III.

V. MIXED RED CELL ADHERENCE ASSAYS

The principle of this technique is that antibodies bound to platelets are detected by means of red cells. Platelet monolayers in the wells of microtiter trays are used and IgG antibodies fixed to these platelets are detected by means of anti-IgG-coated red cells. This technique was found to be sensitive for the detection of HLA and non-HLA platelet antibodies.[4] A similar test, in which low ionic strength medium is used in the sensitization of the platelets, was evaluated as a method for pretransfusion platelet compatibility testing. The results of this test were found to be very well correlated with posttransfusion increment.[35] For details of this technique see Rachel et al.[36]

VI. RADIOIMMUNOPRECIPITATION AND SDS-POLYACRYLAMIDE GEL ELECTROPHORESIS (SDS-PAGE)

The principle of this technique is as follows: platelets are labeled with ^{125}I and sensitized with the antibodies under investigation. They are then washed and solubilized in an NP-40-containing buffer and glycoprotein-antibody complexes are isolated by binding to protein-A or by a second anti-human immunoglobulin antibody. The complexes are dissociated by heat and the labeled glycoproteins are analyzed in SDS-PAGE and visualized by autoradiography.[6,37] The immunoprecipitation technique is described in Addendum IV.

VII. IMMUNOBLOT

In this assay, unlabeled platelets are solubilized in NP-40 buffer and the proteins are separated by SDS-PAGE. The proteins are then transferred from the gel onto nitrocellulose paper (the blot), which is then incubated with the serum under investigation. After washing, antibody bound to the proteins is detected by ^{125}I-labeled antiglobulin and autoradiography or by using enzyme-linked antiglobulin (peroxidase, alkaline phosphatase) and a color reaction (Rock et al.[38]). The immunoblot technique is described in Addendum V.

VIII. ANTIGEN CAPTURE ASSAYS

A. USING ISOLATED GLYCOPROTEINS

The principle of this technique is as follows: platelets are isolated from ethylene diamine tetraacetate (EDTA) blood and membranes are prepared by sonification and differential centrifugation and then solubilized. The glycoproteins are then isolated by means of detergent-phase separation and coated onto the wells of flat-bottomed microtiter plates.[8] This technique was found to be more sensitive for the detection of autoantibodies against platelet-specific antigens and HLA antibodies than assays involving ^{51}Cr, radiolabeled monoclonal anti-IgG binding, and indirect immunofluorescence.

B. USING MONOCLONAL ANTIBODIES COATED ON MICROTITER PLATES

In this assay, glycoproteins are isolated from a platelet lysate by means of monoclonal antibodies coated on the wells of microtiter plates.[39] The plates are then incubated with the serum under investigation and subsequently with radiolabeled or enzyme-linked monoclonal anti-human IgG. In a more recent version of the technique,[9] intact platelets, sensitized with the antibodies under investigation or *in vivo* sensitized platelets are solubilized and the lysate is centrifuged. The supernatant is then incubated with immunobeads coated with monoclonal anti-human IgG. Subsequently, the beads are incubated with ^{125}I-labeled monoclonal antibodies against platelet glycoproteins to detect these in antigen-antibody complexes fixed onto the anti-IgG-coated immunobeads from the lysate.

C. MONOCLONAL ANTIBODY-SPECIFIC IMMOBILIZATION OF PLATELET ANTIGENS ASSAY (MAIPA)

In this assay, target platelets are simultaneously incubated with the serum under investigation and monoclonal antibodies against a particular glycoprotein. The platelets are then solubilized and the lysate is incubated in the wells of microtiter plates coated with polyclonal anti-mouse immunoglobulin. The human antibodies in the complex consisting of antigen, human antibody, and mouse monoclonal antibody are then detected with alkaline phosphatase-labeled anti-human immunoglobulin and substrate. This technique was described by Kiefel et al.[11] and is described in Addendum VI.

The antigen capture assays have the following advantages: they are sensitive and the result automatically defines the glycoprotein against which the antibodies are detected. A further advantage of the MAIPA is, that in contrast, for example, to immunoprecipitation, the conformation of the glycoproteins is not altered. Contaminating antibodies which may be present in the serum under investigation, e.g., anti-HLA class I antibodies, do not interfere in this assay.

Disadvantages of these techniques are that, in a case involving the detection of unknown antibodies, a variety of monoclonal antibodies must be used. Furthermore, false-negative results may be obtained if a human antibody is directed against the same or an adjacent epitope as the monoclonal antibody used in the assay.

IX. METHODS TO DISTINGUISH BETWEEN PLATELET-SPECIFIC ANTIBODIES AND HLA ANTIBODIES

In the diagnosis of neonatal alloimmune thrombocytopenia and posttransfusion purpura (PTP) it is essential to detect platelet-specific antibodies and, if detectable, to establish their specificity. In the serum of mothers of thrombocytopenic infants and of patients with PTP, HLA antibodies are often present which, except in immune precipitation techniques and antigen-capture assays, interfere with the detection of platelet-specific antibodies.

It was shown that by treating platelets with a solution of hypertonic acid chloroquine, the HLA class I antigens are removed from platelets.[40] Platelet-specific antigens appeared not to be affected by this treatment.[41] Further studies have shown that after 20 minutes of incubation of platelets with chloroquine, 80% of the HLA antigens had been removed while there was no effect on GPIIb/IIIa or GPIb/IX. However, after one hour of incubation, approximately 50% of the GPIIb/IIIa had been removed.[42] An alternative method for the removal of HLA antigens from target platelets was described by Kurata et al.[43] It depends on acid treatment of the platelets. The method of chloroquine treatment is described in Addendum VII.

X. METHODS TO ELUTE PLATELET ANTIBODIES

A modification of the ether elution method described by Rubin[44] and a modification of the elution method by lowering the pH[45] are used in our laboratory. For a description, see Addendum VIII.

Selection of appropriate technique — In the detection of platelet autoantibodies, the immunofluorescence test (IFT) on the patient's platelets is used in many laboratories. With this test, autoantibodies can be detected on the platelets of the vast majority of patients with severe idiopathic thrombocytopenia.[46] However, the IFT is relatively insensitive since about 1000 to 2000 antibody molecules must be bound per platelet for the test to be positive.[15] This number is above the minimum number of antibodies capable of causing immune destruction of platelets, although this probably depends on the class and subclass of the antibodies. This number is also well above the number of IgG molecules detected on the platelets of normal subjects, i.e., <450 as measured in the MARIA. Therefore it is advisable if the direct IFT is negative on the platelets of a patient with ITP, to perform the MARIA on the patient's platelets, which, moreover, is a quantitative technique which may prove to be of value in monitoring patients with alloimmune thrombocytopenia (AITP). In our laboratory, we also routinely test the serum from ITP patients and an eluate from the patient's platelets in the IFT. A positive result with the eluate proves the antibody nature of platelet-bound Ig.

XI. DETECTION OF ALLOANTIBODIES

A. NEONATAL ALLOIMMUNE THROMBOCYTOPENIA (NAITP)

In the diagnosis of NAITP it is essential to detect platelet-specific antibodies in the maternal serum. It is convenient to first test the maternal serum in the indirect IFT using paternal platelets or if these are not available, donor platelets. Because a positive result may be due to platelet-specific but also to HLA class I antibodies, distinction between these two possibilities is indicated. This can be done by using chloroquine-treated platelets as described above. If platelet-specific antibodies are detectable, then their specificity must be determined using a panel of phenotyped platelets and if the mother is or has been thrombocytopenic, a direct IFT test and or a MARIA on the maternal platelets is indicated to exclude the presence of autoantibodies.

If the indirect IFT is negative, the presence of platelet alloantibodies has not been excluded, because of the relative insensitivity of the IFT. It has, for example, been shown that many antibodies against the HPA-5^a (= Br^b) and HPA-5^b (= Br^a) antigens are not detected in the IFT, although they are readily detected in the MAIPA.[11] Therefore, further investigation of the maternal serum in the MAIPA or in the MARIA is indicated. The specificity of the maternal antibodies can be confirmed by phenotyping the maternal and paternal platelets.

B. POSTTRANSFUSION PURPURA

For the diagnosis of the classical posttransfusion purpura (PTP), which occurs often about 5 to 7 days after a transfusion, it is essential to demonstrate the presence of platelet-specific antibodies in the serum of the patient. Here, again, it is convenient to first test the serum in the indirect IFT with a phenotyped platelet panel. If positive reactions occur, a distinction between platelet-specific and HLA-class I antibodies is indicated. If no platelet-specific antibodies are detectable in the IFT, the serum should be further investigated in the MAIPA and/or MARIA. During the acute phase of thrombocytopenia, the direct IFT on the platelets of the patients is often positive. The specificity of the platelet-specific antibodies can be confirmed by phenotyping the patient's platelets and by testing an eluate from them.

If thrombocytopenia develops during or immediately after a transfusion, the serum of the donor must be tested for platelet-specific antibodies in the indirect IFT, by which, in the cases described so far, the responsible alloantibodies could be readily detected.

C. CROSSMATCH FOR ALLOIMMUNIZED PATIENTS

If a patient has become refractory to platelet transfusions because of alloimmunization against HLA-class I or platelet-specific antigens or both, the easiest way to solve the problem is to perform a crossmatch with donor platelets to select compatible donors. The number of crossmatches depends on the percentage of donors with whose cells the patient's serum reacts and whether one must depend on platelet concentrates prepared from random donor units or whether thrombocytapheresis can be done. The technique used must be sensitive enough to detect HLA class I and platelet-specific antibodies. In our laboratory we use the ELISA described in Addendum III. A disadvantage of the ELISA is that when anti-IgM is also used in the crossmatch, IgM cold platelet autoantibodies may interfere in the reaction. Good results have also been described with the solid-phase technique described by Rachel et al.[36]

XII. DETECTION OF ANTIBODIES AGAINST GRANULOCYTES

Like techniques for the detection of platelet antibodies, those developed for the detection of granulocyte antibodies depend on different principles and, even more than in the case of platelets, accuracy and reliability of techniques are hampered by the fragile nature of the cells and by the presence of Fc-receptors (both FcRII and III) on their membrane. Again, techniques which have been described depend on a secondary effect of the granulocyte antibody interaction, i.e., agglutination or the binding and activation of complement, on changes in granulocyte functions, on detecting granulocyte-associated Ig (GrAIg) by means of antiglobulin antibodies, and finally on antibody-dependent lysis of sensitized granulocytes by effector lymphocytes.

Techniques based on changes in granulocyte function suffer from the same drawback as those for the detection of platelet antibodies, namely that nonimmunological factors may change the function of these cells *in vitro*. With regard to techniques based on an effect of granulocyte-antibody interactions, a granulocyte cytotoxicity test has been developed and used by several investigators. However, the value of this technique has not been established. In fact, its value is doubtful since McCullough et al.,[47,48] using ^{111}In-labeled granulocytes, found no reduction in intravascular recovery, half-life, or organ localization of granulocytes in patients whose serum reacted positively with these granulocytes in a cytotoxicity test. Reliable techniques based on agglutination have been developed and found to be useful and important in the detection of granulocyte antibodies. Granulocyte agglutination techniques and examples of techniques for the detection of GrAIg will be discussed in this chapter.

XIII. AGGLUTINATION TEST

For this test, it is essential to use pure granulocyte suspensions, because the presence of other cells such as lymphocytes and red cells makes the results less reliable. A macrogranulocyte agglutination test was developed by Lalezari et al.[49] With this test they were able to demonstrate the presence of granulocyte-specific antibodies and to define several granulocyte-specific alloantigen systems.[50] A microagglutination test was developed later[51] and is now in general use.

It is important to realize that two essentially different mechanisms are involved in granulocyte agglutination. First, agglutination may result from crosslinking granulocytes if the antibody reacts with an antigen on two different cells. This type of agglutination is only brought about by IgM antibodies.

Agglutination by IgG antibodies depends on a quite different mechanism. Sensitization of granulocytes with IgG antibodies does not lead to direct agglutination, but appears to activate the cells, which leads to the formation of pseudopods.[52] For this process the cells must be viable. After the formation of the pseudopods the cells move slowly towards each other. Agglutination is then probably established by a reaction of IgG antibodies fixed to their antigen on one cell with Fc-receptors on another cell. The process is temperature dependent,[52] and requires metabolic energy and an intact microfilament system (Verheugt et al.)[53]

A modified microgranulocyte agglutination test in capillary tubes has been described.[54] It is more difficult to perform but it is very sensitive.[55–57] Granulocyte-specific and HLA class I antibodies as well as antibodies against non-HLA antigens shared with other cells, e.g., 5a, 5b, HMA-I and -II, are detected in the granulocyte agglutination test. A distrinction between HLA class I and granulocyte-specific antibodies may be required, e.g., in the diagnosis of neonatal alloimmune neutropenia (NAINP). This can be done by using chloroquine-treated granulocytes.[58] However, our experience with this procedure is that it leads to false-positive reactions. We find absorption of the serum with platelets a better way for this distinction. If, after absorption, a serum still reacts with granulocytes, further distinction between the then still various possible antibody populations must be made. In the diagnosis of NAINP, testing the serum with a typed granulocyte panel is indicated. If that does not solve the problem, further investigations could include testing the serum with monocytes in a newly developed monocyte IFT[59] and further absorption studies. Alternatively, flow cytofluorometry in which fluorescence of the various cell populations is measured separately can be applied (see below). The microgranulocyte agglutination test as used in our laboratory is described in Addendum IX.

The technique "monoclonal antibody-specific immobilization of platelet antigens assay", as described for platelets, can also be applied to granulocytes, using, of course, anti-granulocyte monoclonal antibodies and the same applies for the immunoprecipitation and immunoblot techniques.

Techniques for the detection of granulocyte-bound Ig, based on the use of labeled antiglobulin reagents, have been described and they will now be discussed.

XIV. IMMUNOFLUORESCENCE TEST (IFT)

A fluorescence test for the detection of granulocyte allo- and autoantibodies was described by Verheugt et al.[60] The principle of the technique is, of course, the detection of bound Ig by means of FITC-labeled antiglobulin reagents. Important steps in this technique are the fixation of the granulocytes used to detect free antibody with 1% paraformaldehyde and the use of F(ab′)2 parts of FITC-labeled antiglobulin reagents, both measures to reduce non-specific binding of IgG to Fc-receptors.

It should be realized that immune complexes present in a patient's serum may cause positive reactions in the granulocyte IFT. Tetanus-anti-tetanus and DNA-anti-DNA complexes were shown to give positive results.[61] In some cases it will therefore be necessary to distinguish between bound immune complexes and antibodies. One way to solve this problem is to prepare an eluate which, in the case of immune complexes, will be negative. Another approach is to block Fc-receptors with monoclonal antibodies.[59] The immunofluorescence test is described in Addendum X.

A microtiter modification of the granulocyte IFT has been described by Press et al.[62] The advantage of this assay is that it requires small quantities of reagents and low numbers of cells.

XV. FLOW CYTOFLUOROMETRY

It was shown by Verheugt et al.[63] that both allo- and autoantibodies against granulocytes can be quantitatively determined by flow cytofluorometry. The detection of alloantibodies against granulocytes using flow cytofluorometry was also described by Veys et al.[64] Using a Coulter Epics system, cell populations are separated by analysis of their light-scattering properties. Thus, fluorescence of each cell population, granulocytes, monocytes, and lymphocytes, can be measured. This is helpful in detecting the cell specificity of antibodies. Similar results have been obtained by Robinson et al.[65]

Using an EPICS Flow Cytometer (Coulter Electronics, Hialeah, Florida), Minchinton et al.[66] compared the results obtained with the granulocyte IFT and with flow cytofluorometry. The techniques demonstrated equivalent simplicity, specificity, sensitivity, and reproducibility. However, it was difficult, using the FACS (fluorescence-activated cell sorter) reading method, to distinguish between a negative and a weakly positive granulocyte IFT test due to considerable variation in background fluorescence for the neutrophils of different donors. The FACS method was superior for use on chloroquine-treated granulocytes. Thus, before the FACS can be used, interpretation of the results must be standardized by reference with the manual technique.

XVI. PROTEIN A ASSAY

A technique in which use is made of the binding of IgG to staphylococcal Protein A (SPA) has been developed.[68] The disadvantage of this technique is that only IgG antibodies can be detected and that IgG3 antibodies, which may well be the most important from a clinical point of view, are not detected.

XVII. ENZYME-LINKED IMMUNOSORBENT ASSAY (ELISA)

Although ELISAs have been found satisfactory in the detection of platelet antibodies, they are not satisfactory for use on granulocytes. This is due to the numerous intrinsic granulocyte enzymes which interfere in the reaction. No solution for this problem has been found so far.

XVIII. ELUTION OF GRANULOCYTE ANTIBODIES

Four different elution methods were compared by Helmerhorst et al.[45] It was found that elution by lowering the pH was the best method — better than ether, DMSO, or heat.

The acid elution method is the same as the method for platelets (see Addendum VIII), except that the granulocytes are suspended in phosphate-buffered saline (PBS)/0.1% BSA (bovine serum albumin) and that after incubation the granulocytes are centrifuged at 200 *g* for 5 minutes.

XIX. DETECTION OF MONOCYTE REACTIVE ANTIBODIES

Monocyte serology is particularly difficult because of the presence on the monocyte membrane of high-affinity Fc-receptors (FcRI): nonspecific binding of IgG to these receptors has made the application of techniques based on the antiglobulin principle impossible. So far, therefore, only cytotoxicity assays have been applied: a cytotoxicity test using monocytes, isolated by adherence to plastic and labeled with carboxy-fluoresceine diacetate,[68] and a two-color fluorescence test.[69] Disadvantages of these cytotoxicity assay are first, that only complement-binding antibodies are detected in them and second, that their reproducibility is poor. This is due to nonspecific cell death and to binding of complement-binding immune complexes to Fc-receptors.[70]

Recently, a new fluorescence test, using flow cytofluorometry, has been developed by Kuijpers et al.,[59] and it can be applied to monocytes. In this technique, the nonspecific adherence of IgG to FcRI is prevented by down modulation of FcRI. This is done by incubation with monoclonal anti-FcRI followed by incubation with goat anti-mouse IgG. After this treatment, FcRI is no longer detectable on the monocytes. However, HLA class I and class II antigens, the monocyte-specific antigens HMA I and II, as well as the antigen of the 5-system and LFA-1, remain detectable.

The reproducibility of this technique proved to be excellent. It can be applied for the detection of antibodies against monocyte-antigens not shared by other blood cells, such as monocyte-specific antigens and antigens shared by monocytes and endothelial cells and to detect noncomplement-binding anti-HLA class II antibodies, which cannot be detected in the lymphocyte fluorescence test. Such monocyte-reactive antibodies may be important with regard to organ transplantation and blood transfusion reactions. The technique is described in Addendum XI.

Furthermore, the technique "monoclonal antibody-specific immobilization of platelet antigens assay", described for platelets, can also be applied to monocytes, using, of course, monoclonal anti-monocyte antibodies; the same is true for the immunoprecipitation and immunoblot techniques.

ADDENDUM I
Monoclonal Antibody Radioimmunoassay (MARIA)

Materials

- EDTA buffer (PBS/EDTA): stock solution(10×):

0.175 *M* disodium hydrogen phosphate ($Na_2HPO_4 \cdot 2H_2O$)	156.5 g
0.089 *M* $Na_2EDTA \cdot 2H_2O$ (sequestrine = complexon)	166.5 g
1.541 *M* NaCl	450 g

  Distilled water to 5000 ml

  Dilute stock solution before use: 9 parts H_2O + 1 part stock solution. Correct pH, if necessary, with 4 *N* NaOH to 6.8–7.0
- EDTA buffer/BSA 0.2% (w/v) (PBS/EDTA/BSA)
- 20% Sucrose (w/v), 0,2% BSA (w/v) in EDTA buffer
- ^{125}I-labeled monoclonal anti-human IgG, IgG1, IgG2, IgG3, IgG4, and anti-human IgM (CLB-MH16-1M, MH161-1M, MH162-1M, MH163-1M, MH164-4M, and MH15-1M, respectively). Purified monoclonal antibody IgG is ^{125}I-labeled by the Iodogen according to standard procedures followed by separation of unbound ^{125}I from the antibodies by gel filtration. A stock solution of ^{125}I-labeled McAb is prepared at a concentration of 1 mg/ml and stored at −70°C.

Direct MARIA on patient's platelets

- Centrifuge EDTA-anticoagulated blood for 10 minutes at 400 *g* without braking, place the PRP in a plastic tube and centrifuge for 7 minutes at 1500 *g*. Wash 3 times with PBS/EDTA/BSA at 1500 *g* for 7 minutes and make up a suspension of 40 × 10^6/ml
- Incubate 250 μl of the platelet suspension (i.e., 10 × 10^6 platelets) with 75 μl ^{125}I-monoclonal anti-Ig (6.6 μg/ml: dilute stock solution 1:20 in PBS/EDTA/BSA) and 74 μl PBS/EDTA/BSA. Also incubate 250 μl of the platelet suspension with 75 μl of diluted ^{125}I-monoclonal anti-Ig and 75 μl nonlabeled, undiluted, purified monoclonal anti-Ig. This is the control to measure the nonspecific binding of the monoclonal anti-Ig to platelets. Then incubate for 60 minutes, mixing carefully every 20 minutes.
- Put 750 μl sucrose solution in an Eppendorf tube.
- Place 100 μl aliquots from each incubation mixture (in triplicate) on top of the 750 μl sucrose in the Eppendorf tubes and centrifuge at 13000 *g* for 5 minutes. After removal of the sucrose solution, cut off the tip of the tube and collect in a RIA tube for gamma counting.

Indirect test

- Centrifuge EDTA-anticoagulated blood for 10 minutes at 400 *g* without braking, collect the PRP and determine the cell concentration. Incubate 20 × 10^6 platelets suspended in 100 μl autologous plasma for 60 minutes at room temperature (RT) with 400 μl of the serum under investigation (to which, previously, 7.5 μl 0.5 *M* EDTA has been added). Wash 3 times with PBS/EDTA/BSA, centrifuge at 1500 *g* for 7 minutes, make up a suspension containing 40 × 10^6 platelets/ml, and continue as for the direct test.

Calculation

The number of IgG molecules detected per platelet is determined as follows:

$$\text{No. of molecules/platelet} = 4 \times 10^{12} \times A/B \times C$$

A, the number of counts per 20 seconds measured in the tip of the Eppendorf tube; B, specific activity (counts/20 seconds/μg) of the labeled monoclonal, on the day of the experiment; C, number of platelets in the tip of the tube. (By means of double-labeling experiments, it has been shown that the binding ratio of the various monoclonal anti-IgGs and human IgG is 1:1. Based on this, 1 μg monoclonal anti-IgG binds 4 × 10^{12} molecules IgG, calculated using Avogadro's number and molecular weight.)

Notes:

- Sera and monoclonals (diluted in PBS/EDTA/BSA) are cleared before use by centrifugation in an Eppendorf centrifuge at 13000 *g* for 15 minutes.
- Nonfixed platelets are used.
- Determining the exact number of platelets before incubation with the monoclonal antibody is very important.
- Beware of low counting efficiency when glass tubes are used.
- The sucrose solution must be removed right to the surface of the pellet.
  The tips of the tubes must then be cut off as soon as possible to prevent radioactivity-containing fluid, stuck to the wall, from reaching the platelets.
- Beware of differences in counting efficiency between gammacounters.

ADDENDUM II
Microimmunofluorescence Test on Platelets

Materials

- Phosphate-buffered saline (PBS):
  140.3 m*M* NaCl 8.2 g
  10.9 m*M* $Na_2HPO_4 \cdot 2H_2O$ 1.9 g
  1.8 m*M* $NaH_2PO_4 \cdot 2H_2O$ 0.3 g
  Distilled water to 1000 ml
  pH 7.4
- Pbs/EDTA/BSA .02% (see Addendum I)
- NH_4Cl solution:
  154 m*M* NH_4Cl 8.3 g
  10 m*M* $KHCO_3$ 1 g
  0.098 m*M* EDTA ($Na_2EDTA \cdot {}_2H_2O$) 0.33 g
  Distilled water to 1000 ml
  pH 7.2
- 1% Paraformaldehyde (PFA) solution in PBS (w/v)
- FITC-labeled anti-Ig, IgG, etc. (Dakopatts F202, CLB-KH16, F, etc.), appropriately diluted in PBS/EDTA/BSA
- 33.3% Glycerol in PBS (v/v)
- Round-bottom microtiter plates (Greiner)

Isolation of platelets

- Centrifuge 10 ml EDTA-anticoagulated blood for 10 minutes at 400 *g* without braking; remove PRP and place it in a plastic tube; centrifuge for 7 minutes at 1500 *g*; remove supernatant plasma and place it in a separate tube.
- Pipet 1 ml PBS/EDTA/BSA on the pellet and resuspend the platelets, fill the tube with PBS/EDTA/BSA and centrifuge 7 minutes at 1500 *g*.

Note: If there are many red cells in the suspension, they should be lysed by resuspending the pellet in 2.5 ml NH_4Cl solution and incubating for 5 minutes on ice.

- Wash the platelets twice with PBS/EDTA/BSA and make up a suspension containing 3×10^8/ml.

Fixation of the platelets

- Add 2.5 ml PFA solution to the pellet, resuspend, and incubate for 5 minutes at RT, wash the cells twice with PBS/EDTA/BSA, and make up a suspension containing 3×10^8 cells/ml in PBS/EDTA/BSA.

Direct test

- Place 20 μl patient's platelet suspension in the wells of a round-bottom microtiter plate.
- Add 20 μl FITC-labeled antiglobulin reagent, mix or shake, and incubate 30 minutes at RT in the dark. Add 150 μl PBS/EDTA/BSA, suspend, and centrifuge at 400 *g* for 5 minutes and wash twice with 150 μl PBS/EDTA/BSa. Then add 10 μl 33.3% glycerol to the pellets, mix, and place the suspension on a slide. Let the platelets settle for 15 minutes and then read with a fluorescence microscope.

Indirect test

- Place 20 μl of a suspension of PFA-fixed platelets and 20 μl serum in the wells of a round-bottom microtiter plate, mix on a shaker, and incubate 30 minutes at RT. Add 150 μl PBS/EDTA/BSA with force and wash three more times. Then proceed as for the direct test.

ADDENDUM III
ELISA for the Detection of Platelet Antibodies

Materials

- PBS/EDTA buffer (see Addendum I)
- PBS (see Addendum II)
- PBS/Tween 20: 500 ml PBS + 1 ml 25% (v/v) Tween 20
- PBS/Tween/BSA: 50 ml 20% (w/v) BSA + 200 ml PBS + 125 μl 25% (v/v) Tween 20
- Conjugate: F(ab′)2 — goat anti-human IgG-HRP from Cappel (no. 3301-0121): 27 ml PBS/Tween/BSA + 3 ml normal goat serum inactivated at 56°C for 30 minutes + 15 μl Cappel anti-IgG
- Phosphate-citrate buffer: 24.3 ml 0.1 *M* citric acid (1.92 g/100 ml distilled water) + 25.7 ml 0.16 *M* Na_2HPO_4 solution (2.84 g/100 ml distilled water) + distilled water to 100 ml. Adjust pH to 5.0 with 10.9 m*M* $Na_2HPO_4 \cdot 2H_2O$ solution
- OPD solution (prepare just before use and keep in the dark): 4 tablets OPD + 12 ml phosphate-citrate buffer (see above) + 5 μl H_2O_2 (add just before use)
- 4 *N* H_2SO_4: 80 ml distilled water + 10 ml concentrated H_2SO_4
- 5 *N* NaOH: 20 g NaOH in 100 ml distilled water
- Microplates: Nunc Maxisorb
- ELISA reader: Titertek Multiscan MC

Preparation of the platelet suspension

- Collect 10 ml of EDTA-anticoagulated blood, centrifuge 10 minutes at 400 *g* without braking, remove the PRP and place it in a plastic tube. Add PBS/EDTA to 10 ml, centrifuge for 7 minutes at 1500 *g*. Wash the platelets three times with PBS/EDTA (10 ml) and make up a suspension in PBS/EDTA with a concentration of 1×10^8 cells/ml.

Method

- Place 50 μl of the platelet suspension in wells of a microtiter plate, centrifuge the plate for 5 minutes at 300 *g*, incubate the plate for 15 minutes in a 37°C incubator with 100% humidity and 5% CO_2, wash 4 times with PBS-Tween. Dilute the serum under investigation 1:2 in PBS/Tween/BSA (200 μl serum + 200 μl dilution fluid) and pipet 50 μl of the diluted serum in each well and incubate for 60 minutes at 37°C. Wash the plates 4 times with PBS/Tween and add 50 μl of conjugate per well in an appropriate dilution in PBS/Tween/BSA. Incubate 30 minutes in the 37°C incubator, wash the plate 4 times with PBS/Tween and subsequently once with PBS. Add 50 μl OPD-substrate-solution per well, incubate for 5 to 10 minutes at RT in the dark, shaking the plate every 5 minutes. Add 50 μl 4 *N* H_2SO_4 per well to stop the reaction. Mix and read the optical density with the ELISA reader at 492 nm.

ADDENDUM IV
Immune Precipitation of Platelet Antigens

Materials

- CGSE (citrate-glucose-saline-EDTA) buffer:

0.12 *M* NaCl	7.01 g
0.0129 *M* NaCitrate	3.79 g
0.03 *M* Glucose	5.4 g
0.005 *M* Na_2EDTA	1.85 g
Distilled water to 1000 ml	
pH 7.4	

- Wash buffer:

0.01 *M* Tris	1.2 g
Nonidet P-40 0.5% (v/v)	5 ml
150 m*M* NaCl	9 g
Distilled water to 1000 ml	
pH 6.8	

- Lysis buffer — 10 ml wash buffer supplemented with

5 m*M* *N*-Ethylmaleimide	12.5 mg
2 m*M* PMSF (phenyl-methyl-sulfonyl-fluoride) (from a stock solution of 100 m*M* PMSF in ethanol)	200 μl
Soy bean trypsin inhibitor (20 μg/ml)	200 μg

- TENA (Tris-EDTA-NaCl) buffer:

0.154 *M* NaCl	9 g
0.01 *M* Tris	1.2 g
0.001 *M* Na_2EDTA	0.37 g
Distilled water to 1000 ml	
pH 7.4	

- PBS/EDTA/BSA (see Addendum I)
- SDS sample buffer stock (5× concentrated):

10% (w/v) SDS	2 ml
88% (v/v) Glycerol	1 ml
0.1% (w/v) Bromophenol Blue	0.5 ml
Distilled water	0.25 ml

- Protein A sepharose 10% suspension v/v in wash buffer

Method

- Prepare PRP from EDTA-anticoagulated blood by differential centrifugation (see Addendum II). Platelets from PRP are ^{125}I-labeled as follows: wash the platelets once with CGSE buffer and twice with TENA buffer, resuspend in TENA buffer at a concentration of 1 to 2 × 10^9/ml. Cell-surface iodination is performed following the Iodogen method according to standard procedures. Wash platelets 3 times with TENA buffer.
- Incubate 1 × 10^8 platelets with 100 μl antibody-containing serum or eluate for 1 hour at RT. Then wash the platelets 5 times with PBS/EDTA/BSA. Lyse the platelets in 100 μl freshly prepared lysis buffer.
- Centrifuge the lysates at 13000 *g* for 15 minutes and preclear 3 times with Sepharose CL4B in total for 24 hours.
- Incubate precleared lysates with 50 μl 10% suspension of rabbit anti-human IgG, coupled to protein A-sepharose according to manufacturers instructions, by tumbling overnight at 4°C.
- Wash the Sepharose beads twice with the washbuffer and place the beads on a discontinuous sucrose gradient (250 μl 10% sucrose and 750 μl 20% sucrose in 0.01 *M* Tris HCl, pH 6.8). Centrifuge for 5 minutes at 13000 *g* and wash the beads once with 0.01 *M* Tris/HCl. Elute the bound glycoproteins by boiling in 50 μl SDS sample buffer diluted 1:4 in Distilled water before use. Then analyze the samples on polyacrylamide slot gels according to Laemmli under non-reducing conditions; follow by autoradiography.

ADDENDUM V
Immunoblot Technique

Materials

- Lysis buffer:
  10 m*M* Tris HCl
  1% (v/v) Nonidet-P40
  5 m*M* Na_2EDTA
  5 m*M* *N*-Ethylmaleimide
  2 m*M* PMSF
  Soy bean trypsin inhibitor 20 μg/ml
  pH 8.0
- Towbin transfer buffer:

0.912 *M* Glycine	72 g
0.02 m*M* Tris	12 g
20% Methanol	1000 ml

  Distilled water to 5000 ml
  pH 8.3
- SDS sample mix (5× concentrated): see Addendum IV
- Block buffer:
  PBS (see Addendum II)
  Fetal calf serum 10% (v/v)
- Protein A sepharose 10% (v/v)

Method

- Isolate platelets as described in Addendum II. Solubilize for each cm on the slot gel (width 1.5 mm) 10^9 platelets on ice for 30 minutes in 200 μl of lysis buffer. Remove undissolved material by centrifugation at 13000 *g* for 30 minutes at 4°C and preclear the lysate with 200 μl of a 10% suspension of protein-A sepharose for 30 minutes at 4°C.Mix the supernatant with 100 μl concentrated sample buffer and heat for 5 minutes at 95°C. Subsequently, SDS-PAGE is performed according to Laemmli.
- Transfer the glycoproteins to a nitrocellulose sheet at $6V/cm^2$ for at least 8 hours at 4 to 8°C in Towbin transfer buffer; immerse the nitrocellulose sheet immediately after transfer in blocking buffer and incubate for 90 minutes with gentle shaking. Then incubate strips of the sheet with platelet antiserum diluted 1:25 or platelet eluate in PBS containing 0.2% (w/v) gelatin and 0.05% (v/v) Tween-20 for 3 hour at RT. Wash the strips twice in PBS containing 0.2% (w/v) gelatin and 0.1% (v/v) Tween-20 for 60 minutes. Then add 1×10^6 cpm of ^{125}I-labeled anti-human Ig/ml in the same buffer for 1 hour at RT. Wash again (two times during 60 minutes). Blot briefly with filter paper and air dry before exposure (Kodak X-omat-RP film using a Dupont Cronex Lighting Plus AH intensifying screen at −70°C).

ADDENDUM VI
Monoclonal Antibody Immobilization of Platelet-Antigen Assay (MAIPA)

Materials

- Affinity-purified goat anti-mouse IgG (Jackson, MS)
- Flat-bottom, 96-well microtiter plates (Nunc, maxisorb)
- PBS/EDTA/BSA 0.2% (see Addendum I)
- 50 m*M* $NaHCO_3$ buffer, pH 9.6
- Solubilization buffer:
  10 m*M* Tris 1.21 g
  0.15 *M* NaCl 9 g
  Distilled water to 1000 ml
  Adjust pH to 7.4
  Add NP-40 (final concentration 0.5% [v/v]) 5 ml
- MAIPA (Tris) incubation buffer:
  10 ml Solubilization buffer supplemented with 0.5 ml Tween 20 (final concentration 0.05% [w/v]) and 0.5 ml 1 *M* $CaCl_2$ solution (final concentration 0.5 m*M*)
- ELISA wash buffer:
  PBS/0.05% (w/v) Tween 20
- Murine monoclonal antibodies against platelet glycoproteins (GP) of any specificity available, e.g., CLB-thromb/1 (C17) (CD46), against GPIIIa; CLB-thromb/4 (CD49b), against VLA2-chain; CLB-thromb/CD42b against GPIbα
- Affinity-purified alkaline phosphatase-labeled monoclonal goat anti-human IgG or -IgM (Jackson, West Grove, PA)
- Alkaline phosphatase-substrate buffer:
  1 *M* diethanolamine 52.6 g
  0.5 m*M* $MgCl_2$ (0.250 ml 1 *M* $MgCl_2$)
  Distilled water to 500 ml
  Adjust solution with 4 *N* HCl to pH 10
- Alkaline phosphatase substrate tablets: Sigma 104. Each tablet contains 5 mg substrate. Use 1 table per 2.5 ml substrate buffer
- Eppendorf centrifuge
- 37°C Incubator
- The use of an automated ELISA washer is preferred
- ELISA reader

Method

- Coat microtiter plates with goat anti-mouse (GAM) IgG: per well 50 μl GAM 3 μg/ml diluted in $NaHCO_3$ buffer, pH 9.6, one day or more before use.
- Freshly isolated platelets: centrifuge 10 ml EDTA-anticoagulated blood for 10 minutes at 400 *g*. Remove PRP and wash platelets 3 times in PBS/EDTA/BSA and once in NaCl 0.9%/BSA 0.2% (w/v). Make up a suspension containing 1×10^8/l in NaCl/BSA.
- Place 0.5 ml of the nonfixed platelet suspension in Eppendorf tubes, centrifuge 2 to 3 minutes at 13000 *g* in an Eppendorf centrifuge, remove the supernatant and place on the pellet 50 μl PBS/BSA, 50 μl of a monoclonal antibody dilution and 40 μl of the serum under investigation (inactivated at 56°C and 30 minutes); mix and incubate for 30 minutes at 37°C in an incubator, wash 3 times with 750 μl (ice-cold) NaCl/BSA, centrifuge for 2 to 3 minutes at 13000 *g*, add 50 μl solubilization buffer (ice-cold) to the pellet, resuspend, and incubate 30 minutes at 4°C; centrifuge the lysate for 30 minutes at 13000 *g* at 4°C to remove insoluble material. In the meantime, wash the GAM-coated microtiter plates 5 times with PBS/Tween (in the ELISA-washer), incubate the plate for 1 hour at 4°C with 300 μl MAIPA incubation buffer/BSA (50 ml incubation buffer + 0.5 ml BSA 20%) per well to block the plate. Prepare glass tubes with 150 μl cold MAIPA incubation buffer/BSA per tube.

• Carefully remove 37.5 μl supernatant and add this to the 150 μl MAIPA incubation buffer in the tubes, mix, empty the microplate, place 50 μl diluted lysate into wells (in triplicate). Use MAIPA incubation buffer/BSA for lysate independent background determination; incubate overnight at 4°C. Dilute the alkaline phosphatase-labeled GAH-IgG or -IgM 1:4000 in MAIPA incubation buffer/BSA. Wash the ELISA-plate 5 times with PBS/Tween to remove unbound glycoproteins. Add 50 μl GAH conjugate per well and incubate 2 hour at 4°C; wash the ELISA plate 5 times with PBS/Tween to remove excess conjugate. Prepare substrate: 2 mg alkaline phosphatase substrate per ml alkaline-phosphatase substrate buffer. Add 50 μl substrate solution per well and incubate at 37°C in the dark. Measure the extinction at 405 nm (titertek).

ADDENDUM VII
Chloroquine Treatment of Platelets

• For preparing the platelets see Addendum II.
• Place 2.5 ml chloroquine (200 mg/ml PBS, pH 5.0) on a pellet containing about 10×10^8 platelets; resuspend carefully, and incubate for 1 hour at 37°C (incubator); wash the cells twice with PBS/EDTA/BSA 0.2% and resuspend carefully.

ADDENDUM VIII
Methods to Elute Platelet Antibodies

Ether Elution

• Mix washed, packed, sensitized platelets obtained from 30 ml EDTA-anticoagulated blood by differential centrifugation (see Addendum II) with one part PBS-BSA 0.2% and 2 parts ether by vigorous shaking for 2 minutes; incubate the mixture for 30 minutes at 37°C in a waterbath, often repeating the shaking. Centrifuge for 10 minutes at 2800 *g*. This results in three layers: ether, stroma, and eluate; remove the eluate with a Pasteur pipette.

Acid Elution

Materials

• Acid buffer:
  76 m*M* Citric acid $[C_3H_4OH(COOH)_3H_2O]$ 16 g
  300 ml PBS (see Addendum II)
  Distilled water to 1000 ml
  Adjust pH to 2.8 with about 40 ml 1 *N* NaOH
• Alkaline buffer:

214 m*M* Tris	25.7 g
22 m*M* Na_2HPO_4	3.8 g
0.5% BSA (w/v)	5 g
Distilled water to 1000 ml	

Method

• Prepare 500 μl of platelet suspension (3×10^8/ml, see Addendum II). Centrifuge for 10 minutes at 400 *g*. Remove supernatant and add 250 μl acid elution buffer dropwise to the pelleted platelets. Resuspend and incubate for 7 minutes at RT and centrifuge 10 minutes at 1500 *g*. Add the supernatant to 250 μl alkaline buffer. The pH should be 7.2.

ADDENDUM IX
Microleukocyte Agglutination Test

Materials

- 1% Methylcellulose (w/v)/PBS
- PBS/BSA 0.2% (see Addendum II)
- NH_4Cl solution (see Addendum II)
- Medinol 195
- RPMI/BSA 0.2%, normal AB serum (negative control), polyspecific serum (positive control)
- 50-μl Hamilton syringe

Isolation of granulocytes

- Place 2.5 ml 1% methylcellulose in a glass tube (150 × 115 mm), add 10 ml EDTA-anticoagulated blood, mix, and incubate 30 minutes at an angle of 45° at 37°C. Transfer the leukocyte-rich supernatant to a glass tube (110 × 15 mm) with a Pasteur pipette; centrifuge 5 minutes at 120 *g* and remove supernatant; place 2 ml of ice-cold NH_4Cl on the pellet, resuspend, and lyse the red cells during 5 minutes on melting ice, wash 3 times with PBS (centrifuge 5 minutes at 250 *g*) and make up a suspension of 8.0×10^6 cells/ml in RPMI/BSA.

Technique

- Take 2 μl of undiluted serum and dilute to 1:4 in RPMI/BSA in wells under Medinol; cover the microtiter plate and incubate 1 hour and 45 minutes at 37°C; read under an inverted microscope.

ADDENDUM X
Immunofluorescence Test on Granulocytes

Materials
- 1% Methylcellulose (w/v)/PBS
- PBS/BSA 0.2% (w/v)
- Ficoll Isopaque solution SD 1.077
- 1% PFA (w/v)/PBS
- NH_4Cl solution (see Addendum II)
- 33.3% Glycerol (v/v)/PBS
- FITC-labeled F(ab′)2 or Fab fragments of anti-human Ig, -IgG, or -IgM (CLB S26H17 4F2, K26H16 F1074, or K26H15 21F2, respectively), appropriately diluted in PBS/BSA
- AB serum (negative control)
- Polyspecific serum (positive control)

Isolation of granulocytes
- Place 2.5 ml 1% methylcellulose in a glass tube (150 × 15 mm), add 10 ml EDTA-anticoagulated blood and incubate the tube at an angle of 45° for 30 minutes at 37°C; place 2.5 ml Ficoll Isopaque in two glass tubes and place the leukocyte-rich plasma on top of the Ficoll Isopaque; centrifuge 20 minutes at 1000 *g*, remove the ring fraction containing the lymphocytes and monocytes and subsequently the Ficoll Isopaque. Add 2 ml NH_4Cl to the pellets and lyse the red cells during 5 minutes on melting ice. Wash the cells 3 times with PBS/BSA (5 minutes at 250 *g*), fix the granulocytes in 2 ml PFA for 5 minutes at RT, wash twice in PBS/BSA, and make up a suspension containing 10×10^6 cells/ml in PBS/BSA.

Direct rest
- Centrifuge a 40-μl suspension of the patient's granulocytes (5 minutes at 250 *g*) and remove the supernatant. Add 50 μl FITC-labeled antiglobulin and incubate 30 minutes at RT in the dark, wash twice with PBS/BSA, centrifuge 5 minutes at 250 *g*, remove the supernatant, add 20 μl glycerol, resuspend, and transfer to a slide; cover, let the cells settle for 15 minutes and read under a fluorescence microscope.

Indirect test
- Incubate 50 μl granulocyte suspension with 50 μl serum for 30 minutes at RT, wash 3 times with PBS/BSA, centrifuge 5 minutes at 250 *g*, add 50 μl FITC-labeled antiglobulin, incubate 30 minutes at RT in the dark; continue as for the direct test.

ADDENDUM XI
Immunofluorescence Test on Monocytes

Materials

- CD64 monoclonal antibody against FcRI (e.g., McAb 10.1)
- Goat anti-mouse Ig
- RPMI 1640/10% FCS (v/v)
- FITC-labeled F(ab′)2 of anti-human IgG (CLBK26H16 F1074), appropriately diluted in PBS/BSA
- PBS/BSA 0.2% (w/v)
- 1% Paraformaldehyde solution (w/v)/PBS
- Isotonic solution of Ficoll Isopaque S.D. 1.074 at 20°C
- Isotonic solution of Percoll S.D. 1.062 at 20°C, pH 7.4
- Flow cytometer (FACS, Becton and Dickinson)

Isolation of monocytes

- Centrifuge ACD-anticoagulated blood for 20 minutes at 2200 *g*, collect the buffy coat, and place it on a layer of Ficol Isopaque. Centrifuge again for 20 minutes at 2200 *g*.
- Wash the cells from the ring fraction twice with RPMI/FCS and resuspend them in the Percoll solution. Centrifuge for 15 minutes at 1000 *g* and collect the monocytes from the interphase. *Note:* Further purification of the monocytes may be achieved by elutriation.
- Make up a suspension in RPMI/FCS containing 2.5×10^6 cells/ml.

Preparation of FcRI-modulated cells

- Place 0.05 ml of the monocyte suspension and 0.05 ml monoclonal anti-FcRI (McAb 10.1 diluted 1:500 in RPMI/FCS) in wells of a microtiter plate, incubate at RT for 30 minutes, then wash three times with RPMI/FCS and resuspend the cells in a solution of 0.10 ml unlabeled goat anti-mouse Ig (the reagent GM17-01F from the CLB is used diluted 1:2000 in RPMI/FCS). Incubate 30 minutes at 37°C in a humidified atmosphere with 5% CO_2. Wash the cells three times with PBS/BSA, fix the cells for 5 minutes in 1% PFA, wash twice with PBS/BSA, and resuspend in 0.05 ml PBS/BSA.

Method

- Incubate the modulated monocytes suspended in 0.50 ml PBS/BSA with 0.01 ml of the serum under investigation, or a dilution thereof, for 30 minutes at RT and wash the cells again three times with PBS/BSA; then incubate the cells with 0.05 ml FITC-labeled conjugate for 30 minutes at RT, wash three times with PBS/BSA, and measure the intensity of the fluorescence in a flow cytometer.

REFERENCES

1. **Soulier, J. P., Pareteau, C., and Drouet, J.,** Platelet indirect radioactive Coomb's test. Its utilization for PL^{A1} grouping, *Vox Sang.,* 29, 253, 1975.
2. **Von dem Borne, A. E. G. Kr., Verheugt, F. W. A., Oosterhof, F., Von Riesz, E., Brutel de la Riviere, A., and Engelfriet, C. P.,** A simple immunofluorescence test for detection of platelet antibodies, *Br. J. Haematol.,* 39, 195, 1978.
3. **Tate, Y., Sorensen, R. L., Gerrard, J. M., White, J. G., and Krivit, W.,** An immunoenzyme histochemical technique for the detection of platelet antibodies from the serum of patients with idiopathic (autoimmune) thrombocytopenic purpura, *Br. J. Haematol.,* 37, 265, 1977.
4. **Shibata, Y., Juji, T., Nishizawa, Y., Sakamoto, H., and Ozawa, N.,** Detection of platelet antibodies by a newly developed mixed agglutination with platelets, *Vox Sang.,* 41, 25, 1981.
5. **Kelton, J. G.,** Platelet-associated IgG, in *Immunologic Aspects of Platelet Transfusion,* American Association of Blood Banks, Publications, Arlington, VA, 1985, 21.
6. **Mulder, A., van Leeuwen, E. F., Veenboer, J. G. M., Tetteroo, P. A. T., and von dem Borne, A. E. G. Kr.,** Immunochemical characterization of platelet specific alloantigens, *Scand. J. Haematol.,* 33, 267, 1984.
7. **Huisman, J. G.,** Immunoblotting: an emerging technique in immunohematology, *Vox Sang.,* 50, 129, 1986.
8. **Collins, J. and Aster, R. H.,** Use of immobilized platelet membrane glycoproteins for the detection of platelet-specific alloantibodies in solid-phase ELISA, *Vox Sang.,* 53, 157, 1987.
9. **McMillan, R., Tani, P., Millard, P., Berchtold, L., Renshaw, L., and Woods, V. L., Jr.,** Platelet-associated and plasma anti-glycoprotein autoantibodies in chronic ITP, *Blood,* 70, 1040, 1978.
10. **Millard, F. E., Tani, P., and McMillan, R.,** A specific assay for anti-HLA antibodies: application to platelet donor selection, *Blood,* 70, 1495, 1987.
11. **Kiefel, V., Santoso, S., Weisheit, M., and Mueller-Eckhardt, C.,** Monoclonal antibody-specific immobilization of platelet antigens (MAIPA): a new tool for the identification of platelet-reactive antibodies, *Blood,* 70, 1722, 1987.
12. **Mueller-Eckhardt, C., Schultz, G., Sauer, H. K., Dienst, C., and Mahn, I.,** Studies on the platelet radioactive antiglobulin test, *J. Immunol. Meth.,* 19, 1, 1978.
13. **LoBuglio, A. F., Court, W. S., Vinogur, L. B. S., Maglot, G. A. B., and Shaw, G. M.,** Immune thrombocytopenic purpura. Use of a ^{125}I-labeled antihuman IgG monoclonal antibody to quantify platelet-bound IgG, *N. Engl. J. Med.,* 309, 459, 1983.
14. **Shulman, N. R., Leissinger, C. A., Hotchkins, A. J., and Kantz, C. A.,** The non-specific nature of platelet-associated IgG, *Trans. Assoc. Am. Physicians,* 14, 213, 1982.
15. **Tijhuis, G. J., Klassen, R. J. L., Modderman, P. W., Ouwehand, W. H., and von dem Borne, A. E. G. Kr.,** Quantification of platelet-bound immunoglobulins of different class and subclass using radiolabelled monoclonal antibodies: assay conditions and clinical applications, *Br. J. Haematol.,* 77, 93, 1991.
16. **Helmerhorst, F. M., Smeenk, R. J. T., Hack, C. E., Engelfriet, C. P., and von dem Borne, A. E. G. Kr.,** Interference of IgG, IgG aggregates and immune complexes in tests for platelet autoantibodies, *Br. J. Haematol.,* 55, 533, 1983.
17. **Vos, J. J. E., Huisman, J. D., van der Lelie, J., and von dem Borne, A. E. G. Kr.,** Platelet-associated IgG in thrombocytopenia: a comparison of two techniques, *Vox Sang.,* 53, 162, 1987.
18. **Schneider, W. and Schnaidt, M.,** The platelet adhesion fluorescence test: a modification of the platelet suspension immuno-fluorescence test, *Blut,* 43, 389.
19. **Lazarchick, J. and Hall, S. A.,** Platelet-associated IgG assay using flow cytometric analysis, *J. Immunol. Meth.,* 87, 257, 1986.

20. **Rosenfield, C. S., Nichols, G., and Bodensteiner, D. C.,** Flow cytometric measurement of antiplatelet antibodies, *Am. J. Clin. Pathol.,* 87, 518, 1987.
21. **Dunstan, R. A. and Simpson, M. B.,** Heterogeneous distribution of antigens on human platelets demonstrated by fluorescence flow cytometry, *Br. J. Haematol.,* 61, 603, 1985.
22. **Nel, J. D. and Stevens, K.,** A new method for the simultaneous quantitation of platelet-bound immunoglobulin (IgG) and complement (C_3) employing an enzyme-linked immunosorbent assay (ELISA) procedure, *Br. J. Haematol.,* 44, 281, 1980.
23. **Doughty, R., James, V., and Magee, J.,** An enzyme linked immunosorbent assay for leukocyte and platelet antibodies, *J. Immunol. Meth.,* 47, 161, 1981.
24. **Gudino, M. and Miller, W. V.,** Application of the enzyme linked immunospecific assay (ELISA) for the detection of platelet antibodies, *Blood,* 57, 32, 1981.
25. **Hedge, U. M., Powel, D. K., Bowes, A., and Gordon-Smith, E. C.,** Enzyme-linked immunoassay for the detection of platelet associated IgG, *Br. J. Haematol.,* 48, 39, 1981.
26. **Horai, S., CLaas, F. H. J., and van Rood, J. J.,** Detection of platelet antibodies by enzyme-linked immunosorbent assay (ELISA) on artificial monolayers of platelets, *Immunol. Lett.,* 3, 67, 1981.
27. **Folea, G., Mandrand, B., and Dechavanne, M.,** Simultaneous enzyme-immunologic assays for platelet associated IgG, IgM, and C3. A useful tool in assessment of immune thrombocytopenia, *Thromb. Res.,* 26, 249, 1982.
28. **Saleem, A., Banez, E. J., and Sitters, B.,** Enzyme labeled immunosorbent assay (ELISA) for detection of platelet-antibodies, *J. Clin. Lab. Sci.,* 12, 68, 1982.
29. **Schiffer, C. A. and Young, V.,** Detection of platelet antibodies using a micro-enzyme-linked immunosorbent assay (ELISA), *Blood,* 61, 311, 1983.
30. **Tamerius, J. D., Curd, J. G., Taini, P., and McMillan, R.,** An enzyme-linked immunosorbent assay for platelet compatibility testing, *Blood,* 62, 744, 1983.
31. **Yesus, Y. W., Scrivner, D. L., Mitchell, M. A., and Ranashir, M.,** A simplified micro ELISA procedure for the measurement of platelet-associated IgG (PAI gG), *Am. J. Clin. Pathol.,* 81, 81, 1984.
32. **Yam, P., Petz, L. D., Scott, E. P., and Santos, S.,** Platelet crossmatch test using radiolabelled staphylococcal protein A or peroxidase anti-peroxidase in allo-immunized patients, *Br. J. Haematol.,* 57, 337, 1984.
33. **Howe, S. E., Lynch, D. M., and Lynch, J. M.,** An enzyme-linked immunosorbent assay for the quantification of serum platelet-bindable IgG, *Transfusion,* 24, 348, 1984.
34. **Lynch, D. M., Lynch, J. M., and Howe, S. E. A.,** Quantitative ELISA procedure for the measurement of membrane-bound platelet-associated IgG (PAIgG), *Am. J. Clin. Pathol.,* 83, 331, 1985.
35. **Rachel, J. M., Terri, C., Summers, B. S., Sinor, L. T., and Plapp, F. V.,** Use of a solid phase red red blood cell adherence method for pretransfusion platelet compatibility testing, *Am. J. Clin. Pathol.,* 90, 63, 1988.
36. **Rachel, J. M., Sinor, L. T., Rawfik, D. W., Summers, T., Beck, M. L., Bayer, W. L., and Plapp, F. V.,** A solid-phase red cell adherence test for platelet cross-matching, *Med. Lab. Sci.,* 42, 194, 1985.
37. **Santoso, S., Kiefel, V., and Mueller-Eckhardt, C.,** Human platelet alloantigens Br^a/Br^b are expressed on the very late activation antigen 2 (VLA-2) of T lymphocytes, *Hum. Immunol.,* 25, 237, 1989.
38. **Rock, G., Decary, F., Tittley, P., and Fuller, V.,** Electroblotting and immunohistological staining and identifications of platelet antibodies, *Br. J. Haematol.,* 67, 437, 1987.
39. **Woods, V. L., Oh, E. H., Mason, D., and McMillan, R.,** Autoantibodies against the glycoprotein IIb/IIIa complex in patients with chronic ITP, *Blood,* 64, 156, 1984.
40. **Blumberg, N., Masel, D., Mayer, T., Horan, P., and Heal, J.,** Removal of HLA-A,B antigens from platelets, *Blood,* 63, 448, 1984.

41. **Nordhagen, R. and Flaathen, S. T.,** Chloroquine removal of HLA antigens from platelets for the platelet immunofluorescence test, *Vox Sang.*, 48, 156, 1985.
42. **Langenscheidt, F., Kiefel, V., Santoso, S., Nau, A., and Mueller-Eckhardt, C.,** Quantitation of platelet antigens after chloroquine treatment, *Eur. J. Haematol.*, 42, 186, 1989.
43. **Kurata, Y., Oshida, M., Take, H., Furubayashi, T., Mitzutani, H., Tomiyama, Y., and Tarni, S.,** Acid treatment of platelets as a simple procedure for distinguishing platelet-specific antibodies from anti-HLA antibodies: comparison with chloroquine treatment, *Vox Sang.*, in press.
44. **Rubin, H. L.,** Antibody elution from red blood cells, *J. Clin. Pathol.*, 16, 70, 1963.
45. **Helmerhorst, F. M., van Oss, C. J., Bruynes, E. C. E., Engelfriet, C. P., and von dem Borne, A. E. G. Kr.,** Elution of granulocyte and platelet antibodies, *Vox Sang.*, 43, 196, 1982.
46. **von dem Borne, A. E. G. Kr., Vos, J. J. E., van der Lelie, J., Bossers, B., and van Dalen, C. M.,** Clinical significance of positive platelet immunofluorescence test in thrombocytopenia, *Br. J. Haematol.*, 64, 767, 1986b.
47. **McCullough, J. J., Weiblen, B. J., Clay, M. E. et al.,** Effect of leukocyte antibodies on the fate in vivo of indium-III-labeled granulocytes, *Blood,* 58, 164, 1981.
48. **McCullough, J. J., Clay, M. E., Richards, K. et al.,** Leukocyte antibodies: their effect on the fate in vivo of indium-III labeled granulocytes, *Blood,* 60(Abstr.), 80a, 1982.
49. **Lalezari, P., Nussbaum, M., Gelman, S. et al.,** Neonatal neutropenia due to maternal isoimmunization, *Blood,* 15, 236, 1960.
50. **Lalezari, P. and Bernard, G. E.,** Improved leukocyte antibody detection with prolonged incubation, *Vox Sang.*, 9, 664, 1964.
51. **Lalezari, P., Jiang, A., and Lee, S.,** A microagglutination technique for detection of leukocyte agglutinins, in NIAD Manual: A Tissue Technique, Ray, J. G., Hare, D. B., Pederson, P. D. et al., Eds., Publ. No. (NIH) 77-545, National Institutes of Health, Department of Health, Education and Welfare, 1976, 4.
52. **Lalezari, P.,** The granulocyte: function and clinical utilization, in *Progress in Clinical and Biological Research,* Greenwalt, T. J. and Jamieson, G. A., Eds., Alan R. Liss, New York, 1977, 209.
53. **Verheugt, F. W. A., von dem Borne, A. E. G. Kr., van Noord-Bokhorst, J. C., van Elven, E. H., and Engelfriet, C. P.,** Serological immunochemical and immunocytological properties of granulocyte antibodies, *Vox Sang.*, 35, 294, 1978.
54. **Severson, C. D., Greazel, N. A., and Thompson, J. S.,** Micro-capillary agglutination, *J. Immunol. Meth.*, 4, 369, 1974.
55. **Thompson, J. S. and Severson, C. D.,** Granulocyte antigens, in *A Seminar on Antigens on Blood Cells and Body Fluid,* Bell, C. A., Ed., American Association of Blood Banks, Washington, D.C., 1988, 151.
56. **Thompson, J. S.,** Antileukocyte capillary agglutinating antibody in pre- and post-transplantation sera, in *Manual of Clinical Immunology,* Rose, N. R. and Friedman, H., Eds., American Society of Microbiology, Washington, D.C., 1976, 868.
57. **Smith, W. K., Mold, J. W., Tseng, S. L. et al.,** Microcapillary agglutination assay for detection of specific antileukocyte reactivity in neutropenic patients, *Am. J. Haematol.*, 7, 329, 1979.
58. **Minchinton, R. M. and Waters, A. H.,** Chloroquine stripping of HLA antigens from neutrophils without removal of neutrophil-specific antigens, *Br. J. Haematol.*, 57, 703, 1984.
59. **Kuijpers, R. W. A. M., Dooren, M. C., von dem Borne, A. E. G. Kr., and Ouwehand, W. H.,** Detection of human monocyte reactive allo-antibodies by flow cytometry following selective down modulation of the Fc receptor I, *Blood,* 78, 2150, 1991.
60. **Verheugt, F. W. A., von dem Borne, A. E. G. Kr., Decary, F. et al.,** The detection of granulocyte alloantibodies with an indirect immunofluorescence test, *Br. J. Haematol.*, 36, 533, 1977.

61. **Engelfriet, C. P., Tetteroo, P. A. T., van der Veen, J. P. W. et al.,** Granulocyte specific antigens and methods for their detection, in *Advances in Immunobiology: Blood Cell Antigens and Bone Marrow Transplantation. Progress in Clinical and Biological Research,* McCullough, J. and Sandler, S. G., Eds., Allan R. Liss, New York, 1984, 121.
62. **Press, C., Kline, W. E., Clay, M. E. et al.,** A microtiter modification of granulocyte immunofluorescence, *Vox Sang.,* 49, 110, 1985.
63. **Verheugt, F. W. A., von dem Borne, A. E. G. Kr., van Noord-Bokhorst, J. C. et al.,** Autoimmune granulocytopenia: the detection of granulocyte autoantibodies with the immunofluorescence test, *Br. J. Haematol.,* 39, 339, 1978.
64. **Veys, P. A., Gutteridge, C. N., Macey, M., and Ord, A. C.,** Detection of granulocyte antibodies using flow cytometric analysis of leucokyte immunofluorescence, *Vox Sang.,* 56, 42, 1989.
65. **Robinson, J. P., Duque, R. E., Boxer, L. A., Ward, P. A., and Hudson, J. L.,** Measurement of antineutrophil antibodies by flow cytometry: simultaneous detection of antibodies against monocytes and lymphocytes, *Diagn. Clin. Immunol.,* 5, 163, 1987.
66. **Minchinton, R. M., Rockman, S., and McGrath, K. M.,** Evaluation and calibration of a fluorescence-activated cell sorter for the interpretation of the granulocyte immunofluorescence test (GIFT), *Clin. Lab. Haematol.,* 11, 349, 1989.
67. **Boxer, G. J., Boxer, M. A., and Boxer, L. A.,** The identification of antiplatelet and antineutrophil antibodies by ^{125}I-staphylococcal protein A, in *Immune Cytopenias,* McMillan, R., Ed., Churchill Livingstone, New York, 1983, 87.
68. **Thompson, J. S., Severson, C. D., Goeken, N. E., and Rhoades, J. R.,** Granulocyte and monocyte antigens and antibodies, in *HLA Typing: Methodology and Clinical Aspects,* Ferrone, S. and Solheim, B. G., Eds., CRC Press, Boca Raton, FL, 1982, 35.
69. **Jager, M. J., Claas, F. H. J., Gratama, J. W., de Lange, P., Zwaan, F. E., and van Rood, J. J.,** 9a: A risk factor in bone marrow transplantation, *Tissue Antigens,* 32, 100, 1988.
70. **Baldwin, W. M., III, Claas, F. H. J., van Rood, J. J., and Van Es, L. A.,** All monocytes antigens are not expressed on renal endothelium, *Tissue Antigens,* 21, 254, 1984.

Chapter 17

PLATELET CROSSMATCHING

J. Freedman

TABLE OF CONTENTS

ISBN 0-8493-4938-9

I. INTRODUCTION

This chapter will describe the background, value, and limitations of platelet crossmatching and will attempt to estimate the clinical importance of the technology at the present time.

The transfusion of platelets to patients with thrombocytopenia induced by chemotherapy began in the early 1960s. Platelet transfusions used therapeutically and prophylactically in the management of thrombocytopenic patients have significantly reduced the incidence of hemorrhagic complications. In recent years, platelet utilization has increased ten times more than red blood cells. Transfusions of either whole blood or red cells increased 58% between 1971 and 1980. During the same period, platelet utilization increased 598%, from 0.4 to 2.8 million units.[1] The growing demand brought an increased awareness of problems associated with platelet transfusion therapy. A major problem has been the detection and management of platelet alloimmunization. It was soon observed that, in patients who had received multiple transfusions, random donor platelet transfusions became ineffective in increasing the platelet count; this was due to development of antibodies which shortened the survival of the transfused platelets.

II. ALLOIMMUNIZATION AND THE REFRACTORY STATE

Platelet transfusions are generally administered as a pool of 6 to 10 individual concentrates collected at random. As a result of exposure to foreign antigens in transfused platelets and other blood products, up to 50% of patients with acute myeloblastic leukemia, almost 100% of patients with aplastic anemia, and 10% of patients with solid tumors will develop platelet alloantibodies.[2–4] The frequency of alloimmunization in acute leukemia has been estimated to range from about 40 to 60%;[4,5] the former figure is more likely correct, although the incidence of alloimmunization is probably at least partially dependent on the patient population and the immunosuppressive therapy administered. Immune destruction of transfused platelets is perhaps the major problem faced by the blood bank in the transfusion management of patients with marrow aplasia due to leukemia, chemotherapy, and aplastic anemia. As HLA or platelet-specific antibodies develop, posttransfusion platelet increments diminish because of immune destruction and recipients derive little or no benefit; such recipients are called refractory. The clinical effect is a progressively shortened survival of the transfused platelets and failure of the transfused platelets to produce hemostasis. In this clinical state of refractoriness to subsequent random-donor platelet transfusion, the patient fails to respond appropriately to transfusions of random platelets in the absence of nonimmune factors known to cause platelet consumption, such as infection, fever, splenomegaly, consumptive coagulopathy, amphotericin, active bleeding, etc.

Alloimmunization to platelets is characterized clinically by the failure to recover adequate numbers of circulating platelets following transfusion of platelets which have been prepared and stored properly. Although shortened platelet survival may be the earliest sign of alloimmunization, it is usually impractical to measure survival accurately and determinations of platelet recovery are used instead. There was no uniformity in the early literature as to the minimum recovery which constituted a satisfactory platelet transfusion, but over recent years, it has been recognized that it is appropriate and necessary to use a corrected count increment (CCI) after transfusion in order to standardize for transfusions of differing dosages of platelets to recipients of different size. The method described by Daly et al.[6] is frequently utilized. Usually CCI is evaluated 1 hour and/or 24 hours after transfusion, although it was recently suggested that a 10-minute CCI may be equivalent to the 1-hour CCI.[7] Using the formula of [(posttransfusion − pretransfusion platelet count)/number of platelets administered $\times$ 10^{11}] $\times$ body surface area in m^2, a satisfactory posttransfusion CCI at 1 hour and at 24 hours are $>7500/\mu l$ and $>4500/\mu l$, respectively.[6]

Measurement of platelet increments 1 hour after transfusion has been suggested to be a reliable way of distinguishing clinically between alloimmunization (very low 1-hour increments) and other causes of platelet destruction (near-normal increments at one hour with subsequent rapid fall in counts).[6] A number of studies have, however, reported alloimmunized patients with no evidence of other causes of platelet consumption who have good 1-hour posttransfusion CCI but poor increments at 24 hours.[7–11] This may relate to antigen-antibody affinity, or state of activation, suppression, or saturation of the reticuloendothelial system. Consequently, we believe that it is preferable to evaluate patients using both the 1-hour and the 24-hour CCI.

When alloimmunization and the refractory state begin to develop, patients who continue to receive repetitive pooled platelet products experience progressively decreasing platelet increments. The length of time before refractoriness occurs is variable and may be influenced by the disease process and its therapy, the frequency of transfusions, and possibly host genetic factors.[2,5,12,13] Typically, the refractory state begins within weeks or occasionally months of repetitive transfusions.[14] Substitution of single-donor platelets from HLA-identical donors will provide normal increments in approximately 60 to 70% of these patients (see below). With time, however, even HLA-identical platelets may become ineffective. Patients are frequently broadly immunized, i.e., immunized to virtually all donors, and the probability of choosing a purely random donor whose platelets will not be destroyed is very low. There is, however, usually a group of potential donors against whom the patient is not alloimmunized. The problem is defining the antigenic profile of the donor population to which the patient is not alloimmunized. When the cause (i.e., the alloantigens to which the patient is immunized) of the immunologic refractory state is not known, the use of sensitive crossmatching procedures to select compatible donors may be the only available recourse. Routine crossmatching has, however, been expensive, logistically complex, and places additional time burdens on volunteer donors.

There is no well-defined relationship between the number of donor exposures and the extent of antibody formation, although it has been suggested that there may be a lower incidence of alloimmunization in patients exposed to platelets derived by apheresis from fewer donors.[15,16] It remains unclear whether multiple exposures are necessary for alloimmunization, although patients with acute leukemia usually develop antibodies 2 to 6 weeks after beginning platelet therapy. In contrast to the report of Pegels et al.,[17] the findings of Freedman et al.[7] and Dutcher et al.[14] suggested that immunization is not dose dependent.

Close attention must be paid to the clinical state of patients receiving platelet transfusions. It has become evident that a number of patients who develop limited and/or broad-spectrum HLA antibodies may lose these antibodies over a couple of weeks, with or without continued exposure to platelet transfusion.[13,18,19] This may be due to development of antiidiotypic antibodies.[20,21] Antibody specificities may change over time and, in some cases, narrow alloantibody specificities may broaden while in others, antibodies may actually disappear.[13] Frequent serum samples should therefore be taken for antibody detection and crossmatching.

III. PLATELET ANTIGENS

Several antigenic systems are present on the platelet surface. These include blood group determinants such as the ABO system, HLA determinants (the antigens expressed by the major histocompatibility complex), and platelet-specific antigens that appear to be alloepitopes on integral platelet membrane glycoproteins.

The clinical significance of transfusing platelets and plasma that are ABH incompatible with the recipient has been a controversial issue.[22–29] Although ABO matching was considered to be of relatively little importance in platelet transfusion, it is now believed that it is preferable to transfuse patients with ABO-compatible platelets.[29] Heal et al.[30] evaluated the frequency in which ABH compatibility could be detected in an IgG platelet crossmatch using an antiglobulin solid-phase kinetic enzyme-linked immunoabsorbent assay (ELISA). It was concluded that increased IgG binding occurs in a majority of platelet crossmatches when group O recipients are tested against group A donors; transfusions of group B platelets to incompatible recipients may be more likely to result in satisfactory increments than incompatible transfusions of group A platelets, but this remains to be proven. The authors found that chloroquine failed to remove ABH antigens from the platelet surface (in contrast to its effect on HLA antigens), but that the use of a chemically synthesized human blood group A trisaccharide antigen covalently linked to insoluble crystalline silica (Synsorb-A) may be a useful adjunct to platelet serologic testing when group O serum needs to be tested against group A platelets.

The clinical significance of reduced platelet recovery in patients receiving ABO-incompatible platelet transfusions is subject to a diversity of opinion. Heal et al.[30] suggested that giving group A platelets to group O recipients is serologically and probably clinically distinct from giving group B platelets to group O or A recipients. This may, in part, explain previous reported variations in patients' responses to ABO-mismatched transfusions. The authors suggested that in thrombocytopenic patients who are refractory to random-donor platelet transfusions, and in whom platelet support with HLA-matched platelets is only marginally effective, ABH compatibility may, in selected instances, play an important role.

Incompatibility within the HLA system appears to be responsible for a major portion of the alloimmunization against platelet antigens and for the subsequent clinical refractoriness to platelet transfusions. Platelet membranes contain HLA class I A and B antigens; HLA C antigens are poorly represented on the platelet and are not considered important for matching, and the platelet does not express HLA class II antigens. The biochemistry and serology of the HLA system are complex and there is considerable polymorphism within the system. Briefly, the HLA antigens consist of a polymorphic chain (α) and nonpolymorphic smaller chain (β_2-microglobulin). Either of two loci on chromosome 6 (the A or B locus) codes for the α-chain which has a polymorphic, a nonpolymorphic, and an oligopolymorphic portion. The oligopolymorphic portion results in expression of "public" antigens which are shared with several specific "private" antigens, the commonly determined HLA antigens. The private HLA antigens are presumably on the polymorphic portion of the molecule; they all group into "cross-reactive groups" or CREGS, based on the presence of public antigens. Broad alloimmunization in the refractory state is usually caused by alloantibodies induced by public epitopes.[33]

HLA antigens on platelets may arise intrinsically or may be absorbed from the plasma. The amount of HLA antigen detectable on platelets may vary from one antigen to another and from one patient to another.[34–38] It has been suggested[39] that adsorbed antigen is less important *in vivo* and may be less detectable by certain assays.

Platelets also have allomorphic antigenic structures which are specific to the platelet. These include serologically defined alloantigens, e.g., Pl^{A1}/Pl^{A2}, Bak^a/Bak^b, Pen^a/Pen^b, Br^a, etc.[40] Some of these are defined biochemically in terms of the specific platelet membrane glycoprotein on which the antigen resides. There may be other platelet-specific antigens which, as yet, remain unidentified, since, in highly alloimmunized patients, in the absence of detectable antibodies to platelet-specific antigens, HLA-identical platelets may not survive on transfusion. Overall, however, the most important antigenic determinants for platelet compatibility appear to be represented by, or closely linked to, the HLA locus.

IV. HLA MATCHING

Since Yankee et al.[12,41] showed that, of the various platelet alloantigens, HLA markers are most likely to provoke a humoral immune response, investigators have attempted to provide refractory alloimmunized patients with HLA-compatible single-donor plateletpheresis products. Initially, related donors were used; subsequently, unrelated matched donors have been shown to be suitable and easier to procure. While HLA-matched platelets are beneficial in many cases, HLA matching is expensive and a large pool of registered donors is required.[41–45] Furthermore, the high degree of polymorphism in the HLA system makes it difficult to provide HLA-identical (''A''-matched, in which all four A and B antigens of the HLA locus are the same between donor and recipient) platelets for many alloimmunized patients. In addition, HLA matching does not reliably predict platelet transfusion response in all patients. Even when ''A''-matched platelets are administered, in about 18 to 35% of the cases, the transfusion does not result in an appropriate posttransfusion platelet count increment.[24,25,46–49] While the reason for these failures is unclear, a possible explanation is the presence of antibodies directed against platelet-specific antigens; such antibodies have been detected in the sera of 22 to 25% of alloimmunized patients.[17,50] It is possible that the lack of response may be due to the presence of anti-drug antibodies or autoantibodies.

It is also well recognized that there may be differing expression of HLA antigens on different cells, as in the case of HLA-B12, which is strongly expressed on the lymphocytes but which can have a highly variable difference in quantitative expression on platelets from the same individual.[36] Successful transfusions have been reported to occur in 35% of alloimmunized patients receiving HLA-mismatched donor platelets;[11,46] this phenomenon has been explained by restricted alloimmunization,[51] immunogenicity,[38,48,52] impaired reticuloendothelial cell function,[53] coincidental matched platelet-specific antigens, poor platelet HLA antigen expression, and decreased immunologic competence of the recipient.[4]

The principles of compatibility testing in platelet transfusion are similar to those used in transfusion of red cells, i.e., antibody detection and antigen matching. Antigen matching is particularly applied to selection of potential donors on the basis of ''private'' HLA antigens. However, a major disadvantage of this approach is the cost of establishing and maintaining a necessary panel of several thousand HLA typed apheresis donors. Several studies have indicated that relatively small numbers of perfectly matched donors are available per patient.[44,45,54] In a random population, the odds of providing a full ''A'' match range from about 1:50 for the most common phenotypes to 1:100,000 for less common phenotypes.[45] In a study examining the frequency of compatible donors in HLA alloimmunization,[45] for 100 patients and 2470 donors, each patient had an average of only 1.3 donors who were perfectly matched (range 0 to 14). More donors were identified for patients with common genotypes, but 25 patients with unusual HLA phenotypes had no perfect matches. HLA-identical platelets are thus frequently unavailable. Because of such difficulties, studies have been performed which have indicated that it may not be necessary to select donors for private HLA antigens and that public HLA antigens may be more important;[31–33] it has been confirmed that it may be useful to transfuse platelets within "cross-reactive" groups in which platelets bear common public antigens.[46] Although a number of studies have demonstrated the value of HLA matching in providing histocompatible platelet support for alloimmunized patients, this approach extrapolates the results of histocompatibility testing done on lymphocytes to platelet and it does not take into account the possible influence of quantitative differences in antigenic expression on platelets or of antibodies to platelet-specific antigens. It appears that, since some HLA antigens are poorly expressed or not expressed at all on the platelet, matching for all of the HLA antigens may not be necessary. Platelets may thus be selected on the basis of serologic similarity to the recipient, but approximately 40 to 50% of platelets selected on serologic cross-reactivities are ineffective.[11] As noted above, 28 to 35% of alloimmunized patients have excellent posttransfusion CCI despite major HLA mismatches[25,55] and, therefore, HLA matching may result in the exclusion of valuable donors for alloimmunized patients. Findings such as these have indicated a need to develop techniques other than HLA matching that can predict and select compatible platelets for alloimmunized patients.

V. PLATELET CROSSMATCHING

Pretransfusion platelet crossmatching is a more direct approach to identifying compatible donors for alloimmunized recipients. A direct crossmatch would eliminate the guesswork inherent in HLA matching. By performing a compatibility test with patient's serum against intended platelet donors in a manner analogous to the major crossmatch used in selecting red blood cells for transfusion, one would be able to detect any antibody directed against an antigen present on the platelet. By relying on HLA matching, the degree of matching is limited to HLA antigens alone. It is still uncertain how important antigens other than HLA are in causing antibody-mediated refractoriness. Nonetheless, the failure of 20 to 35% of HLA-identical platelet transfusions suggests that non-HLA antigens play a significant role in platelet refractoriness.

The availability of simple accurate platelet crossmatch techniques should enhance the efficacy of platelet transfusions. The optimum platelet crossmatch method would ideally predict poor transfusion responses. A number of assays have been tested as potential platelet crossmatch methods. Compatibility testing has been difficult in platelet transfusion because of the problem of unidentified antibodies to platelet antigens, the difficulties in working with platelets compared to red cells (requiring more sophisticated and laborious techniques than reading of agglutination), the short life span of platelets, and the lack of predictive value (particularly the high incidence of false-negative results) of a number of the methods examined. In general, the techniques which have been used to detect antiplatelet antibodies in the serum are (1) those examining antibody-mediated changes in platelet function or chemistry, (2) those which detect antibodies against HLA antigens by lymphocytotoxicity, and (3) those which detect antibodies against platelet antigens (HLA and other).

A satisfactory platelet crossmatch should be capable of detecting both HLA and platelet-specific antibodies. It is important that the test supplies results quickly enough to meet demands for platelets in alloimmunized patients and within the relatively short outdating period for plateletpheresis products. Ideally, the techniques would utilize a stored bank of donor platelet samples to select the appropriate donor for subsequent plateletpheresis. The assay should be rapid and simple, yet have good sensitivity, specificity, and predictive value. Techniques used to detect antiplatelet antibodies may be characterized as follows: (1) inhibition of platelet function;[56] (2) platelet aggregation;[57,58] (3) antibody-induced platelet injury;[59] (4) platelet migration inhibition;[60] (5) complement fixation;[61,62] and (6) measurement of serum antibody by binding assays. Binding assays include those measuring platelet-bound IgG following platelet lysis or solubilization, e.g., Fab/anti-Fab assay[63] which is accurate but complex and requires radioisotopes, radial immunodiffusion[64] and rocket electrophoresis[65] which are simple but require a large number of platelets and are lengthy, and nephelometry[66] which is quantitative and rapid but false positives occur from particulate matter in the solutions. The complement lysis inhibition[67,68] and the two-stage immunoradiometric[69] assays are quantitative but are complex, time-consuming, and difficult to calibrate. The above binding assays have been mainly applied to detection of platelet-associated IgG rather than for circulating antibodies.

The direct ligand-binding assays which measure serum antibodies seem to have the most potential for use in platelet crossmatching. Examples of such binding assays include radiolabeled antiglobulin tests,[70,71] enzyme-linked antiglobulin tests,[72-74] staphylococcal protein A,[75] and immunofluorescence.[76-79] Advantages of such techniques include simplicity, speed, standardization, and objectively quantifiable endpoints. In addition, many of these methods, e.g., the platelet suspension immunofluorescence technique (PSIFT) or the platelet radioactive antiglobulin test (PRAT) can detect cell-bound complement as well as immunoglobulin. Recently a solid-phase red cell adherence assay has been described.[80] These assays will permit detection of anti-HLA antibodies, platelet-specific antibodies, auto- and drug-induced antibodies.

All the above techniques have been applied to the direct detection of incompatibility of platelets in alloimmunized patients by testing recipients' serum against donors' platelets. The early reports were discouraging, probably due to the relative insensitivity and nonspecificity of the techniques. More recently, with newer reagents and techniques, there appears to be general agreement that crossmatch methods are able to predict the outcome of transfusion with good accuracy and sensitivity.

A. EARLY STUDIES

Initially, to predict platelet compatibility in alloimmunized patients, the lymphocytotoxicity crossmatch was utilized. This test proved, however, to be nonreproducible and insensitive and the detection of anti-HLA antibodies by lymphocytotoxicity alone has proven to be inadequate for predicting success in platelet transfusion in alloimmunized individuals. Filip et al.,[81] Pogliani et al.,[82] and Wu et al.[83] were among the early investigators who indicated that lymphocytotoxicity was not highly predictive of transfusion results, with both false-positive and false-negative results being frequent. While lymphocytotoxic antibody measurement may correlate well with responsiveness to random donor transfusion[84] and may be a useful screening test, it is limited in that it detects only HLA antibodies; a false-negative rate of 40% was reported by Herzig et al.[85] and an overall error rate of 35% was reported by Kickler et al.[10] Consequently, assays detecting antibodies reacting with platelets themselves were developed. These included those measuring platelet damage, functional alteration, or thrombocytotoxicity. Early tests included platelet aggregation, platelet factor (PF)-3 release, chromium release, complement fixation, and serotonin release; all these proved insensitive, nonreproducible, unpredictive, and technically difficult. Later, the platelet migration inhibition test was shown to be sensitive, predictive, and reproducible but time-consuming, requiring up to 12 to 18 hours.[86] Few of the early studies were prospective analyses. Wu and co-workers had suggested that platelet aggregometry may be useful in selecting compatible donors for patients refractory to random platelet transfusion,[87] but subsequent prospective crossmatching, using platelet aggregometry, PF-3 and serotonin release, and lymphocytotoxicity test, was relatively insensitive and unreliable.[83]

Although the above studies were generally unsatisfactory for platelet compatibility testing, they suggested that similar approaches might be helpful in selecting donors for refractory patients. In the early studies, in particular, differences in technique and differing patient populations with differing definitions of alloimmunization and response, precluded comparison of the studies. Although it was clear that positive crossmatch tests generally predicted transfusion failure, it was often difficult to determine from the reports how much preselection of donors by HLA typing was done and therefore difficult to assess the accuracy of negative tests in predicting compatibility if crossmatch was used as the only test of donor selection. There were few direct comparisons of different platelet crossmatching tests in the same donor-recipient pairs and it remained unclear whether the role for platelet antibody testing was to supplement, as opposed to replace, HLA typing. Until the early 1980s, given the state of the art, it was felt that centers with a large demand for selected platelets were still best served by developing capabilities for HLA typing. The advances in platelet crossmatching in the past 5 to 6 years, however, have been impressive and definitive approaches should be forthcoming in the next few years. More recent methods have utilized ligand binding to antibody; this group of assays includes anti-IgG labeled with radioactive iodine, fluorescent probes, enzymes, or staphylococcal A protein labeled with iodine or an enzyme. Ligand-binding assays, using polyclonal or monoclonal anti-IgG labeled with a marker, have been found to be superior to other assays in detecting antibodies which may be important for compatibility testing in platelet transfusion.

B. MORE RECENT STUDIES

Brand et al. in 1978[48] reported a 93% success rate in predicting platelet transfusion compatibility, using a combination of lymphocytotoxicity and fluorescent antibody crossmatch techniques. These results were supported by a number of investigators in the early 1980s. Pegels et al. in 1982[17] suggested that platelet crossmatching should include both the indirect PSIFT and the lymphocytotoxic test. Myers et al.[88] used a quantitative immunofluorescence technique to detect immunity to platelets in multitransfused patients; the method predicted platelet survival results in 88% of transfusions, whereas comparative platelet aggregation, serotonin release, and lymphocytotoxicity testing showed correct predictions for only 41 to 59%. A good agreement between an indirect platelet immunofluorescence test crossmatch and posttransfusion platelet recovery was shown by Waters et al.,[89] but few patients were studied. The radiolabeled antiglobulin test was shown by Kickler et al.[10] to be highly effective for crossmatching platelets. Freedman et al.[7] also evaluated the indirect PRAT and PSIFT for platelet crossmatching in 29 patients and confirmed the observations of others. In contrast to previous studies which used single-donor platelets, the study of Freedman et al. used platelets from multiple random donors for prospective crossmatching and transfusion and suggested that, using the PRAT in particular, it may be practical to screen random donor platelet concentrates to select compatible platelets for alloimmunized patients. The PRAT successfully predicted the outcome of transfusion in 90% of cases. In all patients, transfusion of crossmatch-compatible platelets resulted in a significantly higher 24-hour CCI than was obtained following transfusion of random or incompatible platelets. Mean $\pm$ SEM 24-hour posttransfusion CCI was 17.79 $\pm$ 2.01 in 26 patients who received crossmatch-compatible pooled random-donor platelets, 1.19 $\pm$ 0.56 in 21 patients who received crossmatch-incompatible platelets, and 4.42 $\pm$ 0.97 in 25 patients who received random unmatched platelets. There was an 83% correlation of results with PRAT with those obtained by PSIFT.

The same authors recently compared four techniques, the standard lymphocytotoxicity (LCT), a Biotin-Avidin enzyme immunoassay (ELISA), the

PSIFT, and the PRAT, in prospective crossmatching for selection of compatible random-donor platelets for transfusion.[90] Patients with nonimmune causes for refractoriness were excluded; 107 episodes of pooled random donor platelet transfusions were evaluated in 26 patients. There was good reproducibility of results by individual techniques, but concordance of results by the different methods was only 40 to 60%. Using a rank scoring system, the relative efficiency of predictiveness for all transfusions was PRAT > LCT > PSIFT > ELISA. Mean posttransfusion CCI ($\times 10^9$/l) following PRAT-compatible platelets was 13.9 ± 12.7 at 1 hour and 7.3 ± 6.9 at 24 hours. In contrast, following PRAT-incompatible platelets, the CCI was 5.7 ± 7.8 at 1 hour and 2.1 ± 4.1 at 24 hours. Results were similar for the LCT. A limited evaluation of a radioimmunofiltration modification of PRAT suggested that it was a simple, fast, efficient, and inexpensive alternative. The efficiency of individual techniques was similar to that described by others.[14,16–18] The efficiency of combinations of techniques was evaluated and a combination of PRAT and LCT afforded the best predictability; sensitivity was higher than for either PRAT or LCT alone (93% vs. 79% and 63%, respectively). The combined use of LCT and PRAT had a sensitivity of 93% using the 1-hour CCI and 85% using the 24-hour CCI, i.e., about 10% of alloimmunized refractory patients tested by these methods gave false-negative results. This was similar to the success rate reported by others using a combination of crossmatch techniques.[9,14,18,48] However, a low specificity (47%) was obtained using the LCT and PRAT, indicating that many compatible platelets may give false-positive results and the platelets will thus unnecessarily not be transfused. Nonetheless, in compatibility testing, the aim is to prevent poor transfusion responses. Consequently, sensitivity is more important than specificity and we prefer to have few false negatives and will therefore tolerate some false-positive results. There remains however a need for improved platelet crossmatch methods. Most reports have evaluated platelet crossmatch methods using single-donor apheresis platelets. Thrombocytapheresis is expensive, requires significant commitment of time from the donor, and the procedure itself is not without risk. The potential to provide alloimmunized patients with effective platelets from random donors may reduce transfusion costs, as well as time spent by, and potential risk to, the donors. However, the use of pooled random-donor platelets may be useful only in selected patients (see below).

The predictive values for platelet crossmatches have been determined for virtually all methods.[91,92] Studies selecting platelets by HLA matching and platelet crossmatching had 75 to 95% higher predictive values for platelet crossmatching[11] than 60 to 80% with HLA-matched donors.[55] The predictive values, sensitivities, and specificities of the platelet crossmatch tests using labeled-immunoglobulin binding were similar and the methods appeared to be, in general, comparable. Brubaker et al.[91] reemphasized that posttransfusion platelet survival and/or platelet recovery evaluation are extremely important in the analysis of platelet crossmatching techniques. Most studies have used the CCI to measure platelet survival, but predicted count increment and survival of radiolabeled transfused platelets have also been used. The level of posttransfusion platelet increments considered to be satisfactory has varied considerably from study to study. Patient evaluation is also critical in the analysis of data. The patient's underlying disease and cause for bone marrow insufficiency (chemotherapy vs. radiation therapy, aplastic anemia, marrow transplantation, etc.), should be reported; a number of studies provided no patient disease information. In general, the studies did account for common pathologic causes of decreased posttransfusion platelet survival (e.g., sepsis, fever, splenomegaly, etc.). There are additional pathological factors affecting posttransfusion platelet survival that are not included in most studies, e.g., dysproteinemias, liver disease, acute renal transplant rejection, collagen vascular disease, administration of antilymphocyte globulin or IV IgG.

The number of crossmatches per patient is not included in most studies. The data reported by Brubaker et al.[91] included only five patients who averaged about six single-donor transfusion crossmatches and one patient who averaged 22 crossmatches. The authors indicated that the number of crossmatches performed in various studies varied from 33 to 230, with most studies averaging four to six crossmatches per patient, while three studies averaged less than two crossmatches per patient. The number of crossmatches per patient and the total number of crossmatches are important in choosing proper statistical methods. The statistical data indicated patient variation. Comparing results of each patient using weighted averages, the sensitivity decreased from 85 to 71%. Weighted average sensitivity indicated some patients who had more false negatives than others. Sensitivity is dependent on false negatives, i.e., a compatible crossmatch with unsatisfactory posttransfusion CCI; this might be due to causes other than immune.

McFarland and Aster[93] compared four platelet compatibility assays (PSIFT, ^{51}Cr release, microlymphocytotoxicity, and a radioactive monoclonal anti-IgG assay, MAIA). The MAIA was most predictive of platelet transfusion outcome with an approximately 75% predictability for posttransfusion platelet recovery at 1 hour and 2 hours. The only other assay to reach statistical significance was PSIFT (63% predictability for a 1-hour posttransfusion recovery). The degree of HLA compatibility between donor and recipient (exact matches vs. those utilizing cross-reactive associations) was unrelated to the ability of the MAIA to predict transfusion results. This study of 55 transfusions separated them into those occurring in the absence of nonimmune causes of platelet destruction (35 transfusions from 25 donors administered to 17 patients) and those in whom one or more nonimmune causes of platelet refractoriness were present. In those who had no nonimmune causes for platelet destruction, the sensitivity of the MAIA was 75 and 69% for 1-hour and 24-hour recovery, respectively, specificity was 73 and 100%, and predictability was 74 and 76%. Results with the LCT showed a sensitivity of 24 and 30%, specificity of 73 and 88%, and predictability of 47 and 45% for 1- and 24-

hour CCI, respectively. The PSIFT had a specificity of 40 and 31%, specificity of 93 and 88%, and predictability of 63 and 44%. The chromium release assay had a sensitivity of 12 and 10%, specificity of 100 and 100%, and predictability of 48 and 32%, respectively. An advantage of the MAIA assay is that it may be performed on frozen donor cells. In contrast to this study, others have found the PSIFT to be more sensitive;[48] possible explanations are the differences in serum: cell ratio in different studies, and the fact that in the study of McFarland and Aster all transfusions were matched or only slightly mismatched for class I HLA antigens. It may be that more extreme HLA incompatibilities are necessary to demonstrate positive reactions in the PSIFT. The lack of predictiveness of the LCT in this study is probably due to the fact that closely HLA-matched donors were used for these patients. It is important to note that even with the MAIA, occasional false-positive and, more commonly, false-negative reactions were noted, particularly when the 1-hour CCI was examined. The false-positive reactions for 1-hour recovery predictions may reflect the high sensitivity of the technique in detecting platelet-bound IgG, i.e., it may be capable of detecting amounts of IgG insufficient to cause poor 1-hour recoveries, but sufficient to cause platelet destruction in 24 hours. False-negative reactions might be explained by the inability of this monoclonal antibody to detect immunoglobulins other than IgG; alternatively, clinically inapparent nonimmune factors causing platelet consumption may have affected recoveries in some patients.

Harvard et al.[94] also compared lymphocytotoxicity and radioimmunoassay for detection of alloantibodies to platelets. Platelet-specific antibodies (antibodies reacting with platelets but not lymphocytes) were detected in 6 of 20 sera; the study demonstrated the usefulness of comparing the reactions of antisera with platelets and lymphocytes from the same donors.

The recently described monoclonal antibody-specific immobilization of platelet antigens (MAIPA) technique for identification of platelet-reactive antibodies[95] is not only a sensitive tool for typing of donors for platelet alloantigens, but may also be for detailed analysis of sera with ambiguous serological findings. It may be useful in platelet compatibility testing because it can give information about both HLA-specific (including noncytotoxic) and platelet-specific antibodies and it is the preferred method of detection of low-affinity antibody to the recently described Br antigens.[96] Other recent studies are described below.

C. FALSE-POSITIVE, FALSE-NEGATIVE, AND DISCORDANT RESULTS

False-positive results in the ligand-binding assays may have been due to detection of serum IgG that bound to the platelet surface but did not cause immune clearance. False-negatives may have been the result of high background values in the negative controls or due to nonimmune clearance of the platelets in the recipient, e.g., unidentified hypersplenism, or subclinical consumptive coagulopathy. The lack of concordance between the assays remains disturbing, particularly so for the PRAT, PSIFT, and ELISA assays, as the three techniques are basically similar and differ primarily in how the antibody is tagged. Several comparative studies have noticed significant differences in the predictive value of different platelet crossmatch techniques. A recent study found a 74% predictability for a radiolabeled monoclonal anti-IgG assay and a 63% predictability for the PSIFT.[93] Freedman et al. reported a 40 to 60% discordance between four techniques tested in parallel.[90] Kakaiya et al.[9] found discordant results in 13 of 31 (42%) crossmatches performed simultaneously by ELISA, PSIFT, and LCT. Ware et al.,[97] comparing radiolabeled and fluorescein-labeled antiglobulin platelet crossmatch assays, found that despite similar values for sensitivity and specificity in the two assays, test results were concordant in only 68% of the transfusions. It has been observed that the PSIFT and ELISA may fail to demonstrate low-titer HLA antibodies that do react in the LCT;[48,98] the reactions in the LCT may be caused by non-IgG antibodies or result from variable expression of HLA antigens on platelets compared to lymphocytes. On the other hand, not all the antibody specificities of alloantibodies to public HLA epitopes are detected in the standard LCT assay (a phenomenon referred to as CYNAP) and, for the LCT, it is probably better to use an antiglobulin-enhanced LCT.[99,100]

The review of Brubaker et al.[91] indicated that there are significant differences in the sensitivity of the same techniques performed in different laboratories, as well as between the different immunoglobulin-binding assays. Different techniques usually used antibodies from different sources; the effect of this is unclear, although it is unlikely alone to account for the discordant findings, since the reagents appeared to be both specific and potent. The variability of compatibility results with different crossmatch assays may reflect differences in the ability of particular individual methods to detect antibodies or particular specificity or equilibrium constant. On the other hand, the differences may simply reflect local expertise with the individual methods rather than the intrinsic serologic advantage of any method. We have also observed some patients to have IgM alloantibodies that caused rapid destruction of transfused platelets which were compatible in crossmatch tests using anti-IgG; transfusion of crossmatch-compatible platelets using anti-IgM resulted in good CCI.

It is important to caution that an assay should not be assumed to be uniformly consistant between technologists or between laboratories. In brief, at present there are numerous antiplatelet antibody tests with varying degrees of complexity and reproducibility. Current results suggest that more than one test should be available in any platelet antibody laboratory, since there is significant discordance between results obtained using different techniques. Decary[101] observed that although there was good agreement between 12 laboratories in detection of anti-Pl^{A1} this was not true when the antibody was weak (42 to 82% agreement); the lack of agreement was particularly evident for anti-HLA antibodies.

VI. LOGISTICAL AND TECHNICAL ISSUES

The ideal platelet crossmatch test should meet criteria of reproducibility, simplicity, rapidity of testing, and accurate prediction of posttransfusion response. A difficulty in crossmatching for platelet transfusion relates to the way platelets are obtained, e.g., by apheresis, and to the inability to preserve platelets for a considerable length of time, as for red cells. Apheresis platelets used in a single transfusion cannot be stored for longer than 24 to 48 hours and relatively few donors could be used as a panel from which to select the optimum compatibility. The technique must also take into account that platelets for alloimmunized patients are frequently required on short notice. Because of the relatively short storage time for platelets, these usually are administered shortly after procurement. It is impractical for donors generally to come to be tested for platelet crossmatching and then have to wait to donate if the *in vitro* results are "compatible". A large number of platelet donors may need to be screened. It would be preferable for platelet-related compatibility data to be stored in a form capable of providing immediate information about donor platelet types. HLA typing has this advantage because of the ease of storing such information in computers. However, as indicated above, antibodies to platelet-specific antigens undoubtedly also play a role in some patients, and testing and computer lists for these have not been found practicable at this time.

An alternative approach is to create long-term banks of potential donor platelets by cryopreservation or other methods of membrane preservation. This has been utilized in frozen lymphocyte panels for HLA typing, but has not, as yet, found general application with platelets. Although large-scale platelet cryopreservation can produce a clinically useful product for transfusion[102] platelet injury due to freezing and thawing may interfere with *in vitro* crossmatch testing.

The availability of a convenient platelet storage method should facilitate the general application of platelet crossmatching procedures for alloimmunized patients. All platelet crossmatch techniques have in common the requirement for a convenient and reliable method of storage of donor platelets, both to facilitate performance of the assay and to achieve accurate, reproducible, crossmatch results. Schiffer and Young[103] suggested that platelets stored in suspension may be satisfactory for this purpose. Kiss et al.[104] recently showed that both HLA and Pl^{A1} antigen reactivity can be maintained adequately in liquid-stored platelets when kept at 4°C for up to one year; this has been our experience also with platelets evaluated by flow cytometric testing. The platelets were stored in a modified Hank's buffer solution; we add sodium azide and paraformaldehyde to treat the platelets. To minimize the potential problem of false-negative crossmatches due to antigen loss, it is suggested that the stored donor platelets be updated at 6 to 8 months, since there is some evidence of loss of HLA reactivity in 10% of donor platelets by one year of storage. Alternative storage methods have been examined, e.g., frozen-stored platelets.[93,105,106] Generally, these platelets are desiccated in microtiter wells frozen at −70°C and appear to be suitable as crossmatch reagents, but these platelets require more processing steps and/or equipment than do platelets stored in suspension. Advantages of using frozen platelets are both immediate and potential. They include convenience, in that the platelets are already available, and the ability to establish a stable, standardized donor-platelet system for platelet antibody detection, allowing comparison of results over time. It should be possible to prepare a frozen platelet pool from multiple donors with known platelet-specific and HLA phenotypes that would readily permit assaying for HLA, auto- and allo-specific antibodies. The availability of single-donor platelets of known HLA phenotype would permit a convenient assessment of immunoreactivity *in vitro* and reduce inappropriate use of this blood product. Recently, the use of frozen platelets for platelet antibody testing by flow cytometric analysis was described.[107]

Another problem encountered relates to the fact that measurement of antibody directed against platelets is made more difficult by the tendency of platelets to nonspecifically adsorb plasma constituents, including immunoglobulins and immune complexes, on their surfaces. Platelets are also metabolically responsive to small amounts of residual thrombin in serum. It is important, therefore, to include ABO-compatible negative control sera in the antibody detection and compatibility assays. Essentially all the ligand-binding assays depend on the addition of anti-human IgG antibodies, coupled to marker substances, directed against the patient's platelets or platelets incubated with the test sera, e.g., immunofluorescent-labeled antibodies assessed semiquantitatively, microscopically, or quantitatively by flow cytometry; radiolabeled IgG, which is highly quantitative; radiolabeled staphylococcal A, which binds specifically to IgG (expecting IgG3); immunoglobulin linked to enzyme, usually alkaline phosphatase, and measured spectrophotometrically; IgG linked to horseradish peroxidase and tested in semiquantitative fashion histochemically; and visual semiquantitation of immunoglobulin-coated red cells in the solid-phase red cell adherence assay. Because normal platelets have a baseline level of approximately 0.2 to 0.4 pg of surface IgG, and because the platelet membrane nonspecifically adsorbs immunoglobulins, some of the quantitative techniques, particularly immunofluorescence, require preincubation of the cells with paraformaldehyde to decrease nonspecific binding without affecting platelet antigenicity.[7,77,108] Nonetheless, problems with background fluorescence still remain.

In platelet antibody tests it is often difficult to distinguish between platelet-specific and HLA antibody. As a result, the clinically significant antibody specificity may be unknown, preventing evaluation of donor selection by using antibody specificity. The methods of distinguishing between HLA and platelet-specific antibodies, e.g., absorption of anti-HLA, chloroquine[109] or citric acid pH 3.0[110] stripping of HLA surface antigens, are important, but outside the scope of this paper. Brubaker and Romine[111] evaluated the significance of circulating HLA and platelet-reactive antibodies by using parallel lymphocyte and platelet panels of characterized cells in retrospective analysis. They found platelet-specific antibodies, unrecognized by lymphocytotoxicity, to be important in such patients. They observed that, despite compatible lymphocytotoxicity crossmatches and HLA-matched platelet transfusions, platelet transfusions fail in up to 40% of patients. While several investigators have suggested that platelet-specific antibodies are responsible for unsuccessful recoveries of HLA-matched donor platelets, in general, studies have not determined the clinically significant nature of the antibody specificity. Brubaker and Romine[111] showed that much of the reactivity appeared to be against platelets (100%), and not against lymphocytes (30%); although this level of reactivity appears high, as indicated earlier, other crossmatch studies appear to support this contention. The study showed a lack of correlation between lymphocytotoxicity and an ELISA for predicting platelet survival; the sensitivity of the ELISA has been reported elsewhere to be 86%[91] in comparison to a sensitivity for lymphocytotoxicity of 23 to 57%.[9] The authors suggested that platelet crossmatching be solely used in the selection of platelets for allosensitized patients and that a direct platelet crossmatch test be used rather than lymphocytotoxicity.

HLA-identical platelets are frequently unavailable; therefore platelets selected on the basis of serologic similarity to the recipient are often used. The approach has drawbacks, with approximately 40 to 50% of platelets selected on serologic cross-reactivities reported to be ineffective.[11] In addition, since approximately 40% of non-HLA-identical platelet transfusions may be successful,[11,46] HLA matching may be unnecessarily restrictive and may result in the exclusion of valuable donors for alloimmunized patients, resulting in too few available donors to support a patient. The use of a direct crossmatch technique would eliminate the guesswork inherent in HLA matching. Previous studies showed the utility of platelet crossmatching as an adjunct to HLA matching. Others have shown that platelet crossmatching can be used to select platelets independently of HLA matching. Kickler et al.[112] evaluated the usefulness of crossmatching the patient's serum with prospective platelet donors who were not preselected on the basis of their HLA type. The patients did not have nonimmune causes for platelet transfusion failure and all had demonstrated lymphocytotoxic antibody against at least 30% of lymphocytes tested in the antibody screening; the patients were selected for study because they lacked sufficient HLA-identical donors. Platelets for crossmatch were from five to six plateletpheresis donors who were scheduled each day without regard to HLA type. Using a radiolabeled antiglobulin test, 148 crossmatches were performed to find 48 potential donors for 11 alloimmunized patients who had high levels of HLA alloantibody with unusual HLA types, making provision of HLA-matched platelets difficult. In individual donors, the percentage of negative crossmatches ranged from 0 to 70%; there were two false-negative crossmatches and one false-positive crossmatch. It is noteworthy that although some patients had lymphocytotoxic antibody against all lymphocytes tested, compatible donors were still found by crossmatch, i.e., for the three patients with 100% reactive HLA antibody levels, they were able to find five compatible donors of the 47 screened. For those patients with intermediate levels of HLA antibody (45 to 65% reactivity), an additional 19 donors were found. Thus, despite what appeared to be a high degree of alloimmunization, platelet crossmatching could identify platelet donors who would ordinarily not be considered as feasible donors on the basis of their HLA type. This selection procedure (independent of HLA matching) identified sufficient donors to maintain the patients through prolonged periods of thrombocytopenia. Hence, fewer donors have to be HLA typed and a smaller pool of typed donors needs to be maintained. Often, many donors are typed because they have uncommon phenotypes and they are rarely recruited to donate platelets. Other donors, with common phenotypes or homozygous antigens, may be asked to donate with sufficient frequency to develop immune dysfunction. If prospective crossmatching can be shown to be equivalent to, or better than, HLA matching, the cost of a platelet support program may decrease. Further prospective trials of HLA-matching vs. platelet crossmatching in a large population of alloimmunized patients are warranted.

A major impediment to widespread use of crossmatch methods has been that several hours are required to complete even small numbers of tests and, sometimes, finding compatible donors for broadly alloimmunized patients may require extensive crossmatching. Rachel et al.[113] used a rapid solid-phase red cell adherence (SPRCA) technique in retrospective examination in 20 patients (80 transfusions) and indicated that 63% of crossmatch-compatible transfusions had been successful. More recently, the same authors reported that using the SPRCA for prospective platelet antibody detection and crossmatching showed an overall correlation of platelet crossmatch results with transfusion outcome of 97%.[114] The patient's sera were tested in the antibody screen against 12 group O donors selected at random with no knowledge of their HLA or platelet antigens. A total of 2878 crossmatches were performed for 87 patients, of which only 17% were compatible. When the patients were grouped according to whether their sera showed positive results in the antibody screen against some, but not all, of the 12 test platelets, 31% of the patients' sera were compatible with potential donors. In contrast, for patients whose sera reacted with all 12 test platelets in the antibody screen (indicating broad alloimmunization), only 4% of 2144 crossmatches were compatible. The actual number of compatible donors per patient ranged from 0 to 6. When only transfusions given to patients who did not have nonimmune causes for platelet destruction were examined (N = 32), the sensitivity of the crossmatch was 92%, specificity 100%, predictive value of an incompatible crossmatch 100%, of a compatible crossmatch 95%, and the SPRCA had an efficiency of 97%. Since the SPRCA is comparable in terms of speed and simplicity to methods currently in use for red cell compatibility testing, it potentially can be used in hospital laboratories before most platelet transfusions to detect platelet alloimmunization. Patients with negative antibody screens could then still be transfused with pooled random-donor platelets, whereas alloimmunized patients would be identified earlier and could be supplied with apheresis platelets from crossmatch-compatible donors. Furthermore, the SPRCA method is now available in commercial kit form. In limited studies, we have found the SPRCA to be more predictive than the LCT, ELISA, and PSIFT by microscopy; it had approximately the same predictive value as the PRAT in our hands, although sensitivity and specificity were higher in flow cytometric assays, which also have the advantage of rapidity, but require specialized equipment and expertise.

The reports of Kickler et al.[112] and Rachel et al.[113,114] addressed the question of the ''highly immunized'' patient and emphasized that not all patients who have a poor posttransfusion platelet increment can be managed equally well. Patients often become more broadly alloimmunized during the course of therapy. This suggests that patients should be tested frequently and refractoriness evaluated in terms of degree of severity, i.e., defined on the basis of the extent of reactivity in an immunologic test and/or level of response to platelet transfusion in the absence of nonimmune causes for poor responses. Petz[115] suggested that, immunologically, severity of alloimmunization is probably more accurately defined on the basis of a ligand-binding crossmatch assay against a panel of donors, than on the basis of a lymphocytotoxicity assay. The above papers are the first to address specifically the issue of the broadly immunized patient. In several other studies, 30 to 50% of crossmatch tests were negative,[7,9,90,91,97] suggesting that many of the patients studied were only moderately immunized. These reports indicate that the percent of negative crossmatches may vary considerably from patient to patient. When patients had lymphocytotoxic antibodies against 100% of the panel, Kickler et al.[112] found that 11% were crossmatch-negative; similarly, Rachel et al.[114] found that only 4% of potential donors were crossmatch-negative when patients were broadly immunized. Both groups reported that there were some patients for whom no compatible donors could be found. Nevertheless, for all but a few patients, compatible platelets were found.

Finally, it should be noted that many of the binding assays in particular require equipment and/or reagents not commonly found in routine blood transfusion laboratories, e.g., spectrophotometers (ELISA), gammacounters, radioisotopes (PRAT), fluorescent microscopes/flow cytometers, fluorochrome-labeled antibodies (immunofluorescence assays), etc.

A. WHY HAS PLATELET CROSSMATCHING NOT BEEN MORE WIDELY USED?

A lack of uniformity of methodology is not the issue, since various ligand-binding assays can be used with similar efficacy. The time required to provide crossmatch tests is not a major problem with newer assays. The main impediment has been that one must obtain platelets from a number of potential donors, perform the crossmatches, and then select the donor or donors. This problem has not as yet properly been addressed. Kickler et al.[112] scheduled five to six apheresis donors each day, but this would be insufficient for highly immunized patients. Rachel et al.[114] organized ''mass phlebotomies'' of potential donors, a logistically difficult approach. The most practical solution to this problem is to establish a large group of apheresis donors whose platelets can be stored and crossmatched as necessary against patients' sera. This is feasible if the platelets can be stored for long periods. Although some reports have indicated suitability of frozen-stored or liquid-stored platelets for crossmatch tests, more data are needed.

B. WHAT THEN IS THE ROLE FOR PLATELET CROSSMATCHING?

It seems clear that platelet crossmatching is effective for moderately immunized patients and should probably be more widely implemented to prevent unnecessary ineffective platelet transfusions, and as an alternative to maintenance of a large file of HLA-typed donors. While more data are needed to establish the role for platelet crossmatching in highly or broadly immunized patients it appears that at least some compatible donors can be found for most patients. A crossmatch technique that allows for the rapid performance of numerous crossmatches is preferable because the patients who most need selected platelets are those most likely to have a low percentage of compatible crossmatches. Nonetheless, crossmatching seems to allow the best hope for management of these difficult patients. If successful, crossmatching may be less expensive and more reliable than alternative approaches. The logistic and technical problems inherent in providing crossmatch-negative platelets can and should be overcome and platelet crossmatch techniques should be more widely implemented until the goal of actual prevention of alloimmunization is achieved.

It should be emphasized that, as only about one half of the clinically refractory patients have alloantibodies,[9,114] only when the patient has been documented to be refractory to pooled random-donor platelet transfusions in the presence of alloantibodies should consideration be given to the provision of ''selected'' donor platelet products. If this restriction is not applied, selected donor transfusion costs will increase and effectiveness will decrease. The selection of tests to detect antibody may vary depending on local expertise. Freedman et al.[90] suggested a combined approach, using a lymphocytotoxicity test along with a test that employs platelets as the target cell; as long as the tests can be performed reliably and have documented ability to predict transfusion responses in the local laboratory, any one of the variety of assays can be used. It is probably important to establish assays which err on the side of prevention of false-negative results to protect against ineffective platelet transfusion.

VII. COST CONSIDERATIONS

Once alloantibodies to random-donor platelets are documented in the refractory patient, the next question becomes the provision of the best platelet support. Effective platelet support for refractory patients may be provided by one of the following products: (1) crossmatch-compatible, pooled random-donor platelets; (2) crossmatch-compatible single-donor platelets; (3) HLA-matched single-donor platelets; or (4) crossmatch-compatible, HLA-matched, single-donor platelets. It is likely that no single approach will be adequate in all patients and it is possible that a selective step-by-step approach using the various options may be the optimal way to manage refractory patients. Among considerations for appropriate management should be the cost effectiveness of different approaches. The economic aspects of medical therapy or surgical procedures have become an accepted element in the overall health care evaluation procedure. New strategies aimed at providing blood products more effectively and efficiently should include evaluation of program costs.[116,117] Freedman et al.[116] attempted to determine the most cost-effective approach to obtaining compatible donors for refractory patients. The study followed certain assumptions to perform detailed cost analyses and to provide comparative cost-effectiveness data for platelet transfusion support strategies in alloimmunized refractory thrombocytopenic patients. While prospective studies are needed to determine the validity of these assumptions, this evaluation attempted to provide blood centers with an approach and tools with which to draw their own conclusions of costs, using local data regarding compatibility rates and optimum HLA pool size.

It appears clear that, at least for immunized patients with narrow alloantibody specificities, it is possible to use the crossmatch to identify compatible, less costly random donors; the crossmatch-compatible units would then be pooled as a transfusion dose. Although an attractive approach, practically it is difficult, since it would require the ready availability of appropriated technicians to perform the tests, completion of the tests in a short period of time, and the storing of the units being tested until the compatible platelet concentrates are identified. It would be easier to do the crossmatch on frozen-platelet samples available from a panel of previously recruited apheresis donors. This might allow non-HLA-typed apheresis panels to be used as the most cost-effective approach, since this strategy would avoid the two major costs associated with HLA-typed apheresis panels, i.e., HLA-typing and the requirement to recruit and maintain the large HLA-typed donor pool.

It remains, however, unclear how often limited antibody specificities may be expected in a clinically refractory population, in comparison to broadly reactive antibodies. Recent studies have indicated that 34% of patients referred for apheresis platelets have broadly reactive alloantibodies and, for those highly immunized patients, only 4 to 11% of random donors were crossmatch-compatible.[112–114] The frequency with which long-term platelet support can be achieved using crossmatch-compatible random donors remains to be determined; some data suggest that 65% of alloimmunized patients can be supported by HLA-matched transfusions.[48] Freedman et al.[116] demonstrated how the degree or frequency of crossmatch-compatibility dramatically influences cost. The likelihood of finding compatible donors is likely quite different among leukemics undergoing initial induction, where it might be 50%, than it is in other refractory patients. Compatibility rates tend to drop as patients are exposed to subsequent transfusions. Using sensitivity analysis, the authors varied the compatibility rate and documented that cost will double if compatibility falls from 50 to 10%. Sensitivity analysis was also performed to investigate the effect of HLA donor pool size on cost. Schiffer et al.[45] reported that for 100 consecutive alloimmunized patients, an average of only 1.3 A-matched donors were found in a pool of 2470 HLA-typed individuals. Duquesnoy et al.[46] reported that a pool of 5000 HLA-typed donors provided an average of only 1.5 perfect matches for 48 patients. More recently, it has been suggested that success rates of "B" HLA matches are better than previously described and smaller donor pools can be used.[118–120] The above cost-effectiveness evaluation demonstrated that, in order to produce a fixed number of HLA-compatible donors for the study population, an HLA-typed donor pool of 3000 is 1.5 times as expensive to operate as a pool of 1000. The calculations did not, however, consider how often donors will actually donate. It has been suggested that combined crossmatching and HLA matching may be required for optimal platelet transfusion support. This study suggested that, from a cost-effectiveness viewpoint, the increase in efficiency of adding HLA matching to crossmatching is counterbalanced by significantly increased costs. The crossmatching procedures were shown to be fairly expensive; clearly, reduction in the cost of crossmatch assays would enhance their cost effectiveness. While this analysis favored the crossmatch strategy, ideally with single donors, a number of the assumptions made still need to be tested prospectively. Not evalulated in the study were the costs of failed platelet transfusions in refractory patients, costs of increased patient morbidity, hospital stay, loss of time from work, and earnings.

VIII. ALTERNATIVE APPROACHES TO THE REFRACTORY PATIENT

Refractoriness to platelet transfusions remains a serious problem in patients who need continued platelet support. A number of strategies have been used in an attempt to prevent, circumvent, and reverse the refractory state. Prevention and reversal of alloimmunization to platelets are beyond the scope of this paper. In an attempt to circumvent alloimmunization, a variety of approaches other than matching have been used. Massive platelet transfusions[121] have only marginal effectiveness and are expensive. Similarly, plasma exchange[122] has proven to be of marginal effectiveness and is expensive. The same may be said for the use of IV gammaglobulin.[123,124] Steroids[125] and splenectomy[126] are ineffective in alloimmunization. Slichter et al.[127] attempted to reverse preexisting platelet alloimmunization in a small number of dogs by treatment with antithymocyte globulin and procarbazine hydrochloride; while reversal (or partial reversal) are achieved, it is hard to be enthusiastic about the use of such agents in man. The most common and useful approaches remain single-donor HLA-matched platelets and/or platelet crossmatching. Strategies to prevent the development of alloimmunization are likely to be the most successful and cost-effective approach in the long run.

IX. CONCLUSIONS

Platelet transfusions have permitted major advances in the treatment of leukemia, aplastic anemia, and many malignancies, by reducing the risk of thrombocytopenic hemmorhage that occurs particularly with intensive chemotherapy. Platelet transfusions may result in alloimmunization, most commonly due to antibodies to HLA antigens, causing refractoriness to subsequent platelet transfusion.

Consequently, HLA matching has been the standard method of selecting platelets for patients immunized to platelet antigens. Despite the use of HLA-matched platelet transfusion, immune transfusion failures still occur and 20 to 35% of HLA-identical platelet transfusions may be unsuccessful. Consequently, the platelet crossmatch approach to select platelets for transfusion of alloimmunized patients has developed. A number of studies have shown the utility of platelet crossmatching as an adjunct to HLA matching. More recent reports suggest that crossmatching may be useful to select platelets independently of HLA matching. Platelet crossmatching, now feasible because of the availability of rapid methods with enhanced sensitivity, is the most obvious approach to solving the problem of accurately selecting platelets for transfusion, since it should detect antibodies to platelet-specific antigens in addition to anti-HLA.

It has become recognized that it is important that studies to determine the efficacy or predictive value of platelet crossmatching, in the investigative setting at least, should be performed only in alloimmunized patients who have no other cause for increased platelet destruction. Therefore, many of the recent reports of platelet crossmatching have been evaluated specifically in patients who do not have sepsis, bleeding, splenomegaly, etc., that would interfere with the interpretation of the effectiveness of the test. However, on a practical basis, it is almost impossible for blood centers and hematologists to be able to assess accurately all the factors which may interfere with a successful platelet transfusion. More work needs to be done to assess platelet crossmatch tests in clinically ill, as well as clinically stable, patients, to determine the true efficacy of platelet crossmatching for all alloimmunized refractory patients who may benefit for selected platelet donor transfusions.

Platelet crossmatching is likely to be necessary in relatively few patients who receive platelets, i.e., only those who demonstrate strict refractoriness to random platelets. There are clear potential benefits from application of such a technique. Development of simple sensitive reliable methods for providing alloimmunized patients with compatible platelets should result in a decreased need for apheresis HLA-typed platelets, decreased use of random donor platelets, fewer adverse reactions, and decreased patient morbidity. Such an approach may reduce costs of platelet transfusion programs and be important for the optimal logistical use of platelet donors.

REFERENCES

1. **Surgenor, D. M. and Schnitzer, S. S.,** The Nation's Blood Resources: A Summary Report, Publ. 85:2028, National Institutes of Health, Bethesda, MD, 1985.
2. **Howard, J. E. and Perkins, H. A.,** The natural history of alloimmunization to platelets, *Transfusion,* 18, 496, 1978.
3. **Schiffer, C. A., Lichtenfeld, J. L., Wiernik, P. H. et al.,** Antibody response in patients with acute nonlymphocytic leukemia, *Cancer,* 37, 2177, 1976.
4. **Holohan, T. V., Terasaki, P. I., and Deisseroth, A. B.,** Suppression of transfusion-related alloimmunization in intensively treated cancer patients, *Blood,* 58, 122, 1981.
5. **Dutcher, J. P., Schiffer, C. A., Aisner, J., and Wiernik, P. H.,** Long-term follow-up of patients with leukemia receiving platelet transfusions: identification of a large group of patients who do not become alloimmunized, *Blood,* 58, 1007, 1981.
6. **Daly, P. A., Schiffer, C. A., Aisner, J., and Wiernik, P. H.,** Platelet transfusion therapy. One-hour posttransfusion increments are valuable in predicting the need for HLA-matched preparations, *JAMA,* 243, 435, 1980.
7. **Freedman, J., Hooi, C., and Garvey, M. B.,** Prospective platelet crossmatching for selection of compatible random donors, *Br. J. Haematol.,* 56, 9, 1984.
8. **Schiffer, C., Dutcher, J., Hogge, D., and Aisner, J.,** Histocompatible platelet transfusion for patients with leukemia, *Plasma Ther. Transfus. Technol.,* 3, 273, 1982.
9. **Kakaiya, R. M., Gudino, M. D., Miller, M. V. et al.,** Four crossmatch methods to select platelet donors, *Transfusion,* 24, 35, 1984.
10. **Kickler, T., Braine, H., Ness, P., Koester, A., and Bias, W.,** A radiolabeled antiglobulin test for crossmatching platelet transfusions, *Blood,* 61, 238, 1983.
11. **Kickler, T. S., Braine, H., and Ness, P. M.,** The predictive value of crossmatching platelet transfusion for alloimmunized patients, *Transfusion,* 25, 385, 1985.
12. **Yankee, R. A., Grumet, F. C., and Rogentine, G. N.,** Platelet transfusion therapy: the selection of compatible platelet donors for refractory patients by lymphocyte HLA typing, *N. Engl. J. Med.,* 281, 1208, 1969.

13. **Lee, E. J. and Schiffer, C. A.,** Serial measurement of lymphocytotoxic antibody and response to nonmatched platelet transfusion in alloimmunization patients, *Blood,* 70, 1727, 1987.
14. **Dutcher, J. P., Schiffer, C. A., Aisner, J., and Wiernik, P. K.,** Alloimmunization following platelet transfusion: absence of a dose-response relationship, *Blood,* 57, 395, 1981.
15. **Sintnicolaas, K., Sizoo, W., Haije, W. G. et al.,** Delayed alloimmunization by random single donor platelet transfusion, *Lancet,* 1, 750, 1981.
16. **Gmur, J., von Felton, A., Osterwalder, B. et al.,** Delayed alloimmunization using random single donor platelet transfusions: a prospective study in thrombocytopenic patients with acute leukemia, *Blood,* 62, 473, 1983.
17. **Pegels, J. G., Bruynes, E. C. E., Engelfriet, C. P., and von dem Borne, A. E. G. Kr.,** Serological studies in patients on platelet and granulocyte substitution therapy, *Br. J. Haematol.,* 52, 59, 1982.
18. **Bowen, T. J., Berman-Wong, E., Dawson, D. et al.,** Comparison of three crossmatch techniques to immunofluorescence test, and enzyme-linked immunoabsorbent assay, *Curr. Stud. Hematol. Blood Transfus.,* 52, 47, 1986.
19. **McGrath, K., Wolfe, M., Bishop, J. et al.,** Transient platelet and HLA antibody formation in multitransfused patients with malignancy, *Br. J. Haematol.,* 68, 345, 1988.
20. **Reed, E., Hardy, M., and Lattes, C.,** Antiidiotypic antibodies and their relevance to transplantation, *Transplant. Proc.,* 17, 735, 1985.
21. **Suciu-Foca, N., Reed, E., Rohowsky, C., King, P., and King, D. W.,** Anti-idiotypic antibodies in anti-HLA receptors induced by pregnancy, *Proc. Natl. Acad. Sci. U.S.A.,* 80, 830, 1983.
22. **Aster, R. H.,** Effect of anticoagulant and ABO incompatibility on recovery of transfused human platelets, *Blood,* 26, 732, 1965.
23. **Pfisterer, H., Thierfelder, S., and Stich, W.,** ABO, Rh blood groups and platelet transfusion, *Blut,* 17, 1, 1968.
24. **Lohrmann, H. P., Bull, M. I., Decter, J. A., Yankee, R. A., and Graw, R. G.,** Platelet transfusion from HLA compatible unrelated donors to alloimmunized patients, *Ann. Intern. Med.,* 80, 9, 1974.
25. **Tosato, G., Appelbaum, F. R., and Deisseroth, A. B.,** HLA-matched platelet transfusion therapy of severe aplastic anemia, *Blood,* 52, 846, 1978.
26. **Duquesnoy, R. J., Anderson, A. J., Tomasulo, P. A., and Aster, R. H.,** ABO incompatibility and platelet transfusion of alloimmunized thrombocytopenic patients, *Blood,* 54, 595, 1979.
27. **Brand, A., Sintnicolaas, K., Claas, F. H. J., and Eernisse, J. G.,** ABH antibodies causing platelet transfusion refractoriness, *Transfusion,* 26, 463, 1986.
28. **Heal, J. M., Blumberg, N., and Masel, D.,** An evaluation of crossmatching. HLA, and ABO matching for platelet transfusions to refractory patients, *Blood,* 70, 23, 1987.
29. **Lee, E. J. and Schiffer, C. A.,** ABO compatibility can influence the results of platelet transfusion, *Transfusion,* 29, 384, 1989.
30. **Heal, J. M., Mullin, A., and Blumberg, N.,** The importance of ABH antigens in platelet crossmatching, *Transfusion,* 29, 514, 1989.
31. **Oldfather, J. W., Ahmed, P., and Rodey, G. E.,** The use of the antiglobulin-augmented lymphocytotoxic cross-match in predicting the outcome of single-donor platelet transfusions, *Blood,* 64(Abstr.), 229a, 1984.
32. **Oldfather, J., Anderson, C. B., Phelan, D., Cross, D., Luger, A., and Rodey, G. E.,** Prediction of crossmatch outcome in highly sensitized patients based on the identification of serum HLA antibodies, *Transplantation,* 42, 267, 1986.
33. **MacPherson, B. R., Hammond, P. B., and Maniscalco, C. A.,** Alloimmunization to public HLA antigens in multi-transfused platelet recipients, *Ann. Clin. Lab. Sci.,* 16, 38, 1986.

34. **Aster, R. H., Szatkowski, N., Liebert, M., and Duquesnoy, R. J.,** Expression of HLA-B12, HLA-B8, W4 and W6 on platelets, *Transplant. Proc.*, 9, 1695, 1977.
35. **Janson, M., McFarland, J., and Aster, R. H.,** Quantitative determination of platelet surface alloantigens using a monoclonal probe, *Hum. Immunol.*, 15, 251, 1986.
36. **Liebert, M. and Aster, R. H.,** Expression of HLA-B12 on platelets, on lymphocytes and in serum: a quantitative study, *Tissue Antigens,* 9, 199, 1977.
37. **Szatkowski, N. S. and Aster, R. H.,** HLA antigens of platelets. IV. Influence of ''private'' HLA-B locus specificities on the expression of Bw4 and Bw6 on human platelets, *Tissue Antigens,* 15, 361, 1980.
38. **Kao, K. J., Cook, D. J., and Scornik, J. C.,** Quantitative analysis of platelet surface HLA by W6/32 anti-HLA monoclonal antibody, *Blood,* 68, 627, 1986.
39. **Santoso, S., Mueller-Eckhardt, G., Santoso, S., Kiefel, V., and Mueller-Eckhardt, C.,** HLA antigens on platelet membranes. In vitro and in vivo studies, *Vox Sang.*, 51, 327, 1986.
40. **Evatt, B. L. and Stein, S. F.,** Platelet structure and function, in *Platelets,* Smith, D. M. and Summers, S. H., Eds., American Association of Blood Banks, Arlington, VA, 1988, 1.
41. **Yankee, R. A., Graff, K. S., Dowling, R., and Henderson, E. S.,** Selection of unrelated compatible platelet donors by lymphocyte HLA-matching, *N. Engl. J. Med.*, 288, 760, 1973.
42. **Lee, E. J. and Schiffer, C. A.,** Management of platelet alloimmunization, in *Immunologic Aspects of Platelet Transfusion,* McCarthy, L. J. and Menitove, J., Eds., American Association of Blood Banks, Arlington, VA, 1985, 1.
43. **Menitove, J. E. and Aster, R. H.,** Transfusion of platelets and plasma products, *Clin. Haematol.*, 12, 239, 1983.
44. **Duquesnoy, R. J., Vieira, J., and Aster, R. H.,** Donor availability for platelet transfusion support of alloimmunized thrombocytopenic patients, *Transfusion,* 9, 519, 1977.
45. **Schiffer, C. A., Keller, C., Dutcher, J. P. et al.,** Potential HLA-matched platelet donor availability for alloimmunized patients, *Transfusion,* 23, 286, 1983.
46. **Duquesnoy, R. J., Filip, D. J., Rodey, G. E., Rimm, A. A., and Aster, R. H.,** Successful transfusion of platelet 'mismatched' for HLA antigens to alloimmunized thrombocytopenic patients, *Am. J. Hematol.*, 2, 219, 1977.
47. **Gmur, J., Felten, A., and von Frick, P.,** Platelet support in polysensitized patients: role of HLA specificities and crossmatch testing for donor selection, *Blood,* 51, 903, 1978.
48. **Brand, A., van Leeuwen, A., Eernisse, J. G., and van Rood, J. J.,** Platelet transfusion therapy: optimal donor selection with a combination of lymphocytotoxicity and platelet fluorescence tests, *Blood,* 51, 781, 1978.
49. **Slichter, S. J.,** Selection of compatible platelet donors, in *Platelet Physiology and Transfusion,* Schiffer, J. C., Ed., American Association of Blood Banks, Washington, D.C., 1978, 83.
50. **Murphy, M. F. and Waters, A. H.,** Immunological aspects of platelet transfusion, *Br. J. Haematol.*, 60, 409, 1985.
51. **Duquesnoy, R. J., Filip, D. J., and Aster, R. H.,** Influence of HLA-A2 on the effectiveness of platelet transfusions in alloimmunized thrombocytopenic patients, *Blood,* 50, 407, 1977.
52. **McElligott, M. C., Menitove, J. E., Duquesnoy, R. J., Hunter, J. B., and Aster, R. H.,** Effect of HLA Bw4/Bw6 compatibility on platelet transfusion responses of refractory thrombocytopenic patients, *Blood,* 59, 971, 1982.
53. **Kelton, T. G., Carter, C. J., Rodger, C. et al.,** The relationship among platelet-associated IgG, platelet lifespan, and reticuloendothelial cell function, *Blood,* 63, 1434, 1984.

54. **Opelz, G., Mickey, M. R., and Terasaki, P. I.,** Unrelated donors for bone marrow transplantation and transfusion support: pool sizes required, *Transplant. Proc.*, 6, 405, 1974.
55. **Tomasulo, P. A.,** Management of the alloimmunized patient with HLA platelets, in *Platelet Physiology and Transfusion*, Schiffer, C. A., Ed., American Association of Blood Banks, Washington D.C., 1978, 69.
56. **Freedman, A. L., Barr, P. S., and Brody, E. A.,** Hemolytic anemia due to quinidine: observations on its mechanisms, *Am. J. Med.*, 20, 806, 1956.
57. **Harrington, W. J., Sprague, C. C., Minnich, V. et al.,** Immunologic mechanisms in idiopathic and neonatal thrombocytopenic purpura, *Ann. Intern. Med.*, 38, 433, 1953.
58. **Deykin, D. and Hellerstein, L. J.,** The assessment of drug-dependent and isoimmune antiplatelet antibodies by the use of platelet aggregometry, *J. Clin. Invest.*, 51, 3142, 1972.
59. **Cimo, P. L., Pisciotta, V. A., Desai, R. G., Pino, J. L., and Aster, R. H.,** Detection of drug-dependent antibodies by the ^{51}Cr platelet lysis test: documentation of immune thrombocytopenia induced by diphenylhydantoin, diazepam, and sulfisoxazole, *Am. J. Hematol.*, 2, 65, 1977.
60. **Duquesnoy, R. J., Lorentzen, D. F., and Aster, R. H.,** Platelet migration inhibition: a new method for detection of platelet antibodies, *Blood*, 45, 741, 1975.
61. **Aster, R. H., Cooper, H. E., and Singer, D. L.,** Simplified complement fixation test for the detection of platelet antibodies in human serum, *J. Lab. Clin. Med.*, 63, 161, 1964.
62. **Svejgaard, A. and Kissmeyer-Nielsen, F.,** Complement-fixing platelet iso-antibodies. I. A quantitative technique for their detection, *Vox Sang.*, 14, 106, 1968.
63. **Luiken, G. A., McMillan, R., Lightsey, A. L. et al.,** Platelet-associated IgG in immune thrombocytopenic purpura, *Blood*, 50, 317, 1977.
64. **Morse, B. S., Giuliani, D., and Nussbaum, M.,** Quantitation of platelet-associated IgG by radial immunodiffusion, *Blood*, 75,809, 1981.
65. **Kunicki, T. J., Koenig, M. B., Kristopeit, S. M., and Aster, R. H.,** Direct quantitation of platelet-associated IgG by electroimmunoassay, *Blood*, 60, 54, 1982.
66. **Morse, B. S., Giuliani, D., and Nussbaum, M.,** A rapid quantitation of platelet-associated IgG by nephelometry, *Am. J. Hematol.*, 12, 271, 1982.
67. **Dixon, R., Rosse, W., and Ebbert, L.,** Quantitative determination of antibody in idiopathic thrombocytopenic purpura. Correlation of serum and platelet-bound antibody with clinical response, *N. Engl. J. Med.*, 292, 230, 1975.
68. **Kelton, J. G., Moore, J., Gauldie, J. et al.,** The development and application of a serum assay for platelet-bindable IgG (S-PBIgG), *J. Lab. Clin. Med.*, 98, 272, 1981.
69. **Kelton, J. G., Denomme, G., Walker, C., Horse-wood, P., and Gauldie, J.,** The measurement of platelet-associated IgG using an immuno-radiometric assay, *J. Immunoassay*, 4, 65, 1983.
70. **Mueller-Eckhardt, C., Schultz, G., Dienst, C., Mahn, I., and Mayer, B.,** ^{125}I-Anti-immunoglobulin test: a new tool for the detection of drug allergic platelet antibodies, *Vox Sang.*, 34, 43, 1978.
71. **Mueller-Eckhardt, C., Mahn, I., Schulz, G., and Mueller-Eckhardt, G.,** Detection of platelet autoantibodies by a radioactive anti-immunoglobulin test, *Vox Sang.*, 35, 357, 1978.
72. **Tate, D. Y., Sorenson, R. L., Gerrard, J. M., White, J. G., and Krivit, W.,** An immunoenzyme histochemical technique for the detection of platelet antibodies from the serum of patients with idiopathic (autoimmune) thrombocytopenic purpura (ITP), *Br. J. Haematol.*, 37, 265, 1977.
73. **Borzini, P., Tedesco, F., Greppi, N. et al.,** An immunoenzymatic assay for the detection and quantitation of platelet antibodies: the platelet beta-galactosidase test (PGT), *J. Immunol. Meth.*, 44, 323, 1981.

74. **Gudino, M. and Miller, W. V.,** Application of the enzyme linked immunospecific assay (ELISA) for the detection of platelet antibodies, *Blood,* 57, 32, 1981.
75. **Kekomaki, R.,** Detection of platelet-bound IgG with ^{125}I-labelled staphylococcal protein A, *Med. Biol.,* 54, 112, 1977.
76. **van Boxtel, C. J., Oosterhoff, F., and Engelfriet, C. P.,** Immunofluorescence microphotometry for the detection of platelet antibodies. III. Demonstration of autoantibodies against platelets, *Scand. J. Immunol.,* 4, 657, 1975.
77. **van der Schans, G. S., Veehoven, W. A., Snijder, J. A. M., and Nieweg, H. O.,** The detection of platelet isoantibodies by membrane immunofluorescence, *J. Lab. Clin. Med.,* 90, 4, 1977.
78. **von dem Borne, A. E. G. Kr., Verheugt, F. W. A., Oosterhof, F. et al.,** A simple immunofluorescence test for the detection of platelet antibodies, *Br. J. Haematol.,* 39, 195, 1978.
79. **Rosenfeld, C. A. and Bodensteiner, D. C.,** Detection of platelet alloantibodies by flow cytometry: characterization and clinical significance, *Am. J. Clin. Pathol.,* 85, 207, 1986.
80. **Rachel, J. M., Sinor, L. T., Tawfik, O. W. et al.,** A solid-phase red cell adherence test for platelet cross-matching, *Med. Lab. Sci.,* 42, 194, 1985.
81. **Filip, D. J., Duquesnoy, R. J., and Aster, R. H.,** Predictive value of cross-matching for transfusion of platelet concentrates to alloimmunized recipients, *Am. J. Hematol.,* 1, 491, 1976.
82. **Pogliani, E., Deliliers, G. L., Ferrari, R. et al.,** Platelet aggregometry and anti-platelet isoantibodies, *Haemostasis,* 4, 23, 1975.
83. **Wu, K. K., Hoak, J. C., Koepke, J. A., and Thompson, J. S.,** Selection of compatible platelet donors: a prospective evaluation of three crossmatching techniques, *Transfusion,* 17, 638, 1977.
84. **Hogge, D., Dutcher, J., Aisner, J., and Schiffer, C.,** Lymphocytotoxic antibody is a predictor of response to random donor platelet transfusion, *Am. J. Hematol.,* 14, 363, 1983.
85. **Herzig, R. H., Terasaki, P. I., Herzig, G. P., and Graw, R. G.,** The relationship between donor-recipient lymphocytotoxicity and the transfusion response using HLA-matched platelet concentrates, *Transfusion,* 17, 657, 1977.
86. **Levine, S. L. and Brubaker, D. B.,** Detection of platelet antibodies using the migration inhibition assay, *Am. J. Clin. Pathol.,* 80, 43, 1983.
87. **Wu, K. K., Hoak, J. C., Thompson, J. S., and Koepke, J. A.,** Use of platelet aggregometry in selection of compatible platelet donors, *N. Engl. J. Med.,* 292, 130, 1975.
88. **Myers, T. J., Kim, B. K., Steiner, M., and Baldini, M. G.,** Selection of donor platelets for alloimmunized patients using a platelet associated IgG assay, *Blood,* 58, 444, 1981.
89. **Waters, A. H., Minchinton, R. M., Bell, R., Ford, J. M., and Lister, T. A.,** A cross-matching procedure for the selection of platelet donors for alloimmunized patients, *Br. J. Haematol.,* 48, 59, 1981.
90. **Freedman, J., Garvey, M. B., Salomon de Friedberg, Z., Hornstein, A., and Blanchette, V.,** Random donor platelet crossmatching: comparison of four platelet antibody detection methods, *Am. J. Hematol.,* 28, 1, 1988.
91. **Brubaker, D. B., Duke, J. C., and Romine, M.,** Predictive value of enzyme-linked immunoassay platelet crossmatching for transfusion of platelet concentrates to alloimmunized recipients, *Am. J. Hematol.,* 24, 375, 1987.
92. **Sinor, L. T. and Plapp, F. V.,** Platelet antibody detection methods, in *Platelets,* Smith, D. M. and Summers, S. H., Eds., American Association of Blood Banks, Arlington, VA, 1988, 56.
93. **McFarland, J. G. and Aster, R. H.,** Evaluation of four methods for platelet compatibility testing, *Blood,* 69, 1425, 1987.

94. **Harvard, R. A., Jr., Rosse, W. F., and Reisner, E. A.,** A comparison of lymphocytotoxicity and radioimmunoassay for the detection of alloantibodies to platelets, *Blood,* 66(Abstr.), 278a, 1985.
95. **Kiefel, V., Santoso, S., Weisheit, M., and Mueller-Eckhardt, C.,** Monoclonal antibody-specific immobilization of platelet antigens (MAIPA): a new tool for the identification of platelet-reactive antibodies, *Blood,* 70, 1722, 1987.
96. **Kiefel, V., Santoso, S., Katzmann, B., and Mueller-Eckhardt, C.,** Neonatal alloimmune thrombocytopenia (NAIT) caused by a new platelet specific alloantibody Br(a), *Blood,* 70(Abstr.), 340a, 1987.
97. **Ware, R., Reisner, E., and Rosse, W.,** The use of radiolabeled and fluorescein-labeled antiglobulins in assays to predict platelet transfusion outcome, *Blood,* 63, 1245, 1984.
98. **Taaning, E.,** Microplate enzyme immuno-assay for detection of platelet antibodies, *Tissue Antigens,* 25, 19, 1985.
99. **Oldfather, J., Duffy, T., Fuller, T., Fuller, A., and Rodey, G.,** Sensitivity of AHG-CDC and flowcytometry is comparable in detecting HLA alloantibodies, *Hum. Immunol.,* 14(Abstr.), 154, 1985.
100. **Rodey, G. E.,** Prevention of alloimmunization in thrombocytopenic patients, in *Platelets,* Smith, D. M. and Summers, S. H., Eds., American Association of Blood Banks, Arlington, VA, 1988, 93.
101. **Decary, F.,** Summary of the First Canadian Workshop on platelet serology, *Curr. Stud. Hematol. Blood Transfus.,* 52, 6, 1986.
102. **Schiffer, C. A., Aisner, J., and Wiernik, P. H.,** Frozen autologous platelet transfusion for patients with leukemia, *N. Engl. J. Med.,* 299, 7, 1978.
103. **Schiffer, C. A. and Young, V.,** Detection of platelet antibodies using a micro-enzyme-linked immunosorbent assay (ELISA), *Blood,* 61, 311, 1983.
104. **Kiss, J. E., Salamon, D. J., Wilson, J., Ramsey, G., and Duquesnoy, R. J.,** Suitability of liquid-stored donor platelets in platelet compatibility testing, *Transfusion,* 29, 405, 1989.
105. **Kickler, T. S., Salamon, J., Welsh, F., Ness, P. M., and Braine, H.,** A microtiter plate technique for the detection of platelet antibodies and platelet antigen typing, *Transfusion,* 24, 247, 1984.
106. **Tamerius, J. D., Curd, J. G., Tani, P., and McMillan, R.,** An enzyme-linked immunosorbent assay for platelet compatibility testing, *Blood,* 62, 744, 1983.
107. **Lazarchick, J., Das, P. C., Jones, T. J., Russell, R. J., and Hall, S. A.,** Utility of frozen platelets for a platelet antibody assay using flow cytometric analysis, *Diagn. Clin. Immunol.,* 5, 338, 1988.
108. **Helmerhorst, F. M., Bossers, B., de Bruin, H. G., Englefriet, C. P., and von dem Borne, A. E. G. Kr.,** Detection of platelet antibodies: a comparison of three techniques, *Vox Sang.,* 39, 83, 1980.
109. **Blumberg, N., Masel, D., Mayer, T., Horan, P., and Heal, J.,** Removal of HLA-A,B antigens from platelets, *Blood,* 63, 448, 1984.
110. **Kurata, Y., Oshida, M., Take, H. et al.,** New approach to eliminate HLA class I antigens from platelet surface without cell damage: acid treatment at pH 3.0, *Vox Sang.,* 57, 199, 1989.
111. **Brubaker, D. B. and Romine, M.,** Relationship of HLA and platelet-reactive antibodies in alloimmunized patients refractory to platelet therapy, *Am. J. Hematol.,* 26, 341, 1987.
112. **Kickler, T. S., Ness, P. M., and Braine, H. G.,** Platelet crossmatching: a direct approach to the selection of platelet transfusions for the alloimmunized thrombocytopenic patient, *Am. J. Clin. Pathol.,* 90, 69, 1988.
113. **Rachel, J. M., Goodrich, T. J., Summers, T. C., Sinor, L. T., and Plapp, F. V.,** Prospective use of the solid phase red cell adherence method to select platelet donors for alloimmunized recipients, *Transfusion,* 26(Abstr.), 556, 1986.

114. **Rachel, J. M., Summers, T. C., Sinor, L. T., and Plapp, F. V.,** Use of a solid phase red blood cell adherence method for pretransfusion platelet compatibility testing, *Am. J. Clin. Pathol.*, 90, 63, 1988.
115. **Petz, L. D.,** Platelet crossmatching, *Am. J. Clin. Pathol.*, 90, 114, 1988.
116. **Freedman, J., Gafni, A., Garvey, M. B., and Blanchette, V.,** A cost-effectiveness evaluation of platelet crossmatching and HLA matching in the management of alloimmunized thrombocytopenic patients, *Transfusion,* 29, 201, 1989.
117. **Welch, H. G., Larson, E. B., and Slichter, S. J.,** Providing platelet for refractory patients, *Transfusion,* 29, 193, 1989.
118. **Jorgensen, D. W., McFarland, J. G., Hillman, R. A., and Slichter, S. J.,** Plateletapheresis program. II. Computer selection of HLA compatible donors, *Transfusion,* 24, 292, 1984.
119. **McFarland, J. G., Larson, E. B., Hillman, R. S., and Slichter, S. J.,** Cost-benefit analysis of a plateletapheresis program, *Transfusion,* 26, 91, 1986.
120. **Takahashi, K., Juji, T., and Miyazaki, H.,** Determination of an appropriate size of unrelated donor pool to be registered for HLA-matched platelet transfusion, *Transfusion,* 27, 394, 1987.
121. **Nagasawa, T., Kim, B. K., and Baldini, M. G.,** Temporary suppression of circulating platelet-antiplatelet alloantibodies by the massive infusion of fresh, stored or lyophilized platelets, *Transfusion,* 18, 429, 1978.
122. **Bensinger, W. I., Buckner, C. D., Clift, R. A. et al.,** Plasma exchange for platelet alloimmunization, *Transplantation,* 41, 602, 1986.
123. **Schiffer, C. A., Hogge, D. E., Aisner, J. et al.,** High dose intravenous gammaglobulin in alloimmunized platelet transfusion recipients, *Blood,* 64, 937, 1984.
124. **Zeigler, Z. R., Shadduck, R. K., and Rosenfeld, C. S.,** High dose intravenous gammaglobulin improves responses to single donor platelets in patients refractory to platelet transfusion, *Blood,* 70, 1433, 1987.
125. **Slichter, S. J. and Harker, L. A.,** Thrombocytopenia: mechanisms and management of defects in platelet production, *Clin. Haematol.*, 7, 523, 1978.
126. **Hogge, D. E., Dutcher, J. P., Aisner, J., and Schiffer, C. A.,** The ineffectiveness of random donor platelet transfusion in splenectomized alloimmunized recipients, *Blood,* 64, 253, 1984.
127. **Slichter, S. J., Weiden, P. L., Kane, P. J., and Storb, R. F.,** Approaches to preventing or reversing platelet alloimmunization using animal models, *Transfusion,* 28, 103, 1988.

Chapter 18

TRANSFUSION-TRANSMITTED INFECTIONS: EPIDEMIOLOGY RELEVANT TO BLOOD SAFETY

John A. J. Barbara

TABLE OF CONTENTS

ISBN 0-8493-4938-9

I. INTRODUCTION

An obvious precondition of acceptance of any blood donor is that he or she should be fit and well and not be showing any obvious signs of illness. Although this is partly for the donor's benefit, it is also of vital importance in minimizing the risk of acute microbial infections being transmitted to the transfusion recipient. Exclusion of candidate blood donors who are undergoing overt acute infection, together with appropriate history taking, are the first lines of defense for assuring the quality of blood accepted for transfusion purposes. Careful history taking is important because the vast majority of infectious agents that are transmitted by transfusion are those that cause inapparent or subclinical infections in blood donors. The value of restricting blood donation to volunteer, nonremunerated donors therefore becomes immediately apparent. If the financial incentive is removed from a candidate donor who has a relevant clinical history that would debar from donation, there is less likelihood that this history would be concealed.

II. CHARACTERISTICS OF TRANSFUSION-TRANSMITTED INFECTIONS

The different characteristics of microbial agents that predispose them to transmission by blood transfusion have been reviewed by Barbara.[1] They can be summarized as follows:

1. Presence of the agent in either cellular or plasma fractions of blood, or both, in sufficient titer to make contamination of blood or blood components a distinct likelihood

2. Stability of the agent in blood or its components under the various conditions and periods of storage prior to transfusion
3. Resistance of the agent to any virucidal or antimicrobial effects of anticoagulants or methods of processing; the latter is of special significance for products fractionated from pools of plasma
4. Infections that are mild or asymptomatic, leaving the donor feeling and appearing fit enough to donate blood
5. Having a long incubation prior to the development of any symptoms that may subsequently appear
6. Establishment of a persistent, nonresolving state of infection, either by virtue of a carrier state (e.g., hepatitis B virus, HBV) or a latent infection (e.g., cytomegalovirus, CMV), or both, as appears to be the case with the human immunodeficiency virus, HIV

Examples will be discussed of microbial agents that individually reflect many or all of these properties and which thereby pose a significant threat to the safety of blood transfusion. One agent, the human parvovirus (B19), although usually causing only mild (often inapparent) infections, and lacking any state of persistent infection, may still infect a large proportion of hemophiliacs receiving pooled plasma products that have not been subjected to inactivation procedures. Despite the short-lived viremia lasting only a few days, virus titers in the region of 10^{12} particles/ml enable occasional infected donors to contaminate pools of plasma. This example highlights the amplification of risk afforded by the need to pool large numbers of plasma donations (up to 15 to 20,000 units) for efficient fractionation of products such as Factor VIII. Fortunately, this risk appears to be largely eliminated by current procedures for inactivation of viruses in pooled plasma products. This topic will be discussed in detail in a later chapter.

III. THE RANGE OF AGENTS THAT MAY BE TRANSMITTED BY TRANSFUSION

A wide range of microbial agents can be transmitted by transfusion of blood and its components. The extent of risk of transmission of the different agents and subsequent disease depends on a variety of factors, including:

1. Incidence of the infection in a particular geographical area (in relation to carrier *and* immunity rates)
2. Type of blood component transfused (whether cellular or plasma), depending on whether the agent is cell or plasma associated or both
3. Level of immune competence of the transfusion recipient in certain cases

The agents that are associated with potential transmission by transfusion are shown in Table 1 below.

TABLE 1
The Range of Infectious Agents Potentially Transmissible by Transfusion

1. Bacteria

   - Endogenous — bacteremias, persistent or transient: syphilis (*Treponema pallidum*), brucellosis, and others such as *Yersinia* or *Salmonella* species
   - Exogenous — rare contamination during collection or processing of blood (e.g., pseudomonads, achromobacters, and coliforms)

2. Rickettsiae

   - Q fever (*Coxiella burnetii*)
   - Rocky Mountain spotted fever (*Rickettsia rickettsii*)

3. Parasites

   - Malaria (*Plasmodium* species)
   - Chagas' disease (*Typanosoma cruzi*)
   - African trypanosomiasis
   - *Toxoplasma gondii*
   - Nantucket fever (*Babesia microti*)
   - Visceral leishmaniasis (kala-azar)

4. Viruses

Plasma borne	Cell associated
Hepatitis A (HAV — on rare occasions)	Cytomegalovirus
Hepatitis B (HBV and variants)	Epstein-Barr virus
Delta agent (HDV)	
Non-A, non-B hepatitis	HTLV-I/II
Hepatitis C	
Others ?	
HIV-1 } also cellular	
HIV-2 } also cellular	
Parvovirus B19	
Colorado tick fever virus	

Epidemiology is defined as the study of the factors that influence the frequency and distribution of infectious diseases. The general characteristics that predispose agents to a potential for transmission by transfusion have already been discussed. Specific agents will now be considered in terms of their epidemiology as it relates to the risk they pose for transfusion, concentrating on some of the infections that are not usually emphasized in reviews of posttransfusion infection.

From Table 1, it becomes apparent that several of the transfusion-transmitted infections are also sexually transmissible. Because of their blood-borne nature, several are also common in intravenous drug (IVD) users.

Syphilis, a truly venereal disease, was once an important potential complication of transfusion. Other sexually transmissible infections include the human immunodeficiency viruses, HIV-1 and HIV-2, the hepatitis B virus (HBV), and probably the human T cell leukemia virus, type I (HTLV-I). Cytomegalovirus can also be transmitted sexually. The evidence for sexual transmission of hepatitis C virus (HCV), the major agent of non-A, non-B hepatitis (NANBH) is conflicting,[4,42] although it had been assumed that this route would be epidemiologically significant. Even hepatitis A virus (HAV) has been reported to be transmitted by certain homosexual practices which pose a risk of fecal-oral contamination.[5]

The transfusion-transmitted infections that can be spread by IVD use include HBV, HCV, HDV, HIV, and HTLV-II.

A person who has been exposed by sexual activity or IVD use to one of the above agents is also likely to have been exposed to others transmitted by the same route. It is therefore vital to educate donors as to which behaviors debar them from blood donation so that they may exclude themselves appropriately if they are at risk of contracting the relevant infections. Donor selection is thus the first, vital step in maintaining a safe blood supply, and the prime aspect of donor selection is the exclusive use of volunteer blood donors. By avoiding financial incentives for blood donors, an important reason for the withholding of relevant "risk" histories is removed.

IV. BACTERIA

A. SYPHILIS (*TREPONEMA PALLIDUM*)

Historically, syphilis presented a serious risk following transfusion but refrigerated storage of blood and blood components has virtually eliminated the problem in developed countries. Transmission is extremely rarely reported and the widespread use of antibiotics following treatment involving transfusion renders any potential risk minimal. In countries with a high syphilis incidence, 2 megaunits of penicillin G or its equivalent should be administered to recipients by injection.[2]

Syphilis was transmissible by transfusion not only because donors might be infectious during the incubation period, but also because untreated, asymptomatic donors with latent syphilis could transmit the spirochete.[3] *Treponema pallidum* is unlikely to survive for more than 72 hours at 4 to 6°C in citrated blood but there is a close relationship between the number of treponemes added to donor blood and survival times determined by assay in rabbits.

Other treponemal infections (nonvenereal) — Since infections with yaws (*Treponema pertenue*) and pinta (*Treponema carateum*) are often asymptomatic and have a spirochetemic phase, there is a possibility in endemic areas (the tropics, the West Indies, Central and South America) of transfusion transmission, although this has never been recorded.

B. LYME DISEASE (*BORRELIA BURGDORFERI*)

This is another spirochete disease of worldwide distribution which is being studied currently as a potential transfusion risk. Aoki and Holland[6] recently reviewed the possible significance of Lyme borreliosis in a transfusion context. At least four Ixodid ticks carry the bacterium and transmission to humans can cause a chronic disease. Although *B. burgdorferi* is still viable after storage in blood for 60 days at 4°C, no instance of spirochetemia in the absence of clinical symptoms has yet been reported. Exclusion of overtly infected potential donors should prevent transmission and no case associated with transfusion has yet been documented.

C. BRUCELLOSIS (UNDULANT FEVER)

Brucella abortus can survive for more than a month in stored blood. Tabor[7] has reviewed the transfusion significance of this microorganism. Several transfusion cases of symptomatic infection with *B. abortus* have been reported, the majority in children and splenectomized patients, although none have been from the U.S. The risk is small except in immunosuppressed recipients, since the concentrations of bacteria in infected donor blood are very low. The incubation period in infected recipients can range from 1 to 24 weeks.

A history of brucellosis excludes potential blood donors in many countries, but the majority of infections are asymptomatic. However, the level of risk for recipients is too low to warrant routine specific antibody screening of blood donors, despite the chronic nature of the infection.

D. OTHER BACTERIAL OR RICKETTSIAL INFECTIONS

The occasional transfusion-associated infections from asymptomatic bacteremic donors are often associated with prolonged storage of platelet preparations at room temperature. Heal et al.[8] reviewed nine fatal transfusion septicemia reports to the Food and Drug Administration in the U.S. between 1980 and 1983; six were due to contaminated platelet concentrates. Chronic low-grade bacteremia (e.g., due to *Salmonella* infection) is a potential risk and transmission may also occur during the incubation or convalescent phases of infection. Transient acute bacteremia after dental extractions has also been identified as a further potential risk factor.

Psychrophilic bacteria that can grow in citrated blood stored at 4°C add a further dimension to the problem. Transfusion of blood from donors with subclinical *Yersina enterocolitica* bacteremia has caused fatal septicemia and several cases have been reported in the world literature (see review by Jacobs et al.,[9] which includes information on *Salmonella* transmission by transfusion and a case of *Campylobacter jejuni* septicemia, probably caused by transfusion). It is noteworthy that, unlike other contaminating organisms, *Y. enterocolitica* does not cause visible hemolysis of stored blood,[10] thereby circumventing the safety measure of inspection of blood prior to transfusion.

Rickettsial infections are rare causes of transfusion complications. Q fever (*Coxiella burnetti*) has been reported to have been transmitted via blood transfusion,[11] as has Rocky Mountain spotted fever (*Rickettsia rickettsii*),[12] from donors incubating these infections. The rarity of such transmissions is probably due to the severity of symptoms deterring sufferers from donating blood.

Rare exogenous contamination of blood during collection or processing has been reported as the cause of transmissions of bacteria such as pseudomonads, achromobacters, and coliforms. Blood packs in which bacterial proliferation occurs nearly always contain cold-growing bacteria such as Gram-negative rods from the families Pseudomonaceae or Enterobacteriaceae.[13]

V. PARASITES

In certain areas of the world, parasites pose a considerable potential risk for transfused patients.

A. MALARIA (*PLASMODIUM* SPECIES)

Blood transfusion provides an ideal artificial "vector" for the transmission of malarial parasites from an asymptomatic donor to a recipient. An inoculum of as few as 10 parasites can transmit malaria and therefore any blood component containing even small numbers of red cells is a potential hazard if prepared from an infected donor. Fresh plasma, cryoprecipitate, and platelet and granulocyte concentrates have all been incriminated on occasion; even red cells in transplants such as a kidney or bone marrow have been reported to have transmitted *Plasmodium falciparum*.

1. Stability of Parasites in Stored Blood

All species of malarial parasite can stay viable in blood stored at 4°C for at least one week. We have reported one case of transfusion-transmitted *P. falciparum* where the parasite remained viable for 19 days prior to transfusion.[14] Bruce-Chwatt[15] reviewed a large number of cases of *P. malariae* transmitted by transfusion; in most cases blood had been stored for under one week and transmission after two weeks of storage was very rare. However, the organisms do survive well in frozen blood. In contrast, frozen or freeze-dried plasma has not been associated with malarial transmission.

2. Incubation Period and Infectivity

Four species of malarial parasites infect man, namely *P. falciparum, P. vivax, P. malariae,* and *P. ovale*. The severity of illness they cause varies considerably. *P. falciparum,* which can invade circulating red cells of all ages with a consequent severe parasitemia, causes the most serious infections, often fulminating and fatal in a nonimmune recipient. *P. vivax* and *P. ovale* favor young red cells and *P. malariae,* aged ones. The extent of parasitemia and hemolysis, together with the severity of their infections, is limited for these three species.

P. falciparum has no secondary phase outside the red cell and infections are resolved within three years of infection (usually within one year). In contrast, the other malarial parasites may remain dormant in the liver for longer, so that true relapses may occur after long periods. In most cases, *P. vivax* and *P. ovale* do not relapse beyond three years, but *P. malariae* is more persistent. Transmissions of the latter have occurred as long as 10 to 53 years after initial exposure in the donor, especially after splenectomy; the spleen appears to play a part in preventing maturation of parasites, thereby avoiding reinfection.[16] Because of its prolonged latency, *P. malariae* is therefore the most common cause of transfusion malaria in nonendemic areas, whereas *P. vivax* and *P. falciparum* are the most common causes of malaria worldwide.

Bruce-Chwatt[2] has estimated the frequency of posttransfusion malaria as varying from less than 0.2 cases per million units of blood transfused in nonendemic countries to 50 or more per million in certain endemic countries. The incubation period of transfusion malaria depends on the numbers and strains of parasites transfused. It also depends on the host and on the use of antimalarial prophylaxis. With *P. falciparum* and *P. vivax,* incubation is between one week and one month, but it may be several months for *P. malariae.*[15]

B. CHAGAS' DISEASE (*TRYPANOSOMA CRUZI*)

Several reviews have dealt with Chagas' disease and the other parasites that will be discussed later. For detailed references, these reviews should be consulted.[1,16–18]

Trypanosoma cruzi, the causative agent of Chagas' disease is estimated to infect between 16 and 18 million people in South and Latin America, where it may frequently be transmitted by blood transfusion. The infection is prevalent in rural areas where transmission to humans, usually in childhood, is by insect bites (triatomial insects, a genus of arthropods in the order Hemiptera). The parasite is ingested by the insect and is deposited on the skin of humans in a fecal pellet. This is then scratched into the skin or rubbed onto the eye, causing infection of the host, with characteristic lesions at the site. Transmission is not a problem in areas of hygienic housing conditions where the insects do not thrive or feed on animals living with the households.

The minimum incubation period of *T. cruzi* is one to two weeks. Death occurs in 10% of acute cases, but acute infections can be treated, with a 50 to 90% success rate. Most acute infections are, however, subclinical and approximately 50% of patients with chronic disease are asymptomatic. Between 5 and 40% of untreated patients may eventually develop serious chronic complications (cardiomiopathy, megaesophagus and megacolon) after 10 or more years and no treatment is available for patients with chronic disease.

T. cruzi parasites can survive for more than 10 days in blood stored at 4°C. They can be transmitted by plasma even if it is frozen at −20°C for 24 hours but not if lyophilized. In the various regions of South and Latin America, the prevalence of seropositive donors ranges from 1 to 22%. Approximately 12% of recipients of seropositive blood become infected. The addition of 125 mg of crystal (gentian) violet to the unit of blood kills the parasite within 24 hours at 4°C without damaging the red cells or causing toxic reactions in the recipients if the transfusion involves only a small number of units of blood.

Factors contributing to transmission-transmitted Chagas' disease include:

- Stability of the parasite in stored blood
- High prevalence in endemic areas of chronic asymptomatic patients with latent infection
- Migration from high-prevalence rural areas to urban areas

The risk of transfusion transmission by migrants from high to low endemic areas has been reviewed recently[19] in the light of two such cases in Canada and the U.S. These cases occurred as a result of transfusion of blood donated by asymptomatic Latin American immigrants chronically infected with *T. cruzi*. Various serological tests are available which may be used in nonendemic areas to screen donors from endemic areas.

African trypanosomiasis is a disease caused by trypanosomes found over a wide area of sub-Saharan Africa, transmitted by the bite of tsetse flies (*Glossina* species). Two species of these trypanosomes cause human sleeping sickness, fatal if untreated. *T. brucei rhodesiense* is usually symptomatic so that transmission by blood transfusion is extremely rare. *T. brucei gambiense* causes a more chronic form of illness and in the asymptomatic phase transmission by blood transfusion may occur. This risk is poorly documented and only a few cases have been reported.

C. TOXOPLASMOSIS (*TOXOPLASMA GONDII*)

The prevalence of antibodies to *Toxoplasma gondii* varies widely in different geographical locations. In the U.K. (North London) a prevalence of 36% in plasmapheresis donors[20] has been found. In the U.S., prevalence varies from 20 to 80%, with 18% of seropositive subjects having IgM antibody, a marker of active infection.[7] The parasite has been isolated from donors' blood as long as four years after the onset of infection. As an obligate intracellular parasite, *T. gondii* will persist in white cells and can survive storage at 4°C for up to 7 weeks.[7]

The risk of severe toxoplasmosis after transfusion is restricted to immunosuppressed patients receiving leukocyte concentrates. It may therefore be prudent to collect leukocytes for nonimmune immunosuppressed recipients only from donors without antibody to toxoplasma.

D. NANTUCKET FEVER (*BABESIA MICROTI*)

Nantucket fever is caused by an intraerythrocytic protozoal parasite (*Babesia microti*) transmitted by tick bites. *B. microti* is limited to the northeastern coast of the U.S., Wisconsin, and Minnesota, but can survive for more than two weeks in blood stored at 4°C. The disease is normally mild and often asymptomatic. Transmissions by transfusion have occasionally been reported. Bruce-Chwatt[2] has therefore recommended that individuals from endemic areas who have had a recent febrile illness or who have high levels of antibody to *B. microti* should be excluded as blood donors.

E. VISCERAL LEISHMANIASIS (KALA-AZAR)

Leishmaniasis has only rarely been transmitted by transfusion, even in endemic areas.[7]

VI. VIRUSES

In developed countries, viruses are the microorganisms that present the most serious risk in the context of transfusion-transmitted infection. Furthermore, unlike several of the previously discussed agents, virus infections are not amenable to curative treatment and effective antiviral agents have only recently begun to show promise.

A. HEPATITIS A VIRUS (HAV)

This common infection of worldwide distribution is spread by the fecal-oral route. In areas of poor hygiene and sanitation, most infections occur in childhood. Viremia is transient and no viral carrier state exists. Although fecal-oral transmission in homosexual males has been recorded,[5] it is not a significant factor in the cluster of transfusion-transmitted infections associated with this form of sexual intercourse. However, the brief phase of asymptomatic viremia in HAV infection has resulted in a handful of posttransfusion cases. In 1986, Azimi et al.[21] described a case of posttransfusion hepatitis A (PTHA) involving two premature infants, the mother of one of the infants, and an additional 15 nurses. The infants were infected by transfusion of blood from a donor who developed hepatitis A shortly after donating. In all, 18 infections occurred. This case highlights the important epidemiological feature of the diminishing proportion of people infected by HAV in developed countries as hygiene and sanitation improves. Up to 1986, at least 11 incidents of PTHA had been reported in the world literature (see Barbara[1] and Azimi et al.[21] for details).

B. HEPATITIS B VIRUS (HBV) AND THE DELTA AGENT (HDV)

The transfusion aspects of HBV have been extensively reviewed.[1,18,22] The incubation period is from 2 to 6 months; the majority of infections are anicteric and symptoms, if any, are usually mild. These factors, together with the chronic carrier state that develops in approximately 5 to 10% of infections, readily predispose the virus to transmission by blood transfusion. There are estimated to be up to 300 million carriers of hepatitis B surface antigen (HBsAg) worldwide. Approximately one fourth of this total are likely to be hepatitis B *e* antigen (HBeAg)-positive, exhibiting high infectivity in sexual, maternofetal, and percutaneous modes of transmission. Such carriers are also inevitably infectious for nonimmune recipients, by virtue of the large inoculum involved in transfusion. Carriers of HBsAg who have antibody to the *e* antigen (anti-HBe) are much less infectious by all routes except transfusion, where the large inoculum size renders them hazardous to their recipients. Although HBV infection occurs worldwide, the incidence varies dramatically in different areas as in the following broad approximations:

- Asia, Africa, Latin America: 10% carrier rate, 60 to 90% seropositivity (past exposure)
- Mediterranean: 1% carrier rate, up to 30% seropositivity
- Northern Europe: 0.1% carrier rate, 2 to 4% seropositivity

These generalized figures illustrate the need for assessment of the transfusion risk in individual geographical areas before deciding upon optimal policies as regards transfusion safety.

Thus, in the U.K. (anti-HBV prevalence of approximately 2%), the majority of recipients of blood or blood products will be susceptible to HBV. On the other hand, the carrier rate is relatively low. This contrasts with, for example, tropical areas where although 10% of donors are likely to be HBsAg carriers, the majority of the adult population will be immune. In low-prevalence areas, there is a good case for vaccination of nonimmune recipients of pooled plasma products or multiple (regular) transfusions. Pooling large numbers of plasma units multiplies the risk of contaminating the pool with one or more of the plasma-associated viruses. Fortunately, as mentioned earlier, effective methods for inactivating viruses have been developed which greatly reduce the chances of infection in recipients.

In high-prevalence areas, where adequate funding is often most lacking, it is questionable whether HBsAg screening of blood for transfusion to adults is cost effective.[23] Since acquisition of HBV infection is age dependent, infants or children in these areas are at higher risk of HBV infection by transfusion than are adults. Selective screening of donors whose blood is required for infants may therefore be a suitable strategy in certain high-prevalence areas.

Lovric[24] has proposed another strategy for areas of high prevalence which is based on screening of donors for anti-HBs and HBsAg at their first donation. Those who are both anti-HBs-positive and HBsAg-negative require no further HBV testing of subsequent donations. The scheme is, however, dependent on having a significant proportion of regular blood donors and efficient maintenance and retrieval of donor records. Both these requirements may often be lacking and would require considerable resources for implementation.

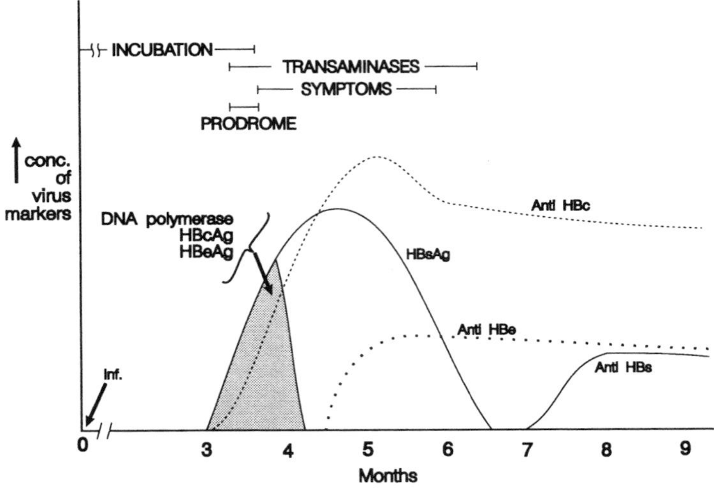

FIGURE 1. Typical time course of markers of acute HBV infection.

In low-prevalence areas, a small number of blood donors may donate blood in the asymptomatic phase of HBV infection prior to appearance of HBV markers (Figure 1).

The actual time course of HBV infection is very variable. If a chronic carrier phase develops, then anti-HBs does not appear and HBsAg persists, often lifelong, although the level does decrease slowly with time. This is why HBsAg-positive blood donors born in high-prevalence areas with a pattern of infection early in life generally have lower HBsAg titers than those from low-prevalence areas. In the latter case, infection will often have been acquired in adulthood (e.g., by sexual transmission or IVD use).

As HBsAg levels decline, anti-HBc may be the only remaining marker of a past HBV infection. A proportion of donors with confirmed anti-HBc positivity and lacking any other HBV markers may therefore be able to transmit HBV by transfusion.

Furthermore, asymptomatic donors may transmit HBV by transfusion during acute infections, as HBsAg declines and before the development of anti-HBs (the "diagnostic-window"). In this situation anti-HBc will, however, be detected. Anti-HBc screening may therefore be of some value as an adjunct to HBsAg screening in the prevention of PTHB.[25,26] The actual benefit of such screening requires assessment locally. In countries where anti-HBc screening is a routine pretransfusion requirement, it may be performed as a surrogate marker for non-A, non-B hepatitis (NANBH) infectivity. In any case, anti-HBc screening should not replace pretransfusion HBsAg testing because development of HBsAg precedes that of anti-HBc (Figure 1).[27]

It appears that largely as a result of donor education to exclude donors at risk of contracting HIV infection, the incidence of PTH in the U.S. has fallen significantly. Large-scale prospective studies prior to the recognition of AIDS indicated that approximately 10% of transfusions in the U.S. resulted in PTH, 10% of which was due to HBV. PTH in the U.S. is now estimated to be as low as 1 or 2%.[28] In developed countries, PTHB is relatively rare. The exclusion of donors at risk of contracting HIV infection may well prove to have a similar value as the exclusive use of volunteer donors.

Any recipient who is affected by PTHB and becomes a carrier of HIV is at long-term risk of developing chronic liver disease and primary hepatocellular carcinoma.[29,30] The latter, if it occurs, usually takes 30 to 60 years to develop, but the delay may be much shorter when neonates are infected.[31]

1. Variants of HBV

Evidence has recently been accumulating for the existence of variants of HBV. A viral infection characterized by the presence of HBsAg in serum in the face of negative findings for anti-HBc has been reported from Senegal.[32] In some instances, HBsAg positivity caused by this virus (designated HBV_2) followed a previous classical HBV infection with a resolving HBsAg phase. Similar findings have also been reported in sera from the Ivory Coast,[33] suggesting the presence of an agent that cross reacts with the pre-S_2 determinants of the HBV envelope.* Another "variant" of HBV has been reported in Greek patients chronically infected with HBV, who possess a mutant translational codon predicted to cause failure of production of HBeAg.[34] Yet another set of variants lacking normal *a* antigen sequences of HBsAg by an amino acid substitution causing a point mutation have caused HBV "break through" in Italian patients who had been previously vaccinated with hepatitis B vaccine and were anti-HBs positive.[35] The exact significance and impact of these different variants is as yet unclear, but they all appear to be detectable by current HBsAg screening assays.

2. The Delta Agent

This virus is a defective RNA virus which relies on HBV as a "helper" virus to provide its surface antigen.[36] It was originally found in Northern Italy. However, antibody to delta has been detected in plasma samples from Europe, Australia, Asia, and America. In the U.S. it is found in 3.8% of HBsAg-positive blood donations,[37] but is rare in British blood donors.[38] The virus multiplies in the liver and is transmissible by blood and body fluids (e.g., via IVD use). Because of its dependence on HBV infection, HBsAg screening prevents the transmission of delta agent by blood and coagulation factor concentrates by which it could otherwise be spread. As delta infection may increase the severity of chronic hepatitis B in HBsAg carriers, it is prudent to avoid transmission to seronegative HBsAg-positive recipients who

* Recent data suggest that "HBV_2" may not be a new variant, but may merely reflect differences in host response in the infected subjects.

should therefore also receive HBsAg-screened blood if they require transfusion.

C. NON-A, NON-B HEPATITIS

Until recently, the epidemiology of NANBH (diagnosed by "exclusion" of other hepatitis viruses) was not amenable to detailed study. However, the cloning of a part of the genome of an RNA virus (designated the hepatitis C virus, HCV) by Chiron Corporation[39] of California has led to the development of an enzyme-linked immunosorbent assay (ELISA) for antibody to this virus.[40] The topic has been recently reviewed[41] and further details may be found therein and in the proceedings of a symposium held to discuss international data obtained with the assay.[4]

The existence of a carrier state for NANBH has long been predicted on the basis of epidemiological data such as the significant prevalance of post-transfusion NANBH in some areas of the world and the continuing infectivity of certain donors capable of transmitting the infection. This carrier state, together with the long incubation period of the infection (up to approximately four months), predisposes the virus to transmission of NANBH by transfusion. Although it was assumed that, like HBV, sexual transmission of NANBH would be a significant route of infection, this has not been borne out consistently in seroepidemiological studies with the anti-HCV assay to date. A study in 259 Danish male homosexuals compared HCV acquisition with that of HIV and HBV, in serial samples stored at −70°C between 1981 and 1989.[42] In contrast to HBV and HIV, sexual transmission of HCV appeared to be a rare event, although HCV seroprevalence was higher in male homosexuals than in Danish male blood donors of the same age range. Our understanding of the significance of sexual transmission of HCV is incomplete, but IVD use has been clearly established as a risk factor worldwide, with rates of seropositivity of approximately 70% being found uniformly in IVD users. Increased prevalence in mentally handicapped patients has also been reported in Brussels (11.1% in one institution and 3.3% in another)[4] and in the U.K. (5.6%),[43] compared with those in blood donors, reported to be between 0.2 and 1.5% around the world.[4] The geographic variation in HCV prevalence is not as striking as with HBV, which is somewhat surprising when compared with the different incidences of PTH worldwide. This may be due to the particular nonstructural antigen that has been cloned and used in the original anti-HCV assays. Structural antigens are becoming available and it will be interesting to see how prevalences of antibody to these antigens compare in different countries. In very small trials on stored African sera, much higher prevalences have been reported[4] with the new assays but it is not clear how much of this reactivity is due to false positivity because of the high levels of IgG present in the samples.*

* Anti-HIV assays incorporating extra antigens — including structural ones — have now superseded the first available ones. It is still necessary, however, to "confirm" ELISA reactivity with supplementary assays because a significant proportion of ELISA reactives remain falsely positive.

Anti-HCV prevalence in New York blood donors (1.2% unconfirmed reactivity overall) increases with increasing alanine-aminotransferase (ALT) levels. Seroprevalance is 8.7% when ALT levels are greater than 65 IU/l, and a striking 55.6%[44] when anti-HBc is present. This is remarkably similar to the correlation of combined surrogate marker positivity with NANBH transmission in prospective studies in the U.S.[45] Similar findings for ALT and anti-HCV have been reported from Australia.[46] On the other hand, in Europe overall, 71% of anti-HCV-positive donors lack surrogate markers for NANBH,[4] but this may reflect lack of specificity of the early assay systems.

HCV seroprevalence in blood donors with a history of hepatitis is also of interest. In Kansas City, where a history of jaundice debars a blood donor, G. Tegtmeier (personal communication) reports a tenfold higher HCV seroprevalence in candidate donors with such a history, compared with donors without this history. In the U.K., where subjects with a history of jaundice are still eligible as donors after appropriate testing, increased HCV seroprevalance has so far not been observed (D. Howell, personal communication).

Maternofetal transmission, as occurs with HBV, would also seem possible for HCV. Data is lacking on this topic, although such transmission concurrent with HIV has been reported from Italy.[47] However, the virus is certainly blood-borne as shown by the high prevalences (>70%) in hemophiliacs[4] and the significant rates of seropositivity in dialysis centers in several countries.[4] Seroprevalence is also high in patients with chronic liver disease, including hepatocellular carcinoma,[48] but the possibility of false positivity in such patients has been raised[50] and supplementary testing of samples with recombinant immunoblot assay (RIBA) and polymerase chain reaction (PCR) are needed to confirm the preliminary findings.

As our understanding of NANBH increases in the light of studies with the anti-HCV ELISA and supplementary tests, it should become clearer whether other "non-A, non-B, non-C" viruses capable of causing PTH do indeed exist.

D. HUMAN IMMUNODEFICIENCY VIRUSES 1 AND 2

These viruses can be transmitted by both cellular and plasma fractions of blood with high efficiency. Although they are causative agents of the acquired immune deficiency syndrome (AIDS), various "pre-AIDS" symptoms can occur and the acute infection is sometimes associated with a glandular fever-like illness. The incubation period to frank AIDS can be very long, with an estimated median for transfusion-associated cases in excess of 8 years.[51] These agents are therefore prime candidates for transmission by transfusion and 90% of HIV seropositive individuals are infectious by this route during the incubation period. The situation is complicated by evidence for the existence of a prolonged seronegative state of HIV infection in a proportion of individuals with continual exposure to the agent.[51] This state of possible "silent" infection is revealed by detecting viral information molecules (RNA sequences) by PCR. The full extent and significance of this phenomenon awaits elucidation.

The degree of infectivity of "silently infected" individuals in relation to transfusion appears to be low, as most cases of transfusion-associated HIV infection can be traced to seropositive donors. In a study by Imagawa et al.,[53] HIV-1 was isolated from 31 of 133 seronegative individuals. Of these 31, 27 remained seronegative during the 7- to 36-month follow-up subsequent to viral isolation. Only four seroconverted after a seronegative period of 11 to 17 months. Presumably virus load or presentation was insufficient to stimulate antibody production; alternatively the phenomenon may be associated with the particular state of the immune system of the infected individuals. In this study, virus was considered to be present in cultures if both reverse transcriptase and the p24 antigen were present in the supernatant. The presence of HIV-1 genetic material was confirmed by PCR. The report of Imagawa et al.[53] is supported by other studies, reviewed by Haseltine.*

As a retrovirus, HIV is capable of producing DNA copies of its genetic material for incorporation into host cell DNA. HIV therefore demonstrates both prolonged latency and a carrier state where virus may be present for long periods of time. It is likely however that there is no totally latent phase when circulating virus is totally absent.[54] This has obvious relevance to transmission by transfusion.

The question of the relative merits of screening for virus antigen as opposed to testing for antibody in relation to the time course of infection will be discussed elsewhere in this book.

An important aspect of epidemiology in relation to all transfusion-transmitted infections is the question of modes of transmission. A clear understanding of HIV transmission allows donor information to be shaped towards efficient self-exclusion by those at risk of contracting HIV infection.

Self-exclusion offers one approach to reducing the risk from seronegative donors during "window" periods or "silent" infections. Its effectiveness will be discussed elsewhere in this book. A clear knowledge of routes of transmission is also a prerequisite for the effective counselling of seropositive donors when discussing ways of limiting the spread of infection.

Now that the risk of HIV transmission by transfusion of blood and its components or products has been reduced in developed countries with efficient donor selection and testing procedures, several other routes of transmission have been identified. Transmission from seropositive mothers to their offspring is known to occur at high frequency, although exact estimates are complicated by passive transfer of antibody across the placenta unless PCR is used. In relation to potential donors, sexual transmission and IVD use are the major factors. Other forms of transmission via skin puncture with contaminated sharp instruments (medical injections, "needle-sticks", tribal scar-

* In a recent update to this report, Imagawa and Detels (HIV-1 in seronegative hemosexual men, *N. Engl. J. Med.*, 325, 1250, 1991), after further follow-up of subjects studied in the first report, feel that "incomplete infection" is a more likely explanation than latent, persistent infection.

ifications) have been more or less implicated, especially in certain countries. Homosexual transmission was initially the main sexual route of infection in developed countries. In contrast, in Africa, roughly equal numbers of men and women are infected through heterosexual transmission. Genital ulceration due to other concomitant, often untreated, sexually transmitted disease has been postulated as the likely explanation for the similar anti-HIV prevalence in men and women. Heterosexual infection is now assuming increased importance in other parts of the world and the situation requires local assessment before donor selection policies are formulated. Numerous studies have estimated the relative risks of different types of sexual exposure and several factors, such as the level of infectivity in different phases of the infection, have been considered potentially significant. A detailed analysis of these considerations is beyond the scope of this chapter but in developed countries it is likely that "bisexual" activity and IVD use have been significant factors in the progression of heterosexual transmission. The significance of HIV transmission by banked breast milk, by tissue or organ transplantation, and by artificial insemination has obvious parallels with blood banking, but is outside the scope of this chapter.

The actual prevalence of seropositive individuals in a given population is of obvious significance to transfusion services even when anti-HIV testing is routine. The absolute number of potential donors who offer their blood during the "window period" of seronegativity is likely to be higher in "high-prevalence" than in low-prevalence populations. This again underlines the vital role of donor education and self-exclusion policies. When formulating exclusion policies, the question then arises: at what time did the "AIDS epidemic" commence? Although HIV infections became recognized when the acquired immune deficiency syndrome was recognized in the early 1980s, most exclusions of risk activity are reckoned to be relevant from approximately 1977. Sporadic earlier cases do come to light, however. The earliest well-documented case in a developed country may be that of an English seaman diagnosed as having an unexplained immunodeficiency with overwhelming pneumocystis and CMV coinfection of the lung.[55] This person was subsequently diagnosed as having been infected with HIV when tissue samples stored after his death in 1959 were subjected to DNA amplification. This detected HIV proviral DNA in kidney, bone marrow, spleen, and pharyngeal mucosa.[56] It is interesting to speculate as to the earliest date at which the Manchester patient may have been infected because of the variable incubation period to the development of frank AIDS. The analysis of incubation period referred to earlier[51] shows that 40% of persons develop AIDS 7 to 10 years after infection.

Prevalence of anti-HIV varies widely, even within the same country.[57] In the U.K., a total of 167 blood donations have been found positive for anti-HIV in 12.6 million tested up to the end of June 1990 (1 in 75,600). The rate in previously untested donors is 1 in 24,500 (V. Rawlinson and H. Gunson, personal communication). In the repository of 200,000 donor sera

TABLE 2
Transfusion-Associated AIDS in the U.K. and U.S., to the End of June, 1990

Cumulative AIDS cases	No. (% of all reports)	
	U.K.	U.S.
All reports	3,433	139,765
Hemophilia/coagulation disorders	207 (6.0)	1,353 (1.0)
Recipient of blood, components or tissue	52[a] (1.5)	3,506 (2.5)
Total, transfusion associated	259 (7.5)	4,859 (3.5)

[a] 28 of these were transfused abroad.

stored between 1984 and 1985 in the Transfusion Safety Study in the U.S.,[58] an anti-HIV prevalence of 1 in 600 donations was detected prior to the initiation of screening. The sera came from the four metropolitan areas with the highest incidence of AIDS cases. It has been estimated that in the U.S. overall, as many as 12,000 HIV infections may have been transmitted by transfusion. Prevalence figures in blood donors are now generally much reduced but will vary in different areas.

The actual numbers of AIDS cases associated with transfusion in the U.S. and U.K. are shown in Table 2.

Transfusion-associated cases of AIDS will continue to occur despite pretransfusion anti-HIV testing introduced in 1985, because of the long incubation period of the disease. However, the proportion of AIDS cases associated with transfusion should fall as the epidemic progresses in the other risk groups.

HIV-2 — What added relevance does the second AIDS virus have to blood transfusion? HIV-2, like HIV-1, is a causative agent of AIDS, with possibly a longer incubation period to the development of symptoms than HIV-1. Antiglobulin-based ELISAs for anti-HIV-1 will detect up to 80% of anti-HIV-2-positive sera, whereas the more specific competitive assays only cross-react in up to 30% of cases. HIV-2 is especially prevalent in West Africa and in countries such as Portugal which have links with West Africa, often through previous colonial associations. The epidemiological principles outlined previously for HIV-1 generally apply to HIV-2 also. Some countries in the developed world have introduced routine pretransfusion screening with combined anti-HIV-1 and anti-HIV-2 assays, although the prevalence of anti-HIV-2 in those countries overall is currently very low. Where combined screening has not been introduced, the safety afforded by screening with an assay demonstrating high cross-reactivity for anti-HIV-2 is considered adequate. It is, however, pertinent to note a recently reported case in the U.K.[49] A 42-year-old British homosexual man who had not had any sexual contacts with West Africa or other HIV-2 endemic regions was found to be anti-HIV-2 positive. Stored sera showed that he had been infected for at least 3 years.

This case reflects the way in which HIV-2 infection could spread into individuals not thought to be currently at high risk.

E. HUMAN T CELL LEUKEMIA VIRUSES

The human T cell leukemia viruses I and II (HTLV-I and -II) are also retroviruses and exhibit extremely long incubation periods to the development of symptoms, which occur only rarely.

1. HTLV-I

The virus is endemic in southwest Japan and in the black populations of the Caribbean islands. It is also endemic in parts of West and Central Africa, South America, and the southern states of the U.S.[60] In parts of Japan, the prevalence of anti-HTLV-I reaches 15% and in the Caribbean it ranges from 2 to 12% (for details of these and other HTLV-I references, see review by Weber[61]).

As a retrovirus, HTLV contains an RNA-dependent DNA polymerase which allows integration of viral DNA into host white cells, resulting in a persistent latent infection with lifelong antibody. Adult T cell leukemia (which gives rise to the alternative abbreviation for the virus, ''ATLV'') only ensues in a small number of cases (approximately 1% of infected persons per lifetime). An alternative manifestation of infection is HTLV-I-associated myelopathy (HAM) — also known as tropical spastic paraparesis (TSP).

HTLV-I can be transmitted sexually, parenterally, and from mother to child (principally through breast milk). Transmission of HTLV-I by cellular elements of blood (but not plasma) can therefore occur, but only at about half the efficiency of HIV. Similarly, it can be spread by IVD use. In areas of high HTLV-I prevalence, such as Japan, blood donor screening programs have been initiated and have been shown to prevent transfusion transmission.[62] Screening of blood donors is also routine in the U.S. Although no case of human T cell leukemia caused by transfusion has yet been reported, a history of blood transfusion can be associated with HAM[63] and cases of transfusion-transmitted HAM have been reported.[64]

The seroprevalence of HTLV-I in 40,000 blood donors in the U.S. was reported as 0.025%, but there is significant geographic variation. The epidemiological background of 51 anti-HTLV-positive blood donors in four major U.S. metropolitan areas has been determined as follows:[65]

- Blood transfusion (themselves or a sexual contact): 31%
- IVD use (themselves or a sexual contact): 24%
- Black, born in the southeastern U.S.: 20%

The most common characteristic was an association with Japan or the Caribbean (61%). Interestingly, four of the male seropositive donors (15%) reported homosexual contact.

Other countries that have reported HTLV seroprevalence figures for blood donors include France (0.011%)[66] and a predicted rate for the U.K. of

0.00036%.[67] However, a recent study of 100,000 U.K. donors detected HTLV infection in 0.005% of donors (M. Brennan, personal communication).

2. HTLV-II

Clinically, HTLV-II has only been associated with a handful of cases of hairy cell leukemia. It is of interest as potentially transmissible by blood transfusion. Current assays for anti-HTLV-I also cross react strongly with anti-HTLV-II, but the significance of the latter to transfusion is not yet clear. In the western hemisphere, a significant proportion of ''anti-HTLV-positive'' blood donors are likely to be positive for anti-HTLV-II. HTLV-II is the commonest HTLV infection found in IVD users.[68,69]

F. CYTOMEGALOVIRUS (CMV)

In contrast with other viruses that pose problems for transfusion safety, the prevalence of CMV seropositivity in donor populations is generally high. Prevalence ranges from 40 to 79% in western Europe, the U.S., and Australia and may approach 100% in developing countries. (For detailed references for this section, see Barbara and Tegtmeier.[70]) CMV seroprevalence increases with age. For example, in Kansas City blood donors, only 24.7% of donors aged 18 to 23 years are seropositive compared with 88.5% of those aged 60 years or older. Interestingly, in all age groups studied, females have significantly higher prevalence than males. Seroprevalence is highest in the lower socioeconomic groups. Fortunately, however, only a minority of recipients of blood are at risk if CMV is transmitted by transfusion and, furthermore, only a small proportion of CMV seropositive blood donations appear to transmit the infection.

Recipients at risk of CMV infection by transfusion are those with reduced immunity. These include low-birth-weight premature infants, patients undergoing immunosuppression to avoid graft rejection after transplantation, and patients with immunosuppression due to underlying illnesses such as AIDS. For babies born to CMV seronegative mothers and for older seronegative patients when indicated, anti-CMV-negative blood or leukocyte-depleted components can be provided (see chapter on prevention of transfusion infections). For transplant patients these special measures are generally only considered justifiable if the transplant donor is also seronegative. Transfusion-transmitted CMV infection in immunocompetent individuals is almost exclusively asymptomatic.

Although only a minority of anti-CMV-positive donations transmit the infection, it is not known which seropositive donors are likely to be infectious. CMV is a DNA-containing member of the herpes group of viruses and, like the others in the group, causes persistent latent infection. Latent CMV resides in the white cells (probably lymphocytes or monocytes) of the host. Granulocyte transfusions therefore enhance the risk of DMV transmission. CMV can cause primary infections, reactivations, or reinfections in humans.

From several studies, one can obtain a range of values for the rate of transmission of CMV by blood transfusion, from 12% in a 1970 study, to 0.2% in 1985. The overall rate appears to be low, at between 1 and 3.5%.

In a Dutch study, the overall number of CMV IgM-positive donors was only 0.16% so that the majority of transmissions are not by recently infected individuals. The figure of 0.16% was consistent with the 0.4% annual incidence of CMV seroconversion found in the Dutch donors which is slightly lower than in other countries. Since CMV latency is cell associated, transfusion risk is restricted to cellular components of blood.

A considerable amount of detailed information has been obtained concerning CMV transmission in newborn infants and considerable variation is noticeable in different studies. There are also different levels of risk related to transplantation of various organs.[70]

CMV infection is spread by a variety of routes including transplacental transmission, breast feeding, and sexual contact. It may be excreted in the saliva, feces, and urine. Specific history taking is therefore not appropriate for donor selection in relation to CMV.

G. EPSTEIN-BARR VIRUS (EBV)

EBV is another of the herpes group of viruses and, like CMV, it causes persistent latent infection in B-lymphocytes of peripheral blood and lymph nodes. Although EBV can cause primary symptomatic infection (infectious mononucleosis or ''glandular fever''), most infections are asymptomatic. Throughout the world, more than 90% of adults are seropositive. At least 1 in 10 million circulating lymphocytes of seropositive individuals contain EBV DNA,[71] but EBV infection after transfusion is rare and symptomatic infection is even rarer. This is presumably related to the large numbers of seropositive recipients. Like CMV, any transfusion risk is restricted to cellular components of blood.

H. HUMAN PARVOVIRUS B19

Infection with the human parvovirus is marked by a short viremia and is not persistent. However, the infection (erythema infectiosum or ''fifth disease'') is mild or asymptomatic and the titer of virus during viremia can be very high. Plasma products made from large numbers of donations can therefore be B19 contaminated because of the occasional viremic donor. Even though 30% of British adults and 25% of French blood donors have antibody to B19, hemophiliacs receiving Factor VIII have a much higher seroprevalence than background, or compared with hemophiliacs treated with cryoprecipitate.[72] Although donations from acutely infected blood donors are estimated to occur at a rate of only 1 in 10,000 to 1 in 50,000,[72] sufficient virus is presumably present to overcome the effects of any neutralizing antibody in the plasma pool. Recently, Williams et al.[73] have confirmed earlier findings and shown that anti-B19 IgG was present in 89% of 45 children in Birmingham, U.K. treated with unheated Factor VIII, compared with 39% in non-transfused controls; 48% of children receiving only cryoprecipitate were seropositive, compared with 41% of untransfused controls. In addition, they also studied seroprevalence in recipients of Factor VIII dry heated at 80°C for 72 hours where only 17% of 12 boys were anti-B19-positive. Less stringent heating methods for treating Factor VIII are not as effective and have been shown to transmit B19 after first exposure.[74] Since B19 is a heat-stable virus, methods of viral inactivation of clotting factor concentrates that successfully prevent transmission to recipients are also likely to inactivate the more heat-sensitive viruses such as HIV. Elimination of B19 transmission is therefore a good index of the efficacy of virucidal procedures.

Because B19 infection is very mild and infrequently transmitted by single blood components, pretransfusion screening is not indicated. However, B19 can precipitate aplastic arises in children with sickle cell anemia and in patients with other types of hemolytic anemia through cytotoxicity for erythroblasts.

I. COLORADO TICK FEVER VIRUS (CTFV)

CTFV is another virus which does not exhibit a true carrier or latent state but which has been reported to have been transmitted by transfusion.[75] The virus is tick-borne and is remarkable for its ability to persist in the end-stage red blood cells of its natural mammalian hosts and in man. Transmission by a blood donor four days after he had removed a tick from his skin and 18 hours before developing fever has been reported.[75]

VII. CONCLUSION

As will be evident from a consideration of the range of microbial agents transmissible by transfusion, a good understanding of the incidence, prevalence, and manifestations of infections and their modes of transmission are essential for maintaining a safe blood supply. Armed with this information, rational approaches can be taken to the education of donors for appropriate self-exclusion, the taking of relevant histories, and the effective counselling of donors found to be infected. A sound knowledge of the epidemiology of transfusion-transmitted infections is therefore a vital aspect of the quality assurance of transfusion safety measures.

ACKNOWLEDGMENT

I am grateful to Dr. Patricia Hewitt for review of the manuscript and to Miss Marina Mobed for secretarial assistance.

REFERENCES

1. **Barbara, J. A. J.,** *Microbiology in Blood Transfusion,* John Wright, Bristol, 1983.
2. **Bruce-Chwatt, L. J.,** Transfusion associated parasitic infections, in *Infection, Immunity and Blood Transfusion,* Dodd, R. Y. and Barker, L. F., Eds., Alan R. Liss, New York, 1985, 101.
3. **Hartmann, O. and Schøne, R.,** Syfilis overført ved blodtransfusion, *Nord. Tidskr. Milit. Med.,* 45, 1, 1942.
4. **Krauledat, P., Ed.,** Proceedings of the First International Symposium on Hepatitis C Virus, Rome, Ortho Diagnostic Systems and Chiron Corp., 1989.
5. **Mindel, A. and Tedder, R.,** Hepatitis A in homosexuals, *Br. Med. J.,* 282, 1666, 1981.
6. **Aoki, S. K. and Holland, P. V.,** Lyme disease — another transfusion risk?, *Transfusion,* 29, 646, 1989.
7. **Tabor, E.,** *Infectious Complications of Blood Transfusion,* Academic Press, New York, 1982.
8. **Heal, J. M., Jones, M. E., Forey, J., Chaudhry, N. A., and Stricof, R. L.,** Fatal *Salmonella* septicaemia after platelet transfusion, *Transfusion,* 27, 2, 1987.
9. **Jacobs, J., Jamaer, D., Vanderen, J., Wonters, M., Vermylen, C., and Vendepitte, J.,** *J. Clin. Microbiol.,* 27, 1119, 1989.
10. **Stenhouse, M. A. E. and Milner, L. V.,** *Yersinia enterocolitica:* a hazard in blood transfusion, *Transfusion,* 22, 396, 1982.
11. Centers for Disease Control, Q fever — California, *Morbid. Mortal. Weekly Rep.,* March 18, 86, 1977.
12. **Wells, G. M., Woodward, T. E., Fiset, P., and Hornick, R. B.,** Rocky Mountain spotted fever caused by blood transfusion, *JAMA,* 239, 2763, 1978.
13. **Braude, A. I., Casey, F. J., and Siemienski, J.,** Studies of bacterial transfusion reactions from refrigerated blood: the properties of cold growing bacteria, *J. Clin. Invest.,* 34, 311, 1955.
14. **De Silva, M., Contreras, M., and Barbara, J.,** Two cases of transfusion-transmitted malaria (TTM) in the UK, *Transfusion,* 28, 86, 1988.
15. **Bruce-Chwatt, L. J.,** Transfusion malaria, *Bull. WHO,* 50, 337, 1974.
16. **Conrad, M. E.,** Diseases transmissible by blood transfusion: viral hepatitis and other infectious disorders, *Semin. Haematol. (Transfus. Probl. Haematol.),* 18, 122, 1981.
17. **Greenwalt, T. J. and Jamieson, G. A., Eds.,** *Transmissible Disease and Blood Transfusion,* The American Red Cross Sixth Annual Scientific Symposium, Washington, May, 1974, Grune and Stratton, New York, 1974.
18. **Mollison, P. L., Engelfriet, C. P., and Contreras, M.,** *Blood Transfusion in Clinical Medicine,* 8th ed., Blackwell Scientific Publications, Oxford, 1987.
19. **Kirchhoff, L. V.,** Is *Tsypanosoma cruzi* a new threat to our blood supply?, *Ann. Intern. Med.,* 111, 773, 1989.
20. **McDonald, C. P., Barbara, J. A. J., Contreras, M., and Brown, S.,** Provision of a panel of anti-toxoplasma-negative blood donors, *Vox Sang.,* 57, 55, 1989.
21. **Azimi, P. H., Roberto, R. R., Guralnik, J. et al.,** Transfusion-acquired hepatitis A in a premature infant with secondary nosocomial spread in an intensive care nursery, *Am. J. Dis. Child.,* 140, 23, 1986.
22. **Cameron, C. H. and Barbara, J. A. J.,** HBV and transfusion, *Prog. Transfus. Med.,* 1, 19, 1986.
23. **Ryder, R. W., Whittle, H. C., Wojiecowsky, T. et al.,** Screening for hepatitis B virus markers is not justified in West African transfusion centres, *Lancet,* ii, 449, 1984.
24. **Lovric, V. A.,** Blood donors: simplified hepatitis B screening in hyperendemic areas, *Transfus. Today,* No. 6, June 1990, 8.
25. **Hoofnagle, J. H., Seef, L. B., Bales, Z. B., and Zimmerman, H. J.,** Type B hepatitis after transfusion with blood containing antibody to hepatitis B core antigen, *N. Engl. J. Med.,* 298, 1379, 1978.

26. **Lander, J. J., Gitnick, G. L., Gelb, L. H., and Aach, R. D.,** Anticore antibody screening of transfused blood, *Vox Sang.*, 34, 77, 1978.
27. **Barbara, J. A. J., Teder, R. S., and Briggs, M.,** Anti-HBc testing alone not a reliable blood donor screen, *Lancet,* i, 346, 1984.
28. **Alter, M. J.,** Disease transmissions: the relationship of blood transfusion to the modes of transmission, in *Autologous Blood Transfusion. Principles, Policies and Practices,* Fairchild, V. D., Holland, N. R., and Lyons, A. R., Eds., American Blood Commission, Alexandria, 1989, 4.
29. **Szmuness, W.,** Hepatocellular carcinoma and the hepatitis B virus. Evidence for a causal association, *Prog. Med. Virol.*, 24, 40, 1978.
30. **Beasley, R. P., Hwang, L. Y., Lin, C. C., and Chien, C. S.,** Hepatocellular carcinoma and hepatitis B virus, *Lancet,* ii, 1129, 1981.
31. **Shimoda, T., Uchida, T., Miyata, M. et al.,** A 6-year-old boy having hepatocellular carcinoma associated with hepatitis B surface antigenaemia, *Am. J. Clin. Pathol.*, 74, 827, 1980.
32. **Coursaget, P., Yvonnet, B., Bourdil, C. et al.,** HBsAg positive reactivity in man not due to hepatitis B virus, *Lancet,* ii, 1354, 1987.
33. **Budkowska, A., Dubreuil, P., Ovatarra, A., and Pillot, J.,** Anti-pre-5_2 as only serum HBV marker: possible relation to HBV-2 infection, *Lancet,* i, 656, 1988.
34. **Carman, W. F., Jacyna, M. R., Hadziyannis, S. et al.,** Mutation preventing formation of hepatitis Be antigen in patients with chronic hepatitis B infection, *Lancet,* ii, 588, 1989.
35. **Carman, W. F., Zanetti, A. R., Karayiannis, P. et al.,** Vaccine-induced escape mutant of hepatitis B virus, *Lancet,* 336, 325, 1990.
36. **Tiollais, P., Charnay, P., and Vyas, G. N.,** Biology of hepatitis B virus, *Science,* 213, 406, 1981.
37. Centers for Disease Control, *Delta hepatitis, Morbid. Mortal. Weekly Rep.*, 33, 493, 1984.
38. **Tedder, R. S., Briggs, M., and Howell, D. R.,** UK prevalence of delta infection, *Lancet,* ii, 764, 1982.
39. **Choo, Q.-L., Kuo, G., Weiner, A. J. et al.,** Isolation of a cDNA clone derived from a blood-borne non-A, non-B viral hepatitis genome, *Science,* 244, 359, 1989.
40. **Kuo, G., Choo, Q.-L., Alter, H. J. et al.,** An assay for circulating antibodies to a major etiologic virus of human non-A, non-B hepatitis, *Science,* 244, 362, 1989.
41. **Barbara, J. A. J. and Contreras, M.,** Non-A, non-B hepatitis and the anti-HCV assay, *Vox Sang.*, 60, 1, 1991.
42. **Melbye, M., Biggar, R. J., Wantzin, P. et al.,** Sexual transmission of hepatitis C virus: cohort study (1981–9) among European homosexual men, *Br. Med. J.*, 301, 210, 1990.
43. **Mortimer, P. P., Cohen, B. J., Litton, P. A. et al.,** Hepatitis C virus antibody, *Lancet,* ii, 798, 1989.
44. **Stevens, C. E., Taylor, P. E., Pindyck, J. et al.,** Epidemiology of hepatitis C virus. A preliminary study in volunteer blood donors, *JAMA,* 263, 49, 1990.
45. **Stevens, C. E., Aach, R. D., Hollinger, F. B. et al.,** Hepatitis B virus antibody in blood donors and the occurrence of non-A, non-B hepatitis in transfusion recipients — an analysis of the Transfusion-Transmitted Virus Study, *Ann. Intern. Med.*, 101, 733, 1984.
46. **Morgan, C., Hyland, C., and Young, C. F.,** Hepatitis C antibody and transaminase activities in blood donors, *Lancet,* 335, 921, 1990.
47. **Giovannini, M., Tagger, A., Ribero, M. L. et al.,** Maternal-infant transmission of hepatitis C virus and HIV infection: a possible interaction, *Lancet,* 335, 1166, 1990.
48. **Kew, M. C., Houghton, M., Choo, Q.-L., and Kuo, G.,** Hepatitis C virus antibodies in southern African blacks with hepatocellular carcinoma, *Lancet,* 335, 873, 1990.
49. **Tremolada, F., Benvegnu, L., and Casarin, C.,** Antibody to hepatitis C virus in hepatocellular carcinoma, *Lancet,* 335, 300, 1990.

50. **McFarland, I. G., Smith, H. M., Johnson, P. J. et al.,** Hepatitis C virus antibodies in chronic active hepatitis: pathogenetic factor or false-positive result?, *Lancet,* 335, 754, 1990.
51. **Kalbfleisch, J. D. and Lawless, J. F.,** Estimating the incubation time distribution and expected number of cases of transfusion-associated acquired immune deficiency syndrome, *Transfusion,* 29, 672, 1989.
52. **Haseltine, W. A.,** Silent HIV infections, *N. Engl. J. Med.,* 320, 1487, 1989.
53. **Imagawa, D. T., Lee, M. H., Wolinsky, S. M. et al.,** Human immunodeficiency virus type 1 infection in homosexual men who remain seronegative for prolonged periods, *N. Engl. J. Med.,* 320, 1458, 1989.
54. **Baltimore, D. and Feinberg, M. B.,** HIV revealed; toward a natural history of the infection, *N. Engl. J. Med.,* 321, 1673, 1989.
55. **Williams, G., Stretton, T. B., and Leonard, J. C.,** Cytomegalic inclusion disease and *Pneumocystis carinii* infection in an adult, *Lancet,* ii, 951, 1960.
56. **Corbitt, G., Bailey, A. S., and Williams, G.,** HIV infection in Manchester, 1959, *Lancet,* 336, 51, 1990.
57. **St. Louis, M. E., Rauch, K. J., Petersen, L. R. et al.,** Seroprevalence rates of human immunodeficiency virus infection at sentinel hospitals in the United States, *N. Engl. J. Med.,* 323, 213, 1990.
58. **Kleinman, S. H., Niland, J. C., Azen, E. A. et al.,** Prevalence of antibodies to human immunodeficiency virus type 1 among blood donors prior to screening. The Transfusion Safety Study/NHLBI donor repository, *Transfusion,* 29, 572, 1989.
59. **Breuer, J., Kenny, C., Shah, N. et al.,** HIV-2 antibody in a low-risk individual, *Lancet,* 336, 384, 1990.
60. **Tajima, K., Kamura, S., Ito, S. et al.,** Epidemiogical features of HTLV-I and incidence of ALT in an ATL-endemic island, *Int. J. Cancer,* 40, 741, 1987.
61. **Weber, J.,** HTLV-I infection in Britain: official recognition of the need for surveillance is overdue, *Br. Med. J.,* 301, 71, 1990.
62. **Inaba, S., Sato, H., Okochi, K. et al.,** Prevalence of transmission of human T-lymphotopic virus type 1 (HTLV-I) through transfusion, by donor screening with antibody to the virus. One-year experience, *Transfusion,* 29, 7, 1989.
63. **Osame, M., Igata, A., Usuku, K., Rosales, R., and Matsumoto, M.,** Mother-to-child transmission in HTLV-I associated myelopathy, *Lancet,* i, 106, 1987.
64. **Petz, L. D., Saxton, E., Lee, H. et al.,** A case of transfusion-transmitted HTLV-I associated myelopathy, *Transfusion,* 29 (Suppl.) (Abstr. S199), 555, 1989.
65. **Operskalski, E. A., Schiff, E. R., Kleinman, S. H. et al.,** Epidemiologic background of blood donors with antibody to human T-cell lymphotropic virus, *Transfusion,* 29, 746, 1989.
66. **Coste, J., Lemaire, J. M., Barin, F., and Courouce, A. M.,** HTLV-I/II antibodies in French blood donors, *Lancet,* 335, 1167, 1990.
67. **Salker, R., Tosswill, J. H. C., Barbara, J. A. J. et al.,** HTLV-I/II antibodies in UK blood donors, *Lancet,* 336, 317, 1990.
68. **Tedder, R. S., Shanson, D. C., Jeffries, D. J. et al.,** Low prevalence in the UK of HTLF-I and HTLV-II infection in subjects with AIDS, with extended lymphadenopathy, and at risk of AIDS, *Lancet,* ii, 125, 1984.
69. **Lee, H., Swanson, P., Shorty, V. S., Zack, J. A., Rosenblatt, J. D., and Chen, S. Y.,** High rate of HTLV-II infection in seropositive IV drug abusers in New Orleans, *Science,* 244, 471, 1989.
70. **Barbara, J. A. J. and Tegtmeier, G. E.,** Cytomegalovirus and blood transfusion, *Blood Rev.,* 1, 207, 1987.
71. **Rocchi, G., de Felici, A., Ragona, G., and Heinz, A.,** Quantitative evaluation of Epstein-Barr virus-infected mononuclear peripheral blood leukocytes in infectious mononucleosis, *N. Engl. J. Med.,* 296, 131, 1977.

72. **Mortimer, P., Luban, N., Keller, J., and Cohen, B.,** Transmission of serum parvovirus-like virus by clotting factor concentrate, *Lancet,* ii, 482, 1983.
73. **Williams, M. D., Cohen, B. J., Beddall, A. C., Pasi, K. J., Mortimer, P. P., and Hill, F. G. H.,** Transmission of human parovirus B19 by coagulation factor concentrates, *Vox Sang.,* 58, 177, 1990.
74. **Bartolomei Corsi, O., Azzi, A., Morfini, M., Fauci, R., and Rossi Ferrini, P.,** Human parvovirus infection in haemophiliacs first infused with treated clotting factor concentrates, *J. Med. Virol.,* 25, 165, 1988.
75. Centers for Disease Control, Transmission of Colorado Tick Fever Virus by Blood transfusion in Montana, *Morbid. Mortal. Weekly Rep.,* 422, 1975.

Chapter 19

TESTING BLOOD FOR INFECTIOUS AGENTS: METHODS AND QUALITY CONTROL

Roger Y. Dodd and William E. Kline

TABLE OF CONTENTS

ISBN 0-8493-4938-9

I. INTRODUCTION

A wide variety of infectious agents may be transmitted from donor to recipient by blood transfusion.[1] In the U.S., the most important of these are the viruses which cause hepatitis and AIDS. In addition, the causative agent of adult T cell leukemia/lymphoma is of concern. There are also a number of parasitic agents which can be transmitted. Of greatest concern worldwide are the malarial parasites and *Trypanosoma cruzi,* the agent of Chagas' disease. Fortunately, however, these parasites represent a very infrequent threat to blood recipients in the U.S. Finally, there are a variety of bacteria which can, on occasion, be transmitted by this route. *Treponema pallidum,* the agent of syphilis, has always been considered to be the most serious threat, although modern collection practice essentially eliminates the risk. Other enteric and environmental bacteria are also an occasional problem.

Although there is considerable public concern about the safety of the blood supply, it is reasonable to suggest that the actual risk of transfusion-transmitted infection is now lower than it has ever been.[1] This reflects the results of a combination of processes designed to increase safety. Measures have been taken to reduce the actual number of homologous transfusions, including reevaluation of the transfusion trigger;[2] implementation of autologous transfusion procedures; the use of hemodilution; and the development and use of recombinant erythropoietin.[3–5] Increasing attention has been paid to the selection of safe donors, by enhancement to the interview and self-deferral processes. Finally, tests of ever-increasing sensitivity have been developed and implemented.

A. NEED FOR TESTING

Although careful donor selection is properly credited as providing the greatest contribution to the overall safety of the blood supply, this process alone cannot prevent the collection of all blood which may harbor infectious agents. A major reason for this is that, in many cases, the infected donor, or patient, is unable to identify any event, exposure, or risk which might have caused the infection. Additionally, there is evidence that some individuals will donate even though they are aware of risk factors,[6] or they may even choose to ignore explicit instructions to avoid giving because of a prior test result.[7] Thus, laboratory testing is complementary to donor selection, but also acts as a secondary line of defense.

Laboratory testing, as currently employed in blood collection, attempts to achieve one of two objectives. First, tests for specific markers of viral infection are used to identify those donations from individuals who are infected with, or infectious for a given agent. Second, surrogate tests are used to identify blood from populations of donors which are thought to offer increased risk of infection; typically, surrogate tests are nonspecific. Because current ethical considerations require that individuals be notified of positive test results, it is essential to confirm all reactive findings.

From a regulatory perspective, laboratory testing for infectious agents represents a process for assuring that the blood products have been evaluated and found safe for distribution. This implies a need for formal operating procedures and rigorous record keeping. In addition, since a donor with a reactive or positive finding is considered to offer risk of transmitting infection, methods must be developed to prevent the acceptance of future donations from such an individual.

B. EXTENT OF TESTING

At the time of writing in late 1990, all whole blood donations in the U.S. are routinely tested for the following specific markers: hepatitis B surface antigen (HBsAg); antibodies to the human immunodeficiency virus, type 1 (anti-HIV); antibodies to the human T-lymphotropic retrovirus, type I (anti-HTLV-I); and antibodies to a hepatitis C virus-derived antigen (anti-HCV). Current tests for anti-HIV-1 also detect 50% or more of HIV-2 infections[8,9] and the test for anti-HTLV-I also detects infection with HTLV-II.[10] In addition, the following surrogate, or nonspecific, tests are performed: a serologic test for syphilis (STS); levels of serum alanine aminotransferase (ALT); and a test for antibodies to hepatitis B core antigen (anti-HBc). The last two tests are thought to identify populations at increased risk of transmitting non-A, non-B hepatitis.[11,12] It should also be noted that increasing attention is being paid to the use of specific, rather than cardiolipin-based, tests for syphilis.[13] Finally, a proportion of donations are tested for the presence of antibodies to cytomegalovirus (anti-CMV), in order to eliminate the risk of serious CMV disease among selected, immunoincompetent patients.

C. QUALITY CONTROL AND QUALITY ASSURANCE

Continued satisfactory performance of testing must be assured and documented. Quality assurance represents the complex of procedures which are designed to reduce variability in testing. This includes activities such as development and review of operating procedures, staff training, proficiency assessment, and inspections programs. Quality control represents the deliberate collection of information to validate the testing process, linked with evaluation of the data and implementation of corrective actions as a result of the data review. Both quality assurance and quality control are important, although it is reasonable to point out that routine quality control procedures for immunoassays are still at an early stage of development.

D. PERSONNEL ISSUES

The quality of testing is dependent upon the availability of well-trained staff. Regulatory agencies often seek to assure this by requiring specific degree levels or credentials for staff. This, however, is not adequate in its own right and institutions must maintain currency among both staff and supervisors. In addition, employers have an obligation to ensure safe working conditions for their staff. The recent promulgation of regulations requiring so-called universal precautions for handling human blood and body fluids should do much to assure the required levels of safety.[14]

II. METHODOLOGY

Although a wide variety of methods is available for detecting viral antigens or antibodies, the enzyme-linked immunosorbent assay (ELISA, EIA) is almost universally used.[15,16] In the U.S., diagnostic and screening tests must be approved by the Food and Drug Administration (FDA) before they can be sold for routine use. Tests used in the preparation of blood, which is classified as a biologic product, are generally classified as "Biologics". Current exceptions to this classification are the STS, the ALT assay, and tests for antibodies to CMV. Tests for anti-HBc are in the process of being reclassified as a Biologic. The regulatory requirements for approval as a Biologic are stringent and data from extensive clinical trials must be provided for review. In addition, the FDA may require that each reagent lot be validated prior to release. Similar approval processes are in place in many developed countries. Table 1 outlines the principal and confirmatory methods for each test and

TABLE 1
Methods Used to Test Donor Blood for Infectious Disease in the U.S.

Agent	Marker	Methods	Confirmation	Regulatory status (U.S.)
CMV	Antibody (total)	Particle agglutination ELISA	NA[a]	Device
HBV	HBsAg	ELISA, RIA	Inhibition	Biologic
	Anti-HBc[b]	ELISA, RIA	NA	Device[c]
HCV	Antibodies to viral encoded protein	ELISA	NA[d]	Biologic
	ALT[b]	Enzyme	NA	Device
HIV-1	Antibody	ELISA, particle agglutination	Western blot	Biologic
HTLV I/II	Antibody	ELISA	Western blot plus RIP	Biologic
Syphilis	Reagin	Particle agglutination	FTA-ABS, etc.	Device
	Treponemal antibody	Particle agglutination, ELISA	FTA-ABS, etc.	Device

[a] Not routinely available.
[b] Regarded as a surrogate for HCV and/or non-A, non-B hepatitis.
[c] Being reclassified as a Biologic.
[d] Research methods only; licensed methods under development.

their regulatory status. A listing of approved tests and their manufacturers may be obtained from: The Director, Center for Biologics Evaluation and Research, United States Food and Drug Administration, Bethesda, Maryland 20892.

A. BLOOD SCREENING TESTS: PRINCIPLES AND PROPERTIES

1. ELISA

a. Basic Principle

Enzyme-linked immunoassays (ELISA) use a chromogenic enzyme-substrate system to detect and partially quantitate the occurrence of an immunologic reaction. In the context of blood screening, such tests are always based upon the use of a solid phase to separate reacted and unreacted components. The fundamental structure of an ELISA procedure requires a solid-phase capture reagent, and an enzyme-labeled detector system. In a direct, or forward assay, the capture reagent is an appropriate antibody if the analyte is an antigen, or an antigen preparation if the analyte is an antibody. The capture reagent is attached to the solid phase by adsorption or, in some cases, by a covalent linkage procedure. Early immunoassays used plastic test tubes as the solid phase. However, essentially all current tests use either a quarter-inch polystyrene bead, or a microplate well. As discussed below, the use of microparticles as a solid phase offers promise and such assays are under development.

The solid-phase reagent is exposed to the sample under test. For tests designed to detect antigens, the sample is often undiluted serum or plasma, but in antiglobulin-based assays for antibodies, the sample may be diluted. Dilutions are generally in the range of ten- to four-hundredfold. After an incubation period of the order of an hour, usually conducted at increased temperature (37 to 45°C), excess sample is removed by washing. Thus, unreacted analyte is removed from that which has reacted and is bound to the solid phase. Some tests, described below, are formatted in such a fashion as to avoid the need for this wash step. Once the capture reaction is complete, the bound analyte is detected by means of a probe, or detection reagent. In a forward ELISA, the detection reagent reacts directly with the bound analyte. Thus, for HBsAg tests, the detection reagent is an antibody to HBsAg. In almost all cases where the analyte is an antibody, the detection reagent is an antiglobulin, which is an antibody that itself reacts with antibody molecules. It is also technically possible to detect antibody by using appropriately labeled homologous antigen. In an inhibition ELISA assay, the detection reagent binds to unoccupied sites on the capture reagent. Thus, in the test for anti-HBc, the capture reagent consists of labeled antibody to the hepatitis B core antigen and anti-HBc in the test sample competes for available antigen on the solid phase.

The detection reagent is labeled with a suitable enzyme; in all available instances, the enzyme is either horseradish peroxidase or alkaline phosphatase. In some cases, the biotin-avidin, or biotin-antibiotin system may be used as an intermediate method to link the enzyme to the actual detection reagent. This step can be exploited to increase the analytic sensitivity of detection. The detection reagent is incubated with the solid phase, again at elevated temperature. Once the reaction is complete, excess detection reagent is washed off the solid phase. The bound probe reagent may then be detected by exposing the solid phase to a substrate appropriate to the enzyme used as the label. This enzymatic reaction is usually performed at room temperature. After a fixed time period, the enzymic reaction is stopped, with acid, alkali, or an enzyme poison. The extent of the enzymic reaction may then be assessed by reading the absorbance of the reaction mixture with an appropriate instrument.

Within certain limits, the optical absorbance of the mixture is a function of the amount of detector reagent bound to the solid phase. There is thus a potential for some degree of quantitation inherent in the ELISA technique. However, the proportional range of most blood screening tests is very limited and in most cases, a typical positive donor sample will generate a maximal response. The ultimate interpretation of blood screening ELISA assays is, in fact a binary one; the result is defined as negative or reactive, depending upon the signal. Thus, the test must incorporate some means of determining a cutoff value.

Typically, the cutoff is calculated from values obtained by testing control reagents included with the test kit. Both positive and negative controls are included and are run in replicate tests. For forward tests, the cutoff is usually defined by taking the mean of negative control absorbance values and adding, or multiplying by, a given constant. In some cases, the cutoff value may be a function of both negative and positive control values. The cutoff value for a test procedure is usually developed, or at least validated, as a result of data developed during clinical trials. The cutoff must be selected to assure an optimal balance of specificity and sensitivity. Routine negative samples generate a distribution of results and it is important to assure that the selected cutoff does not overlap this distribution in such a way as to generate an unacceptable number of false reactive results. If the distribution is normal, for example, the cutoff is usually at least five standard deviations from the mean of negative values.

b. Performance Characteristics

The key performance characteristics for a screening test are sensitivity, specificity, and reproducibility.[16] Sensitivity is the most important characteristic of a screening test inasmuch as more sensitive tests will have the potential to prevent a greater proportion of infections. In the context of these tests, there are essentially two definitions of sensitivity which are related, but not equivalent. Analytic sensitivity relates to the smallest amount of analyte which gives a reactive signal — for example, many tests for HBsAg can detect less than 1 ng/ml of HBsAg. Epidemiologic sensitivity is the proportion of positive test results obtained when the test is performed upon a population known to have the disease or characteristic under test. While analytic sensitivity may be a good guide to the quality of a test procedure, it probably does not have a great impact upon the effectiveness of the test in donor screening, provided the procedure has been approved and licensed by the FDA or an equivalent agency. In addition, it should be pointed out that it is relatively easy to measure the analytic sensitivity of a test for a single analyte, such as HBsAg, by using a dilution series, but that this approach is not necessarily applicable to tests designed to detect antibodies.

Specificity is usually defined as the proportion of negative test results obtained when a population without the disease or characteristic is tested. Thus, the value (1 − specificity) will give the proportion of false-positive results to be expected with a given test. It is often the case that, for a given procedure, improvements in sensitivity may be gained at the cost of losses in specificity. The specificity of a screening test is an important selection characteristic, since poor specificity will result in a higher number of false-positives which must be resolved by repeat and confirmatory testing. In addition, samples with repeatedly reactive screening test results cannot usually be transfused, so the product (and future products from the same donor) will be lost. Experience has shown that manufacturers' claims for specificity of a test are usually reliable, although in many cases, the claims may be conservative, as procedures are continually being improved.

The specificity of a test procedure is dependent upon the nature of the reagents themselves, the nature of the samples to be tested, and the way in which the test components are manipulated. The first of these points will be discussed here, while the others are covered elsewhere. As pointed out above, the selection of the cutoff itself can affect specificity. If the cutoff value is too close to the distribution of negative values, truly nonreactive samples with signals at the outer end of the range may well be classified as reactive. Clearly, the test must be designed in such a way that there is a good separation of the population of negative values from the population of reactive values. In addition to this inherent aspect of specificity, the actual nature of the reagents themselves may impact the test performance. Three examples may illustrate this point. Tests designed to detect anti-HIV have generally used a lysate of HIV grown in tissue culture as the capture reagent. This antigen preparation necessarily includes components of the cells used to grow the virus. In some circumstances, these cellular components included selected HLA antigens which thus detected corresponding antibodies in samples from alloimmunized patients.[17,18] A second example has been noted in homologous sandwich assays in which both the capture and probe reagents were antibodies made in the same animal species. Naturally occurring antiglobulins in donor or patient sera were able to bind the antibody molecules and thus simulate an antigen analyte.[19] Finally, in antiglobulin ELISAs, the final step is detection of immunoglobulins bound to the solid phase. Thus, any bound immunoglobulin would be detected, no matter what its immunologic specificity.

Both sensitivity and specificity are inherent properties of a test which do not generally vary with the sample population being tested. However, specificity is often confused with the positive predictive value (PPV) of a test, which is the proportion of true positive results to test positive (i.e., true positive plus false positive) results. The positive predictive value of a test therefore varies with the prevalence of true positives in a population. A simple example illustrates this. If a test has a specificity of 99.8%, then 0.2% of all negative samples will give a false-positive result. When this test is used on a population with a very low prevalence of true positives — say 0.02%, then the overall rate of reactive findings will be 0.22%. The positive predictive value will be 0.02/0.22, or 9%. In contrast, if the same test is used to evaluate a population with a high prevalence — say 20%, then the overall reactive rate will be 20.2% and the positive predictive value will be 20/20.2, or 99%. As a consequence, even a test with a very high level of specificity may have a poor positive predictive value when used to test a donor population. This also emphasizes the need for confirmatory testing of reactive screening tests to avoid improper donor notification.

Reproducibility of test procedures is the extent to which inter- and intralot variability is controlled. Multiple runs using the same master lot of reagents

TABLE 2
Typical Performance Characteristics of Infectious Disease Tests Used for Donor Blood in the U.S.

Test	Sensitivity[a] (%)	Specificity (%)	Voluntary donor results[b] PPV (%)	% True positives
HBsAg	NA[c]	99.95	50	0.03
anti-HBc	NA	NA	70	2.0
HCV	72–88[d]	99.60	40	0.4
HIV-1	100	99.95	20	0.01
HTLV I/II	NA	99.97	60	0.02
Syphilis (RPR)	NA	NA	40	0.2

[a] Manufacturer's claims.
[b] American Red Cross donor population, as of 1990.
[c] NA: meaningful data not readily available; manufacturer's claims cannot be directly translated to routine practice.
[d] Based upon diagnosed cases of non-A, non-B hepatitis.

should generate the same analytic and epidemiologic sensitivity and specificity, as should runs using different reagent master lots, or runs in different laboratories. Reproducibility of a test kit is a function of both manufacturing and laboratory quality control.[16] Table 2 illustrates typical performance characteristics of blood screening tests when used in a blood center environment.

c. Variables in Test Performance

During the manufacture of test kits, considerable effort is directed towards assuring consistency of test kit performance. Procedural variation in the performance of the tests can have a profound effect upon test results and it is important to understand and control such variability. Of particular importance are sample and reagent volume and dilution; incubation time and temperature; washing techniques; and handling of the conjugate.

Forward ELISA assays are designed so that reagents are in excess and thus variations in the actual volume of the sample have relatively small effects upon the outcome. This is particularly true of negative and strongly positive samples; however, test signals from those samples which are weakly reactive will certainly be proportional to the initial sample volume. Thus, it is important to avoid both inaccuracy and variability in the volume of sample dispensed. In particular, it is critical to avoid a mismatch between the volumes and/or dilutions of the controls relative to the test samples. This is a real concern if the controls are provided in diluted form. It should be noted that, in contrast to forward ELISA tests, inhibition procedures are markedly affected by variations in the volumes of sample and reagents used. The probe reagent is used at a concentration and volume calculated to be less than saturating and the sample competes with the probe. In addition, the cutoff value is generally placed on the steepest part of the response curve. Consequently, technical variations which might have little effect upon a forward ELISA may create significant variation and inaccuracy in an inhibition test.

Physical conditions for the performance of the tests are explicitly defined in the manufacturer's product insert. Good laboratory practice requires that these conditions be met at all times. Thus, the time and the temperature used for each incubation step must be within the required limits. Furthermore, it is necessary to maintain records to show that the conditions have been met. Every effort must be made to avoid a time or temperature mismatch between controls and test samples. This may appear self-evident in bead-based tests, where a single run may include only one set of controls, but samples may be incubated in several reaction trays. However, temperature variations can also occur across a single microplate, especially in an air incubator, so it is important to use the equipment recommended by the test kit manufacturer.

One of the greatest causes of inconsistency in test performance is the process of washing off excess reactants. Incomplete removal of the primary sample (other than in simultaneous-addition formats) may result in loss of sensitivity as a result of competition with the probe reagent. This is particularly true for antiglobulin ELISA tests. Conversely, incomplete removal of the probe reagent will lead to improperly elevated signal levels. This potential for variability is markedly reduced when the recommended automated, or semiautomated, washing devices are used. However, the instrument must be carefully maintained and calibrated on an ongoing basis, since blockage of probes or variations in delivery volume can compromise performance.

The probe reagent is sensitive to a variety of problems. First, care must be taken to preserve the activity of the enzyme component. Heavy metals, azide, and other environmental conditions can affect the enzyme. Thus, the conjugate itself and the substrate solution must be handled with care and the proper diluents must be used. Metallic equipment must not be used for handling the reagent or any component of the substrate. Care may also have to be taken with the source and nature of the water used to prepare the substrate. Second, antiglobulin probe reagents are designed to detect minute quantities of bound immunoglobulins and the reagent is present at an extremely low concentration. Consequently, contamination of the probe reagent with even a minute drop of human serum can block, or inhibit the binding capacity of the reagent, leading to false-negative results. It is essential to avoid any possibility of contaminating the probe reagent; specific pipettes must be reserved only for use with this test reagent, for example.

2. Radioimmunoassay

Radioimmunoassay, or RIA, tests use exactly the same principles and formats as enzyme immunoassays. The only difference is that the probe reagent is labeled with a radionuclide instead of an enzyme. Thus, the test is evaluated using an appropriate nuclear counting instrument. Tests used in blood banking invariably use ^{125}I as the label. This isotope emits relatively low-energy gamma rays and has a half-life of 56 days. Nevertheless, it requires careful handling and is subject to regulation; laboratories must be appropriately licensed before using RIA tests. Since isotope can be detected at a distance, and since the reading instruments can be readily contaminated, extreme cleanliness is necessary, not only for safety, but also for accuracy. It is of interest to note that the RIA procedure does offer additional potential for quality control. Since there is invariably some residual bound reactivity, even in tests with negative samples, it is possible to determine whether probe has been properly added to each test. Given the very infrequent use of RIA in blood collection practice, it will not be discussed further in this chapter.

3. Particle Agglutination

Particle agglutination tests in current use in infectious disease testing in blood collection are designed to detect antibodies. The antibodies react with antigens which are attached or bound to microscopic particles. Because antibody molecules have two or more combining sites, a single antibody can simultaneously combine with two different particles. In appropriate conditions, particles can be linked into a large, macroscopically visible aggregate. In fact, the actual interaction may be somewhat more complex than this simplified description, but this complexity has little practical effect. In direct agglutination tests, the antigen is an inherent component of the particle, as in the case of direct hemagglutination. In indirect agglutination tests, the antigen is attached to the surface of some relatively inert particle. Of the tests in current use, this particle is charcoal, latex, gelatin, or red cells. In the context of blood testing, the serologic test for syphilis represents a special case. A cardiolipin antigen is able to react with antibodies or "reagins" which are generated as a response to infection with *T. pallidum*. In the classic VDRL test, the particles are an emulsion of lipids, including the cardiolipin. In the more frequently used RPR test, the cardiolipin is adsorbed onto charcoal particles.[13]

Particle agglutination tests generally have acceptable levels of sensitivity, which may indeed be comparable to those of ELISA tests, as is the case for a rapid latex agglutination test for antibodies to HIV.[20,21] However, the specificity of agglutination tests is not generally as high as that of ELISA procedures. Frequently, agglutination tests are subject to interference from a variety of biologic factors, most particularly rheumatoid factors and other autoantibodies. In addition, although it is usually very easy to differentiate negative samples from strong positives, intermediate reactions may be very hard to identify or interpret.

Agglutination tests are relatively insensitive to variation in sample volume, but may be profoundly affected by variation in the ionic environment. Thus, it is important to avoid evaporation of samples during testing, particularly when performed upon cards or slides. Care must also be taken to ensure the correct incubation time. Technical staff must be carefully trained in the reading and interpretation of the tests. Since manual tests require that the results be directly transcribed, careful control of record keeping is mandatory. Some method of double checking should be incorporated into this phase. Increasingly, automation is being applied to agglutination tests, as discussed below. This should reduce the risk of error in this area.

B. INDIVIDUAL AGENTS, MARKERS, AND TESTS

1. Tests for HBsAg

HBsAg is a circulating antigen which is associated with active infection with hepatitis B virus (HBV). It is viral coat material which is synthesized in infected cells in great excess; it is released into the circulation as 22-nm diameter particles and tubules. HBsAg itself is noninfectious, as it does not contain nucleic acids. During acute or chronic infection, it may be present at levels of up to 1 mg/ml and several million particles may be present for each infectious virion. Early studies showed that the great majority of blood donations which were infectious for HBV could be identified by simple tests for HBsAg. In fact, the earliest routine methods for detection involved direct precipitation in agarose gel.

Radioimmunoassay for HBsAg was introduced in the mid-1970s but was fairly rapidly supplanted by ELISA. Currently available tests are all of essentially the same format. The capture reagent is antibody to HBsAg, bound to a support, namely a polystyrene bead, tube, or microplate well. The antibody is usually prepared in animals. Sample is added to the tube or well and HBsAg, if present, is bound to the solid-phase antibody. This antigen is detected by a probe reagent which is a labeled antibody to HBsAg, again usually prepared in animals. The label is either alkaline phosphatase or horseradish peroxidase. After incubation, excess probe is washed away and bound probe is detected by an appropriate chromogenic substrate. Because this is a direct sandwich assay, samples which lack HBsAg give low readings and positive samples will give a high reading. Negative and positive controls are included in each test run and are used both for quality control and for the designation of a cutoff value which is used to interpret the results of the test run. Most ELISA tests are able to detect about 1 ng/ml of HBsAg, which is equivalent to about 5×10^5 particles/ml. Current tests are highly specific (better than 99.9%) and appear to be sufficiently sensitive to essentially eliminate the risk of transfusion-transmitted HBV infection.[22]

In some cases, monoclonal antibodies are incorporated into the test. Because of the restricted specificity of these reagents, they do not compete with other antibody components of the test and it is possible to add the sample and the probe simultaneously, thus eliminating one incubation step and one wash step. Some test methods may use a somewhat different approach to labeling, but all current procedures are essentially as described.

Confirmation of HBsAg test results is relatively simple. In essence, the test is performed in the presence or absence of a known preparation of antibodies to HBsAg. If the added antibody inhibits the reaction by at least 50%, then the sample is confirmed to be positive for HBsAg. In some cases, it is necessary to predilute the test sample; instructions for this procedure are provided in the manufacturer's product insert.

2. Tests for Anti-HIV

Infection with HIV stimulates the production of antibodies to HIV gene products and, because HIV infection is persistent, the presence of such antibodies implies infectivity. Following announcement of the recognition and culture of HIV in 1984,[23,24] the HTLV-III isolate and its host cells were made available to a number of selected companies in the U.S. These companies developed commercial versions of an ELISA test designed to detect antibodies to HIV.[25] The first of these tests was licensed in March of 1985. All of the early tests for anti-HIV used a lysate of purified HIV as the capture reagent. The viral lysate is bound to a polystyrene bead or microplate well. Prediluted sample is added and antibodies to HIV, if present, are bound to the viral antigens. Excess sample is washed away and an enzyme-labeled antiglobulin probe is added. Subsequently, excess probe is washed away and adherent probe is detected by a suitable chromogenic substrate. Positive and negative controls are included with each run and are used for quality control and for calculation of the cutoff. A high signal indicates the presence of anti-HIV and negative samples give a low value.

There are a number of variations to this basic format. Most notable has been the use of an inhibition procedure by a British manufacturer. In this test, the capture reagent is viral lysate, but samples compete against an enzyme-labeled anti-HIV probe. Consequently, negative samples generate a high, and reactive samples a low, signal. The other major variation is the use of recombinant,[26] or synthetic,[27,28] HIV antigens as the capture reagent. Such reagents offer the advantages of safety and consistency in manufacture. They may also enhance the sensitivity of the test, since more specific antigen can be loaded onto the solid phase. However, great care must be taken to select appropriate epitopes, so that variations in the antigenic structure of different viral strains does not compromise the ability of the test to detect infection.

The formal sensitivity of anti-HIV tests is assessed in terms of the ability of the procedure to detect individuals diagnosed with AIDS. On this basis, essentially all available tests have a sensitivity of 100%. Perhaps a more important characteristic is the ability of a test to detect HIV infection at the earliest possible time. In general, current tests seem to be quite comparable by this criterion, with only a few days variation in the earliest time of first detection.[29] Some data suggest that certain tests based upon recombinant antigen capture reagents may indeed have increased sensitivity.[30] The specificity of HIV tests is generally better than 99.9% at this time.

In parts of West Africa and its offshore islands, HIV-2 is the predominant AIDS virus.[31] It is clear that this virus is also being introduced into at least some countries in Western Europe, probably as a result of population movements and earlier colonial connections. Tests based upon HIV-1 antigens are able to detect only 50% to 90% of all HIV-2 infections. Consequently, tests designed to detect antibodies to HIV-2 and tests designed to detect both anti-HIV-1 and anti-HIV-2 have been developed.

Confirmation of HIV-1 ELISA tests on donated blood is routinely performed using the Western blot procedure.[32,33] Briefly, a lysate of HIV is subjected to polyacrylamide gel electrophoresis in the presence of sodium dodecyl sulfate in reducing conditions. Each of the polypeptide components of the virus migrates to an extent which is inversely proportional to its molecular weight. After migration, the polypeptide bands are electroblotted onto cellulose nitrate paper. The paper is cut into strips and strips are exposed to test sample. If antibodies to HIV antigens are present, they adhere to the polypeptides on the strip. The adherent immunoglobulins are detected with an enzyme-labeled antiglobulin and may be visualized with an appropriate substrate. Antibodies to the following gene products may be identified: gag — p17, p24, and p55; pol — p31, p53, and p66; env — gp41, gp120, and gp160. A variety of criteria are used to define a positive reaction, but most of these criteria identify the same samples as positive.[33] The Centers for Disease Control and the Association of State and Territorial Public Health Laboratory Directors have endorsed a pragmatic definition, requiring the presence of two of the following bands: p24, gp41, gp120, or gp160. Other criteria call for the presence of antibodies to at least one product from each gene. One Western blot procedure which has been licensed by the FDA requires that the antibodies to p24, p31, and one env glycoprotein be present, whereas another licensed blot procedure requires at least one band from each gene. The absence of any band is evidence that the donor is not infected with HIV-1. Any other pattern is termed indeterminate and must be subjected to additional testing or followup.[32] Western blots for HIV-2 are also available. The World Health Organization has recommended that the presence of two of three env bands be required for a positive reading in such blots.

In the case of HIV testing, it is critical to confirm a reactive test result before notifying and counselling donors. In addition, an FDA-licensed Western blot test may be used to support "reentry" of donors who have had ELISA-reactive test results in the past, provided that two successive samples, drawn six months apart, are negative in both ELISA and Western blot.

Additional methods for confirmation of HIV-reactive ELISA results are available or are under development, but have not yet been licensed by the FDA. Particularly interesting in this context is the use of synthetic peptide-based assays. These procedures will certainly be of value in differentiating between HIV-1 and HIV-2 infection.[34]

3. Tests for Anti-HTLV-I/II

HTLV-I was the first human retrovirus to be recognized and isolated. It is known to be the etiologic agent of adult T cell leukemia/lymphoma and is almost certainly the causative agent of tropical spastic paraparesis. It is transmissible by blood transfusion and is endemic in Southern Japan and parts of the Caribbean; it is present in the North American donor population, with a seroprevalence rate of approximately 0.025%.[35] In order to reduce the risk of primary infection among blood recipients and secondary infection of their family members, testing for anti-HTLV-I was initiated in the U.S. in late 1988. Available test procedures are essentially identical to whole viral lysate-based tests for anti-HIV, with the obvious exception that the capture reagent is prepared from HTLV-I. The closely related HTLV-II is antigenically almost identical to HTLV-I. Consequently, assays prepared from HTLV-I also detect infection with HTLV-II. As yet, this latter virus has not been etiologically linked to a specific disease state. In the U.S., approximately 50% of blood donors identified as positive in the HTLV-I test are actually infected with HTLV-II, with intravenous drug abuse or sexual contact with a drug abuser as the primary risk factor. It has not been possible to establish the actual sensitivity of anti-HTLV-I assays, since there is no gold standard against which to assess this parameter. However, it is reasonable to suggest that current tests are able to identify most, if not all infected individuals who produce antibodies to the virus. At least one of the available tests has a very high specificity, of 99.95% or better.

Confirmation of the HTLV-I/II ELISA test is complex. A Western blot procedure is capable of detecting antibodies to gag and env proteins. A sample which has detectable antibodies to p24 and one env glycoprotein is regarded as positive.[36,37] There is increasing evidence to support the concept that a sample should be considered positive if reactive to either of the gag proteins, p19 or p24, plus an env protein. A proportion of samples which are found, on blots, to have antibodies reactive to p24 but not to an env glycopeptide, may nevertheless have demonstrable glycopeptide antibodies when tested by radioimmunoprecipitation (RIP). Such samples are regarded as positive. Hence, some samples must be tested both by Western blot and by RIP in order to complete the confirmation process.[36,37] It seems likely that the use of ELISA tests derived from synthetic or recombinant HTLV-I env peptide may be used in an algorithm which reduces the amount of blot and RIP testing, however.[37]

Differentiation of HTLV-I and HTLV-II infection has been achieved by amplification of type-specific genome segments. However, it is now becoming apparent that this differentiation can be achieved by the use of ELISA tests prepared from appropriate, viral-specific synthetic peptides.

4. Tests for Anti-HCV

For many years, non-A, non-B hepatitis (NANBH) was considered to be the most frequent transfusion-transmitted infection. However, the agent, or agents of this disease could not be identified and no specific blood screening test was available. Therefore, the identification of an antigenic protein expressed by a cDNA clone (clone 5-1-1) of a segment of the putative viral genome was of extreme importance.[39] It is now clear that Houghton and colleagues had indeed identified the viral agent which causes the predominant and most serious form of transfusion-transmitted NANBH.[40] This virus has now been termed hepatitis C virus (HCV). A recombinant construct has been developed and expressed in yeast. The protein, known as C100-3, consists of a sequence of 363 amino acids coded by the HCV gene and including the original 5-1-1 sequence, linked to human superoxide dismutase. This protein is used as the capture reagent for an ELISA screening test to detect antibodies to the protein. Such antibodies are clearly associated with transfusion-transmitted NANBH, and appear to be a good marker of HCV infectivity among donors.[40] At the same time, antibodies to this particular protein, which is thought to be a nonstructural component of the virus, appear late in infection, may eventually decline, and thus, the test may not be 100% sensitive for detecting infection.

Two ELISA tests for anti-HCV became available during 1990. Both were based upon the C100-3 protein; one uses microplates as the solid phase, the other uses a polystyrene bead. Prediluted sample is added to the capture reagent and incubated. Excess sample is washed off and enzyme-linked antiglobulin conjugate is added as a detector. After incubation and washing, a substrate solution is added to detect adherent conjugate. Positive and negative control samples are included in each run and are used for quality control and to establish the cutoff. The sensitivity of the test procedure is not readily measured. Retrospective analyses of posttransfusion studies suggest that the test will detect 50 to 85%, or more[40,41] of infectious donor samples. Preliminary data, which rely on unproven confirmatory assays, suggest that the tests have a specificity of about 99.6% in donor populations.

At the time of writing, there is no validated confirmatory assay for the anti-HCV ELISA. However, extensive work has been done using a recombinant immunoblot assay (RIBA). This assay, as its name suggests, is similar to a Western blot. Recombinant proteins are applied directly to a nitrocellulose strip, and the strip is used to probe for antibodies in the test sample. The first-generation RIBA has bands consisting of the 5-1-1 protein (expressed in *Escherichia coli*), the C100-3 protein (expressed in yeast), and the superoxide dismutase expression protein. In addition, bands representing high- and low-level reagent controls are present. The RIBA is read as positive if bands to the two viral proteins are present at a density equal to, or greater than, that seen in the low-level control. Positive results in this version of RIBA are clearly associated with other evidence of infection or infectivity. However, it is not yet clear what negative or partial (indeterminate) results signify. A RIBA procedure with additional expressed proteins has been developed and it appears that this may be a much more effective confirmatory or diagnostic tool.

5. Surrogate Tests for NANBH

A number of prospective, posttransfusion follow-up studies, performed in the late 1970s, indicated that 7 to 12% of blood recipients showed signs of liver dysfunction which was termed NANBH and attributed to infection with virus(es). These studies showed that there was an association between elevated levels of ALT in donors and recipient NANBH.[42,43] Subsequent re-evaluation of these studies showed a similar association with anti-HBc in donors.[11,12] It was suggested that implementation of donor screening for ALT elevations and anti-HBc would reduce the incidence of posttransfusion NANBH by about 65%. In 1986, donor screening for both of these markers was introduced into routine practice in the U.S., although a few blood centers had initiated ALT testing several years earlier.

The test for ALT levels is a standard, clinical chemistry procedure, performed on a chemistry analyzer. The standard method involves the addition of sample to a reagent solution. The primary substrates for ALT in the assay are alanine and 2-oxoglutarate. Enzyme present in the sample catalyzes the reaction:

$$\text{L-alanine} + \text{2-oxoglutarate} \rightleftarrows \text{pyruvate} + \text{L-glutamate}$$

The substrate concentrations are adjusted so that the reaction follows pseudo-first-order kinetics. The rate of evolution of pyruvate is measured by a linked reaction in which lactate dehydrogenase reduces the pyruvate to lactate:

$$\text{Pyruvate} + \text{NADH} \rightleftarrows \text{lactate} + \text{NAD}$$

The rate of this reaction is measured by observing the rate of change of absorbance of NADH at 340 nm. This rate is ultimately proportional to the quantity of ALT in the original sample. The rate is measured after a lag period, during which endogenous pyruvate is consumed. Measured rates must be checked for linearity; a nonlinear rate usually signifies a technical or sample problem, or substrate exhaustion due to extremely high enzyme levels. Results are expressed as International Units per liter (IU/l), or, in SI units, as microkatals per liter (μkat/l). The conversion factor is 1 μkat/l = 0.01667 IU/l. The results of an ALT test must always be referred to the temperature at which the assay is performed, since the rate of an enzyme reaction is temperature dependent. Assays are conventionally performed at 37°C in the U.S., but elsewhere, may be performed at 30 or 25°C.

The key issue in donor ALT testing is establishing a cutoff level, above which a donation is withheld from transfusion. Original studies suggested that a conventional upper limit of normal (45 IU/l in that study) was an appropriate value,[42] while another study proposed a value equivalent to the 98.4 percentile value.[43] Currently, it has been suggested that a cutoff value equivalent to the

97.5 percentile value for the donor population is appropriate.[44] ALT levels which are two or more times greater than this cutoff may signify a clinical problem and donors with such levels should be permanently deferred and referred to a physician.

By its nature, the ALT test is not amenable to confirmation. However, samples with elevated results are usually retested to validate the initial finding. Standard quality control measures, as used in clinical laboratories, are appropriate for donor ALT testing.

Antibodies to HBc antigen are produced as a result of active infection with HBV. They appear in the circulation shortly after HBsAg and may persist for the lifetime of the individual, whether or not a persistent infection is established. Anti-HBc may, on occasion, be found in the absence of any other markers of HBV infection. This may represent one of three situations: a false-positive test result; acute HBV infection between loss of HBsAg and detection of anti-HBs; or HBV infection which occurred in the distant past, with eventual loss of anti-HBs. It is possible that, in the second of these two situations, the individual could be circulating infectious levels of HBV. For this reason, tests for anti-HBc will be licensed as a Biologic, to be used for additional prevention of posttransfusion HBV infection. However, anti-HBc testing was implemented as a surrogate test for NANBH infectivity.

The anti-HBc test was originally developed as a diagnostic and, as such, lacks some of the desirable properties of a screening test. Currently available tests are formatted as solid-phase inhibition immunoassays. The capture reagent is recombinant hepatitis B core antigen, bound to a polystyrene bead or microplate well. The probe is a labeled anti-HBc and antibody, if present in the sample, competes with the probe. Sample and probe are added to the solid phase and incubated. After reaction, excess sample and probe are washed off and adherent probe is detected by means of an appropriate chromogenic substrate. As with other inhibition tests, high signal levels are found with negative samples, whereas reactive samples generate low values. Positive and negative controls are included in each run. The cutoff for the test is calculated as a function of the negative and positive control values, usually representing approximately 50% inhibition of maximal signal. The sensitivity of the assay appears to be good when referred to populations of patients with diagnosed HBV infection. It is apparent that the specificity of at least one of the available ELISA procedures is not very high. Up to 30% of donor samples which are reactive may fail to be reactive in a second test for anti-HBc, or the donors may not be found reactive on a subsequent visit.[45,46] This would suggest a specificity of perhaps 99.5%. It is possible that newer versions of this test may have greatly increased specificity.[47]

Currently, there is no validated confirmatory assay for anti-HBc. It is appropriate to repeat reactive samples, and some increase in specificity may be obtained by retesting with a second procedure, such as radioimmunoassay.[45,48]

6. Other Tests

The majority of screening tests for syphilis are based upon the agglutination of cardiolipin, or cardiolipin-coated particles.[13] The test is set up manually, usually by mixing a drop of reagent with a drop of serum on a slide. The reaction mixture is agitated on a rotator and agglutination or flocculation is read by eye. Blood is not transfused when the test result is reactive. However, since the antigen is clearly not specific, there is always the potential that a reactive result is a biological false-positive. Consequently, all reactive samples should be confirmed. This is often done by a specific treponemal test, such as the FTA ABS (fluorescent treponemal antibody absorption) procedure.[13] Frequently, samples are referred to public health laboratories for this additional testing. Screening tests based upon treponemal antigens are now becoming available. Passive hemagglutination or ELISA procedures have been described and are in use in some locations, particularly in Europe. In addition, an indirect particle agglutination procedure which is designed for automated performance on a blood typing instrument has been licensed and is likely to receive wide acceptance.

CMV is a herpesvirus which causes persistent infection. It is now clear that this virus is readily transmitted by transfusion and that it may cause serious disease in immunocompromised or gestationally immature patients. Although 50% or more of all donors are CMV seropositive, only a few percent of donors appear to be infectious for CMV. However, it is apparent that all such infections are transmitted from seropositive donors. Consequently, it is routine to use screened, seronegative blood for transfusion of low-birthweight infants.[49] In addition, many physicians use CMV seronegative blood for transfusion of selected transplant recipients and other patient groups. A number of different formats of tests for anti-CMV are available, including conventional antiglobulin ELISA and latex agglutination. The latter procedure is in widest use in the U.S., as it is rapid and effective. Recently, a particle agglutination procedure has been licensed for use on an automated blood typing instrument.

C. SAMPLES AND SAMPLE HANDLING

One of the basic procedures that may be overlooked or at least underemphasized in viral serologic testing is the process used for the proper identification of samples and the absolute requirement for having them associated with the proper donor and unit of blood. All of the testing considerations outlined in this article are of no use whatsoever if the blood collection and labeling procedures allow the possibility of sample mixups. Standard operating procedures must specify exactly the procedures to be used, staff must be trained thoroughly in the importance of properly performing these procedures, and any breach in these systems must be thoroughly investigated and corrective action implemented.

Each manufacturer of reagents used in testing for serologic markers of infectivity or infection carefully specifies the type of sample and handling precautions that must be used. The type of sample appropriate to a particular assay was determined during the licensing process in the clinical and laboratory trials. It is extremely important from a regulatory and scientific viewpoint to use samples that are consistent with those specifications. When writing the standard operating procedures and training procedures for a laboratory that will be screening blood donations, the type of sample that will be collected for screening must be specified and must be that which the manufacturer has specified. Samples that are to be frozen should not be repeatedly thawed and refrozen. Freeze-thaw stresses may significantly degrade some types of antibodies and antigens, resulting in false-negative tests. In addition, freeze-thaw physical forces may result in the formation of certain aggregates that can cause false-positive test results. If multiple testing of frozen samples may be foreseen, freeze the samples in small aliquots that only need to be thawed one time for testing and then do not refreeze the remainder of the sample. Finally, prolonged storage in the freezer (particularly frostless models with automated defrost cycles) can lead to evaporation or sublimation of water from the samples.

Virtually all of the manufacturers have tests that will perform properly with either serum or nondiluted plasma. When using serum samples, the primary consideration is that the sample should have had sufficient time to clot completely. Centrifugation must be sufficient to remove any microclots, which will raise havoc with most types of sampling instruments if not removed completely. In addition, it is important to insure that there are no visible clots or aggregates of platelets and/or white cells that may also interfere with the sampling process. Although most sampling instruments have sensors designed to detect the presence of clots or aggregates that will interfere with the sampling procedures, an undetected blockage may prevent any sample from being distributed into the microplate or testing well. This would result in a false-negative test.

The same considerations for examining serum samples for clots or aggregates that may interfere with sampling also apply to plasma samples. An additional consideration for plasma samples is the effect of dilution. Plasma samples for viral marker testing should be collected directly from the donor into a tube containing either dry ethylene diamine tetraacetate (EDTA) or liquid EDTA with a volume of less than 0.5% of the sample volume. Larger volumes of liquid anticoagulant may decrease the sensitivity of the test so that a very weak positive reaction will be interpreted as a negative result. This is particularly important when samples for viral marker testing are collected from the tubing between the needle and the collection bag. In this procedure the needle is removed from the donor's arm and then inserted into a series of evacuated sample tubes. This tubing contains approximately 11 ml of whole blood from the donor. This sample can be distributed to tubes with or without anticoagulant. However, after the first 10 to 11 ml have been collected, any further blood will be diluted with the anticoagulant from the collection bag. Such diluted plasma should not be used for viral serology testing unless explicity permitted by the manufacturer's product insert. The extent of the dilution of this anticoagulated plasma is approximately 20%. It has been shown that this dilution factor is sufficient to cause false-negative reactions, although such a situation would be extremely rare. The diluted samples are, however, satisfactory for red blood cell typing tests. These considerations also apply to using segments of anticoagulated blood from the units for viral serologic tests. Segments should not be routinely used for testing and when used for specialized situations, the dilution factor should be taken into account.

When using this method of sample collection from the tubing, it is critically important that the testing laboratory be able to positively identify which samples should be used for viral serologic testing and which should be used for red blood cell typing tests. This identification can be accomplished: by labeling the tubes in a prominent manner; by drawing tubes with or without anticoagulant in a specified sequence; or by drawing tubes with different volumes in a specified order. Whatever identification method is selected, it must be foolproof, and the significance of collecting samples in the proper order must be fully and carefully explained to the blood collection and laboratory staff. As pointed out below, it is extremely important to make sure that the sample tube is well mixed immediately after filling, no matter what the source of the sample.

There are other methods for collecting pilot samples without liquid anticoagulant. A special in-line needle may be incorporated into the collection tubing; once the collection container is full, the tubing may be sealed above the in-line needle which is then used to fill evacuated pilot tubes directly from the donor's vein. Alternatively, the collection tubing may be sealed, then cut on the donor side of the seal; blood is then allowed to drip directly into opened pilot tubes. Both of these methods offer actual or potential hazards to collection staff and neither is recommended. Manufacturers of collection equipment are developing alternate methods for the collection of pilot samples.

Storage of samples is also critically important and should be controlled with carefully designed and monitored standard operating procedures. Manufacturers of viral serologic tests specify the storage conditions for samples. These conditions insure that samples are preserved properly so that the antibody or antigen analytes will not be degraded and the samples will perform satisfactorily in the assay systems. It is usually possible to satisfy the specified storage conditions, with two possible exceptions. First, if there has to be an unusual delay between blood collection and testing, such as may occasionally be necessary with remote collections and long holiday weekends, freezing of separated serum or plasma may be necessary. Note, however, the ALT is unstable at $-20°C$, but that it is stable over a relatively long period at room or refrigerator temperatures.[50] Second, in extreme weather conditions (e.g., Minnesota in January or Arizona in August) there is a possibility that samples may be sufficiently degraded to give spurious results if they are not properly insulated during transport.

D. TEST PROTOCOLS

All of the commonly used test reagents for viral serologic markers utilize a similar strategy for interpretation. Tests from all donors are set up and the initial test results are recorded. At this point any test that is interpreted as reactive using the specified criteria of the test manufacturer is classified as initially reactive.

This initially reactive classification should result in two specific actions on the part of the testing laboratory. First, all of the component products from that donation should be collected and placed in quarantine. At this point all of these components should be identified with a "hold for further processing" label. The hospital or blood center should have absolutely foolproof procedures in place to insure that:

1. The suspect units are taken out of the general storage areas where other untested or tested and satisfactory units are located.
2. The suspect units are labeled in such a manner that their distribution or routine labeling is impossible.
3. All of the components produced from that donation are accounted for.
4. The area in which these initially reactive units are stored is clearly labeled and distinctly separate from storage areas where other products are located.
5. Access to these quarantine areas is restricted to authorized individuals.
6. Records of unit histories clearly show that all of the initially reactive products were handled correctly.
7. All necessary repeat and confirmatory testing is fully completed.

All of the donations that are initially reactive should be retested in duplicate. Some blood collection institutions use the originally tested sample for one of the repeat tests and a second sample (from another tube or from a segment) for the second test. This procedure is designed to be an additional safeguard against a sample mixup problem. However, as discussed above, diluted plasma samples may not be acceptable for testing. In any case, if either of the repeat test results is reactive, then the donation is classified as negative for that particular marker and may be released for distribution.

It is very important that the laboratory design a mechanism to resolve a large discrepancy between the initial and the repeat test result, or at least to find a satisfactory explanation for the discrepancy. For example, if the initial anti-HIV test has an absorbance of >2.000 and both repeat tests have an absorbance of .005, this variation is much greater than would normally be expected. It is important to insure that there was nothing significantly wrong with either the first test or the repeat testing runs or that there was no sample mixup. On the other hand, it is very important that test runs not be invalidated without very good reasons and that these reasons are adequately documented.

Repeatedly reactive donations should have all of the component products labeled with a "Biohazard" label that will prevent both further labeling of the products and the distribution of these products. This portion of the testing process may be most susceptible to errors, and every effort must be made to insure that repeatedly reactive units are not released. Samples from these units should be preserved for confirmatory testing so that donors may be properly classified for deferral and notification purposes. It is important to insure that the storage conditions for these samples be such that the antibody or antigen in the sample will not be degraded. This is particularly important since the confirmatory testing for many of these markers take place some time after the initial and repeat testing. As a general rule, these samples should be frozen at temperatures consistently below $-20°C$ and should not be thawed and refrozen more than is absolutely necessary. The blood products themselves from these donations must be properly disposed of and this disposal process must be thoroughly documented.

III. EQUIPMENT

A. SAMPLE HANDLING EQUIPMENT

Many modern blood centers may handle more than 1000 donations daily, resulting in more than 10,000 individual tests. This workload clearly makes the automation of testing necessary and desirable. Instruments can read and record the huge numbers of multidigit sample identification codes more accurately than human beings and this is, of course, a major safety factor in viral serologic testing. Dispensing samples from the identified test tubes into the testing receptacle is another area where humans will make errors, particularly as the number of tests increases. These two factors make the use of modern samplers almost essential to insure that tests are completed accurately, especially in large blood collection centers. On the other hand, automated test processing equipment can lead to complacency; it is dangerously easy to assume that the equipment is performing adequately when that may not be the case.

As described earlier, most of the modern ELISA tests licensed in the U.S. use either a microplate format, or in the case of a single major manufacturer of reagents, a quarter inch polystyrene bead. There are a number of samplers available for microplate-based tests and a few for the bead-based tests.

It is beyond the scope of this article to make an exhaustive listing of these samplers and compare and contrast them, but all of the reagent manufacturers either manufacture or distribute instruments that can be used with their assays. It is important to review some of the basic considerations that apply to all of the samplers that are available and that will also apply to new generations of samplers that will become available in the future.

1. All samplers should have the ability to read the identification number that is used to label the test samples. This is most often accomplished with a laser bar code reader. It is important to verify that the laser correctly interprets the information that is encoded in the bar code.
2. All samplers should have a foolproof mechanism for distributing the aliquots of serum or plasm into a microplate or bead-based well with absolute accuracy. The test results and the identification of the sample number must also be linked with 100% accuracy. This linkage must be verifiable and should be checked upon the installation of the instrument and periodically thereafter. Positioning of the in-test controls in a specified area of the testing plate is one of the quality control measures that the instrument should accommodate.
3. There should be a mechanism that allows the calibration and adjustment of the sample volume and dilution to be distributed. This is controlled by software, but must be manually verifiable. The manufacturer should provide instructions for such calibration and adjustment and local operating procedures should specify the frequency of this action.
4. There must be a mechanism to detect sampler blockage. The sample volume used in modern ELISAs is usually very small and cannot be accurately verified by visual examination. If blockages in the sampler are not detected, it is possible to generate false-negative results because no sample is distributed into the test well, with the obvious potential for a disastrous outcome. This feature is sometimes difficult to verify, but it is important that intentionally clotted samples be tested to validate its operation.

B. PROCESSING AND READING EQUIPMENT

The nature of ELISA is such that a number of washing and reagent dispensing steps must be accurately accomplished. In our experience, washing steps are the most common cause of variability in these tests. Also, the manual addition of reagents is time consuming and it is possible to inadvertently omit this step for occasional samples. For these reasons, instruments for high- and moderate-volume testing centers have been developed that automatically handle these functions. Such instruments cannot be discussed in detail here, but are available from, or through, test kit manufacturers. It is important to review some of the basic considerations that apply to all of the processing equipment that is now, or will be, available.

1. A processor should have the ability to track the progress of the test that it is performing. This should include a record of the incubation time and temperature of the various stages of the assay. In order to track this, the instrument must have a mechanism to identify each plate it is processing, usually by some type of machine-readable designation of the test plate. This identification system must be verifiable upon installation and with each of the tests that it processes.

2. There must be a mechanism to verify the wash steps that the processors utilize. As previously discussed, it is essential that the washing steps be performed accurately and completely.
3. The spectrophotometer used to measure the optical density of the final test must be accurate. There must be a mechanism that allows calibration and monitoring of the spectrophotometer. The in-run controls that are located in particular wells in the test trays can serve as a continuous monitor of these functions.

IV. TEST/REAGENT SELECTION CONSIDERATIONS

A wide variety of commercially prepared test kits is available for most of the infection markers described in this chapter. In general, it is reasonable to assume that all licensed tests will have essentially the same effectiveness in assuring blood safety. Nevertheless, there may be reasons to select a specific test for use in a blood collection facility or system. Such a choice should be made on the basis of a number of factors, including sensitivity, specificity, reproducibility, logistics, operational characteristics, availability of automated equipment, and manufacturer's performance history and technical support.[16]

Logistic aspects of a test may be of considerable importance. For example, the basic format of the test will determine the equipment needs, and it may be important to assure that all testing uses a bead format, or a microplate format. Similarly, the availability of automated equipment may determine reagent choice, either because the equipment is already available, or because a reagent manufacturer supports the optimal configuration. In large-volume operations, automation of sample handling and identification is critical. Sample pipetting stations must be able to read and handle appropriate bar codes and dispense and dilute samples into the appropriate reaction trays. Similarly, reading equipment must be compatible with, and interfaced to, the dispensing equipment.

V. DATA MANAGEMENT

A. HANDLING DATA ELEMENTS

Data management is, at the same time, the single area most critical to blood safety and most susceptible to error. It is important to pay at least as much attention to the processing of test data as to all of the other areas of testing. The importance of comprehensive standard operating procedures and exhaustive training of personnel in the proper management of the data cannot be overemphasized.

It is, of course, extremely important to handle all laboratory testing information carefully and correctly. However, in clinical laboratory medicine, any test result reported on a patient is interpreted by the clinician in the context of other test results and the patient's signs and symptoms. This is not the case with the data generated in testing donor blood. At the time that these test results are generated, the donor has passed all of the history screening, the confidential unit exclusion procedure, and the check for any other disqualifying factor. The testing results are the only piece of information that will prevent potentially infected or infective units from being distributed for transfusion. Because of this fact, this data must be managed absolutely correctly, or all of the testing will go for naught.

1. Input Data

The blood donation, pilot tubes, and all test results are linked by a single identifier, the whole blood number. Wherever possible, this critical item should be in the form of a bar code which is directly read by the sampling or processing equipment. Many blood systems and blood collection centers use a combination of letters to identify the collection site and a sequential number to identify the donation. When manual data entry is used, there is a significant possibility for this information to be misread or misrecorded, and failing other methods to catch the errors, an unsatisfactory unit may be distributed as a result. Ideally, double entry methods should be used when automated sample identification is unavailable.

In mass processing of blood donations, where it is often necessary to have a very fast throughput of testing and labeling of some blood products (notably platelets, apheresis products, granulocyte products, and red cells for neonatal transfusions), testing is done in a very large batch-processing mode. This often results in multiple batches of multiple tests being processed at the same time. Because of this, it is extremely easy to confuse various phases of different batches of tests and fail to provide the proper incubation times, incubation temperatures, washing, and reagent additions that are necessary for the performance of valid tests. This makes the software-controlled instrumentation discussed earlier extremely critical. Properly designed software-controlled instrumentation can document the complete records of testing of each unit for each of the viral markers. In manual systems used in smaller collection facilities, it is necessary to have manual documentation of each of these processes and even more care must be applied to insuring that the tests are properly performed.

2. Test Results

Management of test results is the final link in the chain of information that will determine the disposition of the blood products and information that is transmitted to the donor. For these reasons, it is important that this information be processed with a high degree of accuracy. Each step is managing this data is sufficiently critical for there to be a documented supervisory review to insure that it has been completed accurately. Ideally, the test equipment will associate each result with the whole blood number or other unique identifier and feed this information to a computerized data management system which will issue appropriate reports and identify samples requiring repeat testing. Again, when data must be managed manually, it is essential that multiple checks be made.

It is, in most cases, necessary to have data printouts of the test results after the initial testing so that initially reactive units can be quarantined, proper samples can be selected for retesting, and retests can be set up. After duplicate retests are performed, the laboratory computer normally collates all of the testing results and passes the information on to the mainframe computer system. For the reasons listed above, it is important that this data be processed correctly and completely. Because this transfer is also critical to the proper labeling and subsequent distribution of blood products, it must be included in the process of validating the blood center's computer system.

Some tests will produce output which is not amenable to automation at this time. Specifically, manual particle agglutination for syphilis and CMV fall into this category. Particular care must be given to entering such manually transcribed data into the computer system, especially where the system is set to assume a negative fill in the absence of a positive test result.

B. LABELING FINAL PRODUCTS

Before units or products can be labeled, all of the testing results must be collected, collated, and inspected for accuracy. In addition, it is necessary to document that all of the units with unsatisfactory testing results have been quarantined. Labeling is the most critical part of the process because only at this stage are the markings on the unit changed so that it appears to be a distributable product. Consequently, this is the stage of blood product processing that must be given extraordinary attention when procedures are designed and written and when staff are trained.

C. QUARANTINE

Prior to labeling, it is essential to confirm that all unacceptable units and components have been located and quarantined. This includes all donations with unsatisfactory test results; from donors who are found to have previous test results or health histories that made them ineligible to donate; and from donors with unsatisfactory responses to the confidential unit exclusion procedure.

Each laboratory that processes donations should have two distinct quarantine areas. The first should be an area for suspected blood products. Any blood product that has an initially reactive test result should be located and placed in this initial quarantine area. Because most of these products will be found to be acceptable for transfusion following repeat testing, the initial quarantine areas should provide proper storage temperatures and conditions for the products to be stored there. All products that are placed into this initial quarantine area should be identified with a label that states "Hold for further processing" so that they cannot be inadvertently distributed should they somehow get out of this area. In order to decrease the chances that the wrong product is quarantined, it is ideal to have computer software that monitors which units should be quarantined and which units are quarantined and that the appropriate "Hold for further processing" label has been applied. Removing products from this initial quarantine area should be limited to specially trained personnel, should be controlled by the computer system, and must be done with the utmost caution because of the possibility of removing the wrong unit. The entry of units into initial quarantine and the removal of units should be documented thoroughly.

A separate final quarantine area should also be established. It is reserved for units found to be repeatably reactive and therefore not suitable for transfusion. This can be a single quarantine area and need not be regulated for the temperature and storage conditions of the final blood product since all of the products going into this area will be destroyed. All of the blood products that are placed into the final quarantine should be identified with a "Biohazard" label so that they cannot be distributed should they be accidentally placed back into the processing stream. It is ideal if the computer system has software that will insure that the proper products have been quarantined by requiring that the whole blood number be read with a light pen or laser scanner. The system should also confirm that the "Biohazard" label has been applied. This area should be physically restricted as to who is permitted to enter it. We recommend, wherever possible, that final removal of products from quarantine, and their destruction, be restricted to a single person. Entering products into final quarantine, removing them from final quarantine, and discarding them must be thoroughly and accurately documented. This documentation should define the time and method of destruction (e.g., incinerator batch, autoclave batch). It is also necessary to establish that the destruction was completed satisfactorily. One way to help to insure that this process is carried out accurately is to locate a dedicated computer terminal in close proximity to the final quarantine area so that units must be physically brought to this area in order that the bar coded information can be read with a light wand or laser reader.

After all quarantining has been completed and verified, labeling can then be completed. It is advisable to have a computerized labeling system if at all possible. This system should read the whole blood or donor number on the product being labeled by means of a light pen or laser scanner and then check the unit record to insure that all of the required tests have been performed and that they are satisfactory (i.e., negative). After the correct ABO-Rh label has been applied, the system should again check that the correct label has been applied.

It is advisable to have one final check of all processing records prior to the distribution of any products. In addition, it is highly recommended that the distribution system utilize automated readers to check the whole blood or donor number and then check testing records for that unit to insure that everything is satisfactory.

D. VALIDATION OF DATA MANAGEMENT SYSTEMS

Because of the importance of data management and data processing to the safe handling and distribution of blood products, it is equally important to insure that these systems perform as expected.

If the software for these systems is written in-house, there is a double responsibility to insure not only that the final product performs properly, but that it has been designed to cover all eventualities. Every step of the process must be defined and documented, and each module of the software must perform as expected. This performance evaluation must be extensively documented, and this has been a major thrust of FDA inspections recently. Even if the software is obtained from another source or is an integral part of processing equipment obtained commercially, the end user has the responsibility of insuring that it satisfactorily performs the functions for which it was designed.

Validation of all aspects of the data handling and management system must follow a fully documented valuation plan that is carefully designed to test all of the limits of the system. This has to include the absence of test results, invalid test results, nonsense test results, negative test results, and positive results. The test plan should identify, before the test is actually run, what the computer system is expected to do with each of these results. After the test is run, then the director in charge of the department where the data is generated and processed must verify that the system performed accurately. This test should also be reviewed by the individual responsible for regulatory compliance and the responsible head of the blood collection center. These tests must be thoroughly documented and the records preserved for FDA inspections. Validation of the data processing system must be performed every time that there is a change in the software or hardware.

VI. QUALITY CONTROL

A. INTERNAL TO TEST

Quality control is an ongoing process which must occur at a number of different levels. It is often conventional to think of quality control in terms only of the review of results from special test samples designed solely for that purpose. However, this approach is short sighted and may not always be available, since appropriate controls for blood screening assays are not readily available.

Overall results for each test should always be monitored. The frequency of initially and repeatedly reactive results for each test should be evaluated. Deviations from the normal range should be investigated and corrections in technique made as appropriate. Variations should be reviewed in relation to reagent master lot number, shift, technologist, and workstation. Variations in repeat reactive rates should be evaluated along with confirmed positive rates, in order to determine whether the changes reflect actual variation in the rate of infection.

Over the long term, an increase in the frequency of initial or repeat reactive rates may reflect a number of problems. One possibility relates to equipment: a loss of pipetting accuracy or failure to assure proper cleanliness may be at fault. Changes in the performance of reagents may also be responsible; an issue which should be brought to the attention of the manufacturer. Sudden increases in the rate of initially or repeatedly reactive results should be investigated to determine whether they relate to particular shift, worker, workstation, or reagent lot. For most forward-type ELISA tests, sloppy procedures will have a marked effect on initial reactive rates. In such circumstances, equipment may need to be cleaned or adjusted, or staff may need to be retrained, unless the problem is clearly related to a single reagent lot. Interestingly, there have been instances of very high rates of initial reactivity which appear to have been a result of variations in sample collection and transport: care should be taken to mix pilot tubes well upon collection and to transport them at a reasonable temperature. Finally, it should, of course, be recognized that an unexplained decrease in reactive rates, particularly those for repeatedly reactive and confirmed positive samples, could signify a technical problem. Another measure, which is somewhat harder to obtain and analyze, is the overall distribution of signal levels for nonreactive samples. The characteristics of this distribution should be stable. An increase in the overall variance of the distribution would imply a loss of control in the overall testing process.

Positive and negative controls are included with all test kits, with the exception of the ALT test, for which external quality control samples must be used. For most ELISA tests, the controls serve two explicit purposes. First, they provide assurance that the test run is functioning properly. Second, they provide a means for calculating a cutoff value, used to interpret the results of each sample in a test run. Each reagent master lot contains controls which must only be used with that lot, since reagents and controls are standardized to work together. Thus, excess, or unused controls cannot necessarily be used as a quality control reagent to standardize tests or reagents. The manufacturers' package inserts provide specific instructions on the interpretation of control values and specify conditions required for a run to be valid. If these conditions are not met, the entire run must be discarded. Clearly, the run should not be repeated until the potential causes of the failure have been investigated and corrective action has been taken.

Additional quality control information can be gained from the control values. Ideally, positive controls should give values in the proportional range of the test. Each test run should give a similar result for the positive control, when standardized to the cutoff. Significant variation from this finding should be evaluated. However, as pointed out above, since controls and reagents may be tailored to work together, it is not advisable to use these values for Shewhart chart analyses, or similar formal evaluative procedures. It may not be appreciated that the actual variance of control values within a run may also provide useful information. The coefficient of variation (CV) for control values should approach an ideal minimum value. The CV of both positive and negative control values may be tracked and a major increase in the value above the local norm for the test and control suggests the potential for loss of technique, or instrument variability as a result of minor malfunction or contamination.

B. EXTERNAL CONTROLS

In the practice of clinical chemistry, it is conventional to include one or more external controls with each run. The value obtained by testing each control is compared with an expected range of values, obtained from experience with that sample. As described below, there are sets of formal rules for evaluating the results of the control tests.[51] These rules can be applied to assess the validity of a single test run, run-to-run variability, lot-to-lot consistency of reagents, and long-term drift. It is important that control samples be consistent over long periods and that their design and manufacture be dissociated from reagent production and design. Ideally, controls should be designed to represent the normal outcome of the test and, preferably, a second control should reflect a test response around the decision point or cutoff of a test. These characteristics are generally built into conventional controls for clinical chemistry, and are designed to be used with tests for analytes whose results are distributed as a continuous variable. In contrast, tests which are used to screen blood products are ultimately interpreted as either negative or reactive. Nevertheless, the actual signals which are produced by ELISA tests are themselves distributed as a continuous variable. Hence, the general principles of external quality control are equally applicable to these tests. The evaluation and use of such a control for HBsAg testing has been described,[52] and the National Committee for Clinical Laboratory Standards has designed a specification for anti-HIV control materials.[53] However, at the time of writing, preparations of this type are just becoming widely available. In the absence of commercial products, some large establishments have developed and used run control samples which have been prepared by selection of an appropriate sample detected during routine testing, or prepared by dilution of a known positive. The reader is cautioned that it is not easy to assure the stability of such reagents during storage.

C. EQUIPMENT QUALITY CONTROL

All modern blood collection centers of any size at all are heavily equipped with automated processing instruments. In addition to the significant efficiencies of automation, this equipment is more accurate and can perform repetitive tasks more precisely than technologists performing the same tests manually. Automated processing equipment is significantly more accurate than technologists in reading the donor identification numbers that are used to label sample tubes and connect the unit of blood with the donor identification information. This increased safety margin is most significant when large volumes of tests are performed daily.

Because laboratorians rely so heavily on this automated processing equipment and because accurate test results are so critical to the safety of the blood supply, the equipment must be validated and quality controlled on a regular basis to insure that it is functioning accurately and correctly.

Although the exact functions vary significantly from manufacturer to manufacturer, ELISA processing equipment performs four basic functions: sample sampling and dilution, reagent addition, washing, and measuring optical density. Detailed instructions for quality controlling all of these basic functions are provided in the manuals that accompany the processing equipment. These instructions should be followed carefully and should be performed on a regular basis as specified in the blood centers standard operating procedures. These procedures must be performed regularly and be fully documented to prove that the procedures have been performed and that the instruments are functioning properly.

Quality control of sampling is usually assessed by preweighing reaction trays and pipetting distilled water, using the same software protocols used for the ELISA assay. The trays are then weighed again after the water has been dispensed and the total volume dispensed is calculated and compared to the expected amount. Each manufacturer will specify what the acceptable ranges of variation are permissible. Other manufacturers provide dyes with known optical densities that can be used in place of samples to insure that sample volumes and dilution steps are performed accurately by running the dyes in place of samples and measuring the optical density. Dilutions and sample volumes can be accurately assessed with this method.

Automated systems for reagent addition can also be quality controlled using the same weighing technique. Again, manufacturers will specify what variations are acceptable.

Quality control of the spectrophotometers used for reading test results can be accomplished by several different methods. Using dyes of known optical density values can demonstrate that the spectrophotometer is functioning normally. There are methods, again provided by the manufacturer of the instrument, that utilize known standards and special software packages that can measure other important functions of the spectrophotometer. Linearity checks determine the difference between the absorbance of known standards and the absorbance value predicted by the instrument. Drift tests insure that the spectrophotometer makes consistent readings over time, and repeatability tests verify that the reading system makes consistent measurements.

D. PROFICIENCY PROGRAMS

Proficiency programs are a component of quality assurance, rather than of quality control, although corrective action must be taken if proficiency is not established or maintained. In a typical proficiency program, blinded samples are provided to a laboratory, which must test the samples as a part of a normal run. The results are then returned to the agency which sent the samples out and the results are evaluated against an expected standard of performance. Although such a performance standard could be set, in advance, on the basis of the known properties of the proficiency samples, it is better, and more usual, to rely upon the results provided by reference laboratories which also test the samples. For samples tested in blood centers, the expected results for each sample will be defined as reactive (or positive), negative, or nonconsensus in the event that the results differ between reference laboratories. The expected performance for a blood center or blood bank laboratory is 100% concordance with all except nonconsensus samples. Currently, the most widely used proficiency panel is provided and administered jointly by the College of American Pathologists and the American Association of Blood Banks.[54]

It has long been recognized that the ideal proficiency program should challenge the entire testing chain, from collection and identification of samples to the preparation and distribution of the report. Unfortunately, this is rarely possible, especially in the context of blood collection. As a consequence, proficiency samples may well be recognized as such, thus receiving special attention and negating the objective of assessing routine performance levels. Since it is ultimately in the interest of an establishment to identify and correct performance deficiencies, managers and supervisors should make their best effort to disguise the identity of proficiency samples from bench workers. At the same time, maintenance of credentialling and licensure are dependent upon satisfactory inspections and proficiency, so failure to meet expected performance in a proficiency program may have serious consequences. Proficiency programs in no way substitute for routine, ongoing quality control and assurance programs.

E. MANAGEMENT OF QUALITY CONTROL DATA

1. ALT Tests

Quality control of measurements of ALT levels can be accomplished with standard methods used in clinical chemistry laboratories. One of the widely accepted methods for monitoring the performance of clinical chemistry assays is known as the multirule Shewhart Chart method.[51] This is a statistical method for ongoing monitoring of the results of repeated assays on a stable known sample to insure that test reagents, instrumentation, and performance are all functioning normally.

To utilize this method, it is necessary to perform a number of assays on a control material. It is important that the control material be stable and available in sufficient quantities that it can be aliquoted and used over a long period of time. Control materials for enzyme analyses are commercially available or can be prepared from pooled serum or plasma from appropriate donors. A minimum of two different control materials should be routinely used and they should be selected for their activity level. One is ordinarily within normal limits and the other represents an elevated result. Repeated analyses of each control material should be performed over a period of three weeks or more.

One measurement of the concentration or activity of the control material should be made for each run, with a minimum of 20 determinations. The mean and standard deviation are calculated for these measurements.

A control chart plots the concentration or activity results on the y-axis and time on the x-axis. A horizontal line is drawn corresponding to the mean derived from repeated measurements of the control material and horizontal lines are also drawn at plus and minus one, two, and three standard deviations from the mean. In routine use, control samples are tested with each run or each day that the analyzer that is being monitored is in use. The results obtained are plotted on the chart. If multiple analyzers are used, each one in use should be tested and the results recorded on a separate chart.

The values obtained for the controls should then be examined to determine if they fall within the range that would be expected if the test system was functioning adequately. Suggested rules for evaluation of the results are as follows:

1. Do both of the results fall within plus or minus two standard deviations of the mean? (Yes, accept the run as valid; No, proceed to rule 2)
2. Do either of the results fall outside the range of mean plus or minus three standard deviations? (Yes, reject the run; No, proceed to rule 3)
3. Do both of the controls in the run fall outside of the mean plus or minus two standard deviations? (Yes, reject the run; No, proceed to rule 4)
4. Do the results of one of the control materials on two consecutive control runs fall outside of the mean plus or minus two standard deviations? (Yes, reject the run; No, proceed to rule 5)
5. Does the difference between the controls within a run exceed four standard deviations (i.e., if one is more than plus two standard deviations and the other is more than minus two standard deviations)? (Yes, reject the run; No, proceed to rule 6)
6. Do four consecutive assays of the control material (applied either to four consecutive runs of one of the control materials or to two consecutive runs of both of the control materials) exceed a sum of four standard deviations either above or below the mean? (Yes, reject the run; No, proceed to rule 7)
7. Does the value for one of the controls fall on the same side of the mean in ten consecutive runs or does the value of both of the controls fall on the same side of the mean in five consecutive runs? (Yes, reject the run; No, accept the run)

Random errors are also known as background errors and are normally indicated by violations of rules 2 or 5. Systematic errors indicate that an instrument or reagent has drifted and needs to be recalibrated or otherwise resolved. Systematic errors are normally indicated by violations of rules 3, 4, 6, or 7. Implications of the multirule Shewhart method for indicating potential causes for failure of an instrument to be in control limits are discussed in an excellent review by Westgard et al.[51]

2. ELISA

As discussed above, routine quality control of the performance of ELISA assays is accomplished by two main methods. One is by the use of calibration controls provided by the manufacturer. These known controls and their statistical analysis are the only controls used by the vast majority of blood bank and viral serology laboratories, and are the only controls commonly required by regulatory agencies. Some laboratories, however, have independently elected to use what are known as run controls. Run controls are known positive samples that have been carefully evaluated as to the strength of reactivity that they would be expected to have in a normally functioning run. Run controls should never be samples that show high levels of nonspecific activity. Run control samples are assayed over a period of time of at least two weeks and should be run with ELISA kits that are nearing the end of their shelf life. It is possible to evaluate the results of these run controls in much the same way as the Shewhart chart analysis outlined above. However, formal rules have not been published, so care should be taken to assess the value and implications of any selected criteria.

Thus, each laboratory may devise their own criteria for accepting or rejecting a run based on the results of a run control; however two methods are commonly used. One is to dilute the run control (with human serum shown not to contain the antigen or antibody being assayed) so that the reactivity is close to the cutoff. ELISA results are commonly expressed as a ratio of the optical density of the sample (S) divided by the optical density of the cutoff in the run (C). Since the vast majority of samples containing antibodies or antigens of viral infection in blood donors are very strongly positive, the sample can be diluted so that it has an average S/C ratio of approximately two. Any run in which this sample yields a positive result can be judged to be valid. The second method is to run a known positive sample over a period of at least two weeks and to calculate the mean and standard deviation of the S/C ratio. Then when the S/C ratio of the run control is within the range of the mean plus or minus two standard deviations, the run can be judged to be valid.

Since the manufacturer's controls are normally tested at the beginning of a run, the run control should be placed at the end of the run to insure that nothing has happened during the test that would lead to a false-negative result (e.g., plugging of a reagent dispenser, failure to add conjugate, etc.).

It is critical, from a regulatory standpoint, to insure that when criteria for run controls are developed and implemented, they are rigorously and uniformly applied. Manufacturer's instrumentation software currently does not judge run controls, so they must be manually evaluated. When standard operating procedures specify that the run controls must be in a certain range for the run to be valid, regulators will expect that the procedures are followed faithfully. The results of each quality control sample must be recorded as part of the permanent record for each test run, along with a description of any action taken as a result of the control values. Ideally, a separate record of quality control data should be retained, to permit analysis of variation over time, and by test reagent lots, shifts, instruments or individual technologists.

F. INVALIDATION OF TEST RUNS

When formal quality control measures are implemented as a routine part of the testing process, it is important to establish standard operating procedures defining the conditions in which test runs will be accepted or invalidated. Once such measures are implemented, they cannot be applied in an inconsistent or arbitrary fashion. Decisions on the acceptance or rejection of a test run should, in general, be based only upon the results of the test kit controls, or the external quality control samples.

Great care must be taken to establish that the conditions used to invalidate ELISA runs do not violate the manufacturer's specifications. That is, if the known positive and negative controls are within the specified ranges, it is not usually an option to declare the run invalid without well-documented reasons. Invalidating runs because of unexpectedly high rates of positive results is particularly risky, and should not be done without documentable reasons (e.g., known failure of a washer).

Thus, there must be sufficient reason for deciding that a run is invalid, and this should not be permitted without referring to procedures or reasons which are listed in the standard operating procedures; the express approval of the laboratory director or supervisor must also be obtained and verified by signature.

On the other hand, laboratories should be staffed with trained technologists who are aware of the factors that influence ELISA assays and they should be alert for machine malfunctions that could adversely affect the validity of the testing results. They should then consult with laboratory supervisors and directors and invalidate any run that shows good reasons for doing so. It is least risky to invalidate runs prior to reading them and obtaining results. Once results have been obtained, runs must only be invalidated with the greatest attention to sound scientific principles and clear cut documentation that will be decipherable and understandable years later.

REFERENCES

1. **Dodd, R. Y.,** Will blood products be free of infectious agents?, in *Transfusion Medicine in the 1990's,* Nance, S. J., Ed., American Association of Blood Banks, Arlington, VA, 1990, 223.
2. **Levine, E., Rosen, A., Sehgal, L., Gould, S., Sehgal, H., and Moss, G.,** Physiologic effects of acute anemia: implications of a reduced transfusion trigger, *Transfusion,* 30, 11, 1990.
3. **Goodnough, L. T. and Brittenham, G. M.,** Limitations of the erythropoietic response to serial phlebotomy: implications for autologous blood donor programs, *J. Lab. Clin. Med.,* 115, 28, 1990.
4. **Goodnough, L. T.,** Erythropoietin therapy in autologous blood donors, *Prog. Clin. Biol. Res.,* 338, 105, 1990.
5. **Goodnough, L. T.,** Erythropoietin as a pharmacologic alternative to blood transfusion in the surgical patient, *Transfus. Med. Rev.,* 4, 288, 1990.
6. **Leitman, S. F., Klein, H. G., Melpolder, J. J., Read, E. J., Esteban, J. I., Leonard, E. M., Harvath, L., Shih, J. W.-K., Nealon, R., Foy, J., Darr, F., and Alter, H. J.,** Clinical implications of positive tests for antibodies to human immunodeficiency virus type 1 in asymptomatic blood donors, *N. Engl. J. Med.,* 321, 917, 1989.
7. **Bastiaans, M. J. S., Nath, N., Dodd, R. Y., and Barker, L. F.,** Hepatitis-associated markers in the American Red Cross volunteer blood donor population. IV. A comparison of HBV-associated serologic markers in HBsAg-positive first-time and repeat blood donors, *Vox Sang.,* 42, 203, 1982.
8. **George, J. R., Rayfield, M. A., Phillips, S., Heyward, W. L., Krebs, J. W., Odehouri, K., Soudre, R., De Cock, K. M., and Schochetman, G.,** Efficacies of US Food and Drug Administration-licensed HIV-1-screening enzyme immunoassays for detecting antibodies to HIV-2, *AIDS,* 4, 321, 1990.
9. **Parry, J. V., McAlpine, L., and Avillez, M. F.,** Sensitivity of six commercial enzyme immunoassay kits that detect both anti-HIV-1 and anti-HIV-2, *AIDS,* 4, 355, 1990.
10. **Hartley, T. M., Khabbaz, R. F., Cannon, R. O., Kaplan, J. E., and Lairmore, M. D.,** Characterization of antibody reactivity to human T-cell lymphotropic virus types I and II using immunoblot and radioimmunoprecipitation assays, *J. Clin. Microbiol.,* 28, 646, 1990.
11. **Stevens, C. E., Aach, R. D., Hollinger, F. B., Mosley, J. W., Szmuness, W., Kahn, R., Werch, J., and Edwards, V.,** Hepatitis B virus antibody in blood donors and the occurrence of non-A, non-B hepatitis in transfusion recipients. An analysis of the Transfusion-Transmitted Viruses Study, *Ann. Intern. Med.,* 101, 733, 1984.
12. **Koziol, D. E., Holland, P. V., Alling, D. W., Melpolder, J. C., Solomon, R. E., Purcell, R. H., Hudson, L. M., Shoup, F. J., Krakauer, H., and Alter, H. J.,** Antibody to hepatitis B core antigen as a paradoxical marker for non-A, non-B hepatitis agents in donated blood, *Ann. Intern. Med.,* 104, 488, 1986.
13. **Swenson, S.,** Syphilis serology, cytomegalovirus testing and alanine aminotransferase testing, in *Selection of Methods and Instruments for Blood Banks,* Dixon, M. R. and Ellisor, S. S., Eds., American Association of Blood Banks, Arlington, VA, 1987, 51.
14. Centers for Disease Control, Guidelines for prevention of transmission of human immunodeficiency virus and hepatitis B virus to health-care and public-safety workers, *Morbid. Mortal. Weekly Rep.,* 38(Suppl. 6), 1, 1989.
15. **Fang, C. T. and Dodd, R. Y.,** Immunoassays, in *Understanding Technology New to the Blood Bank,* Vengelen-Tyler, V. and Baldwin, M. L., Eds., American Association of Blood Banks, Arlington, VA, 1988, 17.
16. **Dodd, R. Y.,** Selection of methods for HBsAg, anti-HIV and anti-HBc testing, in *Selection of Methods and Instruments for Blood Banks,* Dixon, M. R. and Ellisor, S. S., Eds., American Association of Blood Banks, Arlington, VA, 1987, 91.

17. **Kühnl, P., Seidl, S., and Holzberger, G.,** HLA Dr4 antibodies cause positive HTLV III antibody ELISA results, *Lancet,* 1, 1222, 1985.
18. **Sayers, M. H., Beatty, P. G., and Hansen, J. H.,** HLA antibodies as a cause of false-positive reactions in screening enzyme immunoassays for antibodies to human T-lymphotropic virus type III, *Transfusion,* 26, 113, 1986.
19. **Zweig, M. H., Csako, G., Benson, C. C., Weintraub, B. D., and Kahn, B. B.,** Interference by anti-immunoglobulin G antibodies in immunoradiometric assays of thyrotropin involving mouse monoclonal antibodies, *Clin. Chem.,* 33, 840, 1987.
20. **Starkey, C. A., Yen-Lieberman, B., and Proffitt, M. R.,** Evaluation of the Recombigen HIV-1 latex agglutination test, *J. Clin. Microbiol.,* 28, 819, 1990.
21. **Quinn, T. C., Riggin, C. H., Kline, R. L., Francis, H., Mulanga, K., Sension, M. G., and Fauci, A. S.,** Rapid latex agglutination assay using recombinant envelope polypeptide for the detection of antibody to the HIV, *JAMA,* 260, 510, 1988.
22. **Dodd, R. Y.,** Screening for hepatitis infectivity among blood donors: a model for blood safety, *Arch. Pathol. Lab. Med.,* 113, 227, 1989.
23. **Gallo, R. C., Salahuddin, S. Z., Popovic, M., Shearer, G. M., Kaplan, M., Haynes, B. F., Palker, T. J., Redfield, R., Oleske, J., Safai, B., White, G., Foster, P., and Markham, P. D.,** Frequent detection and isolation of cytopathic retroviruses (HTLV-III) from patients with AIDS and at risk for AIDS, *Science,* 224, 500, 1984.
24. **Barre-Sinoussi, F., Chermann, J.-C., Rey, F., Nugeyre, M. T., Chamaret, S., Gruest, J., Dauguet, C., Axler-Blin, C., Brun-Vezinet, F., Rouzioux, C., Rozenbaum, W., and Montagnier, L.,** Isolation of a T-lymphotropic retrovirus from a patient at risk for acquired immune deficiency syndrome (AIDS), *Science,* 220, 868, 1983.
25. **Sarngadharan, M. G., Popovic, M., Bruch, L., Schüpbach, J., and Gallo, R. C.,** Antibodies reactive with human T-lymphotropic retroviruses (HTLV-III) in the serum of patients with AIDS, *Science,* 224, 506, 1984.
26. **Thorn, R. M., Beltz, G. A., Hung, C. H., Fallis, B. F., Winkle, S., Cheng, K. L., and Marciani, D. J.,** Enzyme immunoassay using a novel recombinant polypeptide to detect HIV env antibody, *J. Clin. Microbiol.,* 25, 1207, 1987.
27. **Wang, J. J. G., Steel, S., Wisniewolski, R., and Wang, C. Y.,** Detection of antibodies to human T-lymphotropic virus type III by using a synthetic peptide of 21 amino acid residues corresponding to a highly antigenic segment of gp41 envelope protein, *Proc. Natl. Acad. Sci. U.S.A.,* 83, 6159, 1986.
28. **Smith, R. S. and Parks, D. E.,** Synthetic peptide assays to detect human immunodeficiency virus types 1 and 2 in seropositive individuals, *Arch. Pathol. Lab. Med.,* 114, 254, 1990.
29. **Schumacher, R. T., Garrett, P. E., Tegtmeier, G. E., and Thomas, D.,** Comparative detection of anti-HIV in early HIV seroconversion, *J. Clin. Immunoassay,* 11, 130, 1988.
30. **Stramer, S. L., Heller, J. S., Coombs, R. W., Parry, J. V., Ho, D. D., and Allain, J.-P.,** Markers of HIV infection prior to IgG antibody seropositivity, *JAMA,* 262, 64, 1989.
31. **Cabrian K., Shriver, K., Goldstein, L., and Krieger, M.,** Human immunodeficiency virus type 2: a review, *J. Clin. Immunoassay,* 11, 107, 1988.
32. Centers for Disease Control, Interpretation and use of the Western blot assay for serodiagnosis of human immunodeficiency virus type 1 infections, *Morbid. Mortal. Weekly Rep.,* 38 (S-7), 1, 1989.
33. **Dodd, R. Y. and Fang, C. T.,** The Western immunoblot procedure for HIV antibodies and its interpretation, *Arch. Pathol. Lab. Med.,* 114, 240, 1990.
34. **Gnann, J. W., Jr., Smith, L. L., and Oldstone, M. B. A.,** Custom-designed synthetic peptide immunoassays for distinguishing HIV type 1 and type 2 infections, *Meth. Enzymol.,* 178, 693, 1989.

35. **Williams, A. E., Fang, C. T., Slamon, D. J., Poiesz, B. J., Sandler, S. G., Darr, W. F., Shulman, G., McGowan, E. I., Douglas, D. K., Bowman, R. J., Peetoom, F., Kleinman, S. H., Lenes, B., and Dodd, R. Y.,** Seroprevalence and epidemiological correlates of HTLV-1 infection in U.S. blood donors, *Science,* 240, 643, 1988.
36. **Anderson, D. W., Epstein, J. S., Lee, T.-H., Lairmore, M. D., Saxinger, C., Kalyanaraman, V. S., Slamon, D., Parks, W., Poiesz, B. J., Pierik, L. T., Lee, H., Montagna, R., Roche, P. A., Williams, A., and Blattner, W.,** Serological confirmation of human T-lymphotropic virus type I infection in healthy blood and plasma donors, *Blood,* 74, 2585, 1989.
37. Centers for Disease Control, Licensure of screening tests for antibody to human T-lymphotropic virus type I, *Morbid. Mortal. Weekly Rep.,* 37, 736, 1988.
38. **Chen, Y.-M. A., Lee, T.-H., Wiktor, S. Z., Shaw, G. M., Murphy, E. L., Blattner, W. A., and Essex, M.,** Type-specific antigens for serological discrimination of HTLV-I and HTLV-II infection, *Lancet,* 336, 1153, 1990.
39. **Kuo, G., Choo, Q.-L., Alter, H. J., Gitnick, G. L., Redeker, A. G., Purcell, R. H., Miyamura, T., Dienstag, J. L., Alter, M. J., Stevens, C. E., Tegtmeier, G. E., Bonino, F., Colombo, M., Lee, W.-S., Kuo, C., Berger, K., Shuster, J. R., Overby, L. R., Bradley, D. W., and Houghton, M.,** An assay for circulating antibodies to a major etiologic virus of human non-A, non-B hepatitis, *Science,* 244, 362, 1989.
40. **Alter, H. J., Purcell, R. H., Shih, J. W., Melpolder, J. C., Houghton, M., Choo, Q.-L., and Kuo, G.,** Detection of antibody to hepatitis C virus in prospectively followed transfusion recipients with acute and chronic non-A, non-B hepatitis, *N. Engl. J. Med.,* 321, 1494, 1989.
41. **van der Poel, C. L., Reesink, H. W., Lelie, P. N., Leentvaar-Kuypers, A., Choo, Q.-L., Kuo, G., and Houghton, M.,** Anti-hepatitis C antibodies and non-A, non-B post-transfusion hepatitis in the Netherlands, *Lancet,* 2, 297, 1989.
42. **Aach, R. D., Szmuness, W., Mosley, J. W., Hollinger, F. B., Kahn, R. A., Stevens, C. E., Edwards, V. M., and Werch, J.,** Serum alanine aminotransferase of donors in relation to the risk of non-A, non-B hepatitis in recipients. The Transfusion-Transmitted Viruses Study, *N. Engl. J. Med.,* 304, 989, 1981.
43. **Alter, H. J., Purcell, R. H., Holland, P. V., Alling, D. W., and Koziol, D. E.,** Donor transaminase and recipient hepatitis. Impact on blood transfusion services, *JAMA,* 246, 630, 1981.
44. **AuBuchon, J. P., Wilkinson, J. S., Kassapian, S. J., and Edwards, G. C.,** Establishment of a system to standardize acceptability criteria for alanine aminotransferase activity in donated blood, *Transfusion,* 29, 17, 1989.
45. **Schmidt, P. J., Leparc, G. F., and Samia, C. T.,** Comparison of assays for anti-HBc in blood donors, *Transfusion,* 28, 389, 1988.
46. **Caspari, G., Beyer, H.-J., Elbert, G., Koerner, K., Muss, P., Schunter, F. W., Uy, A., Gerlich, W., Thomssen, R., and Schmitt, H.,** Unsatisfactory specificities and sensitivities of six enzyme immunoassays for antibodies to hepatitis B core antigen, *J. Clin. Microbiol.,* 27, 2067, 1989.
47. **Wolf-Rogers, J., Weare, J. A., Rice, K., Robertson, E. F., Guidinger, P., Khalil, O. S., and Madsen, G.,** A chemiluminescent, microparticle-membrane capture immunoassay for the detection of antibody to hepatitis B core antigen, *J. Immunol. Meth.,* 133, 191, 1990.
48. **Parkinson, A. J., McMahon, B. J., Hall, D., Ritter, D., and Fitzgerald, M. A.,** Comparison of enzyme immunoassay with radioimmunoassay for the detection of antibody to hepatitis B core antigen as the only marker of hepatitis B infection in a population with a high prevalence of hepatitis B, *J. Med. Virol.,* 30, 253, 1990.
49. **Tegtmeier, G. E.,** Posttransfusion cytomegalovirus infections, *Arch. Pathol. Lab. Med.,* 113, 236, 1989.

50. **Williams, K. M., Williams, A. E., Kline, L. M., and Dodd, R. Y.,** Stability of serum alanine aminotransferase activity, *Transfusion,* 27, 431, 1987.
51. **Westgard, J. O., Barry, P. L., and Hunt, M. R.,** A multi-rule Shewhart chart for quality control in the clinical laboratory, *Clin. Chem.,* 27, 493, 1981.
52. **Nath, N., Wilkinson, S., and Dodd, R. Y.,** Use of a control serum containing a low level of HBsAg for monitoring proficiency in screening for HBsAg, *Transfusion,* 26, 519, 1986.
53. Human Immunodeficiency Virus Type 1 Reference Material Specifications; Tentative Guideline, Publication I/LA13-T, National Committee for Clinical Laboratory Standards, Villanova, PA, 1990.
54. **Polesky, H. F. and Hanson, M. R.,** Human immunodeficiency virus type 1 proficiency testing. The American Association of Blood Banks/College of American Pathologists Program, *Arch. Pathol. Lab. Med.,* 114, 268, 1990.

Chapter 20

METHODS OF AVOIDING TRANSMISSION OF INFECTIONS WITH TRANSFUSIONS OF BLOOD AND BLOOD PRODUCTS

W. E. St. Clair

TABLE OF CONTENTS

ISBN 0-8493-4938-9

I. INTRODUCTION

Health care professionals, the general public, governmental agencies, and members of the media recognize the need to constantly review and improve the quality and, when necessary, the quantity of our blood supply system. Certainly this emphasizes safety of blood usage. An important aspect of safety is the reduction of (and if possible the elimination of) the transmission of infectious agents when transfusing patients with blood and blood products. While this is only one of the many important aspects of safety to be considered, it has gained the greatest and most visible attention since the transmission of human immunodeficiency virus (HIV) was identified as one of the potential disasters of transfusions. This realization has led to the establishment of many changes in transfusion practices. This on-going process of improvement in the quality and appropriateness of transfusions must be continued. The ominous specter of HIV infection has been pushed back and the risk of transfusion-associated hepatitis (TAH) has been reduced in a most dramatic fashion.

The blood product service industry must also concern itself with the changing legal climate. There has been increased activity holding manufacturers and suppliers responsible for product safety. These product liability cases are primarily related to expectations of reasonable conduct and reasonably safe products. Usually a risk vs. benefit analysis is applied. Therefore, a fail-safe mechanism need not be in place. Cases of risk vs. benefit are usually decided by a jury on a case-by-case basis. While strict compliance with governmental regulations and/or industry custom may be relevant to a certain case, neither is in itself a deciding factor. These procedures have resulted in uneven determinations. Therefore, the health care industry must establish clear evidence of continuing quality care *and* constant effort to improve quality and appropriateness of service and products.

The need to prevent transmission of infectious agents has been made clear. Many agents have been identified as possible sources of transfusion-associated diseases. Included are syphilis, hepatitis B, non-A, non-B hepatitis, human T cell lymphotropic virus (HTLV)-I, and HIV. Bacterial contamination during drawing, handling, or storage also must be considered. Of course, other risks may be identified.

The solution is less obvious. It is multifaceted and will continue to evolve as evidenced by the changes that have occurred in the past decade and are on-going at this time. Solutions must include continuing improvements in donor selection, laboratory testing for infectious agents, sterilization of blood products, development and use of products to substitute for and to enhance the patient's own production of essential elements, and the review of transfusion practices, along with the monitoring and evaluation of the appropriateness of the use of blood products.

II. DONOR SELECTION

Appropriate donor selection essentially revolves around two issues: responsibility toward the recipient to assure safe blood to the degree possible and responsibility toward the donor to assure, to the degree possible, safe procedures, information and counselling, and confidentiality. There is some overlapping of these two in obtaining the necessary medical history, physical examination, and laboratory tests.

The donor has a reasonable expectation that the facility will perform phlebotomy in an aseptic manner with as little discomfort as possible. Also, the medical history and physical examination should adequately address issues that may put the donor in jeopardy. Donors should not be bled more often than every 56 days and of not more than 500 ml, except in unusual circumstances and then only when cleared by a qualified physician. There should be an interval of at least 48 hours after hemapheresis before a whole blood donation is drawn. Any history of prior deferral should be investigated to determine cause and then appropriate actions taken. Heart, lung, or liver disease or a history of cancer should lead to deferral until a qualified physicain determines that the risk to the donor (or recipient) is acceptable. Surgical interventions should defer the donor only until healed, unless the donor received blood for blood products. In this instance the donor should be deferred for six months. Potential donors who are taking drugs must be evaluated for the reasons the drugs are being taken. Most drugs will not necessitate deferral in the majority of cases. There are exceptions and the blood facility should have mechanisms to evaluate each potential donor individually. Pregnancy is a cause for deferral during the course of the pregnancy and for six weeks afterwards. An exception may be made by a qualified physician when a new mother's blood is needed for exchange transfusion of her newborn. Physical exam of the potential donor should include at least blood pressure, pulse, weight, temperature, and general appearance. The blood facility should establish criteria that conform to the requirements of the federal guidelines of the Food and Drug Administration (FDA). Exceptions should be evaluated by a qualified physician.

The potential donor should be assured of the confidential nature of the information being collected; however, the facility must inform donors of the tests that will be performed on the blood and to whom laws and regulation may require reporting of positive findings. The donor should know of possible inclusion on permanent deferral files. Donors also need to know that they will be given positive results and the meanings of the positive results. The facility should be prepared to explain satisfactorily to donors test results that are positive but that may be inconsistent with the donor's sense of well being; workers must be prepared to discuss positive tests with compassion and understanding. The need to have a very sensitive test which may result in a reduction in specificity must be clarified to a person who may be in an extreme state of agitation immediately after receiving information of positive results in a test for a disease that may be life threatening. The possibility of false-positive results may be admitted while sharing information of sources of follow up, needed precautions, altered life style (at least on a temporary basis), and reporting responsibilities of the facility. Certainly, we must continue to work towards improving confirmatory tests. We also should provide for reentry mechanisms to the blood donor community, when this is appropriate.

Duties toward the recipient have received greater attention and publicity since the identification of acquired immunodeficiency syndrome as a disease capable of transmission via transfusions. This has led to more stringent and visible efforts to prevent spread of all contagious diseases via transfusions. General health history questions help identify potential donors who may present a risk for transmission of infectious diseases. The general appearance of the donor should present as healthy and pulse and temperature should be normal. Exceptions should be made in writing by a qualified physician.

Questions about infectious diseases must be very specific. No person meeting certain parameters should be accepted as a donor. The FDA has determined that donors must be free from any disease transmissible by blood transfusion to the degree made possible by history and examination. The blood bank or transfusion facility must translate these rules into policies and procedures and reduce them to day-to-day workable questionnaires and reports. Examples of specific diseases and related questions are given below. There is some overlapping, particularly in relation to viral hepatitis and AIDS.

AIDS and hepatitis — *Have you ever had jaundice or hepatitis*? The American Association of Blood Banks, in its *Standards for Blood Banks and Transfusion Services*, recommends that anyone having viral hepatitis after age 10 years is not suitable as a donor. *Have you had a positive test for AIDS or hepatitis*? *Have you had a test for AIDS for reasons other than to donate blood*? A history of a positive test should result in permanent deferral, after careful confirmation of the historical fact by appropriately trained personnel. *Have you had chronic liver disease, a persistent cough, unexplained night sweats, unexplained weight loss, unexplained fever, unexplained swollen lymph glands, unexplained white spots in the mouth, skin spots that are blue or purple or have you had any symptoms you thought might be related to AIDS*? Any positive response must be carefully and fully explored with the potential donor. Lifestyle and risky behavior or other potential exposures must be explicitly (but not judgmentally) explored. *Have you been sexually active with a person who has AIDS*? *Have you been paid for having sex*? *Have you paid another person for having sex with you*? *Had sex with a homosexual man or a bisexual man*? *Had sex with an IV drug abuser*? *Had sex with a person who has hemophilia*? *Had sex with a person from Haiti or Africa*? *If you are a man, have you ever had sex with another man*? *Have you ever been an IV drug user*? Any positive response, if valid, should result in placement of the respondent on a permanent deferral list. The potential donor should know of the posibility of such placement before completion of the form. *Do you have hemophilia*? Transfusions of blood products do place these individuals at greater risk for infections transmitted by blood and blood products. *Have you ever been deferred, for any reason, as a donor*? The reasons for this must be evaluated. *Have you lived in Haiti or Africa since 1977? Did you enter the United States from Africa or Haiti since 1977*? Positive responses should be explored to determine if the African nation in question is on the current FDA list of areas with increased HIV (1 or 2) risk for transmission. *Have you received hepatitis B immune globulin in the past year*? This is given to individuals at high risk for hepatitis B due to exposure to blood and body fluids. Not all who work in health care are at high risk. The medical director should establish policies concerning deferral of those in health care who are at high risk. *Have you had surgery or a serious illness in the past six months*? *Have you been transfused with blood or blood products in the past six months*? Donors should be fully recovered from illness or surgery. If they had transfusions during surgery or the illness or for any reason, they must be deferred for six months. *Have you had your ears pierced in the past six months*? *Had acupuncture*? These must be reviewed closely. If it cannot be determined that the procedure was done after effective sterilization of the equipment, or preferably with one-time-use equipment, the donor should be deferred for six months. *Have you had a tattoo in the past six months*? If so, defer six months.

Other infections — Some of the general health questions may reveal that the donor has infections with or without a compromised immune system. For example, evaluation of a positive response to fever or night sweats may reveal sepsis or tuberculosis. In addition to the general questions, the donor should be asked specific questions. *Have you had syphilis*? The positive answer should led to deferral for a year. Persons with active infections should be deferred until the infection is cleared. This includes tuberculosis or respiratory tract infections. Residents of nonendemic countries who have traveled in countries considered to be endemic for malaria should be deferred for six months after returning to this country if they remain asymptomatic and have not taken antimalarial drugs. If the prospective donor has taken antimalarial drugs, or has had malaria, there must be a three-year deferral after becoming asymptomatic, departure from the endemic area, and stopping the drug. Prospective donors who have received pituitary growth hormone should be questioned to determine whether the material was from a recombinant process or derived from human pituitaries. Those who have taken growth hormone from human pituitaries must be permanently deferred, since some of these recipients have developed Creutzfeldt-Jacob disease and the responsible virus may be transmitted by blood transfusions. A person who has been bitten by a rabid animal must be deferred for one year.

Immunizations and vaccinations — Prospective donors who have been immunized recently with toxoids or killed vaccines are not deferred if they are asymptomatic. After rubeloa, mumps, yellow fever, and oral polio vaccine, donors are deferred for two weeks. When a donor receives rabies vaccine for reasons other than a bite by a rabid animal, no deferral is necessary. Deferral for four weeks is indicated following rubella vaccine. Prospective donors who receive hepatitis B vaccine are deferred only if there are reasons for deferral related to the indications for the immunization. There is a one-year deferral following hepatitis B immunoglobulin (HBIG), but there is no deferral necessary if the donor has been given immune serum globulin (unless there are concomitant reasons). The donor should be questioned specifically about these issues.

Before the donor completes the questionnaire, suitable and explicit information about the risks of transmission of infections via transfusions of blood and blood products, and descriptions of behavior that put a person at risk must be provided and the donor should be given an opportunity to ask questions. Then there must be a clear and nonthreatening method of self-deferral after the donation, as described previously.

III. COLLECTION AND STORAGE OF BLOOD

The collection of blood should be under the supervision of a qualified physician and should be carried out by trained phlebotomists. There must be no lesions on the donor's skin at the site of the needle stick. There must be only a single venipuncture. If a second venipuncture is necessary, it must be carried out with a completely new collection set and container. The skin must be properly prepared to assure, to the degree possible, an aseptic collection. The collection set, container, and anticoagulant must be sterile. Pilot samples for laboratory tests should be collected at the time of collection of the donated unit. This may be accomplished by filling the integral tubing with anticoagulated blood. The tubing is then sealed. The blood must be stored immediately after storage in an environment that will protect it from harm, in accordance with policies and procedures established by the facility and in conformity with the requirements of the FDA guidelines. There must be daily documented inspections of the blood to assure no hemolysis and no bacterial contamination.

IV. TESTING FOR INFECTIOUS AGENTS

No invasive medical management is at zero risk. Probably none will reach this laudable goal. However, constant effort must be expended. Donor screening is the second line of defense (after education to reduce the incidence of infectious agents in the potential donor pool); testing is the final defense against transmission of infectious agents by cellular components of blood. Sterilization procedures for protein components may offer additional protection for these transfusions. Required testing includes tests for HIV antibodies, HTLV-I antibodies, a test for syphilis, hepatitis B surface antigen, hepatitis B core antibody, ALT liver enzyme, and antibody to hepatitis C. The FDA has some specific requirements relating to qualifications of individuals who perform the tests and which tests are to be performed.

Enzyme-linked immunosorbent assay (ELISA) antibody tests are useful for screening because of sensitivity. However, false-positive tests will occur. Confirmation of reactive tests must be carried out with specific tests such as the Western blot test. Since neither sensitivity nor specificity is absolute, both the donor and the recipient need to be aware of these limitations. Blood banking facilities must be prepared to deal with donors who receive reports that indicate reactive tests that relate to fatal diseases that do not conform to the donor's sense of well being. The recipient must be made aware of the small but real risk of contracting AIDS and/or other infectious diseases.

Prevalence of about 1 to 2 per 10,000 blood donations with positive tests for antibodies has been reported. Estimates of units of blood products infected with HIV-1 antibodies that are transfused have been estimated from 1 in 50,000 to 1 in 250,000. Because of multiple units of blood per transfusion episode, estimates of likelihood of being infected with HIV during any one episode of transfusion have ranged up to as much as 1 in 28,000 episodes.

A test to detect HIV antigen has been developed, but studies failed to demonstrate added benefit when that test was employed by blood banks. HIV viral cultures are difficult to perform and results are disappointing, with false positives ranging in the 10 to 20% range. Other tests to detect viral proteins have been developed; none are universally accepted or used at this time.

The so-called "window period" that exists between initial infection and antibody production has been estimated to be between six weeks and three months. However, some studies have given reason to believe that the window may extend up to as long as three years. In addition to the concern about a "window period", some controversial evidence now seems to indicate that there may be some instances of seroreversion with continued infectivity. Some researchers have questioned whether or not blood from a donor who is in the "window period" between initial infection and antibody development are infectious to recipients during all or part of that lag time. Clearly, continued work is necessary.

Tests for HTLV-I are routinely performed to identify antibodies to this retrovirus, since infections with it will result in a form of leukemia. Infections with other retroviruses that have been identified (such as HIV-2), and likely others that have not yet been identified, are reasons enough for continued vigilance.

Screening for hepatitis has received much greater attention since the risk of transfusion of the AIDs virus was identified. The reduction of transfusion-associated hepatitis (TAH) has been a slow process, but rather successful. Screening methods to reduce HIV transmission have resulted in a marked reduction of donors with hepatitis B since there is such an overlap in these high-risk populations. Effective tests for hepatitis B are available and recently a test for hepatitis C was approved. Tests now being done include tests for hepatitis B surface antigen (HBsAg), hepatitis B core antibody (anti-HBc), hepatitis C antibody, and alanine aminotransferase (ALT). Donor screening along with laboratory testing now avilable is expected to reduce TAH rates to under 2% from the rates of the 1960s, which were as high as 33%.

V. ALTERNATIVES TO TRANSFUSION OF BLOOD COMPONENTS

Plasma expanders have been used with significant success for several years. Efforts to identify alternatives for the cellular components (red cells, platelets, and neutrophils) have met with very limited success so far.

Recombinant erythropoietin is the hematopoietic stimulant that has been approved for use but only for treatment of anemia patients in end-stage renal disease. Studies have clearly shown that use of this product reduces or eliminates the need for transfusions, therefore reducing the risks of transfusion-associated infections. These same patients maintain a near-normal hemoglobin level with concomitant reduction of symptoms and of anemia, and in most cases experience a more acceptable quality of life. No acceptable substitute has been identified for red cells.

No substitutes for platelets or for granulocytes have been developed to the degree that they are yet available for clinical use. Various methods to meet these needs are being actively investigated.

VI. STERILIZATION OF BLOOD PRODUCTS

Devising methods to sterilize blood and blood components has been an area of active investigation, with some success and many challenges being defined. Sterilization of cellular components has not yet been successful. Effective methods will have to sterilize not only free virus but also eliminate intracellular virus and certain viral proteins integrated into cellular structures. Several methods are under active investigation.

Success has been achieved in sterilization of antihemophilic factor (AHF) concentrate. The risk of transmitting hepatitis B or HIV by AHF is almost zero.

Success in sterilizing plasma and cryoprecipitate outside the research laboratory has not yet become a reality; however, there is reason to hope that this will soon become possible.

VII. BLOOD USAGE REVIEW

The last, but not the least, safety factor concerning the transfusion of blood and blood products is the blood usage review carried out by the medical staff. This should be an integral part of the on-going quality improvement activities performed by members of the medical staff and all other health care professionals. Physicians, and others, have long looked at the activities in which they are engaged to help patients; however, only recently have these been organized, systematized, on going, and (especially) documented.

W. Edwards Deming, Ph.D. worked with industry in Japan to develop an effective quality improvement program. In the 1980s, U.S. industry began to adopt some of those ideas. Health care professionals then realized that the concepts were applicable to their endeavors. Voluntary organizations, such as The Joint Commission on Accreditation of Hospitals (now the Joint Commission on Accreditation of Health Care Organizations), consumer organizations, and various levels of government developed requirements related to quality assurance designed to demonstrate the quality of care provided, recognize areas which could be improved, and identify problems when they were present. Of course, the essence of quality improvement is to take action to improve the usage of blood and blood products and/or to correct problems when these are present. When actions are taken, the effectiveness of these actions should be evaluated, improvement documented, and the information reported and disseminated as appropriate.

The review of blood usage should relate to important aspects of the whole process and should at least evaluate:

1. All instances in which blood or blood products are transfused to meet the needs of patients
2. The ordering practices of physicians for blood and blood products
3. The policies and procedures of the transfusion service and the source of blood and blood products, as well as the adequacy of these units or facilities to provide the quantity and quality of product required
4. All confirmed transfusion reactions
5. The adequacy of criteria used for this quality assurance process

Appropriate transfusion of blood and blood products are reviewed against predetermined indications (or criteria) for their use. All criteria should be reviewed on a regular basis to assure conformity with state-of-the-art utilization of resources. This review is a first-line defense against transmission of infectious agents (as well as against other untoward events), since transfusions that are not carried out will not result in unwanted occurrences. As always, the benefits must be weighed against the potential risks. The quality intent would be to reduce unnecessary transfusions only — not those that are justified. Also, criteria should relate to adequate transfusions when indicated. An example may be the criterion that a hemoglobin and/or hematocrit be on the chart within 24 hours of the completion of a transfusion of red cells. Criteria may speak to the correction of signs and symptoms as well as to the correction of abnormal laboratory values.

Policies and procedures should speak to the full range of issues, including at least selection of donors; confidentiality; safety of donors, transfusion personnel, recipients, and others involved; and storage, handling, and distribution of blood and blood products. Laboratory testing should meet or exceed standards of voluntary organizations to which the facility belongs as well as the requirements of the FDA and other regulating agencies as appropriate. Return of unused blood products and other quality control issues also are a necessary part of policies and procedures. The medical staff should be involved in developing and/or review and approval of these guidelines.

VIII. SUMMARY

Blood transfusions are now remarkably safe and becoming more so as a result of efforts of the blood service community — in all of its facets. The work of suppliers, manufacturers, researchers, governmental regulators, and prescribers have contributed to this. These efforts have been stimulated by ethical, professional, and judicial considerations. Efforts have included donor selection, testing, development of alternatives, and monitoring and evaluation of appropriateness of usage. The health care professions must continue these improvements. Ethical and legal determinations should also be expanded to keep pace with technology.

REFERENCES

1. Proceedings From the Workshop on a National Database for Blood Banks and Transfusion Services, the National Institutes of Health, Bethesda, MD, Sept. 25, 1989.
2. *Accreditation Manual for Hospitals,* The Joint Commission on Accreditation of Healthcare Organizations, Chicago, IL, 1990.
3. Proceedings from the Workshop on Safety in Transfusion of Blood and Blood Products, the National Institutes of Health, Washington, D.C., Nov. 1, 1989.
4. *1989 Quality Assurance Data Management: The Next Generation,* Joint Committee for the Accreditation of Healthcare Organizations, Chicago, IL, 1989.
5. **Evans, R. W. et al. and the Cooperative Multicenter EPO Clinical Trial Group,** The quality of life of hemodilysis recipients treated with recombinant human erythropoietin, *JAMA,* 263, 825, 1989.

Chapter 21

DATA PROCESSING AND COMPUTERIZATION IN BLOOD TRANSFUSION

Raymond D. Aller

TABLE OF CONTENTS

ISBN 0-8493-4938-9

I. INTRODUCTION

Although blood banks and transfusion services traditionally think of their primary service as issuance of a unit of blood for transfusion, most of our attention as blood bankers is actually devoted to information processing. Most preventable complications of blood transfusion relate to clerical (information processing) errors, not to technical shortcomings. Therefore, the greatest increase in blood safety will be achieved by devoting attention to improving information-processing methods.

In many fields of human endeavor, the computer has proven to be a useful tool to improve the accuracy of information processing. Like any other tool, the computer will do damage if used improperly. Unfortunately, some blood bankers have failed to use proper caution in use of this tool. Regulators, recognizing these situations, have set requirements for use of computers in blood banking.[1,2] For the most part, the standards promulgated by these regulators are quite reasonable. Unfortunately, in some cases the new regulatory standards have NOT been reasonably applied, with the result that some blood banks have chosen to use manual systems (unsafe by their very nature) rather than computers (unsafe only if mismanaged).[3]

Use of computer systems in blood banks and transfusion services should be considered a standard of practice, to improve the safety and accuracy of transfusion medicine. At the same time, these tools must be used intelligently and accurately, and must be tested for proper operation, just as any other laboratory instrument or methodology is tested before being placed into operation.

This chapter is presented in three sections: (1) understanding blood bank information flow; (2) selecting a vendor; and (3) installing, validating, and maintaining the system.

II. UNDERSTANDING BLOOD BANK INFORMATION FLOW

The blood bank and transfusion service is, as emphasized above, an exceedingly complex information processing environment. An understanding of this environment is best gained by, first, working in the environment; it is far easier to teach an experienced medical technologist, or clinical pathologist, what they need to know about computers than it is to teach an experienced "computer expert" about the complexities of blood bank or laboratory operation.[4] Likewise, it is not practical for this brief chapter to give the reader a complete introduction to the subject; this presentation should be supplemented by reading of other publications.[5-7]

Study of the data elements which comprise the blood bank "active memory", together with how those data elements must be verified and checked against each other, provides a useful framework for understanding of these systems. Some records relate primarily to donor processing (donor service) while others relate to selecting and issuing units for patient transfusion (transfusion service). The data elements are presented in Appendices 1 through 4, in an arbitrary arrangement not representing an actual vendor-supported computer system, but intended to highlight the data elements that may be useful in such systems and describe certain edit checks and look-up options. ALL data elements, when entered at the keyboard, should be checked to ensure only appropriate (e.g., alphanumeric) characters have been entered. More sophisticated checks for internal consistency and validity introduce a further safety factor; examples include alerting the user to a type mismatch between the patient and a selected component, requiring override before an expired product can be allocated or issued, blocking attempts to issue uncrossmatched or unprocessed units, and ensuring compliance with special patient requirements (e.g., patient requires CMV-negative, Kell-negative, and irradiated product — the machine would check that the selected component meets these criteria). The best accuracy of data entry can be achieved through the scanning of bar codes, totally avoiding transcription and transposition entries commonplace in key entry. Therefore, bar code scanning should be used wherever possible.

Appendices 1 to 4 represent operational (active data) files (to record data about donors, units, and patients); Appendix 5 lists important cross indices, allowing rapid retrieval of groups of records from the operational files; Appendix 6 lists useful transaction/audit files; Appendix 7 notes some aggregated information required for management and quality assurance of the service; and Appendix 8 describes dictionaries for relatively fixed information, listing valid choices for donor groups, call codes, patient locations, and so on.

In an ideal design, all database modifications should be logged in a "raw" transaction file, before/as they occur. The preferable approach to accomplish this may be to have all user-interactive and file maintenance functions simply enter a transaction onto the log, and onto a copy of the log kept on a separate disk (or even a separate machine). A "background" process then posts these transactions (in near-real-time) to the database. This permits complete reconstruction of the database in the event of a hardware failure (e.g., disk crash). The complete transaction log is a complete, real-time audit trail, and can be scanned for quality assurance or other purposes. However, some specialized logs of transactions should also be built for more rapid access. Appendix 6 lists some examples.

III. SELECTING A VENDOR

Space limitations preclude a comprehensive description of the vendor selection process. Instead, I will emphasize certain aspects which have proven to be particularly crucial in assuring success of the system. Several of the references[3-5,9,10] describe vendor selection in greater detail.

Selecting an information system vendor is akin to selecting a long-term business partner for your blood bank. Unlike an item of laboratory equipment, the function (or malfunction) of which impacts only a small portion of blood bank operation, the information system becomes intertwined in every aspect of donor recruiting, processing, component preparation, inventory, patient testing, distribution, and management. Information systems must evolve as regulatory requirements and scientific progress dictate. An active, ongoing, cooperative arrangement with the software vendor is crucial to assure appropriate evolution of the system — unless your institution is willing and able to assume maintenance and enhancement of the software by itself.

Therefore, selecting a vendor who will strongly support the evolving mission of the blood bank is more important than choosing the system with the most ''functions''. One of the best ways to choose a supportive vendor is to talk to present clients of the vendor. Ask the vendor to supply a complete list of users. If not complete, a list may have been edited to omit those who are unhappy with the service being provided by the vendor. Call these users — particularly those institutions relatively similar to your own — and ask: Did the vendor provide an adequate training program before the software was installed? Does the vendor respond rapidly to reports of defects or problems with the software (''bugs'')?[11] Do problems that have been repaired recur in future ''releases'' of the software? Are vendor staff available to answer questions about software function and capabilities?

A. VENDOR VIABILITY

Once a system with a reasonable range of functions is found, provided by a vendor who seems committed to excellent and responsive support of the product, the prospective client is well advised to verify that the vendor has the financial staying power and corporate structure to provide this support for the next several years. Corporate credit ratings, such as that available from Dunn and Bradstreet, are a start. However, a warning is in order about small subsidiaries of large corporations; the recent history of such subsidiaries has reminded us that large corporations do not hesitate to spin off, or simply close down, an unprofitable division. In recent years, most of the successful and enduring laboratory and blood bank information systems have been provided by smaller corporations with a focus on (and clear commitment to) health care information systems. On the other hand, a small, focused corporation may not be able to weather the financial setback of a one- or two-year slowdown in system sales.

B. VENDOR AUDIT

The final step in vendor selection, before signature of the purchase contract, is to verify that the vendor has done its ''computer homework''. How are user complaints and requests for bug fixes documented and followed?

Does the vendor maintain a solid change-control system? When a bug is fixed at one user's site, is the same fix provided to other installations? Are the vendor's staff properly trained and supervised? Is there complete and carefully documented testing of new software modules before these are released to user sites? The best method to accomplish this miniaudit is a visit to the vendor's headquarters office, with actual review of the documentation of these activities. The client may wish to hire a consultant (expert in computer project control techniques) to accompany them on this visit. It may be worthwhile to become familiar with the literature on software engineering techniques.[12-15]

C. CONTRACTING

Having selected a vendor of choice, the user will then negotiate a balanced contract with that vendor.[9,10] However, the second- and third-choice vendors should not be told ''no thanks'' until the contract with the vendor of choice is actually signed. There is no negotiating tool more powerful than the ability to walk away from the table and begin discussions with the ''second-choice'' vendor.

IV. INSTALLING, VALIDATING, AND MAINTAINING THE SYSTEM

More attention should be devoted to proper installation of the system than was devoted to its selection. All too often, an excellent system from a reliable vendor has been selected, but the client has failed to devote sufficient resources to its proper configuration and installation. It may be worthwhile to hire staff, or a consultant, who has successfully installed the system elsewhere. Selection of the implementation team, and careful building of the descriptive dictionaries which define the operation of the blood bank to the computer system, are crucial steps. Further detail on implementation approaches is provided in the references.[6-8]

Before a system may be relied upon to store and process donor and patient data, the blood bank staff must validate its proper function. The vendor will provide some suggestions as to how the user might approach validation, but it is important for the client to devise their own test cases, as well. The user may have built the dictionaries in a fashion unanticipated by the vendor, and careful checking of system function, using user-specific cases, may uncover defects in the software that the vendor's ''standard'' validation protocol would not detect. The reader is referred to additional literature on validation.[11-15]

Once the system goes ''live'', continuing attention must be devoted to proper system operation, and to keeping the system up to date with blood bank practice. There must be a designated system manager, who must be allowed adequate time for ongoing system maintenance. Change control logs, security procedures, and periodic revalidations of system performance are essential.

V. CONCLUSION

Blood bank information systems provide important capabilities to promote staff productivity and reduce errors. However, considerable attention must be devoted to vendor selection, system implementation, and ongoing maintenance in order to achieve these goals. Without proper attention, automated systems can propagate errors; in the absence of appropriate personnel management, the systems may be misused, bypassed, or misinterpreted, to the detriment of patient care. As with the more traditional aspects of blood bank operations, careful management of this new tool is the key to success.

APPENDIX 1
Donor File

- Donor name (fixed syntax, automatic check for similar names upon entry, lookup by sound-alike as well as exact match)
  Donor formal title (e.g., Mr., Ms., Miss, Dr.)
- Donor blood bank ID number (may or may not be SSN) — primary key
- Donor social security number (automatic check for duplicates upon entry)
- Birthdate, sex
- Donor maiden name
- Donor mother's maiden name (used in some systems to crosscheck identification)
- Home address, with zip code, and phone number
- Work address, with zip code, and phone number
- Occupation
- Donor organization (e.g., usually donates at X mobile group)
- Usual credit group (distinct from mobile group)
- Deferral codes and dates — MUST allow for recording MULTIPLE temporary and permanent deferral codes and dates (date deferral placed on file AND date from which deferral is being calculated, such as three-year deferral for antimalarial medication) — preferably, eight or more. Most stringent deferral automatically takes precedence
- Total number of donations, by type (whole blood, plateletpheresis, other types)
  - Donations at our blood centers
  - Donations with other blood banks/centers
- Awards given
  - Date
  - Nature of award (e.g., gallon donor)
- Date of first donation
- Date of most recent donation
- Next date eligible to donate, by type (separate date for whole blood, plateletpheresis, etc.)
- Willing to be on callback/emergency call list? — coded entries, including:
  - Rare donor, don't call routinely
  - Don't call at work
  - Positive blood group antibody, don't call
  - Poor veins
  - etc.
- Recording calls to donate — data elements should be captured online, as a byproduct
  - Date and time
  - Employee ID of recuiter
  - Answer?
  - Response?
  - Did call result in a donation?
- How many times per year willing to donate?
- Availability for/interest in special procedures (e.g., plateletpheresis)
- Blood ABO group and Rh type
- Special typings
  - Other RBC antigens
  - HLA antigens
- Known atypical antibodies
- Identification of primary and secondary physicians (e.g., medical clearance, autologous)
- Date and nature of any correspondence sent to donor, or to donor's physician, together with date of reply, resolution
- Coded comments about donor
- Free text comments about donor
- Donation history (unlimited number of donations) — pointers to the Donation Records

APPENDIX 2
Donation/Unit Record

- Donor ID number (permanent number — link to donor records) — these should NOT recycle
- Donation unit number (link to component records) — use a different series of unit numbers for deferred donations (which do not result in an actual unit)
- Date, time, location, of donation, with credit indication
- Medical history flags (complete medical history still recorded and stored on paper)
- Physical exam results (some centers may choose to record blood pressure, hematocrit/hgb)
- Deferral codes — both temporary and permanent (recorded permanently here, and permanently/temporarily in donor record)
- Record of failed collection, reason
- Donor group identification (e.g., recruiting unit — Elks, Ford, etc.)
- Record of donor reaction
- Employee codes for screener, phlebotomist
- Which arm used
- Type of donor — regular, autologous, directed, apheresis, therapeutic
- For directed units:
  - Patient name, hospital, patient ID number intended for
  - Irradiation necessary? (blood relative)
- Type of product — whole blood, plateletpheresis, plasmapheresis
- Type of bag used — single, double, triple, quad
- Lot number of blood bag used (may be batch-entered, for a range of unit numbers)
- Unit volume
- Records of all test results on this unit
  - ABO/Rh
  - Blood group antibody screening
  - Infectious disease testing
    - Required tests
      - Qualitative (e.g., HBSAg pos/neg)
      - Quantitative (e.g., ALT value) with qualitative interpretation
    - Optional tests (e.g., CMV)
  - Other blood group antigen typings
  - Identification of atypical antibodies
  - Status of follow-up/confirmatory testing on this unit
    - Dates/times/destinations to which specimens were sent
    - Results of those investigations
    - Access/inquiry only to staff with special security level
- Comment codes — about the unit
- Free text comments about the unit
- Pointers to all components made from this unit (see Component Record)

APPENDIX 3
Component Record

- Donation unit number — preferably, these should NEVER recycle
- Donor permanent ID number
- Product code/component type (e.g., WB, PC, FFP, platelets, etc.)
- Component sequence number (e.g., for multiple pediatric units of packed cells) Note that complete identification of a component requires three elements:
    - Donation unit number
    - Component type
    - Component sequence number
- Date and time component made, with employee ID
- Volume/weight
- Date and time component labeled, with employee ID
- Expiration date and time
- Current status of this component
- Current location of this component, with date/time it was moved to this location
- Date and time component converted to another component (e.g., FFP made into Cryo, FFP thawed), transfused, or discarded, with employee ID
- Special procedures performed on this component
    - Irradiation
    - Washing
    - Volume reduction

Note: Some blood centers might wish to consider an irradiated component a different component type, but this would rapidly escalate the number of possible component types, and make automated cross-checking difficult (e.g., for patient requiring irradiated unit, automatically checking that "irradiated" flag is on)

- Disposition of this component
    - Converted to component . . . (with component type)
    - Patient identification to whom transfused
    - Patient identification to whom billed, but discarded (not transfused)
    - Pool number into which this was placed
    - Discard/destruction code, if destroyed without transfusion
- Comment codes about the component
- Free text comments about the component

APPENDIX 4
Patient Record

- Patient permanent identification number (hospital medical record number)
- Patient name
- Birthdate, sex
- Maiden name
- Other names used in past (''also known as'')
- Current account/billing number
- Social security number
- Patient address, other billing data (insurance codes, etc.) (if needed by institution)
- ABO/Rh,antibody screening
    - Record of all intermediate reaction results
    - Interpretation of reaction results
    - Testing performed by/interpretation confirmed by (employee ID)
- Atypical antibodies identified, date
- Other transfusion problems/requirements identified, e.g.:
    - History of febrile reactions — leukocyte removal filter required
    - Immunosuppressed — all cellular components must be irradiated
    - CMV-negative (e.g., neonate) — CMV-negative cellular components required
- Primary and secondary physicians
- Other patient history elements
    - Pregnant?
    - Transplant candidate
    - Diagnosis codes (ICD-9-CM, SNOMED)
- Transfusions given — summary, broken down by product types (RBC, platelets, FFP, etc.)
    - Date of first
    - Number
    - Date of most recent
- Crossmatches and unit allocations performed, transfusions given
    - Date and time of allocation/crossmatch
    - Physician ordering allocation/crossmatch
    - Donor unit number
    - Component type and sequence number, volume
    - Intermediate results of crossmatch testing
    - Interpretation of crossmatch
    - Current status of this allocation
    - Date and time released from crossmatch/allocation
    - Date(s) and time(s) issued, by whom (employee ID), and to whom (nurse/physician ID)
    - Date(s) and time(s) returned to blood bank, who accepted back into inventory
    - Date and time of transfusion
    - Reaction?
- Any follow-up testing (e.g., posttransfusion hepatitis workup)

APPENDIX 5
Important Cross-Indices/Pointer Files

- All donor unit numbers for a donor
- All donor unit numbers for a donation group
- All components for a donor unit number
- All crossmatches for a component
- All donors with given additional antigen typings
- All components in a given location (the "active inventory file")
- All transfused products for a given patient, even over multiple admissions

APPENDIX 6
Useful "Extracted" Transaction Files

Each transaction will be recorded with date and time of the transaction, full donor and patient identification, donor unit identification, component type-sequence number, and employee ID responsible for it.

- Each time a component has been moved from one location to another: source and destination locations
- All laboratory testing: new result, plus old result if one is being changed/replaced
- All additions/changes/deletions to donor and unit deferral codes: new code, plus old code if being changed/deleted
- Modifications of "critical fields" in donor/patient records, such as name, date of birth, social security number

APPENDIX 7
Aggregated/Statistics Files and Functions

- Donation statistics
- Rates of positive testing results
- Billing: revenues (charges) and collectibles (receipts)
- Audits of transfusion practice
- Productivity (CAP Workload)
- Cost analysis (personnel, reagent, equipment cost, etc.)

APPENDIX 8
Dictionary Files

For each of the fields and data elements listed above, valid field values and rules pertaining to the processing of these fields are encoded in a series of dictionaries, tables, or control files. The format and layout of these dictionaries is extremely system specific, so no detailed description is attempted here. However, these dictionaries allow the crucial function of checking for valid entries on manual keyboard entry, and cross-checking these entries with other data elements for internal consistency.

For example, one dictionary may list the possible component types, together with the rules for processing and labeling that component — Packed RBCs, with additive solution, requires negative results on tests A,B,C — before labeling, expires N days after drawing, may be converted to X,Y,Z other components, and so on.

Another function of tables/dictionaries is to provide flags that control system operation. Depending on the values of these flags, the software will function differently — different questions may be asked, and varying screen layouts may be used.

REFERENCES

1. Recommendations for Implementation of Computerization in Blood Establishments. Letter to all Registered Blood Establishments, Food and Drug Administration, Bethesda, MD, April 6, 1988.
2. Requirements for Computerization of Blood Establishments, Food and Drug Administration, Bethesda, MD, September 8, 1989.
3. **Aller, R. D., Weilert, M., and Pasia, O. G.,** Blood bank information systems, *CAP Today,* 4(10), 58, Oct. 1990.
4. **Elevitch, F. R. and Aller, R. D.,** The ABCs of LIS — Computerizing Your Laboratory Information System, revised ed., ASCP Press, Chicago, 1989.
5. **Levitt, J. and Steane, S., Eds.,** Standards for Computer Systems in Blood Banking (National Meeting Workshop Manual), American Association of Blood Banks, Arlington, VA, 1989 and 1990.
6. **Steane, S.,** Chariman, AABB Information Systems Committee, Responsibilities in Implementing and Using a Blood Bank Computer System, American Association of Blood Banks, Arlington, VA, 1989.
7. **Steane, S.,** Chairman, AABB Information Systems Committee, Guidelines for Preparing Standard Operating Procedures for Blood Bank Computer Systems, American Association of Blood Banks, Arlington, VA, 1991.
8. **Weilert, M.,** Implementing information systems, *Clin. Lab. Med.,* 11, 41, 1991.
9. **Aller, R. D.,** Information Management, in *Clinical Diagnosis and Management by Laboratory Methods,* 18th ed., Henry, J. B., Ed., W. B. Saunders, Philadelphia, 1991.
10. **Lincoln, T. L. and Aller, R. D.,** Acquiring a laboratory computer system — vendor selection and contracting, *Clin. Lab. Med.,* 11, 21, 1991.
11. **Beizer, B.,** *The Frozen Keyboard — Living With Bad Software,* Tab Professional Books, Blue Ridge Summit, PA, 1988.
12. **Pressman, R.,** *Software Engineering — A Practitioner's Approach,* McGraw-Hill, New York, 1982.
13. Software Engineering Standards (Compendium), IEEE Computer Society, Los Alamitos, CA (800-272-6657), 1990.
14. ASTM: Standards, Vol. 14.01 (particularly Standard on Rapid Prototyping), American Society for Testing and Materials, Philadelphia, PA, 1991.
15. **Meyers, G.,** *The Art of Software Testing,* Wiley-Interscience, New York, 1979.

INDEX

A

B

D

E

I

J

K

L

M

Q

R

S

T